Occupational
Therapy
for children

Occupational Therapy
for children

Pat Nuse Clark, M.O.T., O.T.R.

Occupational Therapist,
Fulton County Schools;
Occupational Therapy Consultant,
College of Health Sciences,
Georgia State University,
Atlanta, Georgia

Anne Stevens Allen, M.A., O.T.R.

Formerly Assistant Director,
School of Allied Medical Professions,
The Ohio State University,
Columbus, Ohio

with 170 illustrations
Illustrations by Jody Fulks, M.S., Medical Illustrator

The C. V. Mosby Company

ST. LOUIS • TORONTO • PRINCETON   1985

MOSBY

A TRADITION OF PUBLISHING EXCELLENCE

Editor: Rosa L. Kasper
Editorial assistant: Cindy Bendet
Editing supervisor: Elaine Steinborn
Manuscript editors: Elizabeth O'Brien, Carol Sullivan Wiseman
Book design: Jeanne Bush
Cover design: Tom Zigrang
Cover photograph: David S. Strickler/Strix Pix
Production: Mary Stueck, Barbara Merritt, Ginny Douglas

The C.V. Mosby Company
11830 Westline Industrial Drive, St. Louis, Missouri 63146

Library of Congress Cataloging in Publication Data

Clark, Pat Nuse.
  Occupational therapy for children.

  Bibliography: p.
  Includes index.
  1. Occupational therapy for children.   I. Allen,
Anne S., 1923-   .   II. Title.   [DNLM: 1. Occupational
Therapy—in infancy & childhood.   2. Handicapped.
3. Child Development Disorders—rehabilitation.
WS 368 015]
RJ53.025C57   1985   615.8′5152′088054   84-19020
ISBN 0-8016-1162-8

C/VH/VH   9   8   7   6   5   4   05/C/606

Contributors

Anne Stevens Allen, M.A., O.T.R.

Formerly Assistant Director, School of Allied Medical Professions, The Ohio State University, Columbus, Ohio

Peggy Barnstorff, M.O.T., O.T.R.

Owner, Pediatric Therapy Associates, Fort Collins, Colorado

Diana P. Burnell, Ph.D., O.T.R.

Private Practice and Consultation, Saratoga, California

Florence Clark, Ph.D., O.T.R., F.A.O.T.A.

Associate Professor, Occupational Therapy Department, University of Southern California, Downey, California

Pat Nuse Clark, M.O.T., O.T.R.

Occupational Therapist, Fulton County Schools; Occupational Therapy Consultant, College of Health Sciences, Georgia State University, Atlanta, Georgia

Ida Lou Coley, O.T.R.

Children's Hospital at Stanford, Palo Alto, California

Christine Bosonetto Doane, M.S., O.T.R./L.

Director, Occupational Therapy Department, St. Joseph Hospital, Atlanta, Georgia

Linda A. Florey, M.A., O.T.R., F.A.O.T.A.

Associate Chief, Rehabilitation Services, Children's Division, UCLA/Neuropsychiatric Institute, University of California, Los Angeles, California

Janet H. Johnson, M.S., O.T.R.

Occupational Therapist, Colerain School, Columbus, Ohio

Katalin I. Koranyi, M.D.

Associate Professor, Department of Pediatrics, The Ohio State University, Columbus, Ohio

Zoe Mailloux, M.S., O.T.R.

Instructor, Occupational Therapy Department, University of Southern California, Downey, California

M. Jeanette Martin, M.Ed., O.T.R., FAAMD

Director, Occupational Therapy, Georgia Retardation Center, Atlanta, Georgia

Mary A. McIlroy, M.D.

Clinical Assistant Professor, Department of Pediatrics, The Ohio State University, Columbus, Ohio

Martha S. Moersch, M.Ed., O.T.R.

Formerly Program Director for Occupational Therapy, Institute for the Study of Mental Retardation and Related Disabilities, University of Michigan, Ann Arbor, Michigan

Alisa Palmeri, O.T.R.

University of Connecticut Health Center, Farmington, Connecticut

Diane Parham, M.A., O.T.R.

Doctoral Candidate, University of California, Los Angeles, California

Judith M. Pelletier, M.S., O.T.R.

University of Connecticut Health Center, Farmington, Connecticut

Nancy J. Powell, Ph.D., O.T.R./L.

Assistant Professor, School of Allied Medical Professions, The Ohio State University, Columbus, Ohio

Susan A. Procter, O.T.R.

Rehabilitation Engineering Center, Children's Hospital at Stanford, Palo Alto, California

Froma Jacobson-Sadacca, O.T.R.

Upward Foundation, Phoenix, Arizona

Karen E. Schanzenbacher, M.S., O.T.R.

Assistant Professor, State University of New York at Buffalo, Buffalo, New York

Susan Denegan Shortridge, M.H.S., O.T.R.

Visiting Instructor, Department of Occupational Therapy, University of Florida, Gainesville, Florida

Betty Scanlan Snow, M.A., O.T.R.

Occupational Therapy Supervisor, California Children's Services, Lokrantz Developmental Center, Reseda, California

Linda C. Stephens, M.S., O.T.R.

Occupational Therapist, Atlanta Public Schools, Atlanta, Georgia

Foreword

Children are a nation's richest resource. How a nation treats its children is a measure of its civility. The authors of this comprehensive textbook have provided a vehicle for occupational therapists to improve and maintain the health of the nation's children and to assist them in achieving their optimal potential in growth and development. The concepts expressed in this book will facilitate learning for students and practitioners and promote high-quality health care for all children: from the presumably well to those who are ill, disabled, and dysfunctional; from birth through adolescence; and through the developmental stages that are critical to their chronological development.

The authors have addressed theory and practice in ways that provide basic understanding for the student who is developing entry-level professional competency and stimulation and challenge for the advanced student and experienced therapist. Occupational therapy practice in pediatrics encompasses case identification, screening, evaluation, treatment or intervention, reevaluation, follow-through, and health maintenance. The settings in which the therapist practices include neonatal units in general hospitals; community preschools; elementary, junior, and senior high schools; neighborhood health centers; high-density housing developments; training schools and halfway houses for delinquent children and youth; special service agencies for adolescents; public health departments; and the home.

The authors have taken into account the reader's need to be aware of developmental principles and theories; the developmental process through adolescence; general pediatric health care; and the areas of illness, disability, and dysfunction that occur with infants, children, and adolescents, whether congenital or acquired. The authors have therefore provided the reader with tools, procedures, and techniques for identifying and assessing pediatric clients. They discuss the clinical reasoning process that assists readers in developing or sharpening the skill to analyze and synthesize data from evaluation and to plan and implement appropriate strategies for direct and indirect intervention. Direct and indirect intervention strategies are presented for working with children and significant others such as parents, teachers, siblings, and caretakers. The occupational performance frame of reference has served the authors well in the organization of many of their evaluation and treatment formulations.

Occupational Therapy for Children provides a state-of-the-art conceptualization of pediatric occupational therapy practice. In addition to the extensive literature synthesis, the contributors to this volume have shared their commitment as pediatric practitioners to the health care of the nation's children.

This book is a long-awaited contribution to the literature in the field of occupational therapy. It will surely advance the level of pediatric occupational therapy practice and the professionalism of the discipline.

Lela A. Llorens, Ph.D., O.T.R., F.A.O.T.A.
Professor, Chair, and Graduate Coordinator,
Department of Occupational Therapy,
San Jose State University,
San Jose, California

Preface

This book is about the practice of occupational therapy with children. To provide a sound basis for discussion of practice methods and modalities, we have included the most pertinent information about developmental theory, learning theory, and pediatric medicine. However, this book is not intended to take the place of good textbooks on development, pediatric medicine, health care delivery systems, or educational methods. We hope it will serve as a detailed collection of current and time-honored theory and practice in pediatric occupational therapy, as well as a guide to practice trends for the future.

We believe that each child has basic developmental needs and matures through a common developmental process. Yet we also recognize that each child is different and proceeds according to an individual timetable through this process. Many of the differences result from the nature of each child's play opportunities and experiences, as well as from the environments in which each child grows. The differences are also a result of each child's individual biological endowment and of the forces that may positively or negatively affect the growing child from embryo to adulthood.

The primary role of the occupational therapist in pediatrics is to help children play, grow, and develop many of the skills that will enable them to enjoy a satisfying adult life. Occupational therapists do this through the knowledgeable selection and use of everyday activities to evaluate and enhance children's development and competence.

We would like to introduce the reader to children, and to occupational therapy practice with them, through a process that is similar in sequence to a student's academic and clinical experiences. *Part I* introduces the general roles and functions of occupational therapy in pediatrics. This is followed by a survey of the different types of service facilities in which pediatric practitioners most frequently work. It will be noted that the trend is toward practice in education-oriented settings and that even medically oriented practice is most often found in outpatient settings. This does not imply that inpatient, hospital-based practice is outmoded or unnecessary. It does reflect significant improvements in pediatric medical and surgical practices that now enable the majority of "problem children" to become medically stable enough to live at home, with due regard to funding constraints.

Part I concludes with a discussion of the people who are important to the child and to the pediatric occupational therapist. It begins with the family and includes professional and technical members of the health care and educational teams.

Part II provides a compilation of the knowledge base for pediatric occupational therapy. This begins with a review of basic developmental principles and theories. The overview of major theories of child development provides a foundation for the discussion of pediatric occupational therapy. These theories are next integrated into a concise description of the developmental process from the prenatal period through adolescence.

Two chapters in this section provide basic information about child health care and the diseases and disabilities that cause problems for the children who are treated by occupational therapists. We have tried to select a broad variety of diagnostic problems and to provide timely information about cause, classification, course and prognosis, and general management. Implications for occupational therapy intervention will help to carry the focus of information from the pathological to the practical.

Part III uses the knowledge base to define the occupational therapy process. This section includes discussion of the parameters of occupational therapy intervention and broadly defines the generic modalities of practice, including occupational activities; human and object relationships; tools, materials, and equipment for activities; and special adaptation techniques. The generic processes of the discipline, activity analysis and activity adaptation, are presented as a framework for occupational therapy programming with children. A sequence for occupational therapy intervention provides a model for planning individual programs for children seen in treatment. We include a number of sample worksheets for organization and analysis of assessment information and program ideas are included throughout the text. This section also includes information about different instructional approaches that can be used with children, as well as contraindications related to particular methods. Collaborative programs and relationships with parents are necessary to develop play, self-maintenance, and schoolwork skills to an optimal level. Guidelines for such interactive programs are presented in general and specific form.

A therapist's first encounter with a child will typically involve assessment of current function. *Part IV* presents information about the variety of assessment methods and instruments available to the pediatric occupational therapist. These range from methods of observation to the specialized procedures used to develop highly detailed understanding of a child's strengths and limitations. Causes of problems are also identified.

There is a growing concern among the members of the profession that occupational therapists often perform exhaustive evaluations that leave little time or resources for the actual treatment program that is to produce change. This book will emphasize assessment tools that use age-appropriate, familiar activities, and we hope that this will bridge the gap from testing to treatment. There are multitudes of tests available that have been designed to be administered to children, and each therapist will find occasion to develop new evaluation materials. However, we believe that the formal evaluation of children should be kept to the minimum necessary to obtain good information and retain the child's interest. Often as much accurate information can be obtained by watching a child play catch with a shadow for 5 minutes as by administering a 3-hour battery of tests. Therapists need to know what to look for and what they are seeing. This knowledge comes from study of child development and activity analysis.

Part V provides comprehensive information about practice methods and modalities that are used in all occupational therapy programming with children. These chapters in Part V present the major domains of activity. We believe that these domains of play, self-maintenance, and schoolwork should be the beginning

and end of each child's program if they are to be described as occupational therapy. The chapters will give detailed information about age-appropriate steps and modifications of basic activities for children. A wide variety of adaptive techniques and devices are presented that will enable children to explore and control their environments more independently.

A final word is pertinent to the content on schoolwork activities in Part V. This section relates to a child's basic readiness and capacities for schoolwork and preadult development. Most of this preparation will come through therapy experiences in play and self-maintenance activities. However, when a child has specific problems identified during the school-age years, the therapist will need to develop additional programming to ensure the child's adequacy in the school environment. More relevant material will be found in Part VI in discussion of occupational therapy services in educational settings.

The chapters in *Part VI* are meant to provide a foundation for study in the specialty areas of pediatric practice. Although no chapter is exhaustive in discussing its topic, therapists should be able to begin working with special populations in a more confident manner as they seek additional resources to obtain specialist competence. Our finding is that most therapists tend to see two or three special populations of children most often as their interests and experience progress.

As in the chapter on diagnostic problems (Chapter 6), we have tried to present information about a broad variety of specialized practices. In addition to tying information into content presented in Parts I through V, each chapter presents the theories, assessment instruments, and treatment modalities essential to its focus. Part VI includes a chapter about the special characteristics of practice in the public school systems because this is where the greatest proportion of pediatric occupational therapy is now practiced. However, the methods and modalities discussed throughout Parts IV and V have been developed through both educationally and medically oriented practice environments and should not be considered extraneous material for the school therapist.

The contributing authors for this book may be recognized as experienced clinical educators who like to write. We looked for the former characteristic in selection of authors to ensure the timeliness and usefulness of practice information. Of course, without the latter quality it would be impossible to complete the book.

As female members of the occupational therapy profession, we and our contributing authors have made conscientious efforts to avoid terminology that might be considered sexist. Whenever possible, we have referred to children in plural form and used clinical examples of both female and male children. However, it is sometimes impossible to present descriptive material in readable style without the use of gender-related pronouns and possessives. In such instances, it is necessary to abide by the general policy of our publishing company to use the universal masculine forms. Please be aware that unless these forms are used in relation to a specific clinical or gender-related example, they are intended to describe characteristics and actions of both female and male children.

The primary purpose of this book is to serve as a basic text for the occupational therapy student who is involved in academic and fieldwork study in pediatrics. We hope it will serve as a continuing resource to that student long after graduation and certification and that it will also provide a basic reference for the experienced practitioner. Our own experiences as students and practitioners of occupational therapy have caused us to wish for, look for, and finally develop such a resource.

No book of this scope can be produced without the assistance and encouragement of many people. We would like to acknowledge the initiating contributions of Don Ladig and Ida Lou Coley, who conceptualized this comprehensive textbook and gave us the idea for its elaboration and production. Rose Hartsook helped establish an outline for the prodigious chapter on diagnostic problems, and Richard D. Sarkin, M.D. reviewed its content. His willingness to share information and resources and his enthusiasm for occupational therapy education were major factors in the completion of that chapter.

Elnora Gilfoyle, Lela Llorens, and Nancy Prendergast read pages and pages of manuscript, giving valuable and insightful comments that improved both content and presentation. Ann Wade, Karen Feltham, Ruth Humphry, and Debbie Russo assisted with the preparation of the chapter on cerebral palsy, as did the staff of the Franklin County Program, Forest Park School, Columbus, Georgia. A succession of therapists at the Colerain School developed several of the assessment instruments used in Chapters 9, 10, and 11: Kathy Campbell, Vera Demeter, Leni Heller, Marilyn Fetters, Janet Johnson, Mary Stover, and Marilee Wilde. Their development and refinement over the years of most useful instruments demonstrate one of the salutary components of occupational therapy practice today. Julie Garvin assisted with the sensory-integration section of Chapter 3; Carol Leaman and Carol Johnson generously provided assessment tools and guidance. We are indebted to the students of Herndon Elementary School, Atlanta, Georgia, for the photographs in Chapters 14 and 24. In addition, the faculty of the occupational therapy program at Ohio State University gave the kind of support that only friends of long standing and kind disposition can give. To all these colleagues who saw a need for this kind of book and contributed so generously to its development, we extend profound appreciation.

A special kind of acknowledgment must be made to Rosa Kasper whose constant grace, good humor, and editorial wisdom were the catalysts that kept the authors and editors working. David Clark and John Allen tolerated the kind of neglect that is induced by projects of this magnitude. Their understanding and nurture were necessary ingredients. And Scott and Stacy Clark modeled, posed, and assisted in many ways so that we could observe and write about what really happens.

Pat Nuse Clark
Anne Stevens Allen

Contents

Appendixes

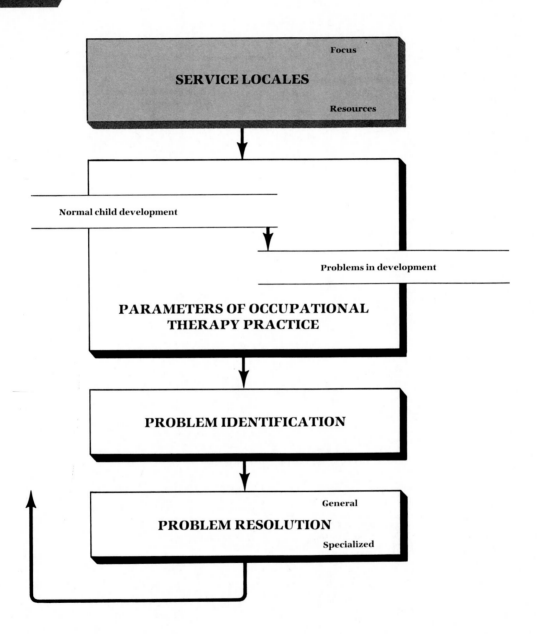

SERVICE LOCALES

Focus

Resources

Normal child development

Problems in development

PARAMETERS OF OCCUPATIONAL
THERAPY PRACTICE

PROBLEM IDENTIFICATION

PROBLEM RESOLUTION

General

Specialized

Introduction

1

PAT NUSE CLARK
ANNE STEVENS ALLEN

The role of occupational therapy in pediatrics

ORGANIZING PRINCIPLES

In 1947 McNary[4] identified the following seven objectives of occupational therapy practice with children:

1. To offer diversional activity to the child when he is undergoing medical treatment,
2. To offer concentrated activity for development of motion of joints, strength of muscles, and coordination,
3. To provide specialized play to teach the elements of self-care,
4. To overcome fears and develop confidence through performance,
5. To encourage normal development in spite of physical, emotional, or intellectual handicap,
6. To provide socializing factors for those who need them and
7. To increase parental understanding of the child's problems through his performance (p. 20).

Thoughtful consideration of the general purposes of current pediatric occupational therapy practice reveals no substantive change in objectives. Certainly, the language of the profession has become more formal and specialized, as have the structure and content of practice. In the early programs the bulk of the occupational therapist's time was spent in actual treatment, namely, teaching children self-care and doing play and recreational activities with them. In contrast, today's therapist may devote longer hours to administrative and supervisory activities and conduct a more formal, comprehensive assessment before initiation of treatment.

The greatest changes in structure and content of occupational therapy practice have resulted from two forces: (1) the overwhelming transformation of contemporary living caused by twentieth century technology

and (2) the resultant, concurrent growth and specialization of the educational process. Adequate discussion of these two forces is beyond the purpose of this text. However, these forces have produced the following six change factors that are pertinent to occupational therapy:

1. The increased life expectancy of children with severe health problems.
2. The expanding scope and variety of publicly supported programs for children.
3. The burgeoning of knowledge in the human sciences, particularly in psychology, the neurosciences, and child development.
4. The impact of modern technology on both diagnostic and treatment aspects of children's programs.
5. The impact of regulatory mechanisms on organization, administration, and documentation of services.
6. The sophistication of methodology for clinical research and its application in occupational therapy.

The purpose of this book is to describe the structure and content of contemporary occupational therapy practice with children and to develop an understanding of the purpose of practice. It is therefore necessary to examine the knowledge that has accrued to the profession, including that resulting from the six change factors described in the preceding paragraph:

1. The current knowledge related to the causes, course, and prognosis of the problems that affect children who are seen by occupational therapists.

2. The focus and variety of settings, agencies, facilities, and service providers pertinent to occupational therapy practice.
3. The principles and processes of child development.
4. The assessment-diagnostic and treatment modalities that have been influenced by the application of research and other technology to occupational therapy practice.
5. The pertinent information related to compliance with regulatory mechanisms governing occupational therapy programs for children.

It is premature to present a detailed discussion of the structure of occupational therapy practice before examination of the knowledge that provides its foundation. However, it will be useful here to present an overall framework that guides, determines, and describes pediatric occupational therapy practice (Figure 1-1). This text essentially duplicates the framework in Figure 1-1 with the exception of the first two chapters, which are introductory and describe service locales, providers, and relationships. In practice, however, one component may never be clearly isolated from the others. It is necessary to have a basic familiarity with the people and places of a child's environments to discuss the child's development and problems in a knowledgeable manner. More detailed information about the dynamics of specialized service settings and mechanisms in relation to occupational therapy practices will be presented later in this book.

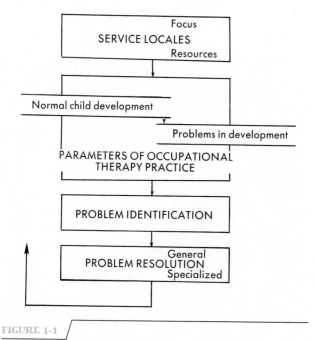

FIGURE 1-1

Organizing framework for comprehensive pediatric occupational therapy.

BASIC METHODS OF SERVICE DELIVERY

Chapman and Chapman[1] outlined a three-dimensional model of health care services that was based on the individual client's right to a healthful, productive life. They categorized services as

1. Life-saving—directed toward prevention of imminent death.
2. Life-sustaining—directed toward health maintenance and prevention of disability.
3. Life-enhancing—directed toward maintenance, restoration, and development of the individual's sense of well-being, social productivity, and self-satisfaction.

It is clear that occupational therapy services are broadly directed toward the life-sustaining and life-enhancing dimensions of health care as described by Chapman and Chapman. In essence, occupational therapy treatment can be said to maintain and enhance the quality of an individual's life. This is an especially important outcome of health services for children with problems, because the biggest part of their lives lies ahead of them. Without life-sustaining and life-enhancing services, such as those delivered by occupational therapists, the future of many children would be less meaningful, less productive, and less satisfying.

A child is likely to receive occupational therapy services at various times during the course of a health problem or handicapping condition. These services may be provided by one or more therapists working through a variety of health care or educational agencies. Occupational therapy services may also differ in method according to the child's status and the agency's objectives. This concept of multiphasic service delivery through a variable course of time, place, and method of intervention constitutes a *continuum of service*.

This chapter will introduce the general methods and settings of occupational therapy services in pediatrics. Discussion of the changes in service over the course of time according to the progression of a child's health status and age will be incorporated into subsequent chapters on pediatric problems and treatment. The service methods described here are a modification of the model developed through the American Occupational Therapy Association (AOTA).[2]

Direct service

Direct service is the most basic method used to provide occupational therapy. This term implies a direct relationship between the child (service recipient) and the therapist (service provider). Usually direct service also denotes face-to-face, hands-on contact between recipient and provider. The usual sequence in direct service is assessment, treatment, and follow-up.

ASSESSMENT

Assessment is an evaluation process that is based on facts (data collected through different formal and informal objective measures of the child's performance) and sound clinical judgment. The latter is the subjective and interpretive component of assessment, and it is the end product of the therapist's individual experiences, namely, the therapist's training, practice, and theoretical frame of reference.

The initial phase of assessment is known as *screening*. In occupational therapy, screening usually includes observation of the child in a natural activity situation and the gathering of some baseline background information about the child. Screening permits the therapist to determine the need for more comprehensive and precise evaluation and subsequent occupational therapy treatment. Occasionally the therapist will decide that occupational therapy intervention is unnecessary or that such services are contraindicated until a later date.

Assessment is a continuing process as the therapist continually thinks through interactions and activity experiences with the child. However, at designated intervals the assessment becomes more structured and is thus recorded. This allows the therapist to

1. Identify present performance
2. Define problems
3. Identify potential performance
4. Develop program objectives and modalities
5. Record and report progress to document change

TREATMENT

Treatment consists of a carefully selected program of change-enhancing activities that are administered by the therapist. The child's response to the activity is guided by the therapist, who is also responsible for changes and outcome of the treatment program. (The terms *treatment*, *therapy*, and *program* are often used interchangeably.) The structure and ramifications of treatment are complex and will be explored in Parts III, V, and VI of this book.

FOLLOW-UP

When the child has obtained the optimal benefits from treatment or has shown no significant change over time (plateaued), therapy is discontinued. The child is assigned to follow-up status. This means that the child is rechecked by the therapist at fixed intervals. Follow-up appointments for children are generally scheduled every 3 to 6 months. This is usually more frequent than follow-up for adults because of the impact of the continuing developmental process on the child's functional level and needs. Frequent follow-up visits allow the therapist to monitor a child's progress and reinstitute therapy in a timely manner when needed.

Eventually the child will be discharged. Parents should always be advised of available resources for future therapy and related needs.

Outreach services

Outreach services are provided by occupational therapists to children who are under the primary care of other agencies. Often these agencies may already employ an occupational therapist. However, special children have special needs, and occasionally more experienced or specialized therapy services are indicated that are beyond the expertise of the agency therapist.

Usually outreach services follow the same assessment and treatment planning sequence as direct service with one important difference. After the assessment has been completed, the visiting therapist develops a *model program* for the child or children. This model program is then demonstrated and described in detail to the agency therapist. The goal is to increase the expertise of the local agency therapist who will continue and carry out the treatment at the agency. The outcome of treatment is a shared responsibility of both visiting and local therapists.

Outreach services are used most frequently to provide specialized services to rural areas. Typically the vis-

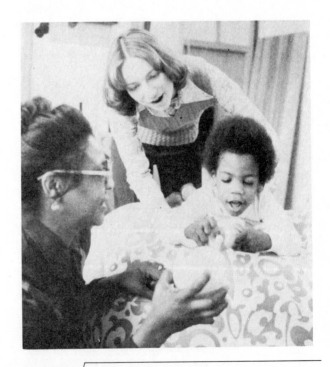

FIGURE 1-2

A visiting occupational therapist works with local staff to bring specialized skills to a small community hospital.

From Allen, A.S., editor: Introduction to health professions, ed. 3, St. Louis, 1980, The C.V. Mosby Co.

iting therapist is employed at an urban, university-affiliated children's center and works with a local therapist whose practice and experience are more general (Figure 1-2).

Indirect service

Indirect service implies that the therapist does not engage in face-to-face, hands-on contact with the child. The concept can be misleading, because usually there is at least one direct contact with the service recipient, and often additional contacts are made at regular intervals. The essence of indirect service is that the bulk of treatment is administered by other direct service providers and based on recommendations made by the occupational therapist. The occupational therapist may or may not be held responsible for the outcome of treatment.

Therapists who work in large agencies with many potential clients, such as school systems, often use *monitoring* as the primary method of service delivery. The therapist directly assesses the child and develops a treatment program. Other direct care staff are then trained by the therapist to carry out program activities on a daily basis. The therapist rechecks the child and the consistency of the program and updates activities and assessment at regular intervals. Using a monitoring system, the therapist is responsible for the outcome of the program.

The responsibility for outcome shifts to the direct care providers in a *consultation* arrangement. The therapist may do direct assessment of individual children and then recommend program methods. Or the therapist may not evaluate directly but instead interview staff members to obtain information about clients and agency procedures. The therapist then discusses and writes down broad recommendations for changes that could facilitate improved services for clients of the agency. The consultation process has its own formal structure and is usually of short duration. The therapist has no direct authority to enforce recommended changes but instead relies on an ability to influence the behavior of staff members.

In practice, most experienced therapists use a combination of direct, outreach, and indirect service methods to provide appropriate occupational therapy services to children. The emphasis on one method of service delivery over another will be influenced by the type of agency in which the therapist is employed.

SERVICE SETTINGS

Almost 15% of all practicing occupational therapists work in the field of pediatrics by providing services to newborns, toddlers, preschoolers, and kindergartners through adolescents. This clientele receives health services in numerous settings, depending on the age of the child, the severity and cause of the problem, and, to some extent, the parents' ability or willingness to pay for services.

Some children with severe problems must be cared for in custodial situations, while others with similar problems may live at home and go to public schools. Maintaining regular school programs for handicapped children among their normal peers is called *mainstreaming* and is mandated by federal law (p. 8).

In all settings the occupational therapist attempts to help children adapt to their physical and emotional surroundings, to assure children the most normal development possible, to assist parents in learning how to understand and deal with their child's needs, and to offer opportunities for daily stabilizing diversion for children under stress.

Neonatal units

Specialized units for the care of newborns at risk are part of the nurseries in teaching hospitals and in specialty hospitals with high obstetrical case loads. These units serve newborns in need of special care, especially those whose survival is in doubt and those who appear to be well but are at risk of serious illness. These newborns are isolated in a sterile, protective environment and handled through sealed apertures in the sides of their bassinets. They are under 24-hour observation because of the rapidity with which life-threatening crises can occur. Nurses, physicians, respiratory therapists, developmental therapists, and other specialized personnel are involved in their care.

The determination of which newborns are to be placed in such units depends on institutional criteria, such as minimal weights, disease categories, or condition of the mother. The components of service are (1) direct observation of the newborn by nursing and medical personnel, (2) physiological and biochemical monitoring by electronic equipment and laboratory personnel, (3) diagnostic and therapeutic procedures, and (4) support of maximal mother-child contact.[3]

In the neonatal setting, developmental therapists, who are often occupational therapists, are involved in these therapeutic procedures by giving sensory stimulation to infants deprived of normal stimulation by the enforced isolation of the unit. These infants are frequently restrained to prevent interference with the tubes and other biomedical devices necessarily attached to them. Sensory stimulation is provided to counteract the negative developmental effects of this isolation and restraint. Splinting is sometimes used to maintain the infant in a safer functional position.

Public health departments and well-baby clinics

Public health departments are financed by city and county governments and offer certain clinical services to residents of the city and region. These services include communicable disease testing, immunization programs, and home health services. Mothers who have no family physician are encouraged to have their infants checked in the well-baby clinic, which is frequently operated under the county's maternal and child health funds, and to participate in the immunization program.

Occupational therapists working in well-baby clinics have the opportunity to develop infant stimulation programs and to teach the mothers about developmental play. This can often mean the difference between a neglected child who fails to develop socially and emotionally and a thriving, happy youngster.

Home health services

Home health services are offered to homebound persons of all ages. These services include bedside nursing, homemaking assistance, hot meals programs, and programs of occupational, physical, and speech therapies.

Home health services provide occupational therapy to children of all diagnoses who cannot be taken to central agencies or schools. Occupational therapy services to homebound children include programs for orthopedic and developmental disabilities. The goals are primarily rehabilitative in nature. Maintenance of health and function, assisting the child to develop in the home environment, and teaching family how to assist or care for the child are also goals of home health services.

Physicians' offices

Most children receive primary health care through the offices of private physicians. Detailed description of their services may be found in Chapter 5.

Occasionally physicians will arrange for therapists to provide assessment and treatment in their offices. Usually such arrangements are made with therapists in private practice. Such an arrangement is convenient for parents because it reduces the need to travel from office to office for services.

Community health centers

Community health centers offer a variety of services to clients from a localized area. The centers usually develop in response to specific needs and as a result of considerable community effort. They are funded in the following ways: by united appeals campaigns, by sliding-scale fee-for-service arrangements, by private endowments, by grants from governmental agencies, and by other sources tapped by enterprising citizens.

The health programs in these centers reflect the community's need for emergency services and general health care. There is usually emphasis on prevention.

Occupational therapy in community health is a diverse practice and often reflects the interests or specialties of the therapists on the staff, for the service potential far exceeds the ability of the center to develop needed programs. Pediatric occupational therapists in community health screen for developmental delay, teach play skills to parents and children, and provide specialized therapy programs for handicapped children.

Health maintenance organizations (HMOs)

Health maintenance organizations (HMOs) are a relatively new type of health agency that provide continuous, coordinated health services to its members. These members enroll individually and prepay their medical expenses with a fixed monthly payment. Under such a system it is to the benefit of the HMO to keep health and medical costs low. One of the ways this is done is to prevent illness and maintain health.

There are two types of HMO. One provides care in a centrally located building with a group of physicians under contract to or employed by the HMO. The other type contracts with community-based physicians to give care in their own offices to HMO members. Occupational therapists seeking to practice in HMO settings find the first type, the so-called group staff HMO, more supportive of their services. Within the central location, occupational therapy programs answering pediatric needs can be developed. The therapist's role in such an agency would include consultation as well as direct service with a great deal of emphasis placed on preventive programs, such as screening for the early detection of developmental problems.

General and children's hospitals

General hospitals are found in small communities and in large cities and constitute the largest classification of hospitals. They accept patients of all ages and diagnoses, but they usually refer complex cases to appropriate specialty hospitals. They serve as the health and emergency center for their surrounding communities.

The occupational therapist in a general hospital provides many services because of the variety of problems and the relatively short stay of most patients. General hospitals require occupational therapists to serve in many capacities, for instance, (1) evaluating patients for physical function and developing therapeutic programs for them and (2) providing cardiac programs, burn care, and stroke rehabilitation. Similar functional services are provided for the pediatric unit but with a greater emphasis on diversional programs and play therapy because of the emotional needs of children separated from their families.

Children's hospitals limit their patient services to the pediatric patient and therefore can usually offer a wider variety of pediatric occupational therapy than can the general hospital with its broader range of needs. In the children's hospital, probably as in no other setting, the seven objectives listed by McNary[4] (p. 2) can each be realized in the same setting. A wide variety of pediatric diagnoses gives rise to a wide variety of treatment objectives. Length of stay is longer in the children's hospital than in the general hospital, which makes emotional and developmental support mandatory. Also found in children's hospitals are functional programs for the development of muscle strength, joint motion, and coordination for the orthopedically and neurologically handicapped child; socializing and developmental programs for all children but especially for those with long hospital stays; and programs that build confidence and positive self-images in children who have experienced either psychological or physical trauma.

As with any program involving children, a second dimension of treating the child is working with the parent. Occupational therapists will teach parents the same skills the child learns and also teach them how to help the child.

Rehabilitation centers

Rehabilitation is defined as a return to the level of function enjoyed before the onset of the disease or injury that has interrupted the client's life. Children who have never attained any degree of independence and who must learn self-care and other basic living skills for the first time are said to undergo habilitation. Agencies that provide habilitative and rehabilitative services are called *rehabilitation centers* and are usually financed by private resources, such as insurance companies, union funds, and united appeals agencies. Payment for services often comes from the state division of rehabilitation services when adults are being served. Children's services are reimbursed by a variety of governmental agencies, both state and federal.

Rehabilitation centers provide the child with a broad range of concentrated corrective programs designed to restore function and advance independence. In addition to medical services, rehabilitation centers provide social and psychological services; occupational, physical, and speech therapies; tutors or classroom teachers; vocational counseling and prevocational testing; orthotic and prosthetic consultation; and other needed services, either in the center or by referral.

As in the children's hospital, the full range of occupational therapy objectives is applicable. Occupational therapists evaluate the children and design treatment programs that promote developmental skills, enhance independence and self-confidence, and develop physical function and coordination. The therapist functions as part of an interdisciplinary team, not only in treatment but also in decision making and problem solving.

Residential programs

Residential programs for the care of handicapped children usually serve the most seriously handicapped population and are usually operated by the state government. Institutions for the profoundly retarded, for the blind, and for the deaf are funded by the states, and the quality of their programs depends on the tax structure and philosophy of the incumbent administration.

Client evaluation, training in adaptive skills, and sensory integrative therapy are the primary concerns of the staff occupational therapists. Because of the residential nature of the institution, diversional programming is also within the purview of occupational therapy planning and of high importance for the stimulation, skill development, and self-confidence of the residents.

Institutions that are primarily custodial will have little to attract a staff of occupational therapists. Occupational therapy is at its best in residential programs when it is closely allied to an educational program with teachers, occupational therapists, physical and speech therapists, and psychologists working together as a team.

Day training centers

Day training centers serve a population of educable mentally retarded and severely physically handicapped persons as an entry point to sheltered or assisted work. Adaptive skills and work skills are taught in these centers, usually to adolescents and young adults. Infants and younger children who are not able to attend public school are also clients of the day training centers. Referral can be made by schools, by the division of vocational rehabilitation, and by other agencies.

Clients go to the day training center on regular schedules three to five times a week. An educational rather than clinical atmosphere is maintained. Occupational therapy programs include evaluation and training in self-care, homemaking, and prevocational skills, including emotional and social skills that are required vocationally. Subcontracted work, such as simple assembly tasks, is sometimes available to be used primarily in client evaluation or training for future assisted placement. Occupational therapists will frequently analyze available jobs in the community to determine their appropriateness for specific clients and to suggest modifications that would enable clients to be successful on the job.

Schools

Occupational therapy services have long been established in specialized schools for handicapped children. Supported by funds from national agencies, service clubs, and other community organizations, both occupational therapy and physical therapy were made available primarily in private schools but also in public schools when the local system was large enough to accommodate a special school for children with special needs.

This imbalance was changed in 1975 through Public Law 94-142. This bill mandated education for all handicapped children within public school systems through programs designed to meet the individual needs of these children. Transportation to the school, special teachers, and occupational, physical, and speech therapies were construed as education-related services necessary to meet these needs, and they were therefore provided by law.

Occupational therapy in public schools has one primary aim—to improve the handicapped student's ability to participate in the special education program. Secondary aims are to consult with parents and teachers, enabling them to understand the needs of the individual child and to assist the child in attaining and applying adaptive skills to classroom and home situations.

Occupational therapists have different roles in private schools, depending on the mission of the particular schools. Those schools that are established to serve children of one handicap group, such as the mentally retarded or the deaf, will often have a staff of therapists to provide services similar to those described previously. These services can also be extended to the prevocational area through prevocational tests, work methods adaptation, job evaluation, and assisted placement.

Private schools are maintained by two primary sources: (1) full tuition and (2) combinations of tuition and charitable endowments. Their programs are not affected by government regulations, so the programmatic quality of these schools varies according to the philosophy of their proprietors and the demands of their clientele. They thus range from being excellent educational and training programs to being mere custodial care centers.

Preschool programs

Preschools are set up in churches and other central locations to provide socialization and environmental stimulation for children younger than kindergarten age. The Head Start program, established under the Economic Opportunity Act of 1964, is an example of such a program developed by public initiative and federal funds. Its purpose was to give disadvantaged children preparation for elementary school programs. Individual grants were made to cities and localities to initiate programs at public locations. Services were later extended to children above the poverty level whose parents were required to pay according to their ability.

Private preschool programs are frequently sponsored by a church or other institution having space available. They depend on parental assistance, partial tuition, and subsidized overhead charges for support. There also are entrepreneurial preschools run for profit in private homes or commercial locations that depend totally on student tuition for support.

Occupational therapy in preschool settings is usually practiced on a consultant basis and is entirely developmental in nature. Screening for developmental delay and evaluation of age-appropriate social and coordinative skills comprise the majority of the assessment in preschool occupational therapy. Developmental and sensory integrative techniques are used in treatment, either at the school or by referral to therapists in private practice.

Private practice

Pediatric occupational therapists in private practice frequently work as consultants to several agencies, preschools, or pediatricians. They may refer children for treatment to other practicing therapists, to staff Certified Occupational Therapy Assistants (COTAs), or to outpatient clinics. Consultants may also combine practice with their consultancies and see patients either at the patient's home or at their own offices.

Consultant, therapist, developmental specialist, prevocational evaluator—all these are roles filled by the occupational therapist in private practice. Services may be reimbursed by individual fees or a combination of patient fees and retainers paid by the employing agencies.

SUMMARY

The organizing principles of occupational therapy have their roots in McNary's original seven objectives.[4] Twentieth century technology and educational specialization produced six change factors that have influenced the practice of occupational therapy. The methods of service delivery and their locales have responded to these factors. At present, occupational therapists may practice in a variety of different settings and give direct, outreach, or indirect services.

REFERENCES

1. Chapman, J.E., and Chapman, H.H.: Behavior and health care: a humanistic helping process, St. Louis, 1975, The C.V. Mosby Co.
2. Gilfoyle, E.M., and Hayes, C., editors: Training: occupational therapy educational management in schools (TOTEMS), Rockville, Md., 1980, American Occupational Therapy Association, Inc. (Supported by Grant #G007801499 U.S. Department of Education, Office of Special Education and Rehabilitative Services, Vol. I to IV.)
3. Korones, S.B.: High-risk newborn infants, ed. 3, St. Louis, 1981, The C.V. Mosby Co.
4. McNary, H.: The scope of occupational therapy. In Willard, H.S., and Spackman, C.S.: Occupational therapy, Philadelphia, 1947, J.B. Lippincott Co.

ANNE STEVENS ALLEN

2

Relationships with others involved in service delivery to children

Children with illnesses and emotional, physical, or mental deficiencies must be treated as "whole persons" within their environments. This is a truism not only in occupational therapy with its long history of concern for the wholeness of the patient, but increasingly in the other helping professions where technological specializations have often divided patient care into units defined by body systems or malfunctioning parts.

It has been suggested that society's present concern for the whole person has generated a need for interprofessional collaboration. Various specialists must learn to work together as one functioning unit to ensure respect for the patient as a whole person and to treat the person as one complex organism rather than treat only separate parts of that person.

Collaborating groups of concerned, helping professionals are usually referred to as teams, and an extensive literature has developed that deals with the formation of teams and their ability to function effectively. Occupational therapists serve on many interprofessional teams and therefore work with many other helping persons. Not all such persons have the training in small group dynamics and interpersonal skills that is part of occupational therapy education. Most occupational therapists find that this part of their education (originally planned for patient interfaces) transfers most helpfully into professional interfaces. Careful attention should be paid to recognition of roles, clear communications, and shared decisions. These are effective tools for establishing relationships with the other persons involved in the care of children—medical and educational personnel and parents. This chapter will discuss the oc-cupational therapist's relationship with medical and educational teams. For a discussion of the occupational therapist's relationship with parents, see Chapter 8.

THE MEDICAL TEAM

The medical team is made up of a variety of persons who are trained in different specialties and who each have different backgrounds, different values, and sometimes different goals. These specialists work together in varying configurations, depending on the needs of the patient. Sometimes the team is made up of a physician and nurse only; sometimes it encompasses the full spectrum of service providers—physician, nurse, social worker, occupational and physical therapists, speech pathologist, and so on. An important aspect of the health team is its ever-changing nature.

Baldwin,[1] one of the leading researchers in team evaluation, has compared teams to traffic on the Los Angeles freeway:

> As with teams, cars (read team members) get on and off for different reasons, at different times, at different places, for different destinations, and with different speeds and sizes (read power and prestige).

Occupational therapists must be aware of the potential contributions of each specialist to the well-being of patients and must be able to adapt to the changing team members with their different "destinations . . . speeds and sizes."

Some occupational therapists have a very close relationship with other members of the medical team, while others practice more separately. A therapist on the staff of a children's rehabilitation unit might interact with the majority of the team members several times a day. A therapist in private practice might not make these contacts more than once a week. In both cases, however, and in situations between these two extremes, interprofessional relationships should be collaborative and understanding.

Good team relationships resolve the problems of overlapping roles among the professions. Informed professionals are aware of the areas of overlap and build cooperative relationships. Horwitz[4] suggests that these relationships can allow practitioners to work at their advanced skill levels for longer periods of time than can the practitioner who does not have access to team support and consultation.

Occupational therapists are trained in skills that sometimes overlap with those of physical therapists, social workers, psychologists, teachers, child developmentalists, and orthotists, to name a few. It is natural to desire autonomy, but this can be counterproductive in professional practice. Keeping open lines of communication; recognizing the skills, overlapping or specific, of other professions; and using those skills to complement one's own are hallmarks of professional competence.

It is the responsibility of each professional to interpret his or her role to others. An occupational therapist can never assume that members of other professions are knowledgeable about the role of occupational therapy in health services for children. A nurse who has experienced occupational therapy as a behaviorally oriented therapy in a clinic for adolescents will be hard pressed to understand the sensory integrative approach used in a school program. A physician who is accustomed to working with child developmentalists in one neonatal nursery must have explained the occupational therapist's role in a different neonatal setting.

Occupational therapists in particular must become experts at explaining their own functions, because their treatment goals are so often hidden within an apparently recreational activity. Any passerby who comments, "Oh, Marty is making a fine wallet!" should be thanked for the compliment but given the significant information that the wallet provides Marty with a means of establishing coordination and strengthening pinch. Group activities especially must be identified as specific treatment goals to other professionals to make the practice credible and desirable.

Physicians

Although occupational therapists can practice without physicians' referrals, in pediatric services the pediatrician is not only a significant source of referrals but also a source of information about the patient and joint planning for the patient. The pediatrician is a medical specialist, having completed medical school and several years of specialized study and practice in children's diseases. Specialists in family practice have a similar length of medical preparation, but they work more broadly with conditions affecting the entire human life span and more intensively with family interactions. Both specialties are considered primary care, for the reason that children may go initially to a pediatrician or to a family care specialist for checkups or when ill. These physicians' offices, therefore, serve as ports of entry to the medical system. Physicians refer patients to other specialties as the need is perceived.

Consulting physicians are usually specialists to whom the child has been referred by the primary care physician; they include orthopedists, ophthalmologists, neurologists, cardiologists, physiatrists, psychiatrists, and pulmonary specialists. It is not uncommon for a seriously ill child or one with multiple handicaps to have several consulting physicians, some of whom must be integral members of the treatment team; others can be more peripheral.

In reference to Baldwin's analogy,[1] the consultants represent the large, fast cars on the freeway, entering quickly and moving on. Occupational therapists should be prepared to relate to them by explaining occupational therapy services and establishing or modifying treatment goals to meet the particular condition. In working with all professional colleagues, these explanations should start with the benefits a particular patient can receive from occupational therapy and the goals to be set and worked toward. From here one can go on to generalities and from generalities to basic theory if the colleague expresses interest. But it is usually desirable to establish interprofessional dialogue by using specific cases.

Nurses

Nurses often serve a coordinating function in the delivery of patient services and can be directly responsible for referrals to occupational therapy and for making it physically possible for the child to go to treatment sessions. It is therefore wise for occupational therapists to acquaint themselves with the nursing staff, make clear to all nurses the role of occupational therapy, and work closely with them in coordinating programs. It is frequently difficult for a nurse who is caring for several patients to allow exceptions to the necessary floor routine for a patient who needs leniency for specific routines prescribed by occupational therapy. Whether a child is allowed to practice feeding skills during the very busy breakfast hour in an institution might very well depend on the relationship between the therapist and the nursing staff.

Nursing was the first of the many undergraduate health professions now in practice, and it has the largest number of practitioners. Student nurses can prepare for the certifying examination and become registered nurses through one of the following routes:

1. Hospital schools that are associated with teaching hospitals, which give classes and practical experience in a program usually 3 years in length. A diploma is awarded.
2. Community or technical colleges that give classes and laboratory experience and arrange for clinical practice with local hospitals. These programs are 2 years in length and award the associate of arts degree.
3. Four-year colleges and universities that offer undergraduate education along with nursing classes and laboratory experience. Clinical practice is arranged with suitable hospitals. The bachelor of science degree is awarded.

Registered nurses can specialize as pediatric nurses through on-the-job training and experience by acquiring specific pediatric nursing skills that other nurses who take general duty jobs do not attain because they transfer from service to service. There is also a classification known as pediatric nurse practitioner, which indicates that the nurse has completed advanced education, usually at the master's degree level, and has acquired advanced skills, particularly in physical assessment. These nurses can establish their own practices within a community but will generally establish a close working relationship with a specific physician or group of physicians.

Licensed practical nurses (LPNs) complete training programs 12 to 16 months in length, usually after high school, and sit for examinations in the state where they will practice. These nurses give bedside care and work under the supervision of registered nurses. Nursing aides are trained in high school vocational programs or on-the-job programs in hospitals. They assist both registered and practical nurses.

The different levels of nurse education make it difficult for newcomers in the health services field to make knowledgeable expectations of nursing staffs. In general, higher levels of education produce nurses with greater theoretical knowledge and therefore higher ability to plan programs, evaluate patients and systems, and make changes; the more technically trained nurses develop high skills in bedside care and the techniques of nursing. As with all generalizations, individual exceptions abound.

Physical therapists

Occupational and physical therapists work closely together in outpatient clinics, hospitals, special schools, public schools, crippled children's agencies, and private practice. Known together as the rehabilitation therapies, occupational therapy and physical therapy have, for the most part, many common goals in patient treatment. But their primary treatment modalities are vastly different. Their goals do overlap, however, and when this happens, the roles of the two professions begin to blur. It is to the advantage of those in both professions to observe the technical differences in one another's practices, even though a good case can be made for eliminating arbitrary boundaries with individual patients, particularly children. Where occupational therapists work with activities and stress adaptability, physical therapists work with physical modalities—for example, heat, ultrasound, mechanics, and water—and stress mobility. These are the foci of their educational programs and the thrust of their practices. Because of their common treatment goals, working relations between the two professions are highly collaborative in most instances. Because of the vagaries of human nature and the economy, the two professions sometimes find themselves competing for patients. When this happens, it must be recognized, and steps must be taken to plan jointly for the good of the patient.

An example of role blurring between occupational therapy and physical therapy can be seen in the treatment goal of establishing trunk stability. The physical therapist must work toward this goal as a prerequisite to sitting and walking; the occupational therapist works toward the same goal as a prerequisite to sitting and using arms for feeding or other activities. Often the exercises that the physical therapist uses in working toward this goal with children look very similar to the activities the occupational therapist uses.

Physical therapy at present is essentially an undergraduate health profession, as is occupational therapy, terminating in the bachelor of science degree. However, physical therapy is officially moving toward establishing all basic education programs at the post-baccalaureate level. Both professions require extensive clinical experience before certification. Whereas occupational therapists can, and do, frequently work without physician referrals, physical therapists do not, a situation that tends to press the physical therapist into the medical model and the occupational therapist into the educational model. It is probably because of their similarities and in spite of their differences that the two professions achieve high degrees of the collaboration and cooperation that Beckhard[2] cites as the essence of health team success.

Speech and hearing specialists

Speech and hearing specialists receive their education at the master's or doctoral level and have studied such topics as speech and hearing disorders, the development of language, the physics of speech, theories and measurements of hearing, and phonetics. Depending on their area of specialization, they are referred to as speech and hearing therapists, speech pathologists and audiologists, logopedists, or phoniatrists.[3] They work only with the body systems having to do with verbal communication (talking and listening), but they see many of the same patients that occupational therapists see. These are primarily the children and youth who are developmentally delayed and children and adults who have suffered brain damage from cerebral vascular accidents, head trauma of various origins, and neurological conditions such as Parkinson's disease and multiple sclerosis.

Occupational therapists in schools for the deaf interact with the entire spectrum of these specialists in verbal communication. In hospitals, schools, and clinics they tend to work mostly with speech pathologists because of the common interest in the developmentally delayed and brain-damaged patients. Frequently occupational therapists will collaborate by incorporating procedures initiated by the speech pathologist into their own treatment time, for example, using pictures to stimulate proper word sounds as part of educational activities with developmentally delayed children. This is an example of combined treatment time made possible through careful planning by the two professionals. It works to the advantage of the patient both in economy and in reinforcement.

Social workers

Social workers are employed by hospitals, clinics, state and local agencies, and sometimes school systems to assist clients and families in their attempts to adjust financially, socially, and psychologically to the problems besetting them. Occupational therapists have frequent meetings with social workers as they each try to help the patient adjust to handicaps of illness, injury, family loss, and vocational stress. While occupational therapists work through activities, social workers employ counseling sessions and assistive negotiations with financial and social agencies.

There are several levels of social work practice, each capable of different contributions to the care of the client. The following levels were established by the National Association of Social Workers, Inc., and published in Standards for Social Services Manpower[5]:

Social service aide No educational requirements, on-the-job training.
Social service technician Completion of a 2-year community college education with an associate of arts or bachelor's degree from another field. This level is sometimes called mental health technician.
Social worker A baccalaureate degree from an accredited program.
Graduate social worker A master's degree from an accredited graduate school of social work.
Certified social worker Certification by the Academy of Certified Social Workers (ACSW) as being capable of the autonomous practice of social work.
Social work fellow Completion of a doctoral degree or substantial practice in a field of specialization following certification by ACSW.

Social workers recognize that social stresses arise from physical and mental illness, and they plan for services to the client that will minimize social dysfunction. Knowledge of agencies and how they operate, of how interagency referrals can be accomplished to the benefit of the client and family, and of cultural and ethnic differences that must be countered or planned for are all part of what the social workers bring to the health team.

Social workers frequently can assist the occupational therapist by finding resources for needed adapted equipment, by helping patients accept or psychologically adjust to various aspects of disabling conditions, and by facilitating interagency communications.

Prosthetists and orthotists

In the field of pediatrics, prosthetists are the person who make and fit artificial limbs. Orthotists make and fit permanent splints and braces. Each specialist works closely with the prescribing orthopedist, physiatrist, or pediatrician to ensure the child's benefit and comfort. They also work closely with the occupational therapist who teaches the child to use the device in the way most effective for that individual's need. During the course of therapy, the occupational therapist may discover a modification that would help the child perform better. This must be discussed with the prosthetist or orthotist because of the possibility of mechanical problems or contraindications and also in recognition of the proprietary rights of the expert. Prosthetists and orthotists were at one time apprentice kinds of specialties where the necessary skills were acquired through on-the-job training. Standards were established in the late 1970s, and a national certifying examination was developed. Current requirements to sit for the examination include graduation from an accredited program and completion of 1 year of experience. At least two universities (New York University and the University of Washington) offer programs leading to the bachelor of science degree.

Child developmentalists

Persons educated in the area of child development have a wide variety of skills and interests. They hold degrees at the bachelor's, master's, and doctoral levels and represent a broad range of special interests and skills: human development, family relationships, child evaluation, infant guidance and care, nursery school, and group care services. Occupational therapists meet these specialists primarily in the infant stimulation, child assessment, and play therapy programs. Depending on interest, level of education, and type of institution, there may be overlap with the occupational therapy program. It is to everyone's benefit to keep the lines of communication open and to discuss common treatment goals and methods.

Technical personnel

For hospitalized children there is an alarming (to the child) array of technical personnel who jab them, prod them, stick things into them, aerate and ventilate them, and perform other incomprehensible and frightening procedures. During planned play periods, which are relatively nonthreatening situations, occupational therapists can often provide comforting interpretations of such treatments and procedures for the child. Cooperation in arranging treatment schedules with laboratory and x-ray personnel, respiratory therapists, and technicians who operate such diagnostic equipment as the electrocardiograph and electroencephalograph can work to the benefit of everyone's schedule by producing a relaxed, unfrightened child at treatment time.

THE EDUCATIONAL TEAM

The educational team is responsible for preparing children with the knowledge and skills essential for productive living in a complex technological society. Occupational therapists have varying degrees of interface with educators, depending in great part on whether occupational therapy is given at the child's home, in a hospital, clinic, private office, or school building. The occupational therapist must be aware of the child's educational achievements and objectives, whether therapy is seen as a separate, medically oriented treatment or as an integral part of the educational curriculum. Gaining this awareness requires communication and often a good measure of cooperation with the educational team. In school settings the occupational therapist is considered one of the educational team members. The following section will describe other members of this team: professional teachers, teacher's aides, other professionals, and support personnel.

Teachers

The teaching profession is made up of persons with specific expertise: kindergarten and elementary school teachers, secondary school teachers, special education teachers, guidance counselors, art and music teachers, teachers of industrial arts, home economics teachers, vocational education and automobile driving instructors, coaches and physical education teachers, and ad-

ministrators. Whatever the specialization of the teacher, all teachers have in common the basic tenets of the profession and the requirements of their particular state regarding certification.

All states require certification for public school teachers, and many require it for teachers in private and parochial schools. The minimal requirement for certification is the bachelor's degree, with the infrequent exception of nursery and kindergarten teachers whose minimal requirement in some states is the associate of arts degree. Many states require teachers to work toward and achieve master's degrees within specified periods of time after employment. The education profession has thus mandated the continuing education that all professions encourage as an essential of continuing professional viability. Guidance counselors and teachers in special education are required to have teaching certificates as well as further qualifications in their special areas.

Occupational therapists often work closely with special education teachers because of their shared interest in handicapped children. These teachers have advanced skills in teaching children who are blind, deaf, emotionally disturbed, mentally retarded, and physically handicapped. They seek the expertise of the occupational therapist in planning for the child's classroom participation through the use of assistive devices, handling techniques, positive self-image and so forth.

The guidance counselor can supplement the prevocational work of the occupational therapist by supplying career information, selected testing services, and counseling with students about vocational, academic, and technical opportunities. The prevocational work that occupational therapists do with handicapped children should be carefully described and demonstrated to the guidance counselor to develop cooperative, effective services for the child. Refer to Chapter 24 for a thorough presentation of occupational therapy in the school system.

Therapists working outside the school system in clinics or other agencies usually familiarize themselves with the educational program of the particular patient as an aid to selecting appropriate and stimulating therapeutic activities. Teachers can be directly approached for conferences concerning the child.

Teacher's aides are trained to assist the professional teacher in the classroom in ways that give the teacher more time to do what he or she is primarily hired to do—teach. Aides will grade papers, monitor hallways, help children with outdoor clothing, and, in general, assist in any classroom or area of the school program. They are sometimes paid employees of the school system; other times they are volunteers. Because of the assistive nature of their job, aides are often directly involved with helping children adjust to the classroom or to feeding themselves or to doing other self-maintenance activities. Occupational therapists should ensure that the aides as well as the teachers are familiar with prescribed routines and equipment.

Other professionals

Others who also join the educational team as needed are speech and language teachers, audiologists, psychologists, and occupational and physical therapists. (See p. 12 for a discussion of physical therapy.)

Speech and language teachers have duties that differ from those of the special educators who are specifically trained to teach academic subjects to the deaf. The speech and language teachers teach communication processes and language skills to all needful children, including the deaf, and are qualified in the area of speech and hearing sciences. Similarly, audiologists evaluate the hearing ability of schoolchildren and recommend hearing aids or other treatments to improve hearing. More is written about speech and hearing personnel on p. 12.

Psychologists relate to the educational team in two ways: (1) as school psychologists hired by the school system and (2) as consulting or clinical psychologists used on a fee-for-service basis by the individual child and family. Licensure requirements vary from state to state, but in general, psychologists may be prepared at the master's or doctoral levels. They will perform services according to their level of qualifications and experience. Most psychologists who serve school systems are prepared to make psychological evaluations, give treatment, and interpret test results.

Support personnel

Bus drivers, maintenance workers, and dietary personnel contribute services to the educational program in their contracted areas and in ways that are not so apparent. The bus driver can have a great influence on the child with a mobility problem, and the dietary worker can influence the child with a feeding problem. All levels of personnel can contribute substantially to the therapeutic and educational programs if the therapists and teachers communicate goals, elicit suggestions, and instruct them in the use of assistive devices and techniques.

SUMMARY

Occupational therapists work with many professionals during their service to children. In health and educational institutions, as well as in the community at large, children are best served if the many persons involved in their treatment communicate and collaborate in goal setting and planning. A variety of professional and technical specialties have been introduced in this chapter to acquaint the reader with the level of knowledge and skills of their colleagues in the helping professions.

REFERENCES

1. Baldwin, D.C., Jr.,: Some conceptual and methodological issues in team research. In Bachman, J.E., editor: Interdisciplinary health care: proceedings of the third annual Interdisciplinary Team Care Conference, Kalamazoo, 1982, Center for Human Services, Western Michigan University.
2. Beckhard, R.: Organizational issues in the team delivery of comprehensive health care, Millbank Mem. Fund Q. **50:**287, July 1972.
3. Black, J.W.: Speech and hearing science. In Allen, A.S., editor: Introduction to health professions, ed. 3, St. Louis, 1980, The C.V. Mosby Co.
4. Horwitz, J.: Interprofessional teamwork, Soc. Worker **38:**5, 1970.
5. Standards for social services manpower, Washington, D.C., 1973, The National Association of Social Workers, Inc.

SUGGESTED READINGS

Ducanis, A., and Golin, A.: The interdisciplinary health care team, Germantown, Md., 1979, Aspen Systems Corp.

Kane, R.A.: Interprofessional teamwork, Manpower monograph No. 8, Syracuse, N.Y., 1975, Syracuse University School of Social Work.

Lawson, D.: Education careers, New York, 1977, Franklin Watts.

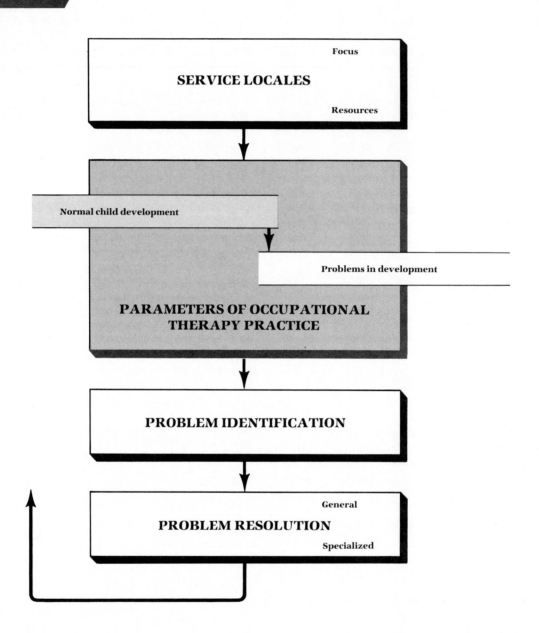

Knowledge base

PAT NUSE CLARK
LINDA A. FLOREY
FLORENCE CLARK

Developmental principles and theories

In the course of studying child development, it is not uncommon to find ourselves reviewing our own life histories by watching children in public and comparing and contrasting events and behaviors with the theoretical models. These mental exercises are inescapable and very appropriate. In fact, this retrospective-observational method gave impetus to the earliest concepts of human development in the past centuries.

In this century, however, developmental concepts have been tested by varying and increasingly sophisticated research methodologies. The end result is a vast amount of information available to occupational therapists and to other providers of children's services. It becomes a formidable task to sort through the literature and determine the most salient theories and findings. This task is further confounded by the continued emergence of new findings, methodologies of child study, and even changing political climates that can call into question, dilute, and even refute long-standing theories.

With these constraints in mind, it is the purpose of this chapter to present a number of durable concepts and theories that can provide a foundation for occupational therapy practice with children. Some recent trends in the study of child and human development will also be considered, since these may well affect the direction of theory development and related practice methods. Chapter 4 will follow this theoretical content with a descriptive narration of the child development sequence. Chapters 3 and 4 should be used as a starting point in the study of child development. The references and recommended journals that follow this chapter should prove useful for the future study and updating of current knowledge.

BASIC PRINCIPLES OF DEVELOPMENT
Maturation and experience

At the core of most developmental theories is an explanation of the interplay between (1) human biological capacity and maturation and (2) the influence of the environment on the behavioral experiences of the individual. In fact, theories tend to be distinguished from each other by the specific weighting of these two factors or by an investigator's emphasis on a particular aspect of human biological function or environment. For example, B.F. Skinner highly values the influence of the environment on human development, whereas Sigmund Freud emphasized biological determinants of behavior. In effect, theorists generally agree that human development is both a process and the product of biological maturation and environmental experiences. *Development* may be defined as the sequential changes in the function of the individual or species. This should be differentiated from the concept of *growth*, which refers to those maturational changes that are physically measurable.

Parameters of development

There are three general parameters of development: biological, psychological, and social. Each parameter has subcategories that will be differentiated later in this section. *Biological development* is primarily related to enzyme systems that stimulate complex metabolic changes. There are two subcategories of *psychological development* that generally refer to those functions we attribute to the cortical operation of the brain: the cognitive and affective (or emotional). In the infant, cognitive psychological function tends to be dominated by neurological maturation and behavioral motivations for survival. As the child develops, cognitive activity is measured by communication skills and the handling of abstract material. Affective development is characterized by the establishment of bonds of feeling and meaning with human and nonhuman objects in the child's environment. *Social development* provides the child with skills to live in a community of others and is a product of both the child's biological capacity to learn and the direct influence of the societal environment on the child's maturation. Learning may be equated with acculturation, that is, the acquisition, internalization, and use of skills necessary to function adequately in one's society.

The parameters of development affect one another. For example, the ancient Chinese custom of foot-binding was socially derived. It was believed that upper-class women should have small feet. However, the practice prevented full development of the bones of the foot. And, because foot-binding limited the mobility of these women, it tended to restrict opportunities for emotional attachments. Another example is that when a person is depressed, there is a subsequent decrease in activity level. Social experiences become limited, as well as the opportunity for physical exercise. A long-term result of depression can be a decrease in muscle tone, strength, and bulk. All social behavior is mediated by the basic biological capacities and psychological needs of the individual and the species and by the changing factors of the environment that impinge on an individual or group. Because of the discipline's continuing concern with the interactions between these three parameters of development as they affect our patients' daily lives, Mosey[28] has proposed that occupational therapy is a "bio-psycho-social" approach to health care.

Dimensions of development

Development is an ongoing process that can be studied in two dimensions: longitudinal and cross-sectional. *Longitudinal development* refers to the chronological sequences of changes throughout the life span: year to year, stage to stage.[23] Investigators of longitudinal development tend to formalize their concepts in stage theories. These theories, such as Erikson's, identify functionally related processes and milestones over the course of time. In contrast, *cross-sectional development* examines discreet areas of function that are occurring simultaneously at any one point in the individual's life.[26] Brazelton,[2] for example, is known for his intensive investigation that focuses on simultaneous development of infant maturation and behavior (Chapters 6 and 15).

Gradients of growth

There are several universal concepts of the directions, or gradients, of growth that have strong implications for treatment. The first principle is that *ontogeny recapitulates phylogeny*, that is, the growth of the individual mirrors the maturational development of the species. This is particularly important to the understanding of the sequential maturation of biological functions. Second, there is a *cephalocaudal progression* of maturation. For example, the purposeful control of motor activity begins with movements of the head (cephalo) and develops gradually in descending order to the caudal (or tail) region of the body. There is a concurrent *proximodistal* gradient of growth from the midline of the body out of the fingers and toes. Finally, there is a change from *mass to specific action* as movement becomes more discriminative and refined.[38]

Stress and adaptation

It is generally agreed that the behavior of living organisms is directed toward maintaining a state of *homeostasis*, or *equilibrium*, that is, a life-maintaining balance of all systems, parts, and forces intrinsic and extrinsic to the individual. *Stress* may be defined as an internal or external force that threatens homeostatic balance. *Adaptation* is the general term for the mechanisms used by the individual to restore homeostasis. The adaptive mechanisms may be physiological or behavioral, used with and without conscious control. The standard example of an unconscious adaptive mechanism is the response of the autonomic nervous system to prepare the body to deal with emergency situations. Similarly, when the child encounters an unfamiliar object, an adaptive pattern may be seen as the child first stands back and then bursts forward to seize the object, as if holding it will restore the sense of equilibrium.

Stress is now generally accepted as having both positive and negative values. The positive result of stress is the initiation of more discriminative, and therefore more mature and adaptive, behavioral responses. This result assumes that the individual has the physiological capacities and maturity to purposefully deal with a stressful situation and learn from it. The negative influence of stress is most likely to occur when stress is multidimensional or beyond the physiological capabilities of the individual, or when it is continuous to the point that the individual is unable to experience intermittent sensations of equilibrium. These distress situations eliminate the discriminative learning aspects of adaptation that ordinarily promote development and allow the person to experience a sense of achievement.

Most theories of interest to occupational therapists attempt to explain the processes that a child uses to adapt to stress, either of a particular type or at different stages. Very often theorists will link the healthy resolution of stressful situations to critical periods or events. The term *critical periods* refers to certain times in an individual's life when a particular type of development or learning can take place most readily or spontaneously.[27] For example, sometime during the sixth year of life, the child's visual and auditory functions, language and social development, and curiosity are at an optimal level for learning to read. This does not mean that the child cannot learn to read 1 year earlier or 10 years later. It simply means that this is developmentally the most opportune period. Other examples of critical periods will be found in this chapter in discussion of various theories and in the developmental sequence presented in Chapter 4.

In contrast, the concept of *critical events* implies more rigid expectations. Critical events may be defined as certain situations that must take place within a given time period or else successful mastery of subsequent developmental tasks will be incomplete. Freud's psychopathological concepts of oral and anal fixation are examples of critical events hypotheses.[27]

It may be hypothesized that theorists who propose critical periods are more inclined to be environmentalists. In contrast, critical events theorists tend to place greater emphasis on biological factors in development. Although such a distinction is not invariant, it is useful as a guide.

General classifications of developmental theories

There may seem to be as many classification systems for theories as there are theories of child development. This section will review several classification systems that should be familiar to occupational therapists because of their relation to practice and research in services for children. Already introduced in this chapter were *stage theories*, which take a longitudinal view of development. The counterparts to these are known as *process theories*, which examine in detail the many variables influencing a particular type or stage of behavior.[26] Many of the elaborate stage theories, such as those developed by Freud and Piaget, demonstrate considerable depth at the process level.

Theories may also be classified broadly by their implicit view of the control of the developmental process. For example, there are *deterministic* and *nondeterministic* theories. The former indicates that the outcome of the developmental process is beyond the control of the individual. Examples of deterministic theory are found in the works of Freud and Skinner. The differences between their theories demonstrate that a determinist may see a human being as a responder to either the environment or to biological nature. In contrast, the nondeterminist view maintains that the individual can rise above biological and environmental destinies. Theorists Carl Rogers and Abraham Maslow were proponents of this view.[29]

Closely allied to the deterministic and nondeterministic perspectives are the preformational and epigenetic classifications. However, these models are associated with specific developmental influences. The *preformational model* was most popular in the last century and has been revived recently by the sociobiological theorists. This model proposes that a human being (or any species) is a product of biological-genetic determinants of behavior and that human functions will develop in a fairly uniform sequence regardless of environmental influences. The *epigenetic model* was favored by theorist Erikson who gave priority to environmental forces. This model proposes that growth and development are continuously shaped by the individual's ongoing experiences and interactions with the environment.[26]

Finally, theories may be classified according to the psychological school of thought that they represent (Table 3-1). The most commonly identified approaches are the psychoanalytic, humanistic, cognitive, behavioristic, and eclectic. In brief, *psychoanalytic theory* proposes that development and behavior are largely inner directed, generally resulting from the will of the unconscious. *Humanistic theory* is generally concerned with the self-actualization process, and the individual is viewed as a purposeful creature of plans, strategies, and choices.[26] A *cognitive theory* concerns the conscious, rational thought of the individual undergoing maturation and how this affects the individual's behavioral repertoire. *Behavioristic theory* is characterized by attention to the environmental stimuli and reinforcements that shape the individual's behavior over time. An *eclectic theory* tends to have a more humanistic view of the individual, but this approach is descriptively or methodologically influenced by one or more of the other schools of thought. Eclectic models appear to be more prevalent among theories of practice and are well represented by the occupational therapy theories described later in this chapter. Table 3-1 illustrates the classification of selected theories according to school of thought.

Although the developmental models that follow will be grossly classified as stage or process theories, each one also reflects some of the thinking represented by the systems of classification discussed in this section. Although it may seem academic at the moment, these varied terms and definitions will most certainly resurface in the therapist's continued study of child development. Perhaps even more important is the fact that the philosophies they represent will be encountered among colleagues in practice settings. Therefore therapists must be familiar with the implied methodologies and approaches to treatment that each classification engenders.

| TABLE 3-1 | Classification of selected developmental theories | | | | |

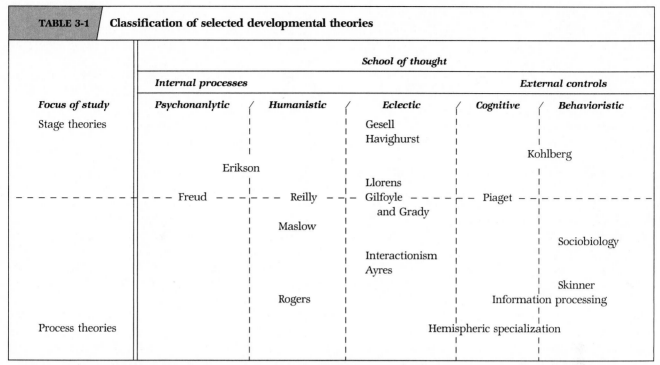

	School of thought				
	Internal processes			External controls	
Focus of study	Psychoanlytic	Humanistic	Eclectic	Cognitive	Behavioristic
Stage theories			Gesell Havighurst		
					Kohlberg
		Erikson			
	Freud	Reilly	Llorens Gilfoyle and Grady	Piaget	
		Maslow			Sociobiology
			Interactionism Ayres		Skinner
		Rogers		Information processing	
Process theories			Hemispheric specialization		

NOTE: This classification assumes that the focus of study in theories falls along a continuum of developmental stages and elaboration of processes. As discussed in the text, theoretical schools of thought tend to be differentiated according to their view of the control of behavior from internal processes to external forces.

STAGE THEORIES
The psychosexual theory of Freud

Discussion of Freud's theory in this chapter will emphasize his model of personality development. Freud proposed that personality arises from the biological, instinctual energy of the individual and that this energy is differentiated through typical environmental experiences at different ages.

The age-related stages that Freud proposed have proved to be the most durable components of his work and have been applied with success to many populations beyond those originally studied (Table 3-2). It should be remembered that most of Freud's patients were upper middle income Viennese women of the Victorian era. Most of his theory was developed through painstaking analysis of the case histories of his patients. He worked with very few children. Therefore the bulk of his data related to childhood was collected from retrospective accounts by use of free association techniques to draw out details of the past hidden in the realms of the unconscious of his adult patients.

Freud was a physician who became interested in neurological disorders, particularly those with no apparent organic base (the hysterical conversions). In keeping with his medical background, Freud assumed that there was a biological determinant for all behavior.

Interestingly, the problems that he encountered most often among his patients are now seen to be reflections of a cultural era that repressed human sexuality. Of course, it is easier for us to identify the heavy environmental influence in the psychopathology that he studied because we are representatives of a different time.

With this background in mind, we can examine the development of the personality according to Freudian psychosexual theory. Structurally the three components of the personality are the id, the ego, and the superego. Each of these parts is engaged in interactive processes with the others, usually characterized by some conflict. Freud longitudinally identified five stages of functional development. Remember that although Freud gave priority to the biological basis of behavior, he also recognized that the outcomes of each personality component and stage were influenced by the environment.

STRUCTURE OF THE PERSONALITY

The initial, motivating part of the child's personality at birth is called the *id*. It represents the psychic energy of the child, the impetus for all behavior. The sole purpose of the id is to rid the person of tension by seeking out pleasurable sensations and avoiding pain. This purpose is called the *pleasure principle*. The id does not think; it only wishes and reacts. If all needs of the id were met, the infant would remain helpless.

TABLE 3-2	Contrasted sequences of selected stage theories

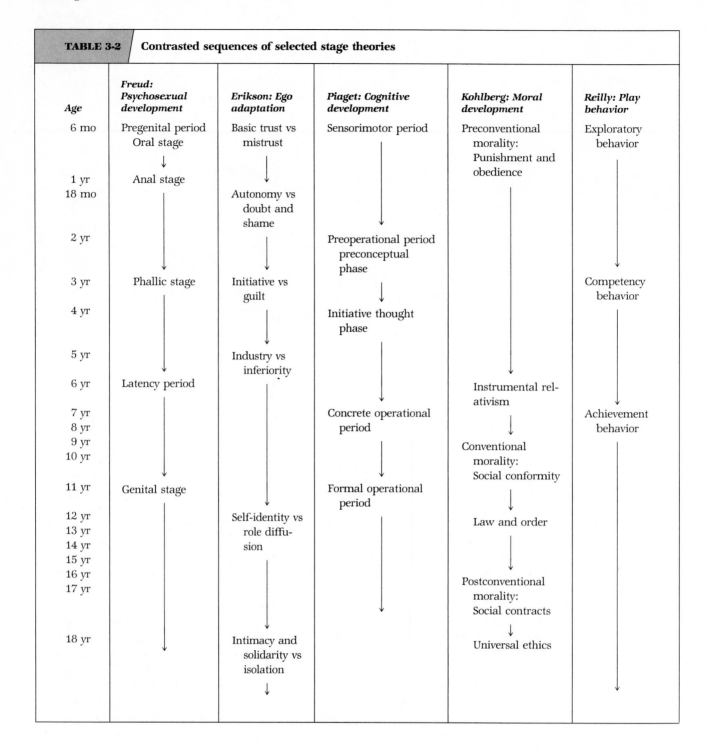

Age	Freud: Psychosexual development	Erikson: Ego adaptation	Piaget: Cognitive development	Kohlberg: Moral development	Reilly: Play behavior
6 mo	Pregenital period Oral stage	Basic trust vs mistrust	Sensorimotor period	Preconventional morality: Punishment and obedience	Exploratory behavior
1 yr	Anal stage				
18 mo		Autonomy vs doubt and shame			
2 yr			Preoperational period preconceptual phase		
3 yr	Phallic stage	Initiative vs guilt			Competency behavior
4 yr			Initiative thought phase		
5 yr		Industry vs inferiority			
6 yr	Latency period			Instrumental relativism	
7 yr			Concrete operational period		Achievement behavior
8 yr					
9 yr					
10 yr				Conventional morality: Social conformity	
11 yr	Genital stage		Formal operational period		
12 yr		Self-identity vs role diffusion		Law and order	
13 yr					
14 yr					
15 yr					
16 yr				Postconventional morality: Social contracts	
17 yr					
18 yr		Intimacy and solidarity vs isolation		Universal ethics	

Freud wrote that the id is able to conjure up mental images of the sensations that repeatedly give it pleasure. Therefore a hungry infant develops mental images of food through repeated satisfaction of the hunger needs. As the infant develops these images, he is able to use the *primary process* of the id, which is the calling up of mental images to satisfy a perceived need in the absence of the real object. The id does not know the difference between the real or the mental image. Satisfying use of either source is called *wish fulfillment.*

The id contains both the life and death instincts of the individual. The *life instincts* include hunger, thirst, and sex drives that ensure the survival of the individual and the species. The source of energy for these drives is called the *libido.* The opposing drives, the *death instincts*, are usually subordinate to life instincts but manifest themselves throughout life in the form of destructive energies and aggressive behaviors.

The *ego* is the part of the personality that starts to develop after birth as the infant comes into contact with the mediating influences of the environment. At present we can consider it as the part of the personality that moderates the id's wishes according to the constraints of the environment.

The ego operates according to the *reality principle*. Nye[29] stated that the ego "attempts to differentiate between what is desired (by the id) and what is actually available (in the environment)" (p. 13). The *secondary process* used by the ego is called *reality testing*. This involves formulating a plan to obtain the desired object and then trying the plan out to see if it works.

The ego modifies libidinal energy through the *displacement process*. This is the transference of energy into alternative actions. The displacement of libidinal energy through a socially acceptable behavior is called *sublimation*. Freud believed that the world's progress toward civilization was dependent on sublimations. For example, if you are hungry and have a visitor, you do not satisfy the libidinal urges of the id by disappearing into the kitchen and eating alone. Instead, because of the mediating influence of the ego, you share the food with your guest.

The third part of the personality is the *superego*. This is the moral component of the personality that reflects the learned values of the culture. Freud believed that the child's parents have the greatest influence on the development of the superego. Operational constructs are the ego-ideal and the conscience. The *ego-ideal* is the child's conception of what other people expect in terms of good behavior. The *conscience* represents what is thought to be bad behavior. The superego uses feelings of pride to reward the moral actions of the ego and guilt to punish bad behaviors. Like the id, the superego is not objective. It responds to mental images as well as to personal actions. Only the ego is realistic as it balances the innate needs of the id with the environmentally molded demands of the superego.

LEVELS OF CONSCIOUSNESS

Freud is best known for his systematic study and organization of concepts related to the unconscious. He constructed a topographical model consisting of the conscious, the preconscious (meaning readily accessible to the conscious), and the unconscious levels. The content of the unconscious realm of the mind is considered to be available at the conscious level with great difficulty. Although only parts of the ego and the superego exist at the unconscious level, all of the id is unconscious. Only small aspects of the ego and the superego are at the conscious level at any one time. The major parts of these two components are stored in the preconscious mind and are called on as needed.

The ego acts as a gatekeeper to the unconscious, channeling through those needs of the id that can be met through socially acceptable ways. Libidinal urges that are in conflict with society (and its mirror the superego) are held back or sidetracked through *defense mechanisms*. There are a variety of defense mechanisms that may collectively be defined as irrational thinking that allows the ego to protect itself from anxiety when rational, adaptive processes are insufficient.

THE PSYCHOSEXUAL STAGES OF DEVELOPMENT

Freud postulated that the impetus for development at different stages of life is centered on obtaining pleasurable sensation in the erogenous zones. Each of his stages is named for the erogenous zone that presumably provided the greatest source of pleasure and contact between the child and environment at that age (Table 3-2).

The *oral stage* is centered around the mouth and lips. Pleasure is derived through sucking, chewing, and feeding. The infant is dominated by the id toward meeting survival needs. The infant develops bonds of loving feelings with parents through their association with oral gratification.

The *anal stage* describes the second and third years of life. Pleasurable sensations are obtained through elimination activities of the anal and perineal sphincter muscles. The most important activity of the anal stage is toilet training. This provides the ego with its first great test of delaying sensory gratification in the face of social pressure.

The *phallic stage*, which covers the period from about 3 to 6 years, was the most controversial part of Freud's theory because of its stress on the child's incestuous feelings toward his or her parents. The centers of sensation here are the external genitalia. Pleasurable activities include masturbation and fantasizing. The latter is an example of the use of mental images to satisfy the libidinal urges of the id. The most important (and criticized) concept is the development of the *Oedipus and Electra* complexes. In essence, Freud hypothesized that children of this age have sexual drives toward parents of the opposite sex and aggressive drives toward parents of the same sex. This conflict signals the emergence of the superego, which in effect punishes the child for such fantasies. The ego responds to this anxiety-producing situation by suppressing the libidinal urges of the id and promoting identification with the parent of the same sex. Through reality testing the ego has realized that it cannot compete with the larger, stronger adult for the affections of the opposite sex parent. So it directs its energies toward becoming more like the larger, stronger, same sex parent.

The oral, anal, and phallic stages were collectively considered the *pregenital period*. Freud believed that the personality was essentially formed through this period. The child develops the ability to survive, to form emotional bonds, to delay gratification, to channel energy into socially acceptable behaviors, and to assume a sex role identity.

The *latency period*, which occurs during the elementary school years, is a time of quiescence and recovery from the turbulent conflicts of the phallic stage. It is essentially devoid of any psychosexual activity. The child shifts his interest from the self to the outside world and increases the quantity of social skills. Because Freud believed that the personality was already formed (through the pregenital period), he did not expect any qualitative changes in social skills to occur thereafter. In other words, although the child might learn to do many more things, the manner in which situations are approached will remain unchanged.

The *genital stage* is characteristic of the teen years, as hormonal changes reawaken the sexual drives of the individual. However, through the socialization process (sublimation and identification) the ego has learned to channel these drives appropriately. The youth seeks heterosexual relationships involving mutual gratification. This emergence of altruistic concerns is characteristic of the adolescent in other areas of life as well. If the ego is successful with sublimation and identification, a healthy adult is the result.

•   •   •

This discussion is limited to a very small portion of Freud's theory. He believed that the mark of the healthy adult is the ability to direct one's energies into love and work. Freud was deterministic in his view that physiological drives give impetus to all behavior. He was also essentially pessimistic about human nature, believing that these drives cause a continual conflict between the individual and civilization. The processes of sublimation and identification were central to controlling drives for the preservation of society.

Although Freud's theory is considered by many to be outdated, it still provides a foundation for subsequent developmental concepts. In addition, many of his concepts are still used in mental health facilities, particularly for diagnostic and analytical purposes. Application of his concepts appears to be more prevalent in private facilities. Freud was a prodigious writer, and many translations of his detailed work are still readily available for those who are interested in exploring his concepts further.[10,14,15,29]

The ego psychology of Erikson

It is almost inevitable to find the theory of Erik Erikson following that of Freud. Erikson began his study of psychology under Freud, and his theory reflects this affiliation. Erikson considered himself a psychoanalyst,

even though he is viewed as the father of ego psychology and a pioneer of the humanistic school of thought.

Erikson took a more optimistic view of human nature and became intrigued with the functions of the ego in response to the environment. Whereas Freud saw the id as the most important aspect of the personality, Erikson gave priority to the adaptive response of the ego in the development of the individual. Much of Erikson's theory crystallized through his studies of the lives of famous people, such as Gandhi and Luther, as he sought to identify what characteristics allow people to go on living in the face of adversity. In addition, he conducted considerable treatment and study with children, including cross-cultural comparisons. He believed that play afforded the best opportunity for observations of adaptive and maladaptive responses of the ego.

Erikson divided the life span into the *eight stages of man*. Each stage is represented by a *personal-social crisis* that gives impetus to ego growth. Erikson accepted Freud's concept of the id as the prime motivator; however, he believed that the ego provided continuity to development. One of Erikson's most important assumptions was that society constitutes itself to provide opportunities for ego growth and identity. As we shall see, the tasks of adulthood direct the individual's attention to facilitating the development of the next generation. All crises recur throughout life, but these particular stages are the critical periods in which crises are best resolved to promote successful living. Erikson viewed development as an autotherapeutic process, that is, the successful resolution of a crisis repairs the wounds of its conflicts and gives the individual a sense of achievement. Erikson prefaced each stage with "a sense of" to refer to the continuing sense of mastery and achievement (Table 3-2). Each stage also results in the acquisition of an abstract personality quality, such as hope or wisdom.

BASIC TRUST VS MISTRUST

The infant from birth to about 18 months must develop psychological trust, the eagerness to approach new experiences without paralyzing fear. Trust develops through the care-giving attentions of the parents, particularly the mother. The initial sense of trust comes from the infant's realization that survival needs will be met and that she can exist in a state of comfort. The most difficult task for the infant is to maintain this trust in the absence of the mother. Erikson believed that the parents must provide gradual opportunities for separation that do not provoke excessive anxiety. *Hope* is the acquired characteristic of this stage.

AUTONOMY VS DOUBT AND SHAME

Autonomy vs doubt and shame is the stage of the 2- to 4-year-old toddler. It is characterized by holding on and letting go and is exemplified by the crisis that occurs through the toilet training process. Erikson specified the relationship of autonomy to the child's increasing control over his body. This permits independent movement into the outer world. Parents must provide opportunities for the child to make choices and develop a sense of self-controlled *will.*

INITIATIVE VS GUILT

The newly autonomous preschooler has mastered basic motor skills and must now build a repertoire of social skills to deal with the outer world. Central to this is the achievement of gender (sex) role identity. Erikson's view of the Oedipus and Electra situations closely parallels that of Freud's, but Erikson's view is more broadly concerned with the child's imitation of the variety of role behaviors. Through imitation the child learns to assume responsibility for himself within the confines of his still limited environment and develops a sense of *purpose.*

INDUSTRY VS INFERIORITY

The elementary school child experiences a period of slow, steady growth. The need for security is transferred from the family to the peer group as the child attempts to master the activities of her age. The peer group is used as a standard of performance against which the child can measure her own skill. The abstract objective of this period is the realization of *competence.*

SELF-IDENTITY VS ROLE DIFFUSION

Erikson studied the period of adolescence in great detail, and the scope of his theoretical formulations for this age is therefore much broader than Freud's. The masterful school child is suddenly shaken by the physiological changes of puberty and must struggle to regain control over his body, identity, and future. During adolescence the prolonged childhood draws to a close, and society asks the adolescent to make choices about adult roles. The teenager experiments with patterns of identity until a sense of continuity and control over the ego is regained and a perspective of the future is acquired. In spite of the often turbulent conflicts between adolescents and their elders, Erikson felt that the actions of both were directed to the same end of helping youth clarify their roles as members of society. Through resolution of the identity crisis the individual gains a sense of *fidelity,* the continuity of the past with the future.

INTIMACY AND SOLIDARITY VS ISOLATION

Earlier relationships have helped the young adult define himself or herself. Now the adult seeks to share that identity through the intimate relationships of marriage and family life. In concert with Freud's view, Erikson saw healthy adulthood as a time of love and work. The abstract capacity derived through this period is *love.*

GENERATIVITY VS SELF-ABSORPTION

The crisis of middle adulthood is to develop the feeling that one's life is meaningful and productive. The person must find a sense of security in the usefulness of his or her chosen personal, social, and economic roles for the continuity and preservation of society. *Caring* is the abstract phenomenon realized during this time of life.

INTEGRITY VS DESPAIR

The stage of integrity vs despair is continuous and largely dependent on a successful sense of generativity. It represents the appraisal of self-worth as the individual faces the physical, economic, and personal losses of old age. It is essentially a case of "it was a very good year" versus "if only." The objective of this stage is the achievement of *wisdom* and the ability to share a satisfying and encouraging philosophy of life with the younger generation.

• • •

It is interesting to note that Erikson began his adult life as an artist, a background that manifested itself in his books through the detailed "life space" portraits he presented in his reports of clinical cases and biographical analyses. His artist's eye as well as his interest in history and anthropology allowed his written work to acquire an insight into and an emphasis on environmental influences, which are lacking in Freud's theories. These factors, as well as the cross-cultural durability of his theories, make Erikson's works especially useful for occupational therapists.[7,15,27]

The cognitive theory of Piaget

Jean Piaget's concept of the child as a little scientist is remarkably reflective of his own youth. By age 10 he had published his first paper in a biology journal, and at 22 he had completed his doctoral dissertation on mollusks. He attended university at the time that Freud, Adler, and Jung were receiving recognition in Europe, and consequently he was influenced to study a good deal of philosophy and psychology. The academic atmosphere in early twentieth century Europe was very stimulating for the study of human nature, and it produced a number of great theorists such as Piaget, Erikson, and Maslow.

By training, Piaget was a zoologist. By vocation, he became a psychologist. His particular interest was in the genesis and theory of knowledge (genetic epistemology). Piaget's first employment was to assist Binet in the standardization of intelligence tests. What interested Piaget most was not the correct responses made by children during testing, but rather the consistency of patterns of incorrect responses at different ages. This interest led him to a research career investigating children's thought patterns. The experimental approach that he developed is called *methode clinique.* This method involved (1) presenting children with familiar objects, such as blocks, pieces of paper, and glasses of water; (2) constructing problem-solving situations with the objects; and (3) asking children to solve the problem *(actions)* and to explain how they had done this *(experience).* The importance of his method lies in the concern for the processes used by the children regardless of the correctness of their problem solving. Although his initial investigations were conducted with his own children, Piaget's studies have since been replicated with several thousand children.

Piaget's work developed a very elaborate theory of the process of cognition as it matures over the span of life from infancy to adolescence. It is necessary to first examine Piaget's major constructs relating to this process in order to understand the sequence of cognitive development periods.

MAJOR CONSTRUCTS

Piaget accepted the biological basis of behavior, but he was more concerned with the developmental *adaptation* of the individual in response to ongoing environmental experiences. He wrote[30] that "the theory of knowledge is . . . essentially a theory of adaptation of thoughts to reality (resulting from) an inextricable interaction between the subject and objects" (p. 24). He examined adaptation through the child's relationships with human and nonhuman *objects, time, and space.* He said that the child organizes his experiences into *mental schemes* (schemata, concepts) through use of mental operations. *Operations* may be defined as the cognitive methods used by the child to organize his schemes and experiences and to direct his actions. The totality of operational schemes available to the child at a given time constitutes the *adapted intelligence,* or cognitive competence, of the child.

The child's quest is for *equilibrium,* a balance between what he knows and can act on and what the environment provides for him. But the child is constantly faced with novel situations and stimuli and in fact would not learn and develop without disequilibrium. Two processes are used by the child to organize novel experiences (and restore equilibrium). *Assimilation* means that the child takes a new situation and bends it to match one of his existing schemes. This may result in some distortion of reality, but it is typically the first cognitive method we all use to confront new situations. For example, a young child who sees a furry, small, four-legged animal tends to call it a *dog.* However, if the child's mother is available and corrects the child with the information that the animal is a cat, the child must then use the process of *accommodation.* That is, the child develops a new scheme in response to

the reality of the situation. Assimilation tends to result in generalization, whereas accommodation improves discrimination. Both are important to the child's development, because although discrimination promotes cognitive maturity, generalization is necessary for organization and continuity.

SEQUENCE OF COGNITIVE PERIODS

Piaget also believed that there was an invariant, hierarchical development of cognition that proceeds from the simple to the complex, from the concrete to abstract, and from personal to worldly concerns. At first, thought is *egocentric,* that is, the child relates all experiences to himself. Through cognitive maturation, thought becomes decentered and *relativistic,* that is, relationships between time, objects, and space assume an importance independent of the child's own experiences. Piaget specified four maturational levels, or periods, of cognitive function: (1) sensorimotor, (2) preoperational, (3) concrete operational, and (4) formal operational.

THE SENSORIMOTOR PERIOD

The child from birth to about age 2 responds to and learns about his environment directly through his sensations and motor responses. The emphasis is on sensory, movement, and manipulative experiences with objects. This period is characterized by the most egocentric thought. Although it is the shortest time period of mental development, it is proportionally the most active.

Piaget differentiated six stages of sensorimotor activity. The *reflexive stage* occurs during the first month. The child's schemes begin in simple biological reflexes that are primitive, general, and related to survival. Piaget felt that the sucking and palmar reflexes, which modify to promote oral and manipulative exploration, are the most critical to early mental development. The baby assimilates sensory experiences, such as the taste of food, with the kinesthetic sensations derived from the reflexive movements of sucking. Through repetition, the child becomes more proficient in the use of reflexes to satisfy basic needs. There is no differentiation between self and object or between sensation and action.

The next sensorimotor stage, occurring in the second through the fourth months, is called *primary circular reactions.* The child repeats reflexive sensory motor patterns merely for the sake of pleasurable repetition. There is still no separation between sensation and action. Essentially the child is establishing primitive habit patterns as the precursors of voluntary movements that are associated with specific sensations.

The third stage, *secondary circular reactions,* evolves during the fifth through eighth months of life. At this time the child begins to show true voluntary movement patterns based on a coordination of vision and hand function. In effect, the child reaches for and grasps everything that is seen. When the action is rewarded by a pleasurable secondary sensation, such as the sound of a bell inside a toy, the infant will repeat the action. The child is beginning to have a primitive awareness of cause and effect.

The fourth stage of *coordination of secondary schemata* completes the baby's first year. This marks exciting changes in the child's operations as the child begins to direct movements in response to stimuli that cannot be seen. The child can respond to and then look for a sound and then look for an object that disappears from view. This marks the emergence of *object permanence*, the awareness that something or someone has continuity beyond the child's direct experience with it. In turn, object permanence signals the beginning of decentered thought.

This phenomenon has implications in affective-emotional development as well. The baby now realizes that when the mother leaves the room, she does not cease to exist. The baby can begin to listen for sounds of his mother in a nearby room and gradually realizes that he can use sound stimuli to find the missing mother (since locomotor development is also progressing rapidly at this age). As shown in Erikson's theory, this awareness is critical to the child's progress toward independence.

The fifth sensorimotor stage, which lasts until about 18 months, is called *tertiary circular reactions*. The child's mental behavior is characterized by searches for new schemes. This development parallels a motor stage when the child is suddenly able to walk and crawl about freely, and parents are hard pressed to keep their youngsters from getting into everything. Although it happens by chance, one of the most important results of this stage is the beginning of *tool use*. The child discovers that he can get more food into his mouth with a spoon or that a distant pull toy can be obtained by pulling on the attached string that previously had no function for him. Prehension patterns become more refined and precise in the process.

The sixth stage of sensorimotor activity, the transitional stage, is marked by *inventions of new means through mental combinations*. It generally occurs during the last 6 months of the second year. This stage is mentally demonstrated through insight and physically characterized by purposeful tool use. The child is looking for alternate means to solve problems. These changes are in large part aided by the child's increasing motor proficiency in speech production and by an expanding receptive vocabulary. The child can now begin to label or symbolically represent mental schemes. Whereas during the previous stages all schemes were represented as sensorimotor experiences, the child is now beginning to represent concepts without direct manipulation.

THE PREOPERATIONAL PERIOD

With the emergence of language and symbolic representation of schemes, the child's cognitive patterns undergo significant changes. Through acquisition of verbal schemes, the child is able to expand his conceptual repertoire more rapidly. In addition, symbolic representation allows the child to organize what he knows and to call on a scheme at will. During the time from 2 to 7 years of age, children learn to systematically manipulate their environments through development of the organizing operations called classification, seriation, and conservation.

Classification is the organization of objects according to similarities and differences. At first, children classify according to one common stimulus characteristic, such as color. Two-year-old children can be seen making little stacks of blocks with each stack a different color. When they have mastered classification according to one common characteristic, children begin to notice other shared characteristics as well as discrete differences. Classification becomes multidimensional. The dog and cat of the example given earlier for assimilation and accommodation become classified as pets. Classifications may be made according to sensory characteristics, spatial arrangements, and readily observable cause and effect relationships.

Seriation is the relationship of one object, or classification of objects, to another. As with classification, this operation is initially exercised at a unidimensional level. Proximity of objects tends to afford the earliest stimulus for seriation. However, as the child matures and vocabulary increases, he can rank-order objects in terms of size, weight, color intensity, and other sensory characteristics.

Conservation is the end product of the preoperational period. It permits the child to recognize the continuities of an object or class of objects in spite of apparent change. A typical Piagetian example would be to show the child a ball of clay. The clay is flattened or rolled out in front of the child who is then asked if the amount is the same. A child who is still unable to conserve sees that the physical appearance is different and would say that the amount is not the same.

The most primitive kind of conservation is by the number of objects (in different spatial arrangements). Later the child begins to conserve mass (as in the clay example), area, length, and volume. The ability to conserve is critical to learning to read and do math, for the child must learn to recognize the sameness of sounds and values in letters and numbers regardless of their arrangements.

The preoperational period is divided into two distinct phases. The 2- to 4-year-old child is considered *preconceptual*. The chief task here is for the child to expand her vocabulary and thus increase the quantity of symbolic representations. Typically classification is the primary operation that develops at this time, although the child is also learning verbal concepts that will promote use of seriation and conservation. Play provides the arena for learning, and the child spends considerable time in verbal play.

The *intuitive thought phase*, from about age 4 to 7, provides the child with substantially more social-environmental contacts. The child uses a tremendous amount of imitation by copying whatever is seen and repeating whatever is heard. Children happily relate all the family secrets in great detail. The child answers questions and solves problems intuitively, not really knowing how conclusions were reached. Seriation and conservation develop during this phase as the child is able to deal with multiple characteristics of objects. Through classification and seriation the child begins to use inductive reasoning to relate parts to the whole. This marks the transition to concrete operations.

THE CONCRETE OPERATIONAL PERIOD

The concrete operational period, which covers the life span from about age 7 to 11, is important for the acquisition of reversibility, spatial concepts, and rules. During this time the child is still stimulus and experience bound; he can only think about things that are at least available for sensory manipulation.

Reversibility is an extension of conservation and allows the child to develop more spatial awareness. Children learn that they cannot only add 2 numbers, but that they can also subtract. They gain an understanding that the constant features of an object, such as the conservation of the clay mass, permit it to be returned to its previous state.

Rules are not new to the concrete operational child, but understanding of rules becomes more realistic and complete, and therefore the child is able to apply them. There are rules of causation that prescribe general cause and effect; rules of attribution, related to social causation, such as custom to outcome or event to event; and moral rules for right, wrong, and situational appropriateness. Mature understanding and application of rules continue to evolve through the formal operations period. For example, the preoperational child knows that he should not hit another child because "Mommy says not to." In the concrete operational period the child will refrain from hitting because "It is wrong." At the formal operational level, the adolescent can explain that hitting is a form of violence that has an impact on society and that it is justified only under certain conditions.

Classification, seriation, conversation, reversing, and rule use allow the child to develop systematic ways of organizing parts to wholes and determining parts of wholes. The child begins to make combinations and elementary permutations (combinations of combina-

tions). The use of concrete operations constitutes *empirico-inductive thinking*, that is, the child is able to solve problems by use of information that is concretely available to him.

THE FORMAL OPERATIONAL PERIOD

The formal operational period, which is the final cognitive period, begins at about 11 years of age and continues through the teen years. It signals the transition to mature thinking. The adolescent begins to think about things that are beyond his experience and manipulative control, and he can begin to use mental, language-based manipulation. A typical characteristic is the developing ability to organize one's time and to relate one's schedule to other people's schedules. The adolescent's thoughts are generally relativistic, that is, he sees relationships of object to object or event to event as having importance regardless of direct personal experiences. An interest in world events and social problems is manifest. The youth internalizes abstract values.

The ability to perform mental manipulations demonstrates the teenager's proficiencies with permutations and the laws of probability. Because of these, the adolescent is able to conceptualize possibilities. Plans can be made and tried out mentally and changed according to mental judgments regarding the soundness of the plan. This ability to analyze problems and to plan possibilities is called *hypothetico-deductive thinking* and is used by adults in most situations that can be dealt with on a cognitive rather than an emotional basis.

Piaget believed that this sequence of development leads to the cognitive maturity of adulthood. The representative of this is a person with values, goals, plans, and an understanding of one's purpose in society. Piaget and Inhelder[31] stated that maturation of cognition is dependent on:

1. Organic growth, especially the maturation of the nervous system and endocrine glands. . . .
2. Experience in the actions performed upon objects. . . .
3. Social interaction and transmission and
4. A balance of opportunities for both assimilation and accommodation (p. 154)

Knowledge of Piaget's theory is critical to occupational therapists who plan programs for children. Regardless of the psychosocial or neurological approaches used in treatment, the therapist in an activity-based situation is interacting with a thinking child. The selection and structure of an activity in accordance with the operational skills and concepts of the child are essential. This can be particularly tricky when a child is in transition from one period to the next. Because most of Piaget's work on children's cognition has been translated from the original French, which has different grammatical structure and often offers no readily available English terminology, his work is often difficult to read.

However, a number of Piaget's colleagues[8,31] have described his theory for the English-speaking reader. Other authors have contributed significant works.[26,27,30]

Other stage theories

KOHLBERG: STAGES OF MORAL DEVELOPMENT

Lawrence Kohlberg[22] was interested in the relationship between Piaget's concepts of cognitive development and the acquisition of moral value schemes. He designed a series of fascinating experiments that presented moral dilemmas to children and young adults of different ages (Table 3-1). Like Piaget, he did not make judgments about the correctness of children's choices, but instead he collected data about the concepts used by the children to make moral decisions. He described three discrete levels of moral development, each having two complementary stages.

The first level is called *preconventional morality.* Obedience is the limit to morality until about 8 years of age. Choices are governed by egocentric concerns. The first stage, *punishment and obedience*, is based on the child's desire to avoid punishment from the larger, parental authority figures. The second stage, *instrumental relativism*, is slightly decentered. Decisions are based on personal needs and occasionally on the needs of others when they can be of help to the individual. In other words, you scratch my back, I'll scratch yours.

Conventional morality, the second level of moral development, emerges around 9 or 10 years of age (late concrete operations) and is characterized by social conformity. Its appearance indicates some internalization of rules of social causation. The third stage, *social conformity*, demonstrates behavior that is pleasing to others. It is easy to see how this follows the patterns of instrumental relativism. This is the age when children become very serious about their responsibilities to help with classroom chores. Concern with *law and order* marks the fourth stage. Moral behavior is very rule bound in response to emerging notions of social order and fairness. A typical behavior of this stage is concern with cheating and other infractions of honor codes.

The third level of moral development, *postconventional morality*, is marked by relativistic thinking. There is an effort to define moral principles (rather than obedience) that are flexible for different situations. This is characteristic of the older adolescent with mature formal operations who can consider many variables and possibilities. In the fifth stage, *social contracts*, the young adult makes moral decisions based on social values, with an awareness of the legal implications. A typical example of social contracts thinking is demonstrated by the conscientious objector who registers to provide humanitarian services as an alternative to serving in the army. Kohlberg believes that only a small percentage of individuals attain the sixth stage of moral thinking, *universal ethics*. This stage is represented by the great humanitarian who demonstates a life commitment to preserving the rights and dignity of man, such as Martin Luther King, Jr.

It is interesting to note that Kohlberg's stages lag behind those of Piaget in a chronological sense. This would indicate that levels of cognition must be fairly mature before an individual can use the higher level operative methods to reexamine abstract issues of morality and obedience. Just as adults tend to use concrete and formal operations flexibly according to the merits of a situation, they also use variable stage moral thinking in dealing with everyday situations. It appears that when a situation is novel and does not readily lend itself to assimilative use of moral schemes, the individual tends to direct a higher level of moral thinking toward the situation.[20,22,38]

MASLOW: HUMANISTIC PSYCHOLOGY

Abraham Maslow[15] is generally considered to be the father of humanistic psychology in the United States. He, like Piaget and Erikson, was profoundly influenced by European philosophical trends during the Age of Enlightenment. He outlined a *hierarchy of basic human needs* that are believed to appear in the following longitudinal sequence.

The *physiological needs*, such as food, water, rest, air, and warmth, are necessary to basic survival. The next level is characterized by the need for *safety*, broadly defined as the need for both physical and physiological security. The need for *love and belonging* promotes the individual's search for affection, emotional support, and group affiliation. The need for a sense of *self-esteem*, which is defined as the ability to regard one's self as competent and of value to society, is evidenced as persons grow. The need for *self-actualization*, which represents the highest level, is attained through achievement of personal goals.

If the lower level needs are not met, the individual is not able to direct his energies toward higher levels. For example, if a girl and her boyfriend have just broken up, it is difficult for either of them to concentrate on their studies. Instead they turn to friends (group affiliation) to reestablish feelings of love and belonging.[15]

GESELL: DEVELOPMENTAL SCHEDULES

Arnold Gesell[21a] was a physician whose work gave impetus to the medical specialty of pediatrics. Through his practice, he accumulated data on children's performance of everyday activities, and he was the first to put a timetable on development through a series of developmental schedules. Most of the items on standard developmental evaluations in use today are based on Gesell's findings. The origins of these developmental behaviors are often taken for granted, and Gesell has received little recognition outside of the health care field.

Most of Gesell's work concerns what to look for, how to find it, and at what ages. It would be impossible to list here all of the ages and items that were identified, but a few key definitions should be useful.

Gesell used the term *behavior* to collectively define all kinds of reactions to stimuli, be they voluntary or involuntary. In contrast, a *behavior pattern* is considered to be a discreet, voluntarily repeatable response of the neuromotor system to a specific stimulus situation. The developmental schedules help chart key categories of behavior patterns that are critical to determining the progress of the child. *Motor behavior* is directed toward postural control and locomotion. *Adaptive behavior* patterns are used to manipulate the environment. *Language behaviors* include vocabulary, articulation, and social communication skills. The *personal-social behaviors* are learned controls of bodily functions, such as hygiene and grooming. *Maturity stages* are chronological periods of development in which certain behavior patterns characteristically appear for the first time.

Adaptation is the coordination of physical maturation with the skill demands of the environment. In his studies Gesell found that this was not a smooth process. Typically, behaviors become less adaptive when the child is in a period of rapid physical growth. When the growth spurt subsides, the child is able to concentrate on coordinating his body in the practice of socially acceptable behavior patterns. This cycle of alternating periods of positive and negative adaptation is called *reciprocal interweaving*.[21a]

HAVIGHURST: DEVELOPMENTAL TASKS

Robert Havighurst, a reknowned American educator, proposed that a person must learn specific groups of skills at different ages to meet social expectations. The acquisition of a particular group of skills enables a person to perform adequately the age-appropriate roles of player, student, worker, or retired person. Havighurst believed that it was the ability of the person to learn, rather than merely respond to situations, that differentiated man from animals.

Havighurst believed that each developmental task had biological, psychological, and sociological bases. Similarly, he proposed that the achievement of each task could be facilitated or inhibited by these three forces. The concept of *sensitive periods* was described as the time at which biological, psychological, and sociological conditions were most appropriate to the achievement of a developmental task. These particularly sensitive times often provided a "teachable moment" when the child or adult is most apt to integrate all previous learning to master the skills of a new developmental task with social guidance. Therefore Havighurst analyzed each task in terms of its biological, psychological,

and sociological bases, as well as its educational implications.

Havighurst's *Developmental Tasks and Education*[18] is easy to read and interesting in its discussions of the cultural variations and programmatic implications of the following tasks.

1. Tasks of infancy and childhood
   a. Learning to walk
   b. Learning to take solid food
   c. Learning to talk
   d. Learning to control the elimination of body wastes
   e. Learning sex differences and sexual modesty
   f. Achieving physiological stability
   g. Forming simple concepts of social and physical reality
   h. Learning to relate oneself emotionally to parents, siblings, and other people
   i. Learning to distinguish right and wrong and developing a conscience
2. Tasks of middle childhood
   a. Learning physical skills necessary for ordinary games
   b. Building wholesome attitudes toward oneself as a growing organism
   c. Learning to get along with age-mates
   d. Developing fundamental skills in reading, writing, and calculating
   e. Developing concepts necessary for everyday living
   f. Developing a conscience, morality, and a scale of values
   g. Developing attitudes toward social groups and institutions
3. Tasks of adolescence
   a. Achieving new and more mature relations with age-mates of both sexes
   b. Achieving a masculine or feminine social role
   c. Accepting one's physique and using the body effectively
   d. Achieving emotional independence of parents and other adults
   e. Preparing for marriage and family life
   f. Preparing for an economic career
   g. Acquiring a set of values and an ethical system to guide behavior—developing an ideology
   h. Desiring and achieving socially responsible behavior
4. Tasks of early adulthood
   a. Selecting a mate
   b. Learning to live with a marriage partner
   c. Starting a family
   d. Rearing children
   e. Managing a home
   f. Getting started in an occupation

g. Taking on civic responsibility

h. Finding a congenial social group

5. Tasks of middle adulthood

a. Assisting adolescents to become responsible and happy adults

b. Achieving adult civic and social responsibility

c. Reaching and maintaining satisfactory performance in one's occupational career

d. Developing adult leisure-time activities

e. Relating oneself to one's spouse as a person

f. Accepting and adjusting to the physiological changes of middle age

g. Adjusting to aging parents

6. Tasks of later maturity

a. Adjusting to decreasing physical strength and health

b. Adjusting to retirement and reduced income

c. Adjusting to the death of a spouse

d. Establishing an explicit affiliation with one's age group

e. Adopting and adapting to social roles in a flexible way

f. Establishing satisfactory physical living arrangements

It is appropriate to conclude this section on stage theories with Havighurst's sequence. Essentially Havighurst's work[18] is a compilation of concepts developed and studied by the previously discussed theorists. The tasks given are self-explanatory and very useful to the therapist to get a quick overview of the social expectations for patients at a particular time of life.

PROCESS THEORIES

This section on process theories is generally limited to Skinner's theory of operant conditioning and Rogers' humanistic theory of the self. This approach was chosen because most of the other process theories are variations of the work of these two men or of the theorists presented in the section on stage theories. Skinner's approach is behavioristic and superficially contrasts sharply with Rogers' ideas. However, it should be recognized at the start that Skinner and Rogers are equally concerned with the individual's opportunity to achieve maximal potential. The difference between the two lies in the school of thought that gives each man his methodological orientation. Skinner's view of man is considerably less mechanistic than that of other behaviorists.

Skinner's theory of radical behaviorism

B.F. Skinner is considered a radical behaviorist, not because he is at the extreme of behaviorism, but be-

cause he leans toward the opposite pole. He acknowledges the importance of genetic endowment; he accepts feelings, thoughts, and other "inner events" as behaviors; and he is concerned with self-knowledge and creativity as cultural essentials. In addition, as will be shown, he believes that the initiation of behaviors involves a voluntary element rather than merely a set of uncontrolled responses to environmental stimuli. In these aspects his thinking is radically different from the traditional school of behaviorist thought. It is precisely these differences that make his theory useful to occupational therapists. It must be added, however, that Skinner is strictly a behaviorist in methodology and insists on identification of behaviors that are measurable. However, the range of behaviors that he sees as being measurable is fairly broad.

The components of Skinner's work that are presented here constitute a theory of behavioral development and learning. Skinner believes that all human behavior is shaped by the environment and that bits of behavior may be randomly emitted in response to an environmental stimulus, that is, the organism tries out a behavior that has worked before. Or, an involuntary, reflexive response is elicited by the environmental stimulus. The bit of behavior is then reinforced in some way by the environmental consequences that follow it. Bits of behavior include genetic traits that have proved useful to the species in a given environment and that have been passed on through generations. This sequence of (1) stimulus situation, (2) behavioral response, and (3) environmental consequence constitutes a *contingency of behavior.* It is the mechanism through which the environment shapes behavior.

Skinner clearly states that the environment selects those behaviors that it will reinforce and ignores or punishes those behaviors that are not adaptive. For example, a young child encounters a dog for the first time. Reaching into his behavioral repertoire, the child emits a reaching-and-touching behavior. If the dog responds by nuzzling, licking the child, and providing the child with a generally pleasant sensory experience, it may be said that the child has been positively reinforced (rewarded) by the environmental consequences. The environmental consequences, or *reinforcements,* of a bit of behavior may be defined as controls that strengthen, weaken, or maintain that particular behavior. If the child comes to associate reaching and touching as a means to obtain a pleasant reaction from dogs, he would tend to repeat that behavior under similar stimulus situations. Thus his behavior would be strengthened and maintained as long as it was generally effective in obtaining positive reinforcement. If, on another occasion the child pets the dog and the dog runs away, the reaching-and-touching behavior might be weakened. In the first instance the behavior was reinforced by the environment. In the latter situation reinforcement was absent, that is, not given and therefore negative. If the dog ran away often enough, it is probable that the child's reaching-and-touching behavior with dogs would be extinguished.

The third type of environmental control, called aversive control, punishment, or a *punitive contingency*, is recognized and defined by Skinner. However, he specifically advocates against its use, because its effects on behavior are unpredictable and generally do not promote adaptation. Punishment has been a common form of behavioral control throughout the ages and is generally expected to eliminate behaviors. If the child reached and petted the dog and was bitten, that would be a form of punishment. If this resulted in avoidance of all future dog encounters, as sometimes happens in this situation, the contingency would be maladaptive. The child still has not learned the most effective behavior to use when approaching strange dogs.

The above example of the child and the dog is also useful for discussion of Skinner's concept of *contingencies of survival*. Certain genetic characteristics, such as having adequate vision to see the dog, a musculoskeletal system that produces a stroking movement, and a neurological system that permits one to approach animals calmly, have proved useful to the survival of the species. These characteristics have enabled humans to domesticate animals through the ages for assistance with food production, transportation, and physical safety. In contrast, the species that did not have these characteristics were forced to rely on their own bodies for sustenance, travel, and security. This has not always proved effective, as witnessed by the great number of species that have become extinct.

To recapitulate, Skinner believes that all behavior is a result of the environmental control of the individual, the culture, and the species. He specified that man, the species, and the culture are part of the environment and therefore control as much as they are controlled. Skinner[34] points out that most of man's environment is man-made and that

> Man has changed himself greatly as a person in the same period of time by changing the world in which he lives. . . .Man has "controlled his own destiny". . .the man that man has made is a product of the culture man has devised. He has emerged from two quite different processes of evolution: the biological evolution responsible for man the species and the cultural evolution carried out by that species (p. 198).

What Skinner rejects is the traditional concept of *autonomous man* who functions with no controls. Skinner provides a number of behavioral explanations for the concepts typically used to support the idea of autonomous man. For example, *aggression* is often said to be part of human nature. Skinner would say that this behavior resulted from contingencies of survival. He also points out that aggressive behaviors are strengthened and maintained by here-and-now contingencies of reinforcement. For example, we tell children that it is wrong to hit another child, but then we encourage them to stand up for their rights or to be tough in sports activities. To use Skinner's example, if a man attacks another man and gets the other man's possessions, the attacker is positively reinforced by the goods he has acquired.[34]

A traditionally humanistic concept is the capacity for *self-awareness*. Skinner says this is largely dependent on language, which has been acquired and shaped by the verbal community. Small children do not verbally describe their feelings as a spontaneous behavior. Instead, they learn to describe their feelings because they are questioned regarding these. Even a simple How are you? helps to shape this behavior. The problem with self-awareness, according to Skinner, is its accessibility. A person's verbal behavior may be incongruent with his nonverbal behavior, so it is more difficult to analyze and control it precisely.

Another characteristic capacity of man that has been described as uniquely human is the ability to *think*. Skinner acknowledges that the ability to think is a complex process with a foundation in the genetic endowment of the species (and therefore evolved through contingencies of survival). A behavioral explanation of thinking is that the culture teaches people to make fine discriminations, to solve problems, and to follow rules, including rules for finding rules. For example, children are taught very early to go to a police officer for help, even if they have had no direct contact with such a person. They can be shown a police officer on television or in a book and be reasonably accurate in subsequent real-life situations that require them to identify this person. Skinner suggests that when a person recalls a concept, it is because something in the present situation elicits a response, in a weakened or altered form, that was acquired on another similar occasion.

Self-identity is readily explained in behavioral terms as a "repertoire of behavior appropriate to a given set of contingencies" (p. 189)[34] Skinner says there are a variety of "selfs" that develop according to the specific contingencies of the varied environments of a person's life. Problems arise when an environment changes and becomes inconsistent with prior contingency patterns. For example, children use one set of behaviors with their families and another set with friends. The first few times that they are in a blended situation with family and friends they are unsure of the environmental consequences and try out both sets of behaviors in a haphazard fashion. Typically, parents will respond by complaining that their child was influenced by the poor behavior of the neighbor's children.

For the purposes of this discussion, the final aspects of human nature to be considered are related to the ability to manipulate the environment. Traditionally, *manipulative ability* has been considered one of the hallmarks of the view of man as autonomous. Skinner explains this characteristic simply as a result of contingencies of survival. Manipulative ability improved man's chances for survival when man emitted eye-hand behaviors that changed the environment. Because these behaviors over time had such a strong impact on the survival of the species, the ability to produce them came to be highly valued. In behavioral terms, manipulative behaviors were increasingly accompanied by positive social-cultural reinforcements. In fact, cultures eventually began to systematically train its members to use manipulative techniques that improved their capacity to change the environment.

The concept of environmental manipulation is coupled with the notion of *industry*. Industry may be defined as the person's rate of emitting behaviors that change the environment. Because such behaviors are highly valued by society, it provides satisfying rewards for higher rates of emitting such behaviors.

A word of caution is in order when reading the works of Skinner. They must be read carefully from start to finish, because he uses logical arguments, and scanning will not provide an accurate picture of radical behaviorism.[29,34-36]

Rogers' self theory

Like Maslow, Carl Rogers believed that people have an inborn need for self-actualization. Rogers took a positive view of human nature that was both deterministic (driven by the actualizing tendency) and epigenetic. Central to Rogers' theory is the individual's *inner experiencing*, that is, how one perceives oneself, one's relationships, and one's environment. Rogers acknowledged the instrumental influence of the environment in the development of the self, but he believed that the individual has the capacity to choose responses to the environment that will maintain a sense of personal control.

Many of Rogers' ideas were developed through his clinical practice and academic career in psychology. He also studied for the ministry, and although he did not complete this course, it provides some explanation for the direction of his thinking. One of his characteristic research methods was the use of the Q-sort. Patients were given cards printed with statements of feelings and personal attributes and then asked to divide the cards into two stacks representing the perceived self and the ideal self. This procedure was repeated at various times throughout the course of therapy to measure changes in the discrepancy between the perceived and the ideal selves.

Rogers is best known for his formulation of *client-centered therapy*. Like Erikson, he believed that each in-

dividual has, and must find within himself or herself the resources for growth, adaptation, and self-actualization. Client-centered therapy was designed to elicit these resources, and the therapist takes a nondirective role that encourages the client to say what he or she really feels and wants to do. The *nondirective approach* is readily applied in occupational therapy, when the therapist urges the child to "show me what you can do" and "tell me what you think." This approach has been described by Knickerbocker.[21]

Concepts of the developmental process. Rogers conceptualized the infant as being essentially a clean slate for the development of the self. The totality of sensations constitutes reality. Likes and dislikes are clearly demonstrated in response to pleasant and aversive stimuli.

The child grows to want the pleasurable sensations experienced through love and acceptance of *significant others*. Initially these significant others are the child's father and mother. This need for positive regard forces the child to examine what he does that pleases and displeases his parents. He learns to view himself through others' eyes and to suppress feelings and other inner experiences. This is believed to occur because the child receives *conditional positive regard* from the parents; love and acceptance are given under certain conditions according to the child's actions.

Through growth and increased contacts with the outer world, the child slowly loses sight of himself. Externally derived values and feelings of self-worth are internalized. This alienation of the self from the natural organismic (innate) experience is called the *basic estrangement* of humans. The degree to which this prevents the individual from following the self-actualizing tendency is dependent on the amount of *unconditional positive regard* the person receives from significant others.

Rogers' developmental goal for an individual was for the individual to become a fully functioning person. In essence, this is an individual with an existential approach to life who deals with each new situation based on its own merits and on the individual's own true feelings about the situation. Such persons are able to use reality testing to improve the quality of life, rather than to put up with a constrained existence. Rogers[33] provided the following description:

> He is able to experience all of his feelings and is afraid of none. . .he is his own sifter of evidence, but is open to evidence from all sources; he is completely engaged in the process of being and becoming himself, and thus discovers that he is soundly and realistically social. . . .He is a fully functioning organism, and because of the awareness of himself which flows freely in and through his experiences, he is a fully functioning person (p. 288).

This discussion of Rogers' theory is to some extent limited by the content of his writing. In contrast to the behavioral tradition of Skinner's work, which is largely descriptive, Rogers' work[33] is primarily prescriptive for clinical psychology, education, and other socializing institutions. The works of Knickerbocker[21] and Nye[29] are also noteworthy.

CURRENT TRENDS IN DEVELOPMENTAL THEORY

Current investigators of child development appear to be more concerned with process than were the earlier theorists who have been described thus far. It may be hypothesized that stage theories have been fairly well defined to this point and are generally accepted for the basic structure that is provided. A review of the literature in child development in recent years reveals four areas of study that are beginning to influence the thinking and practice of occupational therapists: (1) hemispheric specialization, (2) sociobiology, (3) interactionism, and (4) information processing. These terms are from the literature and, though not necessarily parallel, seem to be commonly accepted.

Hemispheric specialization

In the late 1960s it became an accepted practice to "split" the brains of individuals with intractable epilepsy. In simple terms, portions of the interhemispheral connections were surgically cut to reduce the spread and intensity of electrical activity caused by seizures. Although such surgery had been practiced earlier with animals, the use of the techniques with humans provided scientists with a unique opportunity to examine the functions of the brain's two hemispheres.

Earlier it had been believed that the hemispheres were basically similar in function, even though one hemisphere would become dominant in control of fine movements. If the left hemisphere became dominant, then the person would be right-handed. The opposite would hold true if the person was right hemisphere dominant. Dominance was generally believed to be controlled by heredity. In addition, it was clinically well established that individuals who had survived cerebral vascular accidents showed definite signs of hemispheric function asymmetry. After experiencing a lesion in the left hemisphere, patients typically had visual-spatial and affective impairment. In contrast, those individuals whose cerebral vascular accidents had occurred in the right hemisphere demonstrated deficits in language production and motor planning. However, there was no information available from intact human brains to corroborate these findings.

However, researchers have since developed a number of techniques that are used to examine separate functions of the cerebral hemispheres, as demonstrated by those individuals on whom interhemispheric commissurotomies have been performed. Replicated results over the years from such investigators as Sperry, Gazzaniga, Kimura, and Geschwind[11] clearly indicate that there are differences in hemispheric functions. It appears that the right cerebral hemisphere plays a greater role in our perception and association of visual and auditory stimuli that are nonverbal. For example, recognition of music, art, and faces appears to be subject to adequate function of the right hemisphere. In contrast, the left cerebral hemisphere is more critical to perception and association of verbal and other symbolic material. Differences have been shown to be both anatomical and physiological.

In addition to intraindividual differences, there also appear to be interindividual differences. It is now believed that left hemisphere functions are more highly specialized in women and that right hemisphere functions are more highly developed in men. Although researchers warn that socialization may exaggerate these differences to a greater degree, this neurophysiological gender difference tends to account for the greater proficiency of women in language-related subjects and the gravitation of men toward math and visual-spatial subjects such as engineering. Similarly, it appears that people's interests may well be determined by which hemisphere is more highly developed for its specialized functions. Persons with dominant left hemispheres may be more interested in art, architecture, and engineering, whereas persons with dominant right hemispheres would gravitate more toward teaching, sales, and writing.[11]

The impact of hemispheric specialization data on human service delivery is yet to be determined. Research techniques have been incorporated into clinical assessment procedures for patients with known or suspected brain damage (see discussion of dichotic listening tests, Chapter 10). There is a growing trend toward the exploration of adequacy of hemispheric function, specialization, and interhemispheric communication in children with learning disabilities.[40] However, the nature-nurture controversy that has been generated with relation to male-female gender differences appears to have resulted in a reluctance to consider the information on a broader scale with the normal population to date.

Sociobiology

The concepts and speculations generated by sociobiology are even more controversial. Sociobiology is defined as "the application of evolutionary principles to the social behavior of animals . . . and human beings as well" (p. 1).[5] This discipline proposes that much of the behavior of human beings that has heretofore been considered socially derived, and therefore environmentally derived, is actually genetically transmitted. Researchers have sought to identify universal behaviors among species and relate the development of those behaviors through natural selection. They propose that each species develops a unique behavioral repertoire over time through the natural selection of those characteristics that are most adaptive for the species. Their concern is not with the different cultural patterns that are used to refine the behaviors, but rather with the species-specific behaviors that are the bases of the cultural patterns. Barash[5] pointed out that although there are thousands of language patterns used by different humans, the capacity to speak, develop, and learn a language and communicate with others is biologically derived and shared by the entire species. Again, the critical difference that the sociobiologists make is that these capacites are genetically, rather than socially, transmitted.

The concepts of sociobiology have been rejected by some social scientists on the grounds that the theory does not account for individual differences and that it has an aura of determinism that could conceivably be used to support discriminative practices.[39] Selected review of the literature in sociobiology indicates that individual differences are not overlooked but are deemphasized.[5,37,41]

In contrast, Thomas[39] noted that sociobiological concepts provide considerable explanation for the growing evidence of the complexity of infant behavior. The human capacities for reflexive responses, sensory perception, speech, and learning are recognized as biologically determined. What has been questioned until recently is how well developed these capacities are at birth.

Interactionism

The concept of interactionism, as defined by Thomas,[39] includes several components. These include the inborn complexity of infant behavior, the plasticity of the human development, and the variable effects of the child's temperament. Simply stated, interactionism postulates that the child is an active social being who contributes to continuity and change in his developmental environment.

As was alluded to earlier, research data now indicate that infants have definite behavioral patterns at birth, including preferential attention to a variety of auditory, visual, tactile, and gustatory stimuli. Active learning, as evidenced by the rapid manifestation and replication of neurodevelopmental reflexes, begins immediately after birth. Imitative behaviors appear within 2 weeks. These behaviors are now defined as being social rather than reflexive.[39] Whereas it was formerly emphasized that infants learned to respond differentially to their mothers' behaviors, researchers now speak in terms of mothers' increasingly differentiated responses to infants' behaviors.[1]

Similarly, it is becoming clearer that the residual effects of early or traumatic experiences are not as permanent as previously thought. Numerous studies of children from varied early environments who later had the opportunity for enriching experiences have led investigators to conclude that the human capacity for change is as important in child development as is the capacity for steady, continuous maturation. Considerable research is now directed toward understanding the influence of multiple attachments at different ages of life.[39] Equally relevant is information about a child's capacity to recover from traumatic experiences, such as separation from parents through divorce or death, as the child develops. Again, the influence of multiple attachments is considered critical, particularly in relation to the need for adequate gender role models.[19] It appears that a child's adaptive development is best facilitated by a balanced combination of continuity and change, rather than overemphasis on either mode.

Finally, interactionism is concerned with the influence of the child's temperament. As a logical extension to the awareness of the strength of the infant's social behaviors, researchers have begun to look at the way the growing child's temperament affects the behaviors and attitudes of others, as well as how the child's temperament affects her response to others. For example, the child who is perceived as "not caring about schoolwork" may be ignored by teachers. If this perception is accurate, such lack of attention may not be as negative an influence on the child as was formerly believed. However, if the child's attitude is a reflection of fear of failure with schoolwork, then neglect by the teachers could be even more threatening to the child. A long-term study by Thomas[39] indicates that there are clear-cut patterns of consistency of temperament over time, and that these patterns in turn contribute to variations in development.

Information processing

In addition to the concern with physiological and social foundations of behavior, recent study in child development has been directed toward the examination of cognitive behavior. Although Piagetian theory had been generally well accepted as an explanation of the developmental maturation of a child's thought content, it left gaps in the understanding of how cognition takes place. The early development of information processing theory has been attributed to Klahr and Wallace.[9] In essence, information processing is actually a conceptual model of how the brain operates from the information it receives. The development of computer technology has provided researchers with terminology for the processes that are involved in cognition.

Information processing uses a simple input-operations-output model. The input includes any sensory stimuli that are received through the sensory organs and transmitted to the central nervous system. Therefore input is dependent on attention, curiosity, exploration, sensory awareness, and sensory recognition. The operations (or cognitive functions) include storage in long- and short-term memory, concept formation, association, sorting, and retrieval strategies. These operations are subject to physiological variations such as age, level of consciousness, and general well-being. The output of cognition is represented by thought or action as the individual makes a choice, moves, or speaks. Output is modified by concurrent operations related to affect and attention.[26]

The information processing model has been widely adopted in psychology and education, and occupational therapists need to be familiar with its relevance to sensory integrative function (Chapter 19). It is a useful tool for both research and program design because of its simplicity and well-defined terminology.

To summarize, the trend toward identification of universal sequences of development that dominated child study through the 1960s has given way to concern with the processes of development and function that underlie such sequences. There appears to be an increasing tendency to examine how the broad range of social, biological, and psychological influences affect different areas of behavior. This trend is reflected in the theoretical frameworks that have developed in pediatric occupational therapy practice. The frameworks that are presented here have been derived from occupational therapists' studies of the various stage theories of child development. What differentiates the occupational therapists' theories is their concern with integration of these developmental theories to provide an explanation of the process of occupation in purposeful activity.

MAJOR THEORETICAL APPROACHES TO PEDIATRIC OCCUPATIONAL THERAPY
Reilly: an explanation of play
LINDA FLOREY

Children engaged in play spend endless hours in doing things and concentrating on things that for all intents and purposes have no observable value except to the children themselves. What children seem to gain from their involvement in play is an experiential know-how that they use to solve daily living situations. The play of childhood seems to provide individuals with strategies for coping with the unknowns of the here and now and for future life experiences.

Mary Reilly's major focus has been to formulate a theoretical explanation of play that gives substance to clinical impressions that play (1) has an organizing effect on human behavior and (2) is a critical base for adult competence. Reilly proposed that the ultimate service play provides is to give meaning to the complexities of society. She stated[32] that "human adaptation falters when meaning cannot be derived from environmental interactions" (p. 15). The central question she raised is how play enables meaning to be attributed to the events of everyday life.

Reilly speculated that the very obvious and commonplace nature of play does not lend itself to rigorous scientific investigation as a discrete phenomenon. Discussion of the values and functions of play is interspersed among many theories of human behavior; however, play has rarely received prominence as a major construct. Instead, play has been approached through the back door in major theories of evolution, psychology, sociology, philosophy, biology, and anthropology. Although a theory might discuss play, it is generally discussed as a vehicle for the development of some other construct.

Reilly was convinced that play figured importantly in attempts to evoke competency in disabled individuals. Therefore she concentrated on (1) the explanatory framework by which play phenomena are examined, (2) the learning system through which the play process is explained, and (3) the play progression through which the changes in the outcome of the play process can be viewed.[32]

THE EXPLANATORY FRAMEWORK

Our knowledge of play is drawn from biology, psychology, sociology, and anthropology. Anyone attempting to examine or explain play must acknowledge this multidimensional nature of the phenomena. Reilly stated[32] that "existing theories about behavior are limited in their ability to explain multiple dimensions and integrating mechanisms." (p. 118). She addressed the question that what is needed is an interdisciplinary approach to explanation. The vehicle she selected for interdisciplinary examination of play is general systems theory.

*General systems theory** addresses the complexity of phenomena, identifies the limits to which theoretical models explain the actions of a phenomenon, and provides relationships between the various models. For ex-

---

*Discussion of general systems theory here is limited to Reilly's interpretation as presented in reference 33. Similarly, her interpretation is used for discussion of concepts attributed to Vickers, Berlyne, Buhler, White, and McClelland. Primary references for these authors may be found in Reilly's book.

ample, the theoretical model that explains temperature control in the body is not the appropriate model to explain human cognition, and vice versa.

Key concepts within general systems theory are (1) the nature of systems and (2) hierarchy. The nature of systems addresses the relationships of parts to wholes, structure to function, and exchange and array of energy. Systems are described with respect to the degree of complexity in the organization of behavior. Hierarchy specifies the levels of complexity and the rules by which such complexity is ordered. The whole of a system is composed of many parts, or subsystems. These in turn may be part of other subsystems. Hierarchy specifies the ordering of subsystems according to the complexity of each one.

The overall function of a hierarchy is to process change from simple to complex and from lower to higher forms of behavior. It implies a sense of order both in the immediate time frame and also within larger time frames. A hierarchy is composed of stages in which older and simpler forms of behavior are transformed into newer, more complex forms. The first level of a hierarchy is the initial and most simple part of a system. Each succeeding level is more complex than the preceding levels. The higher levels direct the lower ones, although there must be stability at the lower levels for the higher levels to provide any direction.

By use of a general systems framework, Reilly saw play as one system that is part of the larger system of behavior. Within play there are subsystems that are arranged in a hierarchical manner. Play is a subsystem of the imagination system of learning. The subsystems within play are exploratory, competency, and achievement behaviors.

A PLAY SYSTEM OF LEARNING

Reilly speculated that the outcomes of play are learning to symbolize and learning meanings. The play-learning process cannot be conceptualized as a fixed connection between stimulus and response under high-need states. She believed that the traditional, behaviorally oriented learning theories are too simplistic to explain the complex nature of play. Instead, she drew on the appreciative system of learning to support her concepts.

The appreciative system of learning was developed by Geoffrey Vickers, a British lawyer and public administrator. He believed that the task of learning was to find a way to look at and examine the many choices presented by a complex society. Reilly believed that the appreciative system provides a way to interpret and give meaning to information. Learning is "a product of the interaction of external facts of reality with internal values" (p. 131).[32] The tendency of *symbols* (or schemata) to link with values is the key to the learning process and enables the individual to derive meanings. The overall product of the appreciative system is judgment.

Reilly believed that a play system of learning operates in a fashion similar to the appreciative system. However, the assumptions made and the ultimate purposes differ. The appreciative system assumes that a symbol formation process is already in operation. The play system does not hold such a conviction, but instead it asks how the symbol formation and classifying processes of the mind are formed. The appreciative system is designed to explain how reality is evaluated, whereas the play system of learning explains how reality is explored and how the exploratory process teaches meaning.

Reilly viewed the *imagination* as being central to symbol formation. Symbols require meaning within one's imagination. Symbols translate sensation into meaning as they name and describe aspects of reality and provide a shorthand representation of the individual's experiences. By storing meaning and codifying experiences, symbols establish a ground plan for communication. Because symbols speak for reality, the imagination is considered a language domain.

The three subsystems of the imagination that process information into meaning are (1) the myth subsystem, (2) the dream subsystem, and (3) the play subsystem. Each subsystem serves different functions and uses different symbols for expression. The *myth subsystem* uses word symbols to represent reality. This component serves the thinking behavior of human beings, and the ultimate product is the logic of reality. The *dream subsystem* uses visual imageries to represent reality. It serves the feeling behavior of humans. The product of this subsystem is the organization of feelings for social relationships. The *play subsystem* uses rules of action to represent reality. It serves the doing behavior of humans and addresses the technology of reality. The *rule* as a symbol seeks to learn What is this? and What can be done with this? The product of the play subsystem is *skill* configuration. Rules provide a code through which the results of actions are stored. The yield of the code is skill.

All three subsystems serve the imagination system of learning, but the rule as a symbol is most relevant to understanding play. Reilly stated[32] that "the symbol of the rule is a product of the built-in characteristic of a nervous system that asks 'What is this' " (p. 140). Reilly drew on the work of psychologist Berlyne to explain the roles of curiosity and conflict in the rule symbolization process. *Curiosity* is a drive triggered by the external stimuli of novelty, uncertainty, degree of conflict, and complexity of incoming information. These stimuli all entail conflict, and by virtue of the conflict they generate, they serve to increase the arousal of the organism. Excessive arousal is relieved by specific exploration. Exploratory responses resolve conflict by favoring one response over another, by providing additional information, or by allowing time to work out a new response to the stimulus pattern.

Reilly believed that play is energized by curiosity and that, as a consequence, reality is explored to obtain the rules of how objects, people, and events work. The rule as a symbol generates meaning in the course of exploratory action. The rules comes to represent the strategies for knowing (or learning) how to do something with objects, people, and events within the boundaries of time, space, and purpose. Reilly stated[32] that "complex organizations of rules learned specifically from action of experience give rise to the skill configurations upon which the competency of man and the technology of his society are founded" (p. 145).

PLAY PROGRESSION

In the play system of learning, skill configurations are acquired, combined, and recombined into different products over time. Reilly hypothesized a progression of play behavior through three hierarchical stages: (1) exploratory behavior, (2) competency behavior, and (3) achievement behavior (Table 3-1). Each stage expresses a higher level of excitement and requires a greater degree of control. Although curiosity is the underlying force that drives the system, each stage is documented by its own motivational force.

Exploratory behavior in play is usually seen in early childhood or when an event is very new or different. Reilly proposed that exploratory play is motivated by *functional pleasure*, a concept described by Buhler. Because anxiety and pressure from unmet basic needs inhibit exploratory behavior, functional pleasure occurs only when major needs have been satisfied. In this stage children tease and test reality as their imaginations search for rules of how things work and do not work. Exploratory play produces schemata for understanding what something is and what can be done with it. For this to occur, the environment must be perceived as secure. The hallmark of this stage is the search to attribute meaning to motions, objects, and people. If the environment permits, feelings of hope and trust are generated.

Competency behavior is characterized by the need to deal with the environment and the need to be influenced by the environment through feedback mechanisms. Reilly proposed that this stage is motivated by the *efficacy drive*, as described by White. Children learn what effects they can have on the environment and what effects the environment can have on them. Through sensory, social, and other forms of feedback, children learn the results of their interactions and continually attempt to monitor their actions to achieve results. This is when the "do it myself" attitude reigns and children repeat activities over and over again to achieve a goal. Competency behaviors provide schemata, or understanding strategies, by which tasks can be mastered. The hallmark of this stage is persistence, which leads to

task mastery and feelings of self-confidence and self-reliance.

Achievement behavior incorporates the learnings of the two previous stages. The nature of achievement was drawn by Reilly from the work of McClelland. The *achievement motive* that McClelland proposed is guided by sets of expectations that are developed through anticipated or past achievement satisfactions or dissatisfactions. Expectations are formed out of universal experiences with problem solving, such as learning to walk, talk, read, or sew. These expectations involve competition with a standard of excellence. Although standards of excellence can be self-related, they are generally set by someone other than the child. Achievement behavior becomes more extrinsically guided as standards are linked to external requirements for pass, fail, good, and bad. Achievement behavior produces schemata for understanding how one's efforts measure up (or compare) in the public domain. This stage is characterized by competition, which has elements of risk and outright danger. Courage is the hallmark of this stage, and feelings of skillful mastery in a puzzling environment are generated.

• • •

In conclusion, Reilly believed that, in play, individuals acquire different kinds of rules that give meaning to environmental transactions. The rules of sensory motor action provide children with skills necessary to learn the rules of role behavior. In turn, the rules of role behavior equip children with the skills to learn the rules of cooperation and competition. Thus the early manipulation of objects and people and engagement in arts, crafts, and games yield the risk-taking behaviors seen in craftsmanship and sportsmanship. The results of engagement in these risk-taking behaviors are seen as necessary preconditions for engagement in adult workmanship. Reilly saw the play of childhood as the precursor to adult competency. The engagement of disabled individuals in arts, crafts, or games enables them to work and play through the exploratory, competency, and achievement processes by which competency is evoked.

Llorens: facilitating growth and development

Lela Llorens' work[23-25] has been broadly influenced by the developmental theorists who were discussed in prior sections of this chapter. Unlike the other occupational therapy theoretical frames of reference presented here, Llorens' model is designed to apply to adults as well. (It should be noted that the other three theorists are also broadly concerned with a life span approach to occupational therapy; however, their theories as presented here are limited to pediatric practice.)

In her 1969 Eleanor Clark Slagle Lecture, Llorens[23]

proposed that occupational therapists focus on physical, social, and psychological parameters of human life tasks and relationships. Within this context the therapist looks at individual functions and their integration, both during specific periods of life (horizontal development) and over the course of time (longitudinal development). The therapist's role is conceptualized as that of a change agent, facilitating the growth and development of the individual.

The premises of Llorens' theoretical framework are the following*:

1. That the human organism develops horizontally in the areas of neurophysiological, physical, psychosocial, psychodynamic growth and in the development of social language, daily living and sociocultural skills at specific periods of time;

2. That the human organism develops longitudinally in each of these areas in a continuous process as he ages;

3. That mastery of particular skills, abilities, and relationships in each of the areas of neurophysiological, physical, psychosocial, and psychodynamic development, social language, daily living and sociocultural skills, both horizontally and longitudinally, is necessary to the achievement of satisfactory coping behavior and adaptive relationships;

4. That such mastery is usually achieved naturally in the course of development;

5. That the fundamental endowment of the individual and the stimulation of experiences received within the environment of the family come together to interact in such a way as to promote positive early growth and development in both the horizontal and longitudinal planes;

6. That later the influences of extended family, community, social and civic groups assist in the growth process;

7. That physical or psychological trauma related to disease, injury, environmental insufficiencies or interpersonal vulnerability can interrupt the growth and development process;

8. That such growth interruption will cause a gap in the developmental cycle resulting in a disparity between expected coping behavior and adaptive facility and the necessary skills and abilities to achieve the same;

9. That occupational therapy through the skilled application of activities and relationships can provide growth and development links to assist in closing the gap between expectation and ability by increasing skills, abilities, and relationships in the neurophysiological, physical, psychosocial, psychodynamic, social language, daily living and sociocultural spheres of development as indicated both horizontally and longitudinally;

10. That occupational therapy through the skilled application of activities and relationships can provide growth experiences to prevent the development of potential maladaptation related to insufficient nurturance in neurophysiological, physical, psychosocial, psychodynamic, social language, daily living and sociocultural spheres of development both horizontally and longitudinally.

With these 10 statements, Llorens sought to identify factors of development that would guide occupational therapy practice. The skills, abilities, and relationships that are critical to the child's development become the tools of the occupational therapist. As part of the Slagle Lectureship she constructed a life span model of developmental theories and activities. In later work she more specifically defined the critical activities to emphasize their importance as occupational therapy media. The activity categories include the following[25]:

1. *Sensory activities.* These activities provide sensory stimulation to the developing individual and are generally initiated by the self or significant others. These activities are enjoyed for their sensory pleasure and include rolling, tossing in the air, swinging, and being cuddled.

2. *Developmental activities.* The specific object of developmental activities is the learning and acquisition of skills. Most developmental activities involve object manipulation. These activities tend to be specifically age related, although most result in skills that will be upgraded in performance of activities appropriate to a later age. Developmental activities are enjoyed, because they provide a sense of mastery and include arts, crafts, creative and dramatic play, and school readiness activities.

3. *Symbolic activities.* These activities are specifically related to gratification of basic needs and expression of feelings. Although the time to learn different symbolic activities may be age related, performance of the activities generally will continue in a similar form throughout the life span. Symbolic activities include eating, collecting, and leading groups.

4. *Daily life tasks.* These tasks are a reflection of cultural expectations in day-to-day life. Whereas eating is symbolic and universal, the techniques used by the individual to feed himself or herself are culturally determined. Daily life tasks include other routine, age-related activities such as using transportation, working, and cleaning house.

5. *Interpersonal relationships.* Llorens has continually stressed the need to consider human interactions as both developmental and occupational therapy activities. The nature and quality of interpersonal relationships change throughout the life span, and mastery of the skills required for interaction is critical to adequate engagement in the other types of activities. Such relationships include the one-to-one dyad, parallel cooperative work, and nurturing.

Using this theoretical framework, Llorens has de-

---

*From Llorens, L.A.: 1969 Eleanor Clark Slagle Lecture: facilitating growth and development: the promise of occupational therapy, Am. J. Occup. Ther. **24:**93, 1970.

EXHIBIT 3-1

Schematic representation of the influence of activity on life task performance demonstrating theoretical assumptions regarding why occupational therapists use activities, tasks, and occupation

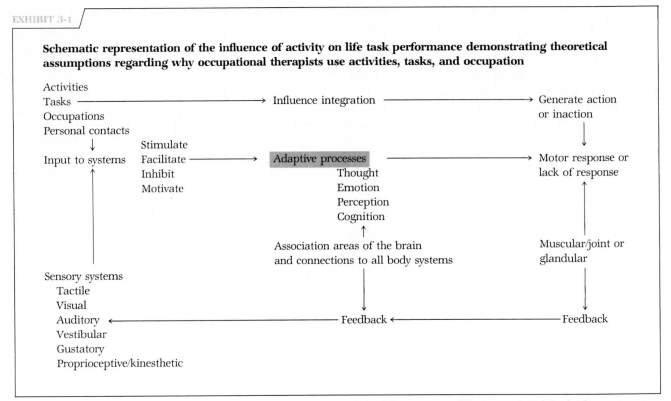

Reproduced with permission of Lela A. Llorens. See also Llorens, L.A.: Occupational therapy: state of the art—potential for development, Proceedings of New Zealand Association of Occupational Therapists Annual Conference, Auckland, N.Z., 1981; and Llorens, L.A., and Burris, B.B.: Development of sensory integration in learning disabilities, Baltimore, 1981, University Park Press.

signed and described a systematic approach to the occupational therapy process that addresses both the horizontal and longitudinal dimensions of development. Through analysis of the developmental tasks, life roles, and expectations of the individual and through analysis of the potential effects of stress, trauma, and disease the therapist is able to identify service needs. Llorens conceived occupational therapy as a problem-solving process that uses a balance of artful caring and consideration with knowledge of the human sciences.[25]

In a more recent, unpublished work,[25a] Llorens explored the meaning of activity within the occupational therapy process. She suggested that the actions of the therapist involve the use of purposeful activity for organized, controlled stimulation of adaptive role behaviors of the patient. Llorens hypothesized that direct and indirect stimulation of the central nervous system can be controlled by the therapist through the activity process (Exhibit 3-1). Activities must be analyzed and selected for their normalizing relation to the physical, psychological, and social components of individual task performance and to the totality of life role requirements.

Because so much of Llorens' work before and since her Slagle Lectureship has dealt specifically with the practice of occupational therapy, it is beyond the scope

of this chapter to provide a complete review. Numerous references to her work will be found throughout the assessment and treatment chapters.[6,23-25]

Gilfoyle and Grady: spatiotemporal adaptation

The theory of spatiotemporal adaptation formulated by Elnora Gilfoyle and Ann Grady is particularly useful as a "normal" development background for understanding the developmental disabilities. In addition to combining concepts from the work of Piaget, Gesell, and Erikson, their approach also draws from the clinical theories of Ayres and the Bobaths (see also Chapters 15 and 19).

Gilfoyle and Grady have used the term *spatiotemporal* to connote adaptation as a process of interactions between the individual and an environment of time and space (Figure 3-1). Adaptation from primitive fetal reflexes to higher levels of function takes place through the maturation of the nervous system. Of primary importance to the adaptive response is the *sensory-motor-sensory (SMS)* process of receiving, integrating, and acting on environmental input. The inborn genetic differences of the child, coupled with environmental variations, produce the unique self-system of the child. Reflex behaviors give way to posture and movement strategies, and these in turn are organized into purposeful behaviors, activities, and skills through the individual's successful experiences with the environment.

There are four components to the adaptation process. *Assimilation* is the sensory reception of stimuli from within and outside the body. The motor response of the body to stimulation is called *accommodation*. The organized process of relating a specific stimulus situation with a discrete motor response is *association*. Through repetition of this SMS pattern, the child is able to apply the process of *differentiation*. This means that the child is able to discriminate between the essential and nonproductive elements of his motor response in the given stimulus situation and can thereafter refine the accommodative pattern.

The SMS process of spatiotemporal adaptation is viewed as a spiralling continuum (Figure 3-1). Development makes up the continuous part of the process, and the interaction between older, undifferentiated SMS behaviors and newer discriminative behaviors promotes the spiralling effect. The following three principles[13] govern the direction of the spiralling continuum:

1. The child's adaptation process with new experiences is dependent upon the past acquired behaviors.
2. With the integration of past experiences with new experiences, the past behaviors are modified in some manner and result in higher level behavior.
3. The integration of higher level behaviors influences and increases the maturity of lower level behaviors (p. 50).

In effect, behavioral maturation and refinement in one activity tend to promote growth in other areas. The totality of functional development reaches higher levels.

Gilfoyle and Grady have defined a sequence for the development of purposeful activity that is useful to occupational therapy practice. In brief, this begins with a primitive phase during which the child visually explores the environment and becomes aware of her hands. Through the transitional phase, which occurs roughly from the fifth through the ninth month, visually guided development of grasp and release leads to the ability to explore objects. During this time also the infant's locomotor development is also significant. With achievement of each milestone toward an upright posture, the function of the infant's hands can be directed less toward maintaining postural stability and more toward exploring objects in the environment. The mature phase of development of purposeful activity begins with the acquisition of fine prehension and progresses through the refined manipulative skill that allows the child to control objects. Gilfoyle and Grady believe that each child develops a set of prehension skills that are both unique to the individual and universally characteristic of the species.

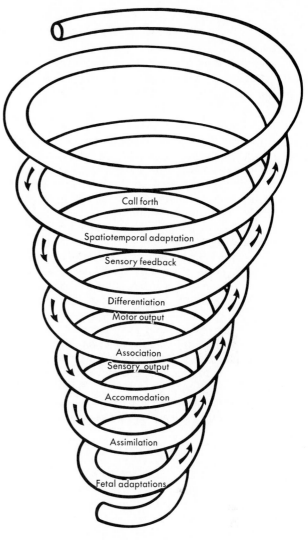

FIGURE 3-1 / **Spiralling continuum.**

From Gilfoyle, E.M., Grady, A.P., and Moore, J.C.: Children adapt, Thorofare, N.J., 1980, Charles B. Slack, Inc.

The positive effects of stress discussed in the beginning of this chapter are detailed by Gilfoyle and Grady and are seen as a challenge to adaptation. However, they differentiate the concept of *spatiotemporal stress*, which means that the adaptive demands of a stimulus situation exceed the functional capacities of the child. In this case, rather than establishing new behavioral patterns, the child "calls up" lower level behaviors to adapt to the new situation. As a temporary measure, this provides the child with the opportunity to "get his bearings" and through association and differentiation of old and new, to determine what elements of the lower level behaviors offer some chance of acting on the new situation. This is a normal process. However, if the spatiotemporal stress continues without respite, either as a result of environmental causes or of an impairment of the SMS integration process, developmental deviation can occur. Then the child experiences *spatiotemporal distress.*

The preceding discussion may be clarified by a review of the theoretical premises of spatiotemporal adaptation, as described by Gilfoyle and Grady*:

1. Development is a function of nervous system maturation which occurs through a process of adaptation.

2. Adaptation is dependent upon attention to and active participation with purposeful events of the environment. Without active participation, the nervous system is deprived of certain forms of sensation (sensory feedback) which, in turn, affects maturation.

3. Purposeful events (behaviors and activities) provide meaningful experiences for enhancement of maturation by directing a higher level adaptive response.

4. Higher level responses result from integration with and modification of acquired, lower level functions, thus adaption of higher level functions is dependent upon a certain degree of association/differentiation of specific components of lower level performance.

5. Adaptation spirals through primitive, transitional, and mature phases of development occurring at the same time within different body segments. The concurrent development of phases considers the adaptation of posture and movement strategies to purposeful behaviors and activities and the linking of behaviors and activities for adaptation to skill.

6. Environmental experiences may present situations of spatiotemporal stress. With stress, the system calls forth past acquired strategies, behaviors, and activities to act upon the demands of the environment and maintain the system's homeostasis.

7. Spatiotemporal distress provokes dysfunction when the adaptation process is interrupted or incomplete resulting in maladaptation. With dysfunction a child repeats purposeless lower level performances. Repetition of purposeless performances results in regression and ultimately leads to developmental disability.

These premises provide a rationale for their approach to treatment. Gilfoyle and Grady give considerable weight to the possibility of establishing new SMS pathways in a young nervous system (see Ayres' theory in the following section). This is achieved through a purposeful activity program that promotes spatiotemporal adaptation through active (as opposed to passive) SMS experiences. They differentiate purposeful activity as that which is initiated and directed toward interaction with objects and events in the environment. (This contrasts with the body-centered actions that Gilfoyle and Grady describe as purposeful behaviors.) The primary role of the therapist is to structure the environ-

ment with stimulus situations that will challenge the child to act through purposeful activity and avoid spatiotemporal distress.[12,13]

Ayres: sensory integration
FLORENCE CLARK

As formulated by A. Jean Ayres, sensory integration theory provides a broad developmental perspective about how the brain develops the capacity to perceive, learn, and organize behavior. Ayres defines *sensory integration* as the organization of sensory input in the brain for the emitting of adaptive responses. Developed through 20 years of research, the theory stands as an elaborate description of how sensory integration develops, how it is enhanced, and how it results in more complex responses. As a developmental theory it has logically evolved from occupational therapy because of the discipline's concern with sensory processing and adaptive responses as foundations of purposeful activity. The uniqueness of sensory integration rests on the depth in which it addresses the neurobiological foundations of behavior.

Ayres' background in occupational therapy and educational psychology has been supplemented by postdoctoral study at the Brain Research Institute of the University of California in Los Angeles. Her early interest in perceptual disorders arose from clinical experiences as an occupational therapist. At that time her caseload of patients included individuals with overt brain damage secondary to cerebral vascular accident (CVA) and cerebral palsy. Gradually her interest extended to the apparently similar perceptual problems of children who seemed to have no upper motor neuron damage and yet were rather loosely called "brain damaged." Largely because of the accessibility and availability of categorical grant funding, most of Ayres' clinical research (through which the theory has been validated) was conducted with children who had perceptual or learning disabilities. Because of this research her theory is commonly identified with learning disability. It must be reemphasized, however, that sensory integration theory has its roots in the study of normal neurobehavioral development. Attention to sensory integrative function is emphasized throughout this text as an integral part of occupational therapy practice. Ayres believed that sensory integrative theory and treatment has application for a wide variety of neurological disorders in children, including mental retardation, autism, and aphasia. In 1979 Ayres published *Sensory Integration and the Child*[4] with hopes that it would correct the bias of overidentification of the theory with learning disorders.

There are many facets to sensory integration theory, not all of which are pertinent to this chapter. What will be emphasized here are Ayres' proposals about the de-

---

*From Gilfoyle, E.M., Grady, A.P., and Moore, J.C.: Children adapt, Thorofore, N.J., 1980, Charles B. Slack, Inc., p. 208.

velopment of the child's capacity to learn, perceive, and organize behavior. Chapter 19 will discuss the research and formulations of the theory related to treatment of children with learning disabilities. Many portions of Chapter 19 will be applicable to children with other neurological handicaps. Other discussions of sensory integrative function as it relates to occupational therapy practice will be found throughout the chapters on assessment and programming.

The key concepts that are used in sensory integration theory are derived from basic research on the vertebrate brain. Therefore comprehension of the theory, as detailed in Ayres' works,[3,4] is dependent on extensive reading of the neurobiological literature and on solid preparation in neuroanatomy and neurophysiology.

THE IMPORTANCE OF SENSORY INTEGRATION

Sensory integration involves the organization of sensations from two or more sensory modalities (such as the tactile and vestibular modalities) for the purpose of emission of adaptive responses. Essentially the theory depicts streams of electrical impulses from a variety of sensory receptors converging in the central nervous system. The net effect is that this multitude of information must be localized, sorted, ordered, and organized so that it becomes meaningful. Collectively the hypothesized neural process that performs these operations is called sensory integration. Because it occurs in the brain, the process is not directly observable. However, some of its posited outcomes, like behavioral organization and adaptive responses, may be observed. Perception, or the ability to attach meaning to sensation, is described by Ayres as one other result of sensory integration.

When sensory integrative function is effective, the adaptive responses that are emitted are defined as successful, goal-directed, purposeful responses to some environmental challenge. A child is considered to have emitted an adaptive response when his actions are appropriate and successfully meet environmental demands. The complexity of adaptive responses varies. For example, at one end of the continuum the child might emit the simple response of being able to hold on and stay put on a stationary swing. The opposite end of the continuum could be the child's complex response of standing on a swing as it rapidly moves while at the same time throwing beanbags at a target. In sensory integration theory the efficiency of adaptive responses and the efficacy of sensory integrative function are believed to be mutually dependent.

Ayres placed great emphasis on the importance of adequate sensory integration as a foundation for normal learning and emotional behavior. She believed that learning occurs in the brain and that learning disorders reflect some irregularity in brain function. She proposed that abstract, complex operations such as reading,

auditory-language processing, and visual processing are dependent on intersensory processing of tactile, vestibular, and proprioceptive, stimuli, particularly the brain stem level. She reasoned that higher cognitive functions that are related to academic learning can be enhanced through better integration of the somatosensory systems when irregularities in those systems can be diagnosed.

Ayres' theory does not place equal emphasis on all the sensory systems. Although initially the visual system was emphasized, research has since suggested the importance of integration of tactile, vestibular, and proprioceptive stimuli as a primary foundation for auditory and visual processing and for the acquisition of language and academic skills. Therefore the tactile and vestibular systems are conceptualized as unifying sensory systems. These systems are believed to provide the sensory input that forms the basic relationship of the individual to gravity and the environment. Ayres believed that vestibular input may prime the nervous system for adaptive function. If the vestibular system is not functioning efficiently, interpretation of other sensations may be distorted.

To support the theoretical postulates that sensory integration underlies behavioral and emotional adaptation, Ayres cited studies by Harlow.[16,17] Harlow's findings indicated that tactile stimulation provides a foundation for emotional attachment to a mother figure. In his studies Harlow discovered that monkeys who were raised with terry cloth surrogate mothers that could be touched, clung to, and hugged showed better adjustment than monkeys who were raised with surrogate mothers made of wire. Contact with the wire mothers did not provide supportive tactile experiences.

Vestibular stimulation and adequate integration of vestibular stimuli are also considered critical to emotional adjustment. Ayres pointed out that all living things must relate to the earth's gravitational pull. Ayres[3] described gravity as "the most constant universal force in our lives" (p. 40). Children are viewed as being endowed with a strong drive to master the force of gravity, which culminates in the assumption of an upright posture and accounts for the appeal of activities that challenge gravity, such as skiing or riding a roller coaster. Efficient integration and modulation of vestibular stimuli are considered by Ayres to be essential for mastery over the earth's gravitational pull. When gravity is experienced as a threat, and a reluctance to move results, children may demonstrate personality disorders associated with the fear of movement. Ayres hypothesized that these children have irregularities in the modulation of vestibular input.

NEURAL STRUCTURES AND RELATIONSHIPS

In her theoretical presentations, Ayres emphasized only those neural structures that are thought to play a major role in sensory integration. These structures include the spinal cord, the reticular formation, the thalamus, and the vestibular nuclei of the brain stem, the cerebellum, and the cerebral hemispheres.

The spinal cord contains many tracts that carry sensations to the brain, and it relays motor messages from the brain to the cranial and peripheral nerves. While some sensory integration is believed to occur within the spinal cord, Ayres proposed that most of the processing is at higher levels of the nervous system.

Ayres postulated that the structures of the brain stem have the greatest role in sensory integration. The reticular formation is composed of neurons that have the capacity to receive multisensory input (convergent neurons). This structure therefore plays a major role in the integration of stimuli from several senses and from the two body sides and in the regulation of attentional mechanisms. The thalamus and the vestibular nuclei of the brain stem are other structures that contribute greatly to sensory integration processes.

The cerebellum is another structure that is believed to play a crucial role in sensory integration. Ayres described it as a processor of all types of sensations, particularly those that are related to the force of gravity and to movement. Finally, the cerebral hemispheres, particularly the cortices, are depicted as the regions that integrate and form associations between all types of sensation. The unique integration that occurs in the cortical association areas is the comparison of present sensory messages to stored past experiences.

The interrelationships among these structures are illustrated when a child feels and observes a puzzle piece. Touch sensations are detected in receptors of the peripheral nerves of the hand, while visual sensations are received in the retinas of the eyes. Via the spinal cord and cranial nerves, these sensations eventually reach the brain stem where attention, localization, and organization begin. In the cerebral cortex details are processed, and the new visual and tactile sensations are associated with past experience. The cumulative effect of neural processing at the various levels leads to a meaningful motor response that is directed by the cerebral cortex and modulated through the cerebellum. This process results in the child's accurate placement of the puzzle piece into the form board.

This example illustrates an important principle of sensory integration theory: higher cortical processes are dependent on adequate organization of sensation in the brain stem. Another principle related to the adequacy of cortical functions is called *lateralization*. In sensory integration theory this is defined as the tendency of specific processes to be handled more efficiently by one side of the brain than the other. The establishment of hemispheric lateralization is viewed as dependent on effective sensory integration, especially of stimuli from the two body sides, at the brain stem level. Ayres posited that when the whole body and all of the sensory systems are working in concert and when sensations are efficiently organized at respective levels of the nervous system, adaptation, learning, and emotional satisfaction are natural outcomes.

THE DEVELOPMENT OF SENSORY INTEGRATION

Ayres' writings[3,4] supply a detailed account of how the child's nervous system develops capacities for sensory integration. The immature nervous systems of newborns have few interconnections between neurons, and they lack appreciable myelination in the cerebral cortices. Consequently, infant behavior is generally stereotypic and regulated by lower neural centers that lack the restraining and modulating influences of the higher brain structures. As the infant interacts with the world, neural interconnections are formed through the increased branching of dendrites (arborization). Sensory stimulation of appropriate kinds and amounts is deemed critical to the development of interconnections at the neural synapses and to the infant's capacity to perceive and adapt to the environment. In the central nervous system the neural flow can be inhibited or facilitated via the interactions of neurotransmitters at the synaptic connections. The result is modulation of sensory reception so that the child can selectively attend to relevant stimuli. Feedback provides the child with continual information about the results of actions and influences ongoing sensory integration. Gradually organization of vestibular sensations helps the infant adapt to the earth's gravitational pull through the achievement of an upright posture. At about 2 years of age the child learns to climb and, through integration of tactile and proprioceptive sensations, she forms a sensory picture of how body parts are related. Sensory integration of visual and somatosensory stimuli is enhanced as the child gains mastery over tool use during the third through seventh years.

In Ayres' theory the status of sensory integration in a child is viewed as a product of genetic endowment and environmental experiences. Within the normal population individual differences will exist in the ability to organize sensation for use. Ayres[3,4] identified the following four principles of brain development that relate to the achievement of each child's maximal potential for sensory integration:

1. *The brain innately seeks out those sensations that will be organizing.* Children are designed to receive pleasure from activities that help to organize their brains. In sensory integration theory it is proposed that neural organization will be optimally promoted if children are encouraged to express this inner drive. The child's choices of play activities are believed to be mo-

tivated by this inner drive to seek organizing sensations. Play activities are therefore regarded as critical to brain development.

2. *The brain must interpret sensory stimuli before it can respond adaptively to those stimuli.* This principle implies that presentation of meaningful amounts and kinds of sensory stimulation will further the developing child's capacity to adapt to environmental demands. For example, rocking a newborn baby will promote better neural processing as long as the frequency and duration of rocking are appropriate to the baby's organizational capacities. This principle proposes that infants and children should be afforded opportunitites to receive stimuli from movement, sight, sound, and touch.

3. *Ontogenetic brain development of the individual is enhanced by many of the same factors that promoted phylogenetic brain development across the species through evolution.* Evolutionary theory suggests that brain development of species occurred in response to environmental demands. The neural processing will be enhanced if growing children are provided with opportunities to successfully adapt to environmental challenges.

4. *As the brain evolved, higher and newer structures like the cerebral cortex remained dependent on adequate functioning of older structures.* The newer structures can process more complex information, but they do so with the benefit of sensory integration that occurs at lower levels of the nervous system. This principle suggests that it is appropriate to emphasize the importance of brain stem sensory integration as a foundation for efficient cortical function.

Principles of sensory integration theory that apply more directly to treatment are described in Chapter 19 and detailed in Ayres' writings.[3,4] It must be emphasized, however, that this theory is continually evolving and modified in accordance with results of ongoing research that is conducted and published by Ayres and other investigators. Therefore serious study of sensory integration theory requires attention to relevant journal articles.

DISCUSSION

Sensory integration theory has transformed many aspects of pediatric occupational therapy. Although Ayres' thinking was broadly influenced by Piaget's description of the sensorimotor stage and by Rood and the Bobaths (Chapter 16) who addressed the relationship of sensory stimuli to motor responses, her sensory integration theory included many new ideas. A critical, differential concept of Ayres' theory is the shift of emphasis from the motor response to its foundations in neural processing. This focus has resulted in a new way of perceiving the sensory-motor dimension of child development.

SUMMARY

Each child who is seen in occupational therapy is in the midst of a dynamic process of growth, maturation, and adaptation. Therefore knowledge of the human development process is critical to the foundation of occupational therapy theory and practice. This chapter has reviewed basic principles of growth and development, as well as selected systems for classification of theories. Stage theories, which examine longitudinal aspects of development, and process theories, which look in detail at one facet of development, make up the most basic classification system.

The best accepted stage theories were developed through the work of Freud, Erikson, and Piaget. Each of these men formulated a series of recognizable stages that correspond to the usual development of one area of human function. Freud's work related to the biologically based psychosexual development of the child as the foundation of emotional and social behavior. Erikson followed much of Freud's thinking but placed greater emphasis on the role of the environment as the moderator of individual adaptation. Piaget concentrated on the cognitive development of the child and formulated a series of periods that are differentiated by the child's use of progressively more elaborate mental operations. He also emphasized the role of environmental experiences as determinants of cognitive and adaptive development.

Other stage theories that are particularly useful to occupational therapy practice include Kohlberg's stages of moral development, Maslow's hierarchy of human needs, Gesell's schedules of adaptive behavioral development, and Havighurst's model of developmental tasks for each major age of human life. Each of these models helps to expand concepts of Freud, Erikson, and Piaget, especially as they relate to age-related activities.

The work of Skinner and Rogers accounts for the most durable process theories. Skinner emphasized the role of the environment in shaping the behavior of the individual and the species. Rogers also recognized the role of the environment but emphasized the importance of a healthy self-concept as a foundation for successful adaptation.

Current trends in developmental theory tend to emphasize process. Scientists are examining the relationship between specialized brain hemisphere functions and human behavior. In addition, they are looking to sociobiology to help differentiate between those human capacities that are derived through the species and those that are environmentally shaped. Current research indicates that many of the social, adaptive, and emotional characteristics of children that were earlier thought to be environmentally shaped may have a greater foundation in inborn capacities. Finally, followers of Skinner's behavioral approach have turned to information processing theory to examine the cognitive functions of the child.

Developmental theories are only useful to occupational therapists if they can be operationalized for practice. This chapter has presented reviews of the theoretical frameworks of Reilly, Llorens, Gilfoyle and Grady, and Ayres. Each of these occupational therapists integrated their studies of developmental theory to formulate an approach to occupational therapy practice in pediatrics. Reilly concentrated on play as the fundamental occupation of the developing child through which the skills that underlie adult competence are shaped. Llorens integrated the developmental theories to propose a model of occupational therapy practice that is related to horizontal and longitudinal aspects of development in the child's life. Gilfoyle and Grady examined the spiralling development of sensory and motor functions of the child as the foundation for purposeful human activity. Ayres studied the role of the brain and its sensory integrative processes that organize and direct observable behavior. No single framework for occupational therapy practice is all inclusive; each must be considered in relation to the others and applied according to the needs of individual children. A derived conceptual model of practice that integrates concepts of the developmental and occupational therapy theories found here will be presented in Chapter 7.

REFERENCES

1. Ainsworth, M.D.S.: Infant-mother attachment, Am. Psychol. **34:**932, Oct. 1979.
2. Als, H., and Brazelton, T.B.: A new model of assessing the behavioral organization in pre-term and full-term infants: two case studies, J. Am. Acad. Child Psychiatry **20:**239, 1981.
3. Ayres, A.J.: Sensory integration and learning disorders, Los Angeles, 1972, Western Psychological Services.
4. Ayres, A.J.: Sensory integration and the child, Los Angeles, 1979, Western Psychological Services.
5. Barash, D.: The whispering within, New York, 1979, Harper & Row, Publishers, Inc.
6. Clark, P.N.: Human development through occupation: theoretical frameworks for contemporary occupational therapy practice, part 1, Am. J. Occup. Ther. **33:**505, 1979.
7. Erikson, E.H.: Childhood and society, ed. 2, New York, 1963, W.W. Norton & Co., Inc.
8. Flavell, J.H.: Cognitive development, Englewood Cliffs, N.J., 1977, Prentice-Hall, Inc.
9. Forman, G.E., and Sigel, I.E.: Cognitive development: a life-span view, Monterey, Calif., 1979, Brooks/Cole Publishing Co.
10. Freud, S.: An autobiographical study. Translated by Strachey, J., New York, 1952, Norton Library.
11. Geschwind, N.: Specializations of the human brain. In Scientific american: the brain, San Francisco, 1979, W.H. Freeman & Co., Publishers.
12. Gilfoyle, E.M., and Grady, A.P.: Posture and movement. In Hopkins, H.L., and Smith, H.D.: Willard and Spackman's occupational therapy, ed. 5, Philadelphia, 1978, J.B. Lippincott Co.
13. Gilfoyle, E.M., Grady, A.P., and Moore, J.C.: Children adapt, Thorofare, N.J., 1980, Charles B. Slack, Inc.
14. Hall, C.S.: A primer of Freudian psychology, New York, 1964, Mentor Books.
15. Hall, C.S., and Lindzey, G.: Theories of personality, ed. 3, New York, 1978, John Wiley & Sons, Inc.
16. Harlow, H.F.: The nature of love, Am. Psychol. **13:**673, 1958.
17. Harlow, H.F.: Love in infant monkeys, Sci. Am. **200:**68, 1959.
18. Havighurst, R.J.: Developmental tasks and education, ed. 3, New York, 1972, David McKay Co., Inc.
19. Hetherington, E.M.: Divorce: a child's perspective, Am. Psychol. **34:**851, Oct. 1979.
20. Kaluger, G.A., and Kaluger, M.F.: Human development: the span of life, ed. 3, St. Louis, 1984, The C.V. Mosby Co.
21. Knickerbocker, B.M.: A holistic approach to the treatment of learning disorders, Thorofare, N.J., 1980, Charles B. Slack, Inc.
21a. Knoblock, H., and Pasamanick, D., editors: Gesell and Amatruda's developmental diagnosis, ed. 3, New York, 1975, Harper & Row, Publishers, Inc.

22. Kohlberg, L.: Stage and sequence: the cognitive developmental approach to socialization. In Groslin, D.: Handbook of socialization theory and research, Chicago, 1969, Rand McNally & Co.

23. Llorens, L.A.: 1969 Eleanor Clark Slagle Lecture: facilitating growth and development: the promise of occupational therapy, Am. J. Occup. Ther. **24:**1, 1970.

24. Llorens, L.A.: The effects of stress on growth and development, Am. J. Occup. Ther. **28:**82, 1974.

25. Llorens, L.A.: Application of developmental theory for health and rehabilitation, Rockville, Md., 1976, American Occupational Therapy Association, Inc.

25a. Llorens, L.A.: Personal communication, 1977.

26. McDavid, J.W., and Garwood, S.G.: Understanding children: promoting human growth, Lexington, Mass., 1978, D.C. Heath & Co.

27. Maier, H.W.: Three theories of child development: the contributions of Erik H. Erikson, Jean Piaget, and Robert R. Sears, and their applications, rev. ed., New York, 1969, Harper & Row, Publishers, Inc.

28. Mosey, A.C.: Meeting health needs, Am. J. Occup. Ther. **27:**14, 1973.

29. Nye, R.D.: Three psychologies: perspectives from Freud, Skinner, and Rogers, ed. 2, Monterey, Calif., 1981, Brooks/Cole Publishing Co.

30. Piaget, J.: Psychology and epistomology: towards a theory of knowledge. Translated by Rosin, A., New York, 1971, The Viking Press.

31. Piaget, J., and Inhelder, B.: The psychology of the child. Translated by Weaver, H., New York, 1969, Basic Books, Inc., Publishers.

32. Reilly, M.: Play as exploratory learning: studies of curiosity behavior, Beverly Hills, Calif., 1974, Sage Publications, Inc.

33. Rogers, C.R.: Freedom to learn, Columbus, Ohio, 1969, Charles E. Merrill Publishing Co.

34. Skinner, B.F.: Beyond freedom and dignity, New York, 1971, Bantam Books, Inc.

35. Skinner, B.F.: About behaviorism, New York, 1974, Vintage Books.

36. Skinner, B.F.: Walden two, ed. 2, New York, 1976, MacMillan Publishing Co., Inc.

37. Smith, J.M.: The concepts of sociobiology. In Stent, G.S., editor: Morality as a biological phenomenon, Berkeley, Calif., 1978, University of California Press, p. 21.

38. Sprinthall, R.C., and Sprinthall, N.A.: Educational psychology: a developmental approach, ed. 3, Reading, Mass., 1981, Addison-Wesley Publishing Co., Inc.

39. Thomas, A.: Current trends in developmental theory, Am. J. Orthopsychiatry **51:**580, 1981.

40. White, J.A.: Selected readings on hemispheric specialization, Phys. Occup. Ther. Pediatr. **1:**71, Spring 1981.

41. Wilson, E.O.: Introduction: what is sociobiology? In Gregory, M., Silvers, A., and Sutch, D., editors: Sociobiology and human nature, San Francisco, Calif., 1978, Jossey-Bass, Inc., Publishers.

RECOMMENDED JOURNALS

American Journal of Occupational Therapy
American Journal of Orthopsychiatry
American Psychologist
Annual Review of Psychology
Child Development
Developmental Medicine and Child Neurology
Journal of Educational Psychology
Infant Development and Behavior
Merrill-Palmer Quarterly
Monographs of the Society for Research in Child Development
Occupational Therapy Journal of Research
Physical and Occupational Therapy in Pediatrics
Scientific American

4

SUSAN DENEGAN SHORTRIDGE

The developmental process: prenatal to adolescence

Development is a continuous process. It proceeds stage by stage in an orderly sequence, despite individual variations. Both biological and psychological development adhere to these rules. Llorens[56] emphasizes the importance of "mastery of particular skills, abilities, and relationships . . . for successful achievement of satisfactory adaptive relationships." According to DiLeo[21] development is:

> a continuum. It advances upward and forward, not in a linear fashion, but more like a spiral, with its downward as well as upward cycle, yet always a bit more upward and a bit less downward, each stage representing a level of maturity whose features are qualitatively different yet derived from and dependent upon earlier stages (p. 3).

Childhood is indeed the magic time in the life span when development blossoms. From the moment of conception through the adolescent years the child passes through many facets of developmental growth. These facets include the physiological, sensorimotor, cognitive, and social-emotional domains.

Periods of growth show great variation; however, for the purpose of clarity, the division of growth periods and their approximate age ranges follow:

Growth period	Approximate age
Prenatal	From 0 to 280 days
Ovum	From 0 to 14 days
Embryo	From 14 days to 8 weeks
Fetus	From 8 weeks to birth
Birth	Average 280 days
Neonate	First 4 weeks after birth
Infancy	First year of life
Early childhood	From 1 to 6 years
Middle childhood	From 6 to 12 years
Adolescence	From 12 to 18 years

PRENATAL PERIOD

Preparation for childbirth begins both biologically and psychologically in the mother before the delivery date. The 280 days following the last menstrual cycle affords ample time to adjust to the developing child.

Biologically the mother's body has been making changes and adjustments in anticipation of the delivery. During the first trimester of pregnancy the adaptive reactions of the uterus greatly influence the developing fetus. Abdominal distention begins to occur because of hyperplasia of smooth muscle fibers, especially in the vicinity of the implantation sites.[80] The preparation of the muscular layer of the uterus is extremely important, because it will open the cervix, help push the baby out, and form ligatures to cut off the blood supplying the lining of the uterus.[89] This hypertrophy continues to keep pace with the growth of the fetus and is largely caused by the increased production of estrogen.

Psychologically pregnancy brings forth sensations that a woman has not known before. The "mystery of birth" becomes less of a fantasy when fatigue, nausea, tenderness of the breasts, or frequent urination occur to remind the woman of her changed state. As pregnancy advances the perception of fetal movement, or quickening, directs the woman's focus even more strongly toward her body and the birth of her child. Before the birth event three distinct phases of development occur in utero. These are the germinal stage, the embryonic stage, and the fetal stage.

The first prenatal stage, which is the period of the ovum, or the *germinal stage*, lasts approximately 2 weeks. This period is initiated from the moment of fertilization to implantation in the uterus. The major emphasis during this period is in the change from a fertilized egg to a complex structure that will consist of 800 billion cells at birth. The structural changes that occur during cell differentiation are seen in the change from a zygote to a blastocyst. The blastocyst is a free-floating sphere that remains in the uterus for approximately 2 days. During this time cells cluster to one side of the blastocyst to form the embryonic disk from which the fetus will develop. The remaining cells form distinct layers. The upper layer, called the *ectoderm*, will become the infant's epidermis and its derivatives, that is, the sensory organs, brain, and spinal cord. The lower layer, the *endoderm*, will later form the digestive system, as well as the liver, pancreas, and salivary glands, and the respiratory system. The *mesoderm*, or middle layer, differentiates into the dermis, muscles, skeleton, and excretory and circulatory systems. The outer cells of the blastocyst, called the *trophoblast*, give rise to the protective and nutritive membranes of the intrauterine environment: the placenta, umbilical cord, and amniotic sac. Once this cell mass is fully implanted in the uterus it is called an embryo.

The second stage of prenatal development, the *embryonic stage*, is swift and lasts from 2 to 8 weeks. Although of short duration, this prenatal period is characterized by rapid growth. The fourth week shows an embryo with a beating heart. Between the fourth and the eighth week the eyes, ears, nose, and mouth become more clearly recognizable, signifying cephalocaudal development. By the end of the first 8 weeks after conception, 95% of the body parts have appeared through the continued process of differentiation. At the end of this prenatal period the embryo is recognizable as a tiny human.

The third prenatal period, the *fetal stage*, lasts from the end of the second month until birth. The appearance of the first bone cells at 8 weeks signals the name change from embryo to fetus. This is the longest of the prenatal stages. At this developmental period almost all of the structures and systems found in the newborn have developed, and many are already functional. These structures are primitive and must be developed further before they can be considered to be completely functional. This is perhaps most clearly seen in the primitive movements of the fetus.

A light touch to the mouth area of an embryo will cause the entire body to convulse, but spontaneous movement does not occur until later (p. 27).[4]

TABLE 4-1	Prenatal development during the fetal stage		
Stage	*Physical development*		*Motor development*
Third month	Length = 3 inches Weight = 1 ounce Eyelids fused Fingers and toes well formed Fingernails growing Sex differentiation*		Kicks, makes fist, turns head, but movement not recognizable by mother
Fourth month	Length = 6 inches Weight = 6 ounces Most rapid growth*		Sucking Pushing with limbs Quickening noted by mother
Fifth month	Length = 12 inches Weight = 1 pound		Sleeps and wakes
Sixth month	Length = 14 inches Weight = 2 pounds Red, wrinkled skin Eyes unfused Taste buds form		Grasp reflex present Slight, irregular breathing Hiccup
Seventh month	Viable* Growth slows		
Eighth and ninth months	Wrinkled skin fills out with fat Weight = ½ pound a week All intrauterine development completed*		Startle reflex present Responds to light and sound Motor action limited because of increasingly tight fit of uterus

Adapted from Annis, L.F.: The child before birth, London, 1978, Cornell University Press.
*Most important characteristic of time period.

These primitive movements continue to refine over the next 7 months. Milani-Comparetti and Giodoni[66] characterized the period from 7 months' gestation to birth in terms of fetal competencies for readiness to be born. These include *fetal locomotion,* which allows the fetus to move around the fetal chamber to find the correct presentation for physiological birth, and *fetal propulsion,* which is the active movement of the fetus involving an extension pattern of thrusting. To understand the tremendous growth and development that occur during this fetal stage, each event should be assessed separately (Table 4-1).

Prenatal influences

The interaction of heredity and environment strongly influences the prenatal period (Table 6-1, p. 80). An ideal environment for the fetus is one that includes an adequate supply of oxygen and nutrients via the functional placenta and umbilical cord, as well as freedom from disease organisms, toxic chemicals, abnormal genes or chromosomes, and maternal stress. Inherited abnormalities make up only a small proportion of birth defects.

> About 20 percent of known birth defects can be traced primarily to hereditary factors. Genetic traits in one or both parents cause a disease or abnormal condition in the child. Another 20 percent or so of birth defects are due to something in the environment of the baby that affects it while it is developing inside the mother. (The remaining 60 percent are caused by the interaction of heredity and environmental factors).[11]

Pregnancy is influenced not only by an after dinner drink, coffee breaks, smoking, and stress of the mother, but also by numerous environmental influences outside the woman's control.

Because of rapid growth during the embryonic period, the unborn child is most vulnerable to environmental insults and disruptions.[61] The effects of many of these prenatal influences depend on the relative stage of development, that is, the point in the developmental sequence when the change in the prenatal environment occurs. Sensitive periods are times during which a particular influence or stimulus from another part of the environment evokes a specific response.[73]

CHILDBIRTH
Labor

At approximately 40 weeks the uterus begins to undergo rhythmical contractions that ultimately lead to the birth of the child. This sequence of events is referred to as labor or parturition.

Labor consists of three stages. The first stage, which entails the major portion of the duration of labor, is dilation of the cervix. The rhythmical contractions signaling pain begin to push the fetus downward while the muscle fibers surrounding the cervical opening are pulled upward by the upper segment of the uterus. The further stretching of the cervix may cause the amniotic sac to burst and release its flow of "waters." These muscular processes of the first stage of labor are involuntary. The maternal abdominal muscles should remain relaxed to allow the uterus to rise during contraction. This rise assists in positioning the fetal head toward the cervix, and it promotes normal dilation.[26] Relaxation resulting from the absence of fear hastens relaxation of the muscle fibers surrounding the cervix and is one of the purposes of childbirth education classes.

Delivery of the infant through the cervical canal and vagina marks the second stage of labor. The physical act of "bearing down" complements the uterine contractions. It is during this stage of delivery that conscious control of breathing and relaxation can facilitate the natural birth process. The birth canal has a tremendous ability to stretch, and, since the bones of the fetus' skull have not yet fused together, the head serves as a pliable instrument for widening the cervix and the vagina. This second phase of labor begins with head-first passage of the fetus into the birth canal. The head-first birth presentation is seen in approximately 95% of the labors; the remaining 5% involve deviation from the cephalocaudal position and are termed malpresentations.[85]

The third stage of delivery consists of expelling the amniotic sac, the placenta, and membranes that are all referred to as the afterbirth.

INFANCY
Physiological development

The neonate comes into the world looking more like a wrinkled old person than a Gerber baby. Typically the physical appearance of the neonate is characterized by reddish skin covered by vernix caseosa. The vernix caseosa is an oily protection against infection that dries in a few days' time.[71] The head appears larger than the body and is usually elongated and bumpy as a result of molding during birth. In addition, the flat, broad nose that is formed of cartilage is often temporarily pushed out of shape by the birth process. Acrocyanosis, caused by sluggish peripheral circulation and mottling in response to cold, may also be present. The neonate's eyelids are usually puffy, making the eyes appear small. The eyes, smoky blue for the first month or two, change gradually to their permanent color. Hair may be abundant or scanty. Often the permanent hair color is different from that at birth. The external breasts and genitals of both males and females may look enlarged. This appearance is temporary and is caused by female hormones that passed to the baby before birth.

The average weight of the neonate is 7 pounds 2 ounces. During the first few days of life most neonates lose 5% to 10% of their body weight because of passage of meconium and urine, as well as delays in feeding.[108] This weight shift is usually regained by 10 days of age. The average length of the neonate is between 19 and 22 inches.

Following birth the full-term neonate must make profound adjustments to his new life. The once totally dependent neonate emerges into an environment where a separate entity must now be responsible for respiration, circulation of the blood, digestion, and temperature regulation.

The traditional cry at birth signals a message to the mother that the baby has arrived and is inspiring air for the first time. Breathing is irregular, rapid, and shallow, involving the abdomen more than the chest. During the first few days after birth the neonate experiences periods of coughing and sneezing. This serves to clear the mucus and amniotic fluid from his airways.[19]

The onset of breathing also marks a significant change in the neonate's circulatory system. A change in the vascular resistance alters the blood flow that once passed via the placenta. Closure of a valve between the right and left atrium (*foramen ovale*) and a vessel that leads from the aorta to the pulmonary artery (*ductus arteriosus*) occurs within the first 10 days of life. In addition, the lungs continue to expand.

Before birth the placenta provided nourishment as well as oxygen for the fetus. After birth the neonate must obtain nourishment from the mother in an external environment. The initial move toward feeding be-

TABLE 4-2	Primitive reflexes
Reflex and onset-integration	*Purpose*
Rooting reflex: 28 weeks' gestation to 3 months	Enables infant to find nipple Allows active contraction of neck muscles
Sucking and swallowing reflex: 28 weeks' gestation to 2 to 5 months	Enables obtainment of nourishment
Moro reflex: 28 weeks' gestation to 5 to 6 months	Breaks up flexion posture to permit extension of trunk and extremities[3]
Traction-grasp reflex: 28 weeks' gestation to 2 to 5 months	Allows reflexive momentary grasp[103]
Crossed extension reflex: 28 weeks' gestation to 1 to 2 months	Used later with positive support to maintain balance on one leg Integration needed for reciprocal movements
Flexor withdrawal reflex: 28 weeks' gestation to 1 to 2 months	Serves as protective response to noxious stimuli
Plantar grasp reflex: 28 weeks' gestation to 9 months	Integration needed for standing[66]
Neonatal neck and body righting reflex: 34 weeks' gestation to 4 to 5 months	Allows log rolling from supine to sidelying
Neonatal positive support reflex: 35 weeks' gestation to 1 to 2 months	Allows weight bearing in upright position
Proprioceptive placing (LE) reflex: 35 weeks' gestation to 2 months	Allows foot to be placed flat on surface, primitive form of ambulation
Proprioceptive placing (UE) reflex: birth to 2 months	Needed for supporting body weight on forearms and on extended arms
Spontaneous stepping reflex: 37 weeks' gestation to 2 months	Precursor to later mature walking
Tonic labyrinthine reflex: birth to 6 months	First manifestations of gravitational influences to head orientation
Asymmetrical tonic neck reflex (ATNR): birth to 4 to 6 months	Enhances supportive framework of voluntary motion
Symmetric tonic neck reflex: 4 to 6 months to 8 to 12 months	Promotes four-point kneeling by breaking up extensor pattern
Palmar grasp reflex: birth to 4 to 6 months	Allows infant to reach out for toy with full palmer grasp[102]

Adapted from Barnes, M.L., and others: The neurophysiological basis for patient treatment, Morgantown, W.Va., 1978, Stokesville Publishing Co.

havior is complemented by hunger contractions, rooting, sucking, and swallowing mechanisms that are present at birth and stimulate physiological maturation.

The neonate's temperature regulation system also gradually changes. Within the uterus the infant's skin was maintained at a constant temperature. The neonate's subcutaneous fat layer is inadequate for insulation, and the large skin surface area contributes to heat loss. Swaddling and heat lamps are frequently used to maintain temperature.

TABLE 4-3	Sequences in gross motor development					
	1 month (4 weeks)	*4 months (16 weeks)*	*7 months (28 weeks)*	*10 months (40 weeks)*	*12 months*	*18 months*
Head control	Supine position: tonic neck reflexes dominate Prone position: rotates head to rest on cheek	Supine position: integration of tonic neck reflexes results in midposition of head Prone position: lifts head in midposition from prone position on elbows	Supine position: lifts head as though trying to sit up Prone position: on hands tries to pivot	Prone position: gets on hands and knees for creeping	Completed	Completed
Sitting	Marked or complete head lag in pull-to-sit position Momentary head righting in sitting Rounded back	Slight head lag in pull-to-sit position Head erect and set forward in sitting position Lumbar curvature	Sits erect momentarily Sits propped up	Sits with good control without support Progresses from sitting to prone position	Sits erect, pivots in sitting position Progresses from sitting to creeping position	Seats self in small chair
Rolling	Partially rolls from supine to side-lying position	Prone to side-lying position	Rolls from supine to prone position, prone to supine position	Completed	Completed	Completed
Locomotion	Absent reflexes dominate	Absent reflexes dominate	Sustains large fraction of weight in standing Bounces actively	Prone position: uses hands and knees for creeping Pulls self to feet Stands and lowers self while holding on Stands supported with hands held	Creeping Pulls to feet while holding railing Cruises sideways Walks with one hand held	Walks alone, seldom falls Runs stiffly Walks upstairs with one hand held Climbs into adult chair

Adapted from Gesell, A., and Amatruda, C.S.: Developmental diagnosis, ed. 2, New York, 1954, Harper & Brothers.

Sensorimotor development

From the moment of birth the neonate shows specific behavioral stages. Wolff[113] was able to separate and identify six newborn behavioral stages: regular sleep, irregular sleep, drowsiness, alert inactivity, waking activity, and crying. These stages have distinct conditions and specific properties. The neonate's response to stimulation depends on this state and on the stimulus.

The neonate's motor responses contribute to his organization of the world and to his survival within its boundaries. The neonate's gross motor activity is developed from movement patterns that began in the intra-uterine environment and from the maturation of reflex behavior that is primarily controlled from the spinal and brain stem level (Table 4-2).

The neonate is capable of more than reflex behavior. He demonstrates orientation, attention, and habituation to visual, auditory, and tactile stimuli.

Following the first month of life the neonate is identified as an infant. At this time of life, motor responses in head control, sitting, rolling, and locomotion continue to develop from simple to complex skills (Table 4-3). At 4 weeks the infant's head position is dominated by the tonic neck reflexes. Head lag is noted in the pull to sitting position; however, the infant is able to lift his head long enough to turn it while he is on his stomach (prone position) to attain a more comfortable cheek-resting posture. By 16 weeks the infant is able to lift his head at a 45-degree angle to the supporting surface. Visual stimulation and an increased ability to deal with gravity allow the infant to attain a more erect head posture. The infant's progression continues so that he is able to support himself propped on his forearms, and, finally, he is able to support himself by extending his arms and resting on the palms of his hands. This developmental sequence of head control is assisted by the emerging righting reactions and the disappearance of the tonic labyrinthine and asymmetrical tonic neck reflexes. The Landau reflex allows the infant to extend his trunk and extremities as he attains pivot prone postures.

Following head control, the infant is able to roll. He first develops the ability to roll from his back (supine position) to his side, then from his stomach to his side, and then from his stomach to his back. The neonatal neck righting reflex allows the trunk to follow the head. By 7 months the infant is able to roll voluntarily from stomach to back, and back to stomach.

The neonate of 4 weeks of age sits with a rounded back and a head that is erect only momentarily. In the infant, however, more muscle extension exists, and the infant's ability to control her head and trunk result in a more upright sitting posture. The 7-month-old can sit with back support provided by a chair or pillow or with arms propped forward in a tripod posture. By 10 months the infant can sit erect and unsupported for several minutes and soon progresses from a sitting to prone posture. By 12 months the infant can sit, rotate, and pivot without losing her balance and attain a creeping position from sitting.

Parents' eager anticipation of their infant's first steps often causes them to regard the spontaneous stepping seen at birth as an advanced motor skill of their "unique offspring." These reflexive stepping movements are visible shortly after birth; however, the complex coordination necessary for walking does not occur until 9 to 15 months of age. Before walking the infant becomes mobile in many ways.

Creeping refers to four-point mobility with only the hands and knees on the floor. This reciprocal limb mo-

TABLE 4-4	Sequences in fine motor development
Action	*Age*
Reflex, automatic hand grasp	0 to 3 months*
Ocular fixation and beginning eye-hand coordination	12 weeks
Reaching, scratching but unable to secure object	16 weeks to 4 months
Precarious ulnar-palmar grasp (fifth and fourth fingers press object against palm)	20 weeks to 5 months
Palmar grasp (all four fingers hold object against palm)	24 weeks to 6 months
Radial-palmar grasp (second and third finger hold object against palm)	32 to 36 weeks to 8 to 9 months
Radial raking at a string	32 to 36 weeks
Radial-digital grasp (object secured by thumb, index finger, and middle finger)	9 to 10 months
Crude release of object	10 months
Plucks string between index and thumb (pincer grasp)	10 to 11 months
Refinement of pincer grasp (neatly plucking from above)	12 months
Builds tower of two 1-inch cubes	15 months
Builds tower of three or four 1-inch cubes	18 months

Adapted from Gesell, A., and Amatruda, C.S.: Developmental diagnosis, ed. 2, New York, 1954, Harper & Brothers.
*All ages are approximate.

tion demonstrates integration of many of the primitive reflexes before engagement in the more complex voluntary process of ambulation. With creeping and crawling come increased trunk flexibility and rotation. The emergence of equilibrium and protective reactions assists the 10- to 12-month-old infant in creeping as fast as others can walk.

The ability to stand is influenced by the emergence of positive support. When her weight bearing is secure, a 7-month-old girl bounces in delight of her new skill and practices the freedom of movement from flexion to extension. She begins to prepare for the upright posture by first attaining a kneel-standing posture, then progressing to a half kneel, and finally to full standing. A 10-month-old boy practices rising and lowering postures by supporting himself on furniture. At this time the infant becomes interested in objects denied him. This interest stimulates an even stronger desire to stand when the objects are moved out of reach. The development of cruising at 12 months of age helps the infant coordinate his high center of gravity and short legs.

The infant's first efforts of unsupported forward movement are often seen in short, erratic steps, unnecessary lifting of the legs, and uncontrollable excitement. By 12 months most infants can walk with help. By 18 months they are able to move throughout their world with the help of a relatively immature balance system, a high protective guard of the upper extremities, and a wide-based gait. When hurried, the infant may regress to the initial creeping pattern. However, with maturational changes in the infant's body proportions and the development of strength and coordination, walking be-

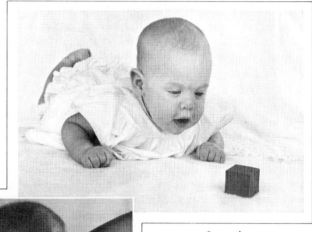

3 months
Looks at cube

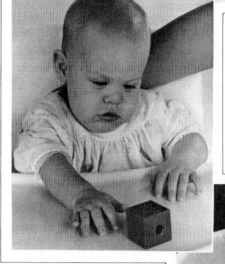

5 months
Looks and approaches

FIGURE 4-1

Developmental progression of prehensile behavior.

From Ingalls, A.J., and Salerno, M.C.: Maternal and child health nursing, ed. 3, 1983, The C.V. Mosby Co.

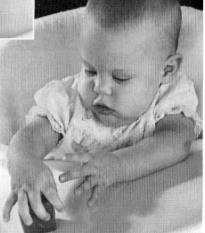

6 months
Looks and crudely grasps with whole hand

comes the primary means of mobility. Walking brings forth new avenues of exploration and a sense of autonomy. The parent must now protect this moving, explorative infant more than previously.

The infant's hands provide a means to reach out to the world and discover it. As in all development, sequences of motor development do not occur independent of each other. The development of mobility and hand function occur simultaneously, each progressing chronologically toward maturation (Table 4-4).

The grasping reflex is present at birth and allows the infant to have automatic contact with anything placed in his palm. The first 12 weeks involve contacting objects more with the eyes than with the hands. Infants look, stare, and grope at objects within their visual fields. By the fourth month infants develop more

voluntary control over their activities. The first voluntary, physical, prehensile activity is swiping at objects. By 5 months reaching toward an object develops, although the grasping skill is limited to a precarious ulnar-palmar grasp. Infants can be observed alternating between looking at their hands and looking at the object (Figure 4-1).

In conjunction with the development of sitting the infant starts to coordinate all the preceding manipulatory skills for grasping activities. The infant still notes the visual and tactile components of manipulation in the visual and oral inspection of most objects.

The development of grasp progresses from an ulnar to a radial posture. Initially objects are held against the palm.

The technique of grasping is improved by the use

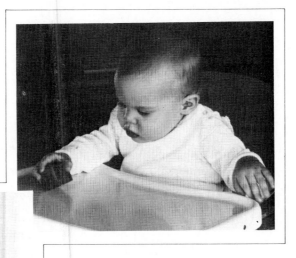

9 months
Looks and deftly
grasps with fingers

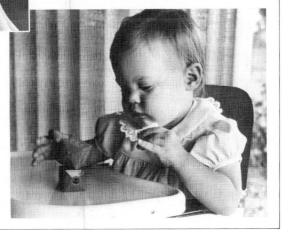

12 months
Looks, grasps with
forefinger and thumb,
and deftly releases

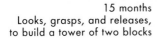

15 months
Looks, grasps, and releases,
to build a tower of two blocks

of the thumb. In the infant of 9 months the thumb envelopes the object by pressing it toward the index finger in a radial-digital grasp. By 10 months the infant uses a crude pincer grasp between the tip of the index finger and thumb. At 1 year the infant places the object between the predominating index finger and the thumb in a superior forefinger grasp that allows opposition. The infant can now build two- to four-cube towers.

The presence of associated movements results in voluntary movement in one limb accompanied by involuntary movement in the other until 5 to 6 years. Voluntary grasp precedes voluntary release, which does not occur until 10 months, and this complements the development of the flexors before development of the extensors.

Cognitive development

The cognitive development of the infant, as described through Piaget's sensorimotor period, has already been discussed in detail in Chapter 3. The cognitive process in this period at first is initiated through reflexive reactions to stimuli and later becomes more purposive as the infant accidentally discovers behaviors that affect the environment. The infant's attention is gradually directed away from his own body as he becomes aware of the results of his activity. This process proceeds to experimentation as the infant tries to produce new events. Through this change the infant's cognitive repertoire that develops includes schemata for the actions of his own body and the concept that objects in the environment are influenced by his body's actions. The infant does not yet understand the effects of other persons on objects.

Although most cognitive development is expressed through sensorimotor exploration, infants are also involved with the development of communication. Prelinguistic speech is a central theme and proceeds through distinct stages. Lennenberg[54] identified seven stages of prespeech that progress from undifferentiated crying to expressive jargon (Table 4-5).

Physiological maturation is central to the development of expressive speech. The pseudocry and cooing are made possible by changes in the infant's vocal equipment. The larynx, which contains the vocal cords, changes as the child grows, allowing the infant to produce a greater variety of sounds. Because the ability to produce different sounds is evidenced in crying, lack of crying ability in the infant may indicate brain damage.[62]

Social-emotional development

The infant's emotional transition from the protective, neutral womb is dramatically changed at the moment of birth. The sense of basic trust or mistrust becomes a primary theme in the child's affective development. The primary concern of the infant is to maintain body functions of the cardiovascular, respiratory, and gastrointestinal systems. As the infant matures the focus then moves to increasing competence in interacting with the environment through his body functions.[57] According to Erikson,[27] "the first demonstration of social trust in the baby is in the ease of his feeding, the depth of his sleep, the relaxation of his bowels." Erikson[27] also included the quality of maternal relationships:

> . . . the amount of trust derived from earliest infantile experience does not seem to depend on absolute quantities of food or demonstration of love, but rather on the quality of the maternal relationship. Mothers create a sense of trust in their children by that kind of administration which in its quality combines sensitive care of the baby's individual needs and a firm sense of personal trustworthiness within the trusted framework of their culture's life style (p. 249).

The basic trust relationship is one that has varying degrees of involvement. Rubin and others[79] believed that feelings of maternal love are not endowed but acquired over time within experiences between two people. This is seen in the progression of contact between mother and infant—first from the mother's fingertips, then with her hands, and lastly with her whole arms as an extension of her body. Klaus and others[50] discussed the

TABLE 4-5	Stages of speech preceding the real word
Stage	*Speech development*
1	Undifferentiated crying: reflexive, produced by expiration of breath
2	Differentiated crying: varied patterns and intensities; pitches signal hunger, sleep, anger, or pain
3	Cooing: chance movement of vocal cords produces simple sounds; first sounds are vowels; first consonant is *h* (6 weeks)
4	Babbling: repetition of simple vowel and consonant sounds (3 to 4 months)
5	Lallation: accidental repetition of what has been heard (6 to 12 months)
6	Echolalia: conscious imitation of sounds (9 to 10 months)
7	Expressive jargon: meaningful utterances that sound like sentences with pauses, inflections, and rhythms (2 years)

Adapted from Lennenberg, E.H.: Biological functions of language, New York, 1967, John Wiley & Sons, Inc.

importance of the en face position and stressed the importance of this early eye-to-eye contact between mother and infant in the attachment process.

The importance of the quality of maternal relationships was demonstrated earlier by Harlow and Zimmerman[40] in their studies of infant attachment relationships among rhesus monkeys. Their research demonstrated that it was not the mere provision of nutrients, but rather the close body contact that was essential to the attachment process.

Ainsworth[2] discussed the attachment process in terms of four stages of attachment. These include undiscriminating social responses (2 to 3 months), discriminating social responses (4 to 6 months), active initiative in seeking proximity and contact (7 months), and goal-corrected partnership or the ability to alter mother's plans to fit better the child's own. Precursors of attachment affect the first two stages of the development of attachment and include both reflexive and early sensorimotor behaviors such as rooting-sucking, looking, listening, smiling, vocalizing, crying, grasping, and clinging.

The role of the father must not be overlooked in the attachment process. Greenberg and Morris[38] identified strong evidence of paternal feelings and involvement with the neonate by new fathers. The father-neonate bond was characterized by engrossment, suggesting that fathers develop feelings of preoccupation, absorption, and interest in their neonate within the first 3 days after birth.

EARLY CHILDHOOD
Physiological development

Preschoolers are much more mobile than infants. They have completed the transition from quadrupedal to bipedal motor skills. In addition, the preschool period is marked by its own special emergents: the development of autonomy, the beginning of expressive language, and sphincter control. The growth rate of the preschooler is less dramatic than that of the infant. The child at this age is still top heavy, and a large cranium and small lower jaw present the characteristic features reminiscent of cherubim and cupids seen in Renaissance paintings.[91] The abdomen sticks out, since a relatively short trunk must accommodate the internal organs. The posture may appear lordotic.

Physiological differences from the mature adult are noted in the characteristic shape, position, and structure of the middle ear. The eustachian tube, which is shorter, more horizontal, and wider than that of the adult, allows free passage to invading organisms and thus increased susceptibility to ear infections in the younger child.[89] The digestive tract also shows lack of full maturation. The shape of the stomach is straight and has less than half the capacity of the average adult stomach. This structural disparity results in frequent stomach upsets in the preschooler.

The special senses demonstrate noteworthy differences as well. The taste buds are more numerous and are located on the side of the cheeks and the throat as well as on the tongue.[89] Because of the immaturity of the macula of the retina, the young child is farsighted.

Significant physiological changes occur in the physiological pathways necessary for sphincter control. Thus the preschooler is capable of entering and successfully completing toilet training. This is evidenced in the change from bulky diapers to training pants.

Sensorimotor development

Preschoolers are amazingly competent individuals. They initially walk with a wide stance and body sway because of their short stature; however, as they physically mature, the preschoolers' repertoire of motor activity steadily advances. The preschoolers' motor development is observed primarily in refinement. Coordination and the ability to voluntarily control movement increase significantly with each yearly advancement.

EXHIBIT 4-1

Activities of daily living

Dressing
2 years: Puts on shoes, socks, and shorts. Takes off shoes and socks.
3 years: Dresses and undresses fully; needs help with buttons, back and front, left or right shoe.
4 years: Can manage buttons completely
5 years: Can dress completely and often tie shoelaces, but cannot do tie.

Feeding
2 years: Has learned chewing and swallowing and can use a spoon well enough to feed self without accidentally inverting it.
3 years: Can feed self with little or no spilling. Can pour out from a jug into cup if not heavy. Feeding skills are now learned and become part and parcel of social skills in accordance with family standards of table manners.

Toilet training
2 years: By this age will tell mother he is "wet" and indicate that he wants to go "potty." Generally clean and almost dry by day.
2 ½ years: Dry at night if "lifted" late in the evening. (Variation is common, and boys tend to be later than girls.)

Adapted from Gesell, A., and Amatruda, C.S.: Developmental diagnosis, ed. 2, New York, 1954, Harper & Brothers.

The 3-year-old who is able to stand on one foot eventually progresses into the 5-year-old who can skip on both feet. The child-directed activity is evidenced in small muscle coordination and activities of daily living (Exhibit 4-1).

Cognitive development

Symbolic representations of the preschooler, particularly in language, are the hallmarks of what Piaget termed the preoperational stage of cognitive development from 2 to 7 years.[74] The child is now able to represent people, objects, and places through the use of words as symbols. Symbols used by children have personal reference for them. The inability to comprehend a general language meaning used in the adult world is demonstrated in a lack of mutually agreed on verbal framework and emphasizes the preconceptual content of the preschooler's speech.[57]

The child's egocentrism, or the belief that everyone perceives and interprets the world in exactly the same way, inhibits the development of such desirable behavior as acceptance of another person's point of view. Preschoolers relish their interactions with the environment through imaginative play; however, they are still not able to share or adhere to "fair play."

Children in the preoperational period still have difficulty distinguishing mental, physical, and social reality. As stated by Pulaski,[76]

> . . . in the preoperational period, the child with his needs and purposes is still the "raison d'être" of the universe; everything is made for man and children according to an established and wise play with the human being at its center (p. 39).

This is displayed in artificialism, animism, centration, and irreversibility.

This cognitive period is divided into two parts: (1) the preconceptual stage, ages 2 to 4 and (2) the intuitive stage, ages 5 to 7. The ability of the child to handle multiple characteristics marks the preconceptual stage. The child's reasoning skills are simple: "the child hasn't had enough experience to understand the relation between representatives of a class and the class itself" (p. 51).[76]

The child between the ages of 4 and 7 years intuitively appears to cope with the physical world, but he continues to be dominated by egocentrism and illogical reasoning: ". . . the child is feeling his way toward logical thinking but is constantly deceived by the perceptual appearance of things . . ." (p. 51).[70]

Psychosocial development

Erikson[27] defined the early psychosocial phase of early childhood as autonomy vs shame and doubt. Autonomy dominates the early part of the preschooler's psychosocial development from 2 to 4 years. The preschooler is adamant about making his or her own decisions. The development of trust in the environment and the improvement in language bring forth control over self and the corresponding strengthening of the preschooler's autonomous nature.

The discovery of the body and how to control it promotes independence in feeding, dressing, and toileting. The success in doing things for himself instills a sense of confidence and self-control in the preschooler.

The negative side of autonomy is a sense of shame or doubt. If the child fails continuously and is labeled messy, inadequate, or bad, shame and self-doubt are learned. Shaming may lead to "secret determination to try to get away with things, unseen."[27] In Erikson's words:[27]

> This stage, therefore, becomes decisive for the ratio of love and hate, cooperation and willfulness, freedom of self-expression and its suppression. From a sense of self control without loss of self esteem comes a lasting sense of good will and pride; from a sense of loss of control and of foreign over control comes a lasting propensity for doubt and shame (p. 254).

Erikson described the latter part of the psychosocial period as initiative vs guilt. Children aged 4 or 5 explore beyond themselves. They seek new experiences for the pleasure of knowing, understanding, and getting projects initiated or started. The child's world entails real and imaginary people and things. If the child's seeking activities are successful, effective, and meet with parental approval, a sense of initiative is developed. This provides a foundation for learning to deal with people and things in a constructive way and provides a method for looking for new solutions, answers, and reasons. As parental voices are internalized via the superego, children may experience guilt. Severe criticism or punishment may teach children to feel guilty. Children need a balance between the initiative to carry out activities and the sense of responsibility for their own actions.

Peer play becomes an important avenue for the preschooler's social development. The preschooler is now able to combine motor, language, and cognitive abilities to become an active participant. Play is essential to the child's continued development in these areas. Although adult-child relationships represent different social interactions, early home experiences are said to influence later peer relations. There is evidence to support that children whose attachments to their mothers are rated as secure tend to be more responsive to other children in nursery school.[68]

Preschool play has a large sensorimotor component, although intellectual growth has progressed beyond this period. Exploration is an important facet of preschoolers' developing initiative; consequently, they are observed manipulating and sensing all aspects of their world of toys.

Play progresses from simple to complex interactions. To separate play from other activities, Garvey[32] proposed that any activity be defined as play if it (1) was engaged in simply for pleasure, (2) had no purpose other than the activity itself, (3) was something the player chose to do, (4) required the player to be "actively engaged" in it, and (5) was related to other areas of the player's life, that is, furthered the individual's cognitive and social development, enhanced creativity, or improved problem-solving abilities. Parten[72] observed the interactions of nursery school children who ranged in age from 2 to 5 years. *Solitary play* was identified in the younger child who tended to play alone, and social interaction was likely to consist of looking at someone else. *Parallel play* was engaged in by those children who were involved in similar activities but who displayed little direct communication. *Associative play* involved shared materials and conversational exchanges but not necessarily play toward a single goal. *Cooperative play* was identified as engagement in a single activity with a commonly accepted set of rules. Much of the past research generated in the area of preschool play has been confirmed in later literature. Recent studies indicate that middle-class preschoolers engage in more associative and cooperative play than lower-class preschoolers.[79]

The development of autonomy provides a foundation for the preschooler's imagination. Now the young child not only explores the world through his senses, but he uses thinking and reasoning to imagine future situations. Play includes fantasy and motor activities that are complemented by words, rhymes, or noises. The power of symbolic thought enables the child to go beyond the immediate perception of objects and react to them in a manner that can be wishful rather than real.

The preschooler's progression to games with rules requires a stronger component of social skills.[75] The child must now conform to established guidelines, and the rule now replaces the symbol. The game presents a real-life situation during which the preschooler tests his newfound social graces. Chapters 3 and 13 discuss play as an essential component of development for all children.

MIDDLE CHILDHOOD
Physiological development

With the continued development of initiative, the school-aged child is seen playing throughout neighborhoods and schoolyards. The middle, or school-age, years, as they are sometimes referred to, stress the relative tranquility between the turmoil of autonomous growth of the preschool years and the identity crisis of the adolescent years.[91] Striking physical differences are noted in growth patterns. Physical development is characterized by slow but steady advances in height and weight that will continue until puberty.[62] The basic pattern of body build, which shows such great variation, also affects motor skills. Problems sometimes arise because the school-aged child wants to copy new things done by friends, but physical limitations prevent success.[12] A wide span of abilities is thus seen: the child may be one who is selected first for participation in sports, or he may be left sitting on the sidelines only to watch. The period of slow growth ends with the onset of the pubescent growth spurt. Although this is generally associated with adolescents, some school-aged children have already entered this phase of development. Growth increases at about age 9 in girls and age 11 in boys.[89] These physical growth differences result in the disparity of height between the sexes. The older elementary school female child is larger than her male counterparts, whereas the younger female child does not show as much variation.[70]

The facial features of the school-aged child have changed by becoming more distinct and individual. The successive losses of baby teeth and the appearance of permanent teeth distinguish the changing face to a greater degree. At almost any time children can display gaps in their smiles, a loose tooth, or a tooth just erupting. The 6-year-old is clearly identified by this toothless grin, while his 8-year-old counterpart is recognized by the tombstone front teeth that loom disproportionately large in his smile.[91]

Organ systems show continued maturation, specifically in the development of keener vision. The digestive system shows added maturity with fewer upsets and longer food retention. Ears are less likely to become infected than they were during the preschool period. The growth of the lower part of the face changes the position of the eustachian tube by making it longer, narrower, and more slanted. It is now harder for disease organisms to invade, and troublesome ear infections are fewer.[89]

Sensorimotor development

Gross motor development during the elementary school years continues to focus on refinement of previously acquired skills. With this refinement, hours of repetition of activity to attain mastery of common interests are seen. Motor capabilities are very diverse for this age group. The skills of the average 8- to 9-year-old include swinging a hammer well, sawing, using garden tools, sewing, knitting, drawing in good proportion, writing or printing accurately and neatly, cutting fingernails, riding bicycles, scaling fences, swimming, diving, roller skating, ice skating, jumping rope, and playing baseball, football, and jacks.[34,91]

Research indicates that children who master a physical skill tend to think better of themselves.[63] Not only does self-esteem improve, but children who have attained mastery of a skill enjoy greater acceptance by other children.[16,69]

It is not uncommon for a child this age to plead for the opportunity to become involved in an activity and then abandon it because of lack of skill or interest. School-aged children's high activity levels provide them with the opportunity to develop strength, coordination, agility, flexibility, and balance. Assessment of readiness is important for parents to consider during the child's quest for increased involvement because of the relative expense of participation and the need to enhance industry rather than inferiority.

Cognitive development

The cognitive period of concrete operation (7 to 11 years) gives the child an opportunity to grasp concepts and relationships in the physical world[74] As stated by Pulaski,[76]

> . . . the operational child is freed from the pull of immediate perception. He is also able to range forward and backward in space and time on the mental level. This speeds up the thinking process immeasurably and gives it much greater mobility and freedom (p. 54).

The middle school child uses reasoning as a primary basis for conceptualizing the world. Older children are now able to weigh several pertinent factors at one time, but their thinking is limited in flexibility. They are still not able to see abstracts, but they deal with concrete objects. The period of concrete operations is highlighted by the addition of two mental operations: reversibility and decentration. Reversibility now enables the school-aged child to try out different courses of action mentally, rather than relying on sensorimotor aspects of the situation. In addition, this mental process results in quicker problem-solving capabilities. The child is also able to decenter or pay attention to more than one physical characteristic at a time. These add to the systematic, logical, concrete thinking of the school aged child. This is seen most clearly in the child's recognition of constancy and his beginning understanding of conservation.

Social-emotional development

During the middle years the child is busy with basic school subjects, perfecting motor skills, and participating in activities with like-sex peer groups. The time of industry vs inferiority is highlighted by building new skills and refining old ones. Middle school children focus on meeting challenges in themselves as well as those presented by the environment. Industry, meaning to build, is evidenced in the child's exploration of the inner workings of things and not just physical appearance. According to Erikson,[27]

> The inner stage seems set for "entrance into life," except that life must first be school life, whether school is field or jungle or classroom . . . . He now learns to win recognition by producing things . . . . He has experienced a sense of finality. There is no workable future within the womb of his family and thus becomes ready to apply himself to given skills and tasks . . . . He develops a sense of industry—i.e., he adjusts himself to the inorganic laws of the tool world (p. 258).

Comparison with peers is increasingly important during this time. A negative evaluation of one's self compared to others or an inability to attain mastery of industrial achievements can result in a sense of inferiority.

The school-aged child is beginning the quest for independence of identity. School-aged children are less egocentric and able to view themselves more objectively. Children at this age have a definite subculture that includes magical rituals and gangs and is exclusively limited to children. This separate subculture is quick to criticize the different sizes and shapes of its members, and it is common for membership to entail a nickname related to these differences as a rite of passage.[91]

Rejection by the child's peers may result from lack of conformity in dressing or physical appearance.[51] Data suggest that social skills are also important determinants of peer acceptance. Children who rarely praised their peers, who had difficulty communicating, and who did not know how to initiate a new friendship were found to be unlikely candidates as friends.[37]

Middle school children may aspire to be teenagers, emulating teenage dress and current slang; however, questions of masculinity and femininity are prominent. Boys associate with boys, and girls associate with girls, each sex pursuing its own separate interests and identities with little communication in between.

Age becomes psychologically important to the middle school child. Both boys and girls tend to associate primarily with peers of the same age.[13] It is not uncommon to add halves or "almost" to age description. The middle school child who is aged 7½ or almost 8 may also declare proudly following school's end that he is in the next school sequence despite a summer's waiting period.[91]

During this age children begin to turn their backs on adults and unite to form a society of children. Values from peers become significantly more important than those of adults. One of the major functions of the peer group involves changing the child's attitudes. The peer group may strengthen existing attitudes, weaken those in conflict with peer group values, or establish new ones.[41] Data indicate that children between 7 and 10 years are highly compliant; they shift consistently in the direction of the peer consensus.[8] Children tend to be less compliant as they approach the adolescent age group.[44]

This society of school-aged children dominates neighborhood streets and backyards with their refreshment stands, bicycle races, clubhouses, and endless explorations of woods, trash cans, and rain-swept streets. Large numbers of school-aged children are seen congregating in group activity, which includes such popular games as hide-and-seek, tag, hopscotch, swing the statue, red light–green light, blindman's bluff, dodgeball, and red rover. Many of the middle school child's games are accompanied by ritualistic chants. The words are often empty of any literal meaning; however, the sense of participation in group ways aids in this repetition.[91]

The child's progression from structured ritualistic games to participation in competitive games with a score is seen in his perception of rules. Piaget identified stages of moral development including rules.[75] Early in the child's thinking (age 4 to 7), rules are viewed as absolute, sacred, and untouchable. Later, children (aged 7 to 10) recognize that rules come from somewhere and they accept what these rule-maker authorities say. Finally, late in the elementary school years (age 10 to 11) children cast aside their belief in the absolute infallibility of rules because they have gained the knowledge that man is the creator of such rules. Children now no longer accept adult authority, rules, or society without questioning them.

ADOLESCENCE
Physiological development

Adolescents are surely identified by the unique circles with which they symbolically identify. However, no formal rite of passage exists for the adolescent in the United States. Various cultural expectations within our society complicate this adolescent time period. States differ in laws concerning when one can consume alcohol, leave school, drive a car, or marry without parental consent.

There is great discussion regarding distinction between physical maturation and culturally defined roles. *Pubescence* refers to the period of time encompassing the physical changes that lead to puberty. These include the physiological growth of reproductive functions and maturation of primary sex organs resulting in secondary sex characteristics. Pubescence lasts an average of 2 years and ends in puberty. According to Ausubel[5] the normal sequence of development during pubescence is as follows:

Girls	Boys
Initial enlargement of breasts	Beginning growth of testes
Straight, pigmented pubic hair	Straight, pigmented pubic hair
Kinky, pigmented, pubic hair	Early voice change
Age of maximal growth	First ejaculation of semen
Menarche	Kinky pubic hair
Growth of axillary hair	Age of maximal growth
	Growth of axillary hair
	Marked voice changes
	Development of the beard

In the male these characteristics include the regular production of sperm by the testes, the development of the penis, growth of pubic and axillary hair, and marked voice changes. The deepening of the voice in the male is a result of the growth of the larynx in ventrodorsal diameter.[12] Female secondary sex characteristics become obvious in the emergence of breasts, a change in bodily proportions, as well as the onset of menstrual periods and the hormonal reactions that accompany them. *Puberty* is the resolution of all "morphological and physiological changes which occur in the growing boy or girl as the gonads change from their infantile to their adult state."[61] The adult state refers to sexual maturation and the ability to reproduce.

The adolescent growth spurt is perhaps the most outstanding physical change that occurs and signifies a time when the velocity of growth doubles. Even to those who live with the adolescent, the growth spurt appears to occur almost overnight. This phenomenon is partially a result of the fact that during the full year that surrounds the point at which peak height growth is measured boys usually grow between 2.8 and 4.7 inches, and girls grow from 2.4 to 4.3 inches on an average.[1] The growth of 5 to 6 inches in a year is not rare. Shuttleworth[88] found that the average age onset of the adolescent growth spurt is 14.8 years for boys and 12.6 years for girls. Much of the growth occurs in the long bones of the legs and arms and is stimulated by the increased output of sex hormones (testosterone in the male and estrogen in the female).[60]

Males and females react differently to their newfound height. Tall females may require reassurance to foster a positive body concept, while tall males are more likely to be pleased with this rapid addition of height. Shorter males are apt to need reassurance, since the timing of the adolescent growth spurt is controlled primarily by genetics.[12]

The process of sexual maturation brings forth many complex social and emotional problems. It is a period of relative sexual maturity in contrast to relative immaturity of social and mental development, and the result of these newfound hormonal changes is confusing.

Personal appearance becomes a source of conflict. There is greater emphasis on the good looks of physical attractiveness and physique than at any other time. The culture's current definition of attractiveness serves as the established norm for bodily proportions and facial features. Adolescent girls tend to be more interested in and concerned about their physical appearance than boys.[23] The adolescent may gaze continually in the mirror, comparing his or her own appearance to the ideal seen in magazines or on television. Marked deviations from idealized norms and cultural stereotypes of masculinity and femininity may adversely influence the adolescent's self-concept and treatment by others.[24] With experience and maturation, some changes in this overwhelming concern about appearance may be expected.

Cognitive development

The development of formal operational thought is a highlight of adolescence. Complex material can now be conceptualized without reliance on concrete schemata. The ability to imagine an infinite variety of options establishes the presence of hypothetical reasoning. The addition of reasoning permits mature understanding of such subjects as mathematics and philosophy. The adolescent's ability to think about his or her own thinking signifies complex mental operations. The mature teenager can now consider all possible relationships that might exist and evaluate these relationships one by one to eliminate the falsity and arrive at the truth.[71] Additional discussion of adolescent cognitive development is found in Chapter 3.

Social-emotional development

Erikson[27] emphasized the role of identity is the adolescent's psychosocial development. During this period society begins to ask the youth to define his or her own role and career aspirations. Erikson believed that to solve one's identity crisis, one must be committed to a role, which in turn means showing commitment to an ideology. The adolescent must define a personal ideology and confirm beliefs, values, and ideals. This commitment, or fidelity, should coincide with prerequisites for the adolescent's desired occupation. The acting out of behaviors, experimentation with new roles, fantasy, self-doubts, and rebellion are seen as the adolescent attempts to establish a firm identity and role that will be most suited to him or her. If a youth fails to integrate a central identity or cannot resolve conflicts between roles and a value system, ego diffusion is the result.

Elaborating on Erikson's theory, Marcia and Freidman[59] evaluated adolescents' levels of crisis and commitment in relationship to occupational choice, religion, and political ideology. They described four iden-

tity statuses. These identity statuses were modes of dealing with the identity issue characteristic of adolescents. Those classified by these modes were defined in terms of the presence or absence of a decision-making period (crisis) and the extent of personal investment (commitment) in two areas: occupation and ideology.

Identity achievers are individuals who have shown a commitment to an occupation and to an ideology. They have experienced a decision-making period. *Foreclosures* are adolescents who have never experienced a crisis. They are committed to occupational and ideological positions but have adopted identities that have been parentally chosen with little or no question. *Identity diffusions* are young people who have no set occupational or ideological direction. They may or may not have experienced crisis, but their defining characteristic is their lack of concern regarding lack of commitment. *Moratoriums* are individuals who are currently in crisis. They have a vague commitment to an occupation or ideology but are in a state of search. Additional studies have provided evidence in support of the existence of these four identity statuses.[60,82,110]

The establishment of ego identity, including occupational identity, is often complex and potentially confusing for the adolescent. Even at the age of 25, one young adult in four is still uncertain what vocation he or she should choose.[94] Decisions concerning occupations interact with other choices in development so that when commitment to the occupational choice is firm, the individual has to some extent fitted himself or herself for it.

There exist a multitude of theories of vocational choice and development. Ginzberg and others[35,36] present a developmental theory proposing movement through three primary psychological periods: a fantasy period, a tentative period, and a realistic period.

Super and others[94,95] present an extensive psychological theory of vocational choice and development. Super differentiates between the adolescent's self-concept and vocational self-concept. The adolescent must translate his self-concept into occupational terms to develop the vocational self-concept. He identifies five vocational behaviors; although ages are typical of the age range, these developmental tasks are not rigidly defined.

Tiedman[99] and Tiedman and O'Hara[100] proposed a theory of vocational development by using Erikson's stages of general personality development as a basis. The emphasis of ego identity is closely intertwined with career development.

Since the central theme of adolescence focuses on identity, the adolescent is in conflict between the emerging responsibility of being an adult and the past classification of being a child. The peer group serves as a support system for the young person who is trying to make this transition from childhood to adulthood. In an attempt to abandon childish modes of behavior and dependence from adults, peers provide a release from the societal pressure for the increased independent behavior that is expected of adults.[5] There is evidence to support the fact that as the adolescent is faced with this pressure, aggressive rebellion may result.[112] This rebellion is often displayed in increased social contact outside of the home. A desire to escape from the demands of parents and community and to retreat to an environment where one's views are appreciated is seen in group attachment.[91] The heightened importance of the peer group increases the adolescent's desire to conform to the values, customs, and fads of the peer culture.[101] This culture often proclaims its differences through symbolism in manners of dress, language, or food fads.

Although the rise of peer attachment introduces an important source of social control into the life of the young person, both peers and parents are important. Data suggest that, depending on the meaning and context of the social relationship, parents *or* peers may be more important. Sorenson found that 88% of the young people surveyed had considerable respect for their parents as individuals, while 48% desired more parental support of their own political and social opinions.[90] These differences in opinion tended to be on finer points of policy rather than on the overall issue. Lerner and Knapp[55] assessed the comparability of parents' and adolescents' attitudes toward societal issues. Their results indicated that although both groups were able to successfully assess the attitudes of each other, "there was a tendency for parents to minimize discrepancies between themselves and their children and a tendency for adolescents to magnify such discrepancies" (p. 35).

SUMMARY

An overview of growth and development, from conception through adolescence, clearly identifies that children are complex individuals. The overt characteristics of physiological, sensorimotor, cognitive, and social-emotional domains are variable for each child. All children, however, must mature through an identifiable developmental sequence to achieve their maximal potential.

REFERENCES AND SELECTED READINGS

1. Adams, W.: Adolescence. In Gabel, S., and Erikson, M.T., editors: Child development and developmental disabilities, Boston, 1980, Little, Brown & Co.
2. Ainsworth, M.D.S.: The development of infant-mother attachment. In Caldwell, B.M., editor: Review of child development, vol. 3, Chicago, 1973, University of Chicago Press.
3. André-Thomas, A.J., and Autgaerden, S.: Locomotion from pre to postnatal life, Clin. Dev. Med. **24:**1963.
4. Annis, L.F.: The child before birth, London, 1978, Cornell University Press.
5. Ausubel, D.P.: Theory and problems of adolescent development, ed. 2, New York, 1977, Grune & Stratton, Inc.
6. Barnes, A., and others: Fertility and outcome of pregnancy in women exposed in utero to diethylstilbestrol, N. Engl. J. Med. **302**(11):609, 1980.
7. Barnes, M.L., and others: The neurophysiological basis for patient treatment, Morgantown, W.Va., 1978, Stokesville Publishing Co.
8. Berenda, R.W.: The influence of the group on the judgments of children; an experimental investigation, New York, 1950, King's Crown Press.
9. Bevling, C.M., and Jacobson, C.B.: Link between LSD and birth defects reported, JAMA **221:**1447, 1970.
10. Bibba, M., and others: Follow-up study of male and female offspring of DES-exposed mothers, Obstet. Gynecol. **49**(1):1, 1977.
11. Birth defects, Pub. No. 59-93, White Plains, N.Y., The National Foundation—March of Dimes.
12. Brophy, J.E.: Child development and socialization, Chicago, 1977, Science Research Associates, Inc.
13. Campbell, J.D.: Peer relations in childhood. In Hoffman, M.L., and Hoffmann, L.W., editors: Review of child development research, vol. 1, New York, 1964, Russell Sage Foundation.
14. Campbell, S.: Fetal growth. In Beard, R.W., and Nathanillsz, P.W., editors: Fetal physiology and medicine, London, 1976, Holt-Saunders, Ltd.
15. Carr, D.H.: Chromosome studies in selected spontaneous abortions: conception after oral contraceptives, Can. Med. Assoc. J. **103:**343, 1970.
16. Clarke, H.H., and Greene, W.H.: Relationship between personal-social measures applied to 10-year-old boys, Res. Q. **34:**288, 1963.
17. Coffey, V.P., and Jessop, J.W.: Maternal influenza and congenital deformities: a prospective study, Lancet **2:**935, 1959.
18. Corner, G.W.: Congenital malformations—the problem and the task. In Morris, F., editor: Congenital malformations, Papers and discussions presented at the first International Conference on Congenital Malformation, Philadelphia, 1961, J.B. Lippincott Co.
19. Craig, G.J.: Human development, Englewood Cliffs, N.J., 1980, Prentice-Hall, Inc.
20. Davids, A., and others: Anxiety, pregnancy and childbirth abnormalities, J. Consult. Clin. Psychol. **25:**74, 1961.
21. DiLeo, J.H.: Child development: analysis and synthesis, New York, 1977, Brunner/Mazel Inc.
22. Drillien, C.M., and Wilkerson, E.M.: Emotional stress and mongoloid births, Dev. Med. Child Neurol. **6:**140, 1964.
23. Dwyer, J., and Mayer, J.: Variations in physical appearance during adolescence. Part 1. Boys, Postgrad. Med. J. **41:**99, 1967.
24. Dwyer, J., and Mayer, J.: Variations in physical appearance during adolescence. Part 2. Girls, Postgrad. Med. J. **42:**1967.
25. Ebbs, J.N., and others: Influence of prenatal diet on mother and child, J. Nutr. **22:**515, 1941.
26. Edwards, M.: Labor and birth. In Tudor, M., editor: Child development, New York, 1981, McGraw-Hill Book Co.
27. Erikson, E.H.: Childhood and society, ed. 2, New York, 1963, W.W. Norton & Co., Inc.
28. Erikson, E.H.: Insight and responsibility, New York, 1964, W.W. Norton & Co., Inc.
29. Foster, J.A.: Physical status and development of the neonate. In Tudor, M., editor: Child development, New York, 1981, McGraw-Hill Book Co.
30. Frazier, T.M., and others: Cigarette smoking: a prospective study, Obstet. Gynecol. **81:**988, 1961.
31. Fricker, H., and Segal, S.: Narcotic addiction, pregnancy and the newborn, Am. J. Dis. Child. **132:**360, 1978.
32. Garvey, C.: Some properties of social play, Merrill-Palmer Q. **20:**163, 1977.

33. Gesell, A., and Amatruda, C.S.: Developmental diagnosis, ed. 2, New York, 1954, Harper & Brothers.

34. Gesell, A., and others: The child from five to ten, rev. ed., New York, 1977, Harper & Row, Publishers, Inc.

35. Ginzberg, E.: Toward a theory of occupational choice: a restatement, Voc. Guide Q. **20:**169, 1972.

36. Ginzberg, E., and others: Occupational choice: an approach to a general theory, New York, 1951, Columbus University Press.

37. Gottman, J., and others: Social interaction, social competence, and friendship in children, Child Dev. **46:**709, 1975.

38. Greenberg, M., and Morris, N.: Engrossment: the newborn's impact upon the father, Am. J. Orthopsychiatry **44**(4):520, 1974.

39. Hanson, J.W., and others: Fetal alcohol syndrome: experience with 41 patients, JAMA **235:**1458, 1976.

40. Harlow, H.F., and Zimmerman, P.R.: Affectional responses in the infant monkey, Science **130:**421, 1959.

41. Hartop, W.W.: Peer interaction and social organization. In Mussen, P.H., editor: Carmichael's manual of child psychology, ed. 3, vol. 2, New York, 1970, John Wiley & Sons, Inc.

42. Herbst, A.L., and others: Adenocarcinoma of the vagina, N. Engl. J. Med. **284**(16):878, 1971.

43. Horrocks, J.E., and Weinberg, S.A.: Psychological needs and their development during adolescence, J. Psychol. **74:**51, 1970.

44. Isoce, I., and others: Modification of children's judgments by a stimulated group technique: a normative developmental study, Child Dev. **34:**963, 1963.

45. Jacobsen, C.: Association between LSD in pregnancy and fetal defects. In Brazelton, T.B., editor: Effects of prenatal drugs on the behavior of the neonate, Am. J. Psychiatry **126**(9):95, 1970.

46. Janerich, D.W., and others: Oral contraceptives and congenital limb-reduction defects, N. Engl. J. Med. **291:**697, 1974.

47. Jones, K.L., and others: Pattern of malformation in offspring of chronic alcoholic mothers, Lancet **1:**1267, 1973.

48. Kaminski, M., and others: Rev. Epidemiol. Sante Publique **24:**27, 1976. (English translation by Little, R.E., and Schnizel, A.: Alc. Clin. Exp. Rep. **2:**155, 1978.)

49. Karelitz, S., and others: Infants' vocalizations and their significance. In Bowman, P., and Manters, H., editors: Mental retardation: proceedings of the international medical conferences, New York, 1960, Grune & Stratton, Inc.

50. Klaus, M.H., and others: Human maternal behavior at the first contact with her young, Pediatrics **46**(2):187, 1970.

51. Kleck, R.E., and others: Physical appearance cues and interpersonal attraction in children, Child Dev. **45:**305, 1974.

52. Kolodny, R.C., and others: Depression of plasma testosterone levels after chronic intensive marijuana use, N. Engl. J. Med. **290:**872, 1974.

53. Landesman-Dwyer, S., and Emanuel, I.: Smoking during pregnancy, Teratology **19:**119, 1979.

54. Lennenberg, E.H.: Biological functions of language, New York, 1967, John Wiley & Sons, Inc.

55. Lerner, R.M., and Knapp, J.R.: Actual and perceived intrafamilial attitudes of late adolescents and their parents, J. Youth Adolesc. **4:**17, 1974.

56. Llorens, L.A.: Application of a developmental theory for health and rehabilitation, Rockville, Md., 1978, American Occupational Therapy Association.

57. Maier, H.W.: Three theories of child development, rev. ed., New York, 1978, Harper & Row, Publishers, Inc.

58. Marcia, J.E.: Development and validation of ego-identity states, J. Pers. **1:**118, 1967.

59. Marcia, J.E., and Freidman, M.L.: Ego identity status in college women, J. Pers. **38**(2):249, 1970.

60. Maresh, M.: Variations in patterns of linear growth and skeletal maturation, J. Am. Phys. Ther. Assoc. **44:**881, 1964.

61. Marshall, W.A.: Puberty. In Falkner, F., and Tanner, J.M., editors: Human growth. Part 2. Postnatal growth, New York, 1978, Plenum Publishing Corp.

62. McCandless, B.R., and Trotter, R.J.: Children: behavior and development, ed. 3, New York, 1977, Holt, Rinehart & Winston General Book.

63. McGowen, R.W., and others: Effects of a competitive endurance training program on self concept and peer approval, J. Psychol. **86:**57, 1974.

64. Metcaff, J.: Association of fetal growth with maternal nutrition. In Falkner, F., and Tanner, J.M., editors: Human growth. Part 1. Principles of prenatal growth, New York, 1978, Plenum Publishing Corp.

65. Milani-Comparetti, A.: Pattern analysis of normal and abnormal development: the fetus, the newborn, and the child. In Seaton, D.S., editor: Development of movement in infancy, Chapel Hill, N.C., 1981, Division of Physical Therapy, The University of North Carolina.

66. Milani-Comparetti, A., and Giodoni, E.A.: Pattern analysis of motor development and its disorders, Dev. Med. Child Neurol. **9:**625, 1967.

67. Montagu, M., and Ashley, F.: Prenatal influences, Springfield, Ill., 1962, Charles C Thomas, Publisher.

68. Moore, S.B.: Correlates of peer acceptance in nursery school children, Young Child. **22:**281, 1967.

69. Nelson, D.O.: Leadership in sports, Res. Q. **37:**268, 1966.

70. North, A., and others: Birth weight, gestational age and perinatal deaths in 5,471 infants of diabetic mothers, J. Pediatr. **90**(3):444, 1977.

71. Papalia, D.E., and Olds, S.W.: A child's world, ed. 3, New York, 1982, McGraw-Hill Book Co.

72. Parten, M.B.: Social participation among preschool children, J. Abnorm. Psychol. Soc. Psychol. **27:**243, 1932.

73. Peterson, W.: General considerations of physical development: growth and maturation. In Tudor, M., editor: Child development, New York, 1981, McGraw-Hill Book Co.

74. Piaget, J.: The origins of intelligence in children. Translated by Cook, M., New York, 1952, International Universities Press, Inc.

75. Piaget, J.: The moral judgment of the child, New York, 1955, Macmillan Publishing Co., Inc.

76. Pulaski, M.A.S.: Understanding Piaget: an introduction to children's cognitive development, New York, 1971, Harper & Row, Publishers, Inc.

77. Rhodes, A.J.: Virus infections and congenital malformations. In Morris, F., editor: Congenital malformations, Papers and discussions presented at the first International Conference on Congenital Malformations, Philadelphia, 1961, J.B. Lippincott Co.

78. Rothman, K.J., and Louik, C.: Oral contraceptives and birth defects, N. Engl. J. Med. **229**(10):522, 1978.

79. Rubin, K.H., and others: Free play behaviors in middle and lower class preschoolers: Parten and Piaget revisited, Child Dev. **47:**414, 1976.

80. Rubin, R.: Maternal touch, Nurs. Outlook **10:**828, 1963.

81. Rugh, R., and Shettles, L.B.: From conception to birth: the drama of life's beginnings, New York, 1971, Harper & Row, Publishers, Inc.

82. Schacter, B.: Identity crisis and occupational procession: an intense exploratory study of emotionally disturbed male adolescents, Child Welfare **47:**26, 1968.

83. Schonfeld, W.A.: Primary and secondary sexual characteristics: study of their development in males from birth through maturity with biometric study of penis and testes, Am. J. Dis. Child. **65:**535, 1943.

84. Schulman, C.A.: Sleep patterns in newborn infants as a function of suspected neurological impairment of maternal heroin addic-

tion, Unpublished paper presented to the meeting of the Society for Research in Child Development, Santa Maria, Calif., 1969.

85. Seeds, J.W., and others: Malpresentations, Clin. Obstet. Gynecol. **25**(1):145, 1982.

86. Shelesynyak, M.C.: Decidualization: the decidua and the deciduoma, Perspect. Biol. Med. **5**:503, 1962.

87. Sherman, A., and others: Cervical-vaginal adenosis after in utero exposure to synthetic estrogen, Obstet. Gynecol. **44**(4):531, 1974.

88. Shuttleworth, F.K.: The physical and mental growth of girls and boys age six to nineteen in relation to age of maximum growth, Monogr. Soc. Res. Child Dev. **4**:3, 1939.

89. Smart, M.S., and Smart, R.C.: Children: development and relationships, ed. 2, New York, 1972, Macmillan Publishing Co.

90. Sorenson, R.C.: Adolescent sexuality in contemporary America: the Sorenson report, New York, 1973, The World Pub. Co.

91. Stone, J.L., and Church, J.: Childhood and adolescence. A psychology of the growing person, ed. 3, New York, 1973, Random House, Inc.

92. Stott, D.H.: Abnormal mothering as a cause of mental abnormality, J. Child Psychol. **3**:79, 1962.

93. Strauss, M., and others: Behavior of narcotics—addicted newborns, Child Dev. **46**:887, 1975.

94. Super, D.E., and Hall, D.T.: Career development: exploration and planning, Annu. Rev. Psychol. **29**:333, 1978.

95. Super, D.E., and others: Career development: self-concept theory, New York, 1963, College Entrance Examination Board.

96. Sutton-Smith, B., and others: Development of sex differences in play choices during preadolescence, Child Dev. **34**:119, 1963.

97. Swann, C.: Rubella in pregnancy as an aetiological factor in congenital malformations, stillbirth, miscarriage and abortion, Br. J. Obstet. Gynecol. **56**:341, 591, 1948.

98. Tanner, J.M.: Physical growth. In Mussen, P.H., editor: Carmichael's manual of child psychology, ed. 3, vol. 1, New York, 1970, John Wiley & Sons, Inc.

99. Tiedman, D.V.: Decision and vocational development, Personnel Guidance J. **40**:15, 1961.

100. Tiedman, D.V., and O'Hara, R.P.: Career development: choice and adjustment, New York, 1963, College Entrance Examination Board.

101. Tuma, E., and Livson, N.: Family socioeconomic status and adolescent attitudes to authority, Child Dev. **31**:387, 1960.

102. Twitchell, T.E.: Attitudinal reflexes, Phys. Ther. **45**:411, 1965.

103. Twitchell, T.E.: Early development of avoid and grasp reactions. In Locke, S., editor: Modern neurology, 1969, Little, Brown & Co.

104. Uchida, I.A., and others: Maternal radiation and chromosomal aberrations, Lancet **2**:1045, 1968.

105. U.S. Congress, Senate, Congress of the Judiciary, Subcommittee to investigate the administration of the Internal Security Act and the internal security laws of the Committee on the Judiciary: Marijuana-hashish epidemic and its impact on United States security, Washington, D.C., 1974, second session of the 93rd Congress (hearing).

106. U.S. Food and Drug Administration: Caffeine and birth defects—tempest in a coffee pot? Pediatr. Alert **5**(19):73, 1980.

107. Versuhalmy, J.: Infants with low birth weight born before their mothers started to smoke cigarettes, Am. J. Obstet. Gynecol. **112**:277, 1972.

108. Vore, D.A.: Prenatal nutrition and postnatal intellectual development, Merrill-Palmer Q. **19**:253, 1973.

109. Watson, E.H., and Lowrey, G.H.: Growth and development of children, ed. 5, Chicago, 1967, Year Book Medical Publishers, Inc.

110. Watterman, A.S., and Waterman, C.K.: A longitudinal study of changes in ego identity status during the freshman year at college, Dev. Psychol. **5**:167, 1971.

111. Weathersbee, P.S.: Heavy coffee intake, miscarriage linked, Muncie Evening Press, p. 19, Oct. 1975.

112. Whiting, B.B.: Six cultures: studies of child rearing, New York, 1963, John Wiley & Sons, Inc.

113. Wolff, P.: The causes, controls and organization of behavior in the neonate, Psychol. Issues (Monogr. 17) **1**:entire issue, 1966.

114. Yamazaki, J.N., and others: Outcome of pregnancy in women exposed to the atomic bomb in Nagasaki, Am. J. Dis. Child. **97**:448, 1954.

MARY A. McILROY
KATALIN I. KORANYI

General pediatric health care

DELIVERY OF HEALTH CARE SERVICES
General aspects

Quality pediatric health care strives toward one primary objective: to enable each individual to pursue childhood and enter adulthood at his or her optimal state, physically, intellectually, and emotionally. Occupational therapists share this objective. In striving toward this goal, occupational therapists must collaborate with parents, physicians, and other resource personnel and therefore understand the various components of pediatric health care and their effective use.

Children receive pediatric health care in various settings, including private offices of pediatricians and family physicians, hospital or community clinics, health department stations, and hospital emergency rooms. Despite differences in locations, staffing, costs, and other amenities, each program offering pediatric care should share the common aim just stated.

Health care needs of children vary over time. The vast majority of professional effort in pediatrics is involved in the delivery of health promotion services and acute episodic care. Smaller amounts of time are given to rehabilitation, the coordination of home health care, and the establishment of educational programs. This chapter will present a description of each of these types of care and detail more thoroughly the most important aspects of preventive care and acute episodic care.

Health promotion

Prevention of illness, screening for disease, and monitoring health through well child checks are accepted goals of pediatrics and are currently in common practice. Presently, interest in *health promotion* is in-

creasing. Health promotion extends beyond prevention and maintenance and attempts to teach patients and families the importance of healthy life-styles.

Health promotion is a long-term process through which patients and families are assisted in accepting the responsibility for health care. It encourages them to take an active role in determining their own health, rather than relying on curative medicine in the future. The development of a mutually satisfying physician-patient-family relationship is important for the success of this process. A constructive relationship allows for better care during acute problems and crises, whether physical or psychosocial, and permits more effective counseling and teaching at routine visits (Figure 5-1). An effective relationship should also help patients and parents develop self-esteem and self-help skills to deal with routine daily problems. The desired result of such efforts in health promotion is to have patients and families establish lifetime goals and patterns that will be beneficial to good health and that will encourage appropriate use of health services.

Preventive and screening services, which are vital parts of pediatric health care and health promotion, will be discussed in detail later in this chapter. The aim of such services is the prevention of mortality and the minimization of morbidity from the many illnesses that afflict children. Early intervention is a necessary part of preventing mortality and morbidity and requires caregivers who are skilled in effective interviewing and the detection of problems. Routine checkups with thorough physical examinations may aid in the early identification of physical problems. Opening the lines of communication about behavior, development, school performance, sex education, and family relationships will assist in early diagnosis and treatment of many of the

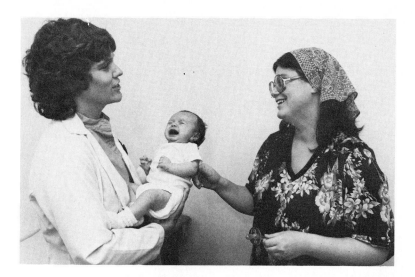

FIGURE 5-1

Effective and constructive physician-family relationships permit better care and counseling and help parents develop self-confidence in dealing with problems.

most common problems in childhood. Parents are often reluctant to begin the discussion about a child's behavior and, in fact, may not recognize a developing pattern of difficulty unless physicians use a developmental approach to health promotion. By using basic knowledge of the stages of development in childhood, the physician can question parents about the most common problems occurring in the child's age group. If the answers indicate that abnormalities exist, treatment programs can be instituted. Often the discussion indicates that the parents need education and understanding of the normal childhood stages, and this aspect of early intervention may prevent potential psychosocial morbidity.

Acute episodic care

Many visits to pediatric health caregivers are for diagnosis and treatment of acute problems, such as infections, minor trauma, or other physical complaints. Upper respiratory tract diseases, otitis media, and diarrheal illnesses account for a large proportion of these visits. In general, acute illnesses are most common between 6 months and 4 years of age. A small peak is often seen in the first 2 years of school, but otherwise the frequency decreases with increasing age. Data from the *National Health Survey*,[7] collected by household interview, indicate that children under age 6 have about 3.8 acute illnesses each year, while children aged 6 to 16 have 2.8 acute illnesses.

Many of the acute illnesses of childhood are mild and self-limited, yet they account for a large part of the demand for physicians' time. Patients with acute illnesses seek care from private offices, community clinics, urgent care centers, and hospital clinics and emergency rooms. The use of scattered services interrupts continuity of care, but it frequently occurs. The education of children and families to deal with minor symptoms by themselves and to use health care services wisely may have great impact on the cost and delivery of health care.

Habilitation and rehabilitation

Children with handicaps have various needs that can best be met through comprehensive care programs. The physician often serves as a coordinator for the various agents of the child's program. More importantly, the physician should be an advocate of the handicapped patient so that the child and family can live more comfortably with long-term disabilities. Children with handicaps need a great variety of experiences that are appropriate for their ages. The physician assists the family in ensuring that the appropriate programs and opportunities for learning, social interaction, and physical habilitation are provided for the child. Encouraging the family to help the handicapped child lead a fulfilling life, where self-discipline rather than overindulgence prevails, is an important aspect of chronic care (Chapter 8).

The physician serves as a referral source for specialists and services available in the community, such as occupational and physical therapists, psychologists, relief caretakers, public health nurses, special schools, and special education classes. The physician also serves as an advisor for decisions about the child's education and residence plans, such as mainstreaming a child with special needs into a regular classroom or placing a previously institutionalized child into alternative living arrangements.

Home health care

Continuing health care in the home for a high-risk child, such as a low birth weight infant, a child who fails to thrive, or a child with multiple handicaps, may be provided by visiting public health nurses. They serve as a liaison between the family and the physician or medical facility.

In addition, homemaker services are available to help families who cannot provide adequate care to a child because of various problems such as maternal illness or insufficient knowledge in child care or homemaking.

Educational programs

Education of children and families constitutes a large part of the pediatrician's efforts. There is little research showing how this is most effectively accomplished. In providing routine care the pediatrician has an excellent opportunity to discuss various health problems, preventive care, anticipatory guidance, and child safety. In addition, teaching materials (videotapes, pamphlets) can be made available in patient waiting areas. Individuals responsible for the care of children can offer group discussion programs regarding health care through organizations such as schools, parents' groups, and churches. Occupational therapists may be called on to participate in this role in community education. Informing the general public regarding important health issues, such as immunizations, health hazards, and safety, can be done through the news media.

PREVENTIVE PEDIATRICS
General aspects

One important part of health promotion, as mentioned previously, is preventive care. Three aspects of preventive care can be identified. First is the prevention of specific childhood illnesses through immunizations. Second is the attempt to prevent disability from asymptomatic diseases by use of screening tests. Early detection of asymptomatic diseases, such as hypothyroidism and phenylketonuria, permits treatment before the disease impairs its victim. Screening of development is also essential because the prevention or minimization of developmental delays and dysfunctions is an important segment of general pediatric health care.

A third aspect of service in preventive care is the promotion of good health through the teaching of healthy life habits and counseling concerning proper diet, exercise, and accident prevention, among other things.

In addition, preventive care is provided in other ways. Physicians try to detect and treat symptomatic diseases as early as possible to prevent secondary complications or sequelae. Habilitative and rehabilitative services are sought to prevent physical and emotional dysfunction from chronic disabling diseases. Both of these aspects are discussed in other chapters of this book.

Well child care

Regularly scheduled health supervision visits for children are important for the assessment of general health, growth, and development. They permit effective administration of immunizations and allow for important screening tests to be performed. These practices will be discussed later in this chapter.

Routine visits also allow for anticipatory guidance in preparing parents for both the certainties and uncertainties of the future.[1,2] (For a more detailed discussion of this topic, see Suggested Readings: Cataldo; Green and Haggerty; and Vaughan, McKay, and Behrman.) For example, when a baby is 2 to 3 months old parents should be informed that the ability to roll over will be developing in the following 2 or 3 months. This knowledge prepares the parent so that the infant is not left unguarded on a surface where he might roll off the edge and fall to the floor. Similarly, since most infants undergo a decrease in appetite at around 1 year of age, parents need to be aware of this change so that they avoid unnecessary conflicts concerning feeding. Uncertainties, for example, a child's reaction at times of stress or crisis, should also be discussed to aid the parent in being prepared to handle such situations.

At these visits the physician can assess the mental and emotional well-being of the patient and the family unit. Although this is not strictly preventive care, it does allow for, if necessary, the early intervention for problems such as behavior abnormalities, discipline difficulties, parental anxieties about normal variations, and toilet training.[1,2,6] These problems, although not causing physical illnesses, lead to psychosocial morbidity, which may have effects throughout an individual's life.[10]

Health care visits for preventive services must be sufficient in number and frequency to meet the individual needs of the child. Determining the optimal number of visits or procedures for all children or parents is impossible. But guidelines and recommendations have been published by the American Academy of Pediatrics[5] "for the care of well children who receive competent parenting, who have not manifested any important health problems and who are growing and developing satisfactorily."

Clearly, many circumstances or conditions may indicate a need for additional visits, and the physician will determine the need and pattern. More frequent visits are indicated for children with low birth weight or with congenital problems that cause no serious difficulties but result in parental anxiety. Also at risk and generally requiring increased professional contact are families with a previous child with an abnormality, those who have lost a child, adoptive or foster parents, and parents who are found to be in greater need of education and guidance, such as teenage mothers.

The current American Academy of Pediatrics recommendations[5] reflect this emphasis on meeting individual needs. They suggest that each health supervision visit should include initial or interval history, measurements of growth, physical examination, sensory screening and developmental appraisal as indicated by age, immunizations and diagnostic tests according to age, discussion of findings, and counseling that concerns problems or anticipatory guidance.

The timing of health supervision visits in the first 2 years has previously been scheduled around the immunization needs of the child, rather than out of concern for the developmental needs of the child and parents. The need for immunizations at certain ages still holds true, but the intervals can be more flexible in an attempt to avoid rigid adherence to providing well child care at specific ages. This attitude also allows for completing a health supervision visit with a visit initiated by a minor acute problem whenever possible.

Six well child visits are recommended as a minimum in the first year, generally at 4 weeks, 2 months, 4 months, 6 months, 9 months, and 12 months. In the second year three health supervision appointments are encouraged at 15 months, 18 months, and 24 months. Each of these visits is important for documenting satisfactory growth and development, discussing dietary and feeding practices, and assessing parental needs for guid-

ance or reassurance. Immunizations are also necessary at the 2-, 4-, 6-, 15- and 18-month visits. The immunization schedule will be discussed later.

Beyond 2 years of age the need for routine health promotion visits is generally diminished, but it will vary according to the health of the particular child and the family conditions. Yearly visits are encouraged from 3 to 6 years of age (Figure 5-2). The American Academy of Pediatrics[5] recommends six routine visits in alternate years for school-aged children 8 to 18 years of age. For the older child and adolescent these visits serve a much different purpose. Very few abnormal conditions will be discovered in asymptomatic children in these groups. Although documentation of normality and the updating of immunizations is important, more pertinent topics for these visits include behavioral concerns, school performance, family and peer relationships, psychomotor development, and sexual development. With adolescents, counseling about drug and alcohol use and about sexual behavior is valuable. (For further reading on this subject, see Suggested Readings: Daniel; Felice and Friedman; and Mercer.)

Screening tests and procedures

Screening procedures are one of the major thrusts of health promotion and are a part of all the routine visits described previously. Various tests are performed at different visits according to age and will be discussed individually in this section. The purpose of the screening tests is to identify illnesses or abnormalities in specific functions that are more likely to respond to corrective treatment while being asymptomatic and that may be more difficult to correct after symptoms are evident or when secondary problems appear. Extremely important, then, to the success of screening for disease is the assurance that programs exist for the treatment of children with abnormalities identified through screening.

Some screening procedures detect diseases that are asymptomatic in early infancy but will lead to damage if left untreated. For example, infants with hypothyroidism appear normal at birth. Over the first few months, characteristic physical signs may occur, but they may be subtle. Mental retardation will occur unless treatment with thyroid replacement is instituted within the first 2 months. A screening test to detect hypothyroidism at birth is now in use in many areas and is valuable in preventing this avoidable retardation.

Developmental screening may help identify treatable diseases and is beneficial for recognizing delays so that appropriate counseling of parents and attempts at remediation can occur. Early therapeutic intervention for the primary developmental problem often leads to a more successful outcome. In addition, the occurrence of secondary developmental difficulties may be prevented by early recognition and treatment programs. Especially

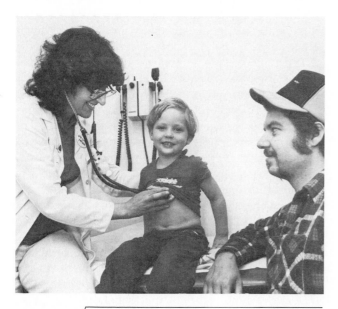

FIGURE 5-2

Routine visits for healthy children document normalcy and allow for discussions of parental concerns about behavior, development, peer relationships, and school performance.

responsive to early attempts at correction are those developmental delays and dysfunctions that result from a patient's major health and environmental problems, such as burns, diabetes, or neglect.

The prevention of secondary problems is important. Aiding a child to develop appropriate adaptive maneuvers or mechanisms to compensate for a primary disability may prevent a later need for extensive rehabilitation.

Most physicians recommend some caution in the use and application of screening tests results. The importance of appropriate identification of a child at risk and the provision of needed services has already been stated. But evidence has shown that children who are labeled as having problems or as being at risk for developing problems have an increased chance of later dysfunction. This effect seems to be related to a child's change in self-image and his expectations as a result of being labeled abnormal.

Occupational therapists should be cognizant of such effects and should be extremely careful in discussing with parents and patients the results of developmental testing and their implications. Significant discrepancies must be communicated to the primary physician, and questions of etiological factors and prognosis should be referred back to the physician for discussion with the family.

MONITORING OF GROWTH

Growth parameters of height, weight, and head circumference aid in screening infants and children for problems that result in abnormal growth. Abnormalities can be either insufficient rate of growth or excessive rate of growth, and either variation may be seen in height, weight, and head circumference. In fact, knowing whether there is an abnormality in only one parameter or in two or all three measurements is important because that knowledge will often suggest different etiological explanations.

Measurements of weight and height (supine length in infants) should be recorded accurately at every visit to the physician or caregiver. Head circumference (Figure 5-3) is most valuable during the first 3 years when the rate of head growth is the greatest. It is generally not recorded beyond that age. Standard curves or growth charts are available and delineate the percentile ranking of any measurement according to age (Figure 5-4). The data obtained from the patient should be plotted on such a graph at each visit. This process provides a visual display of the data and quickly alerts the physician to abnormalities that otherwise might be overlooked.

Single measurements provide little valuable information in most cases, unless they deviate markedly from normal or demonstrate a significant discrepancy between simultaneously obtained percentiles for height,

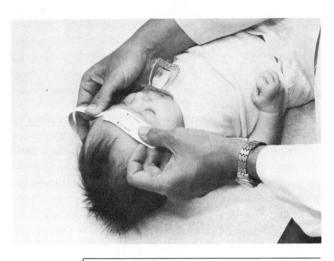

FIGURE 5-3

Occipitofrontal head circumference measures the largest diameter of an infant's head and is vital to detect insufficient or excessive head growth.

weight, and head circumference. For example, if a baby's length and weight at a single examination are at the 50th percentile, but the head circumference is less than the 10th percentile, abnormalities of the skull or central nervous system should be suspected. The subsequent measurement and recording of growth parameters at each visit allow comparison over time, and a change of two or more percentile lines (for example, from 50th to 10th) signifies a need for explanation.

Among the most common abnormal settings is one in which an infant or toddler shows significantly less weight gain than expected while continuing to grow normally in length and head circumference. Generally this picture reflects a nutritional basis for the inadequate growth. The physician must then try to delineate whether there exists a problem in acquiring adequate intake, in losing excessive quantities of calories, or in using food delivered to the body. Insufficient intake may result from poor feeding practices, maternal ignorance or neglect, poverty, or birth defects, such as cleft palate, which may hinder the mechanics of feeding. Excessive loss of calories may be caused by recurrent vomiting or losses in stool from diarrhea or malabsorption. Improper utilization of food may be seen in metabolic disorders such as diabetes, glycogen storage diseases, or cystic fibrosis.

Other patterns of abnormalities should indicate different concerns. Lack of adequate growth in length or height may be seen in metabolic derangements such as renal disease, hypothyroidism, or hypopituitarism. Early excessive growth in height may signify precocious puberty. In severe central nervous system disorders with brain damage, growth curves will often show markedly low values in height, weight, and head circumference. An infant whose head growth is more rapid than ex-

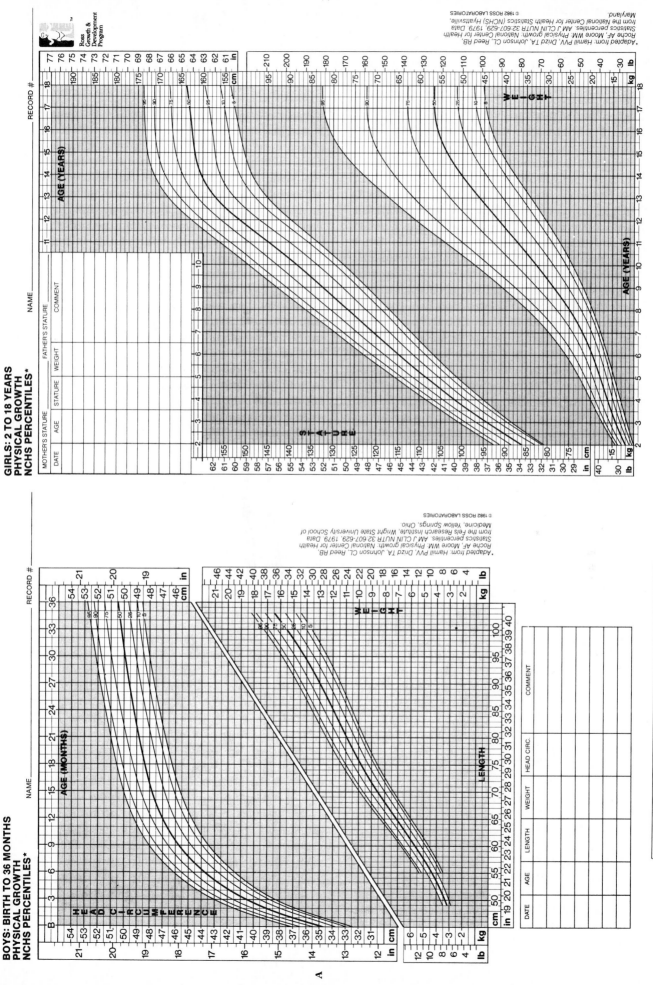

FIGURE 3-4

A, Standard growth curve for plotting lengths and weights of infant boys from birth to 36 months. **B,** Standard growth curve for plotting heights and weights of girls from age 2 to 18 years. Adapted from Hamil, P.V.V., and others: Am. J. Clin. Nutr. **32:**607, 1979.

pected will show a change toward higher percentiles or may have a head circumference greater than the 95th percentile for his age and would likely be evaluated for hydrocephalus.

Accurate and repeated measurements of height, weight, and head circumference are an exceptionally good screening tool for detection of many illnesses and problems. Routine use of these statistics may aid the physician in early detection of diseases, and it also provides other health personnel involved in a patient's care some objective data that may be reassuring with regard to the patient's general health or that may arouse concern, resulting in consultation with or referral back to the physician.

SENSORY EVALUATION

Sensory screening for vision and hearing is mandatory to detect major defects early, to enable development to progress as normally as possible, and to permit maximal rehabilitation before school age for those in whom normal development has been altered.

Children's eyes must be examined for screening purposes in early infancy, before beginning school, and at intervals during the school years. Examination of the infant's eyes should be done several times during the first 6 months. At birth this may consist of only a determination of light perception (blinking in avoidance when a bright light is presented) and visualization of a red reflex by funduscopy. By 3 or 4 months of age the infant should be able to follow a light 180 degrees and therefore demonstrate both visual perception of the light and conjugate movements of the eyes. The eyes should be assessed for alignment by checking to see if light reflects from the same location in both eyes when the patient looks at the light. Further screening procedures can also be done to detect intermittent changes in alignment. This testing is performed by interrupting a patient's conjugate gaze at an object by using a thumb

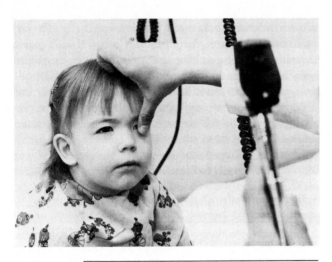

FIGURE 5-5

Screening for intermittent abnormalities in ocular alignment is performed by blocking the vision of one eye and then observing for correction of alignment to return the eye to conjugate gaze when vision is no longer blocked.

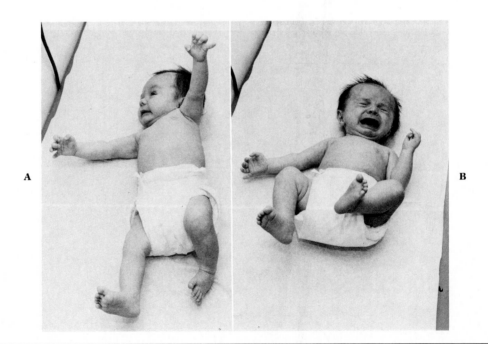

Figure 5-6

The Moro reflex is a normal neurological response in early infancy, often elicited by loud noises or a sudden change in position. **A,** The initial phase involves stiffened extension of arms and legs. **B,** The second phase is flexion and abduction of extremities and, often, crying.

or other block in front of one eye (Figure 5-5). The examiner observes for deviation of that eye away from the object of gaze. Such deviation is readily detected as the interrupted eye moves back into conjugate alignment when vision is no longer blocked.

Visual acuity and muscle alignment should be screened between 3 to 5 years of age and again at other visits during the school years. Acuity can be checked by using standard eye charts or small projection machines. Because this screening is simple and requires minimal equipment, schools and communities will often provide large screening programs. Children with abnormalities of acuity or alignment should be referred for appropriate and thorough evaluation by their physician.

Hearing and language are informally assessed at each visit as the physician interacts with the patient or observes patient-parent communications. The newborn or young infant should respond to a loud noise or clap with blinking of the eyes or a Moro response (Figure 5-6). Normal hearing is demonstrated in 6- to 9-month-olds by their attempts to locate a familiar sound. A bell or rattle can be used to produce sound, and older infants should turn their heads to locate it. The older infant should also be making babbling sounds. At 12 months hearing is indicated by the following of simple directions and the use of two or three meaningful words. Vocabulary continues to expand and the complexity of language increases so that by 3 years of age the child should be able to speak in simple sentences.

Screening of hearing should be done again before the beginning of school so that any loss that might impair classroom work can be dealt with before academic problems are created. Many communities and schools provide hearing screening programs to be certain this service is provided to all children, not just to those who seek professional health care.

Abnormalities in vision or hearing, if detected by occupational therapists in the course of patient evaluation or therapy, should most certainly be communicated to the referring physician to assure that adequate evaluation has been or will be done.

DEVELOPMENTAL ASSESSMENT

Developmental appraisal should occur at every contact between patient and caregiver and is an important aspect of each visit. Initially, simple observation of the infant's motor and social development suffices. As the infant develops, more motor and social skills become obvious, and language and cognitive abilities appear. These capabilities become progressively more complex with age, and the physician must not only observe but also interact with the patient to determine developmental level. Through informal assessment the physician should identify the infant or child likely to benefit from more formal evaluation, whether performed in the of-

fice situation or in a referral system by occupational therapists or other trained personnel.

For screening purposes, the Denver Developmental Screening Test[4] is widely used. It allows establishment of a baseline for an infant's development and can be used repeatedly up to age 6 to help measure progress. It is a brief sampling of abilities and is limited in items tested at very early ages, but it can provide an estimation of a child's developmental course. Concerns noted by informal evaluation or deficiencies noted on the Denver Developmental Screening Test assessment should receive more extensive evaluation by personnel trained in standardized developmental appraisals. The occupational therapist often serves as a resource for evaluation and therapy of noted delays, and the therapist can assist in the establishment of home programs, occupational therapy sessions, or referrals to community programs. In this role the occupational therapist can support the physician-patient relationship and enhance the care given to the child and family.

METABOLIC SCREENING

Several specific screening tests are used routinely in pediatric health supervision. In many states neonates are screened by blood tests for the presence of metabolic diseases such as phenylketonuria, hypothyroidism, or galactosemia. The benefits of early detection of these diseases, which will be discussed in the next chapter, are obvious, since in many cases early treatment can prevent or minimize mental retardation or other pathological consequences of the disease.

HEMATOLOGY TESTING

Hemoglobin or hematocrit testing is a valuable screen for anemia and is usually performed in infants at 9 to 12 months of age. Nutritional anemia from iron deficiency is common at this age among disadvantaged populations. Treatment with iron preparations is fairly simple and will prevent the complications of anemia. Parents of anemic patients also need counseling about proper diet and nutrition for children. The American Academy of Pediatrics[5] suggests hemoglobin or hematocrit testing again at 2 to 4 years of age, during late childhood, and in adolescence. Sickle-cell testing should be done at 9 to 12 months in all black infants. Identification of sickle-cell disease or trait cannot change its presence. However, recognition of the existence of this inherited abnormality can result in effective education of patients and families so that early therapy is received when illness or complications occur and so that genetic counseling concerns are addressed. Also at 9 to 12 months of age, a lead level should be measured if indicated, especially in infants living in older homes in inner city areas. The presence of lead overload should be diagnosed so that any necessary treatment is provided and so that recurrence is prevented.

TUBERCULOSIS SCREENING

Recommendations concerning the use of routine tuberculosis screening tests are currently undergoing change. The risk of tuberculous infection is extremely low for most children in the United States. For this reason nonselective testing of children is not felt to be an efficient public health practice. The American Academy of Pediatrics Committee on Infectious Diseases recommends routine testing at 12 months of age and every 1 to 2 years thereafter, commenting that the test is inexpensive and easily performed and will allow detection and treatment of a few asymptomatic children. The committee report[9] states that in areas where the occurrence of tuberculosis is exceedingly low and screening yield is slight, the physician may wait longer intervals between testing or discontinue routine testing.

URINE TESTING

The benefit of routine urinalysis and urine culture in healthy children is controversial. During preschool and early school years urine cultures of asymptomatic girls may yield positive results in 1% to 2%. But it is unclear what relationship this finding has to the development of chronic renal disease and whether treatment of asymptomatic bacteriuria prevents such complications.

BLOOD PRESSURE SCREENING

Blood pressure screening is recommended[5] for all children 3 years of age and older (Figure 5-7). Previously most childhood hypertension was thought to be secondary to renal disease, metabolic abnormalities, or other pathological causes, and extensive evaluation was warranted. Currently, essential or primary hypertension is becoming increasingly recognized in children, although debate still exists as to what blood pressure levels actually constitute hypertension and at what point treatment is indicated. Prevention of the adult complications of hypertension (heart disease, stroke) seems to be a logical aim and might be aided by the detection of elevated blood pressure during childhood and by effective therapy, where appropriate.

Immunizations

Prevention of childhood illnesses and their morbidity and mortality is one of the proven benefits of pediatric health supervision. Death and disability from poliomyelitis and measles are almost unknown today. Tetanus occurs uncommonly, and deaths and brain damage from pertussis have decreased remarkably.

Immunizations against diphtheria, tetanus, pertussis, poliomyelitis, measles, mumps, and rubella are given routinely during infancy and early childhood. Recommended schedules have been established to provide early and effective protection from these diseases. Table 5-1 displays the schedule as currently recommended.[9]

Known risks and side effects do occur from these immunizations, but the vast majority are very mild (fever, irritability, soreness at the site) and are to be expected. Severe reactions to pertussis vaccine are rare, and even rarer are documented cases of vaccine-related poliomyelitis. The details of these complications have been well described in other texts.[3,8,9] Despite these risks, it is a matter of major concern for the public and individual health and welfare that children receive the recommended immunizations.

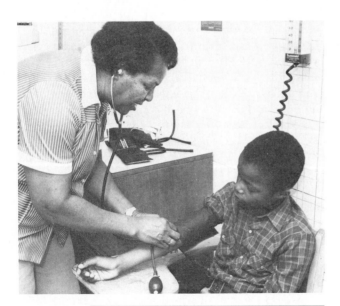

FIGURE 5-7

Blood pressure screening should be performed in all children over 3 years old.

TABLE 5-1	Recommended[9] immunizations and ages for their administration
Recommended age	*Vaccine(s)*
2 months	DTP*, OPV†
4 months	DTP, OPV
6 months	DTP
15 months	MMR‡
18 months	DTP, OPV
4-6 years	DTP, OPV
14-16 years	Td§

Adapted from Report of the Committee on Infectious Diseases, Evanston, Ill., 1982, American Academy of Pediatrics.
*DTP, Diphtheria and tetanus toxoids with pertussis vaccine.
†OPV, Oral attenuated poliovirus vaccine.
‡MMR, Live measles, mumps, and rubella viruses in a combined vaccine.
§Td, Adult tetanus toxoid (full dose) and diphtheria toxoid (reduced dose) in combination.

Nutrition

Nutrition counseling has accrued added significance as people begin to realize that good health is a result of good health practices, not just good medical care. The converse is also true: bad health is not a result of poor medical care, but it may develop from unhealthy lifestyle practices.

Health promotion for children includes the encouragement of better feeding habits and sound nutrition. The trend toward breastfeeding is increasing and should be supported by individuals responsible for child health care. Nutritious and complex infant formulas are available when babies are not nursed, and they are recommended in preference to whole cow's milk or skim milk. Cow's milk products have been shown to be a potential cause of microscopic blood loss from the gastrointestinal tract. Cow's milk has insufficient iron to meet an infant's needs, and it has higher sodium and renal solute content than human milk or commercial formulas.

Introduction of solid foods should be delayed until 6 to 7 months of age. Recent changes in prepared infant foods have markedly decreased the content of salt and sugar, both of which had been added for adult tastes. In addition, attention must be given to supplementation of the diet with vitamins, iron, or fluoride when conditions warrant.

The importance of nutrition extends far beyond the feeding of infants. As pediatric practice moves more into the role of health promotion, increased attention is being given to prevention of illnesses in adulthood. Heart disease, stroke, and cancer cause the majority of deaths of American adults. Many of the habits that contribute to adult morbidity from these problems begin in childhood.

The prevention of obesity in adulthood can probably be aided by the discouragement of obesity in childhood. Advice to parents is important to change the idea that a happy baby has to be a fat baby and to encourage proper nutrition (but not overnutrition) throughout childhood.

Sodium intake is felt to play a role in adult hypertension. It is unclear if control of sodium intake in infancy and childhood will contribute to decreasing the incidence of hypertension. While the answer to that question is being sought, prudent eating practices might include the avoidance of excessive salt.

Obesity and salt intake have been mentioned as contributors to heart disease. Lack of exercise also contributes, and continuing exercise programs should be encouraged by those who provide health care to children.

Smoking has been shown to be associated with the development of lung cancer, and the use of alcohol and drugs contributes to the number of accidental deaths.

The prevention of such problems through education of children and families has not been sufficiently researched to determine effectiveness. But such programs deserve a trial. The aim of health promotion in pediatrics is to keep an individual healthy throughout his or her entire life, not just during childhood.

ACUTE EPISODIC CARE
General considerations in outpatient care of sick children

Ambulatory care services provide for both emergency and nonemergency care of sick children. In recent years there has been a growth of ambulatory services for children. This increase has resulted from several factors, such as the rising cost of inpatient care and the recent advances in diagnostic and therapeutic procedures by which children can now be treated in an outpatient setting.

Acute care cannot be scheduled in advance, so health care facilities must be prepared for urgent calls. Ideally the same physician or group of physicians will provide acute and ongoing care for the child. If the child has been examined periodically at the same office or clinic, it is assumed that a complete personal and family history is available, thus the physician can concentrate on the acute visit. If the child is being seen for the first time by the physician, a brief history regarding factors that may influence the present illness (for example, allergies, chronic illness) must be obtained. A follow-up appointment for a complete history and examination can be arranged. For those children who usually receive only episodic or crisis care, it is important to provide preventive health care during the visit for the acute illness. If a child does not have an established source of continuing health care, it is important to emphasize and encourage the benefits of such service.

The emotional aspects of an illness also deserve consideration. Children seldom understand illness. They often view sickness as a punishment for bad behavior. The physician needs to keep in mind the various ages and levels of understanding of children and direct all explanations in a way that is meaningful to the patient. The child deserves simple but honest explanations regarding the illness, procedures, and expected degree of discomfort. Parents may worsen the situation because they often feel guilty, anxious, and tired, and they may ventilate their frustrations on the child or the health care personnel.

The hospitalized child

Many children are hospitalized at least once during childhood. Because of the emotional stresses for the child and the family and the significant expense, hospital admissions should occur only when diagnostic and treatment procedures cannot be performed on an ambulatory basis.

If it is at all possible, the family should be prepared for the hospital admission so that potential problems can be addressed before they arise and anxieties can be diminished. When children are admitted to the hospital, they often feel that they are being punished; they feel abandoned by their parents and they are afraid. In many hospitals preadmission visits are arranged for the child and the parents to develop a sense of familiarity with the setting, the procedures, and the personnel. Showing one child a patient who is happily eating ice cream after a tonsillectomy could allay that child's fears regarding his own surgery. In addition to the hospital tours, materials such as coloring books, pamphlets, or videotapes can be made available to families.

A child should be allowed to express his fears, whether real or fantasized. Preparation at home and in the hospital by playing out fears (for example, giving a shot to the doll) and by role-playing games (for example, as doctor or nurse) may provide insight to the child's fantasies and help alleviate some of the fear. In case of an emergency admission many of the preparations cannot take place, and the event is often confusing and hectic. Nevertheless, the physician and the nurse should try to answer questions of the parents and the child.

Children should be admitted to a pediatric unit and, if possible, matched with children of similiar ages. A realistic and fair statement as to the estimated length of the hospitalization is important. All personnel need to be aware that children are not little adults and that they have special needs. Before any kind of procedure the physician should talk with the patient and explain what will be done and why it is necessary. For children, terms such as *mend a break, fix up,* or *make well* are preferred over more threatening and confusing medical terms. When it benefits the patient, a support person (parent, nurse, or occupational therapist) should be permitted to accompany the child for procedures, such as radiographs, venipuncture, and even minor surgical procedures.

Care should be taken that children do not witness very agitated or very sick patients; tubes, machines, and bandages can be frightening to them. In the event a child is exposed to a very ill or dying patient, he deserves a sensitive and careful explanation.

Parental attitudes help to allay a child's fears, so parents and hospital personnel need to cooperate and understand each other. The child may view the hospitalization as a rejection or lack of love by his parents. The parents and hospital personnel need to become aware of possible changes in the behavior of a child during or after hospitalization, such as regressive behavior, increased clinging, antagonism, or aggressiveness. Parents should be encouraged to bring to the hospital some familiar object (for example, a favorite toy or blanket) that suggests a tie to the security of home. Frequent visits by parents should be encouraged.

Pediatric units should have age-appropriate playrooms or recreational areas for the children. School-aged children staying for an extended period of time (over 2 weeks) should continue their education through homework or hospital-based teachers. Whenever it is possible, hospitalized children should be allowed to get out of their rooms, go to other hospital areas, or receive passes to leave the hospital for a few hours.

Childhood morbidity

Morbidity is much more difficult to measure than mortality. Most childhood illnesses are minor traumatic injuries and acute infectious diseases that leave no sequelae. However, a portion of these problems will lead to chronic conditions or result in psychosocial difficulties.

The incidence of various illnesses has changed tremendously over the past decades. Diseases that were once prevalent, such as poliomyelitis, measles, tuberculosis, and diphtheria, have disappeared as the leading causes of mortality and morbidity. Currently, after the age of 1 year, accidents (in particular, motor vehicle accidents) are the leading cause of mortality in childhood. The second cause before 4 years of age is congenital malformations, while malignancies are the second cause of mortality from 4 to 18 years of age.

The *new morbidity* is a term frequently used now. In pediatric health care this refers to the recently noted increase in care provided for behavior problems, school difficulties, and family social problems. This has occurred because the incidence of severe illness in childhood has decreased as a result of better technology, the prevention of many childhood diseases, and improved treatment of illness. Childhood health care personnel must keep pace with changing causes of morbidity and mortality, and their efforts must be directed toward prevention and treatment of these problems.

SUMMARY

Occupational therapists are called on to direct or participate in efforts to facilitate a child's development of age-appropriate abilities and to help that child respond to the environment with whatever adaptations are necessary. It is important, therefore, that significant health concerns be identified and properly addressed before treatment is initiated or whenever they appear during the course of therapy.

When appropriate pediatric health care services are

effectively delivered, as described in this chapter, the child in need of occupational therapy should be readily identifiable. The careful monitoring of physical, mental, and psychosocial development through the use of routine health promotion visits and screening procedures will provide the physician with the necessary understanding of the child's primary developmental problem and level of abilities and aid recognition of other health problems. Such background information is of great importance for the occupational therapist designing treatment plans, along with determinations of whether the problems are temporary or permanent, what the expected outcomes and prognoses are, and what influence any health problems may have on both the child's development and therapy. Obvious, then, is the need for maintaining effective communications between occupational therapists and the primary physician to meet the changing needs of the child.

REFERENCES

1. Chamberlin, R.W.: Prevention of behavioral problems in young children, Pediatr. Clin. North Am. **29:**239, April 1982.
2. Christopherson, E.R.: Incorporating behavioral pediatrics into primary care, Pediatr. Clin. North Am. **29:**261, April 1982.
3. Feigin, R.D., and Cherry, J.D.: Textbook of pediatric infectious diseases, Philadelphia, 1981, W.B. Saunders Co.
4. Frankenburg, W.K., and Dodds, J.B.: The Denver Developmental Screening Test, J. Pediatr. **71:**181, 1967.
5. Guidelines for health supervision of children and youth, News and comment, May 1982, American Academy of Pediatrics.
6. Metz, J.R., and others: A pediatric screening examination for psychosocial problems, Pediatrics **58:**595, 1976.
7. National health survey, Series 10, No. 141, Washington, D.C., 1981, U.S. Department of Health and Human Services.
8. Recommendations of the Immunization Practices Advisory Committee, Morb. Mortal. Week. Rep. **28**(43):entire issue, 1979; **30**(32): entire issue, 1981.
9. Report of the Committee on Infectious Diseases, Evanston, Ill., 1982, American Academy of Pediatrics.
10. Starfield, B.: Behavioral pediatrics and primary health care, Pediatr. Clin. North Am. **29:**377, April 1982.

SUGGESTED READINGS

Barnett, H.L., editor: Pediatrics, ed. 15, New York, 1972, Meredith Corp.
Cataldo, M.F.: The scientific basis for a behavioral approach to pediatrics, Pediatr. Clin. North Am. **29:**415, April 1982.
Daniel, W.A., Jr.: Adolescents in health and disease, St. Louis, 1977, The C.V. Mosby Co.
Feldman, K.W.: Prevention of childhood accidents: recent progress, Pediatr. Rev. **2:**75, Sept. 1980.
Felice, M.E., and Friedman, S.B.: Behavioral considerations in the health care of adolescents, Pediatr. Clin. North Am. **29:**399, April 1982.
Green, M., and Haggerty, R.J., editors: Ambulatory pediatrics II, Philadelphia, 1977, W.B. Saunders Co.
Hospital care of children and youth, Evanston, Ill., 1978, American Academy of Pediatrics.
Mercer, R.T.: Perspectives on adolescent health care, Philadelphia, 1979, J.B. Lippincott Co.
North, A.F., Jr., and others: Screening in child health care, Pediatrics **54:**608, 1974.
Paulson, J.A.: Patient education, Pediatr. Clin. North Am. **28:**627, Aug. 1981.
Vaughan, V.C., McKay, R.J., and Behrman, R.E., editors: Nelson's textbook of pediatrics, ed. 12, Philadelphia, 1983, W.B. Saunders Co.

6

KAREN E. SCHANZENBACHER

Diagnostic problems in pediatrics

The focus of this chapter is on diagnostic problems found in pediatric populations that are commonly served by occupational therapists. Some sections of this chapter provide general information of interest to pediatric occupational therapists, other sections are designed to provide specific introductory information for subsequent chapters, while other sections provide data that will serve as background information on conditions not directly treated by occupational therapists but seen in the charts and records of their patients.

PRENATAL PROBLEMS

A normal, healthy baby is the wish of every prospective parent. While that wish is realized in the vast majority of pregnancies, a small percentage present risk factors that jeopardize the developing fetus. These pregnancies necessitate the use of specific diagnostic and intervention strategies that are designed to eliminate or minimize the effects of these factors. If prevention is not possible and birth defects are inevitable, the prospective parents are at least provided with a chance to begin to make the difficult decisions and adjustments surrounding that knowledge.

This section deals with complications surrounding the prenatal period of development. It discusses types of birth defects and their causes, the detection and monitoring of high-risk pregnancies, fetal diagnostic and intervention procedures, and the implications for occupational therapy.

Causes of birth defects

The March of Dimes[15] defines a birth defect "as an abnormality of structure, function, or body metabolism which often results in physical or mental handicap, shortens life, or is fatal." More than 250,000 babies are born with birth defects in the United States each year. These birth defects may be caused by genetic abnormalities, adverse conditions in utero, poor maternal health and nutrition, or a combination of these factors.

One type of genetic abnormality is the single gene defect, or inborn error. The gene is the section of the chromosome responsible for the formation of a specific protein. Occasionally a permanent change in the code of a gene will occur, producing a new character or trait called a *mutation*. Some of these mutations are harmless, while others may, for instance, cause malforming enzymes, as in phenylketonuria and diabetes. In fact, over 2,000 single-gene mutations have been identified, many of which cause serious diseases and birth defects.[11]

Chromosomal abnormalities are caused by three specific mechanisms: (1) deletion, which means that a whole chromosome or section of a chromosome is absent; (2) translocation, which consists of one chromosomal section attaching to another chromosome; and (3) nondisjunction, in which a pair of chromosomes fail to separate during cell division.[11] Exhibit 6-1 classifies some commonly known syndromes with the type of mechanism that causes them.

Other birth defects are caused by adverse changes that take place within the fetal environment. Substances and factors that negatively affect the developing fetus are called *teratogens*. Drugs, intrauterine infections, radiation, chemicals, and industrial wastes are the most common teratogens known to affect fetal development. Table 6-1 lists some common teratogens and their possible effects on the developing fetus. It is important to remember that a number of factors determine whether a teratogen will affect the fetus. The dosage, the gestational stage of the infant, and the specific sensitivity of

Classification of syndromes according to type of genetic abnormality

Single-gene mutations (inborn errors)
Phenylketonuria
Tay-Sachs disease
Juvenile diabetes

Chromosomal abnormalities
Deletion
   Cri-du-chat syndrome
Translocation
   Down's syndrome (partial trisomy 21)
Nondisjunction
   Down's syndrome (trisomy 21)
   Turner's syndrome
   Klinefelter's syndrome

the developing organs at the time of exposure to the teratogen are all factors that contribute to the outcome.[127]

Another cause of birth defects is poor health of the mother. Maternal diseases such as diabetes, anemia, cardiac diseases, and metabolic diseases may cause birth defects.[127] Also, chronic stress is believed to have the potential to cause birth defects, because it reduces the blood flow to the uterus, thus limiting the amount of nutrients and oxygen to the fetus. In addition, stress causes the release of hormones, such as cortisone, that in turn can have a teratogenic effect on the fetus.[132,135]

Maternal malnutrition during periods of fetal growth may be very detrimental to the health of the baby. For example, a reduction in protein and caloric intake between 26 and 32 weeks of gestation can permanently reduce the number of brain cells.[128] Continued poor maternal diet is believed to result in low birth weight, neuromuscular disorders, and, later in life, learning disabilities.[15]

In summary, it is estimated that 30% of all chromosomal abnormalities are related to hereditary factors, and about 50% to developmental and environmental factors.[119] This seems to indicate that a great many chromosomal abnormalities could be prevented through greater public awareness of the risk factors and through the careful monitoring of all pregnancies, especially those that may be considered at risk.

Types of birth defects

There are five major types of birth defects: physical malformations, blood diseases, inborn errors of metabolism, chromosomal abnormalities, and conditions caused by various perinatal high-risk factors.[15] Physical malformations consist of malformations, duplications, and absent body parts. Examples of physical malformations are cleft palate, clubfoot, and spina bifida. Blood diseases are malfunctions resulting from reduced or missing blood components, or the reduced ability to perform specific functions. Sickle-cell anemia, hemophilia, and thalassemia are examples of blood diseases. Inborn errors of metabolism prevent the body from producing an enzyme or from converting certain chemicals into other chemicals. Diseases such as cystic fibrosis, muscular dystrophy, phenylketonuria, and congenital hypothyroidism fit into this classification. Chromosomal abnormalities usually result in specific patterns of multiple structural and organic abnormalities such as those found in Klinefelter's disease, Turner's syndrome, and Down's syndrome. Finally, many birth defects are caused by factors that negatively affect the fetus during the birth process itself or during the neonatal period when so many adjustments to extrauterine life must be made. Conditions falling into this last category will be discussed further in the section on perinatal complications.

Identifying the high-risk pregnancy

Early identification of the high-risk pregnancy is of utmost importance to ensure the best results for the greatest number of mothers and infants.[91] This requires the establishment of a network of professionals, paraprofessionals, and lay people concerned with prenatal and postnatal care. Counselors, teachers, therapists, social workers, nurses, and others who come in contact with pregnant women should provide education and counseling geared toward the prevention of the high-risk pregnancy and toward the early referral of any pregnancies that may be at risk. Organizations and agencies concerned with public education should be identified and their activities encouraged. Finally, for those pregnancies that will require special diagnostic and intervention strategies, a highly trained and well-equipped obstetrical care team must be available.[91]

Several studies[62,70,97] have described assessment systems that help distinguish the high-risk patient from the low-risk patient. These systems provide uniform record-keeping of specific factors that have been identified as determinants of perinatal morbidity and mortality. These factors include maternal age, socioeconomic status, race, nutritional status, past medical and obstetrical histories, and current medical and pregnancy problems.[70] The assessments are designed to systematically gather data during the first pregnancy care visit, the third trimester, early in labor, later in labor, and during the postnatal period.[91] Once the high-risk pregnancy is identified, specific diagnostic and intervention strategies may be initiated.

TABLE 6-1	**Effects of common teratogens on developing fetus**

Substance or factor	Effect on fetus
Drugs	
Alcohol	Intrauterine growth retardation; mental deficiency; stillbirth. Babies born to chronic alcoholics may have fetal alcohol syndrome or withdrawal symptoms.
Aspirin	In large amounts may be fatal or cause hemorrhagic manifestations.
Cortisone	Possible relation to cleft palate.
Caffeine	Increased incidence of miscarriage; limb and skeletal malformations.
Dilantin	Fetal hydantoin syndrome (growth and mental deficiency; abnormalities of the face; anomalies of the hands.
Heroin, codeine, morphine	Hyperirritability; shrill cry; vomiting and withdrawal symptoms; decreased alertness and responsiveness to visual and auditory stimuli. Can be fatal.
LSD	Spontaneous abortions; chromosomal changes; suspected anomalies.
Lead	Spontaneous abortion; intrauterine growth retardation; congenital anomalies; anemia. Can be fatal.
Tetracycline	Stains teeth, inhibits bone growth.
Thalidomide	Phocomelia; hearing loss; cardiac anomalies. Can be fatal.
Tobacco	Intrauterine growth retardation.
Tranquilizers	All may cause withdrawal symptoms during the neonatal period.
Intrauterine infections	
Toxoplasmosis	Blindness; mental retardation; cardiac anomalies.
Syphilis	Prematurity; congenital syphilis; anomalies.
Rubella	Rubella syndrome (deafness; blindness; cardiac defects; mental retardation).
Cytomegalic inclusion disease	Intrauterine growth retardation; jaundice; microcephaly.
Herpesvirus	Neonatal infection; microcephaly; retinal dysplasia. Can be fatal.
Hormones	
Diethylstilbestrol (DES)	Cancer of reproductive system in females (20 years later); reproductive anomalies in males.
Chemicals and industrial wastes	
Methylmercury	Congenital abnormalities; growth retardation. Can cause abortions.
Pesticides (some types)	Congenital anomalies.
Social factors	
Maternal stress	Increased fetal anomalies; premature labor; mongoloid birth.
Poor nutrition	Prematurity; toxemia, anemia; intrauterine growth retardation; lower levels of intellectual performance.
Radiation	Congenital anomalies; growth retardation; chromosomal damage; mental deficiency; stillbirth.

Adapted from Klaus, M.H., and Farnaroff, A.A.: Care of the high-risk neonate, Philadelphia, 1979, W.B. Saunders Co.; and Schuster, C.S., and Ashburn, S.S.: The process of human development: a holistic approach, Boston, 1980, Little, Brown and Co.; and Shortridge, S.D., unpublished material.

Evaluation of the fetus

Various biochemical, hormonal, and physical approaches now allow many fetal complications to be diagnosed. The approaches discussed here are the ones most often encountered by occupational therapists in reviewing both research literature and the charts and records of their patients. Included are the following procedures: ultrasonography, amniocentesis, fetoscopy, and selected laboratory procedures.

Ultrasonography has replaced radiography as the preferred method of measuring fetal development, because it is believed to be a safer procedure.[141] With ultrasonography, short pulses of low-intensity, high-frequency ultrasound waves are transmitted through the woman's abdomen to the uterus and the fetus.[23] These signals are reflected back from tissue mass, creating a two-dimensional picture of the fetus, placenta, uterine wall, and amniotic fluid. Types of problems commonly diagnosed from this procedure include multiple pregnancy complications, fetal structural abnormalities, uterine and placental problems, and intrauterine growth problems.

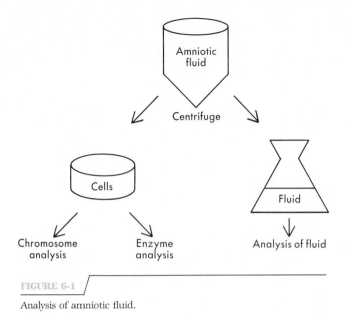

FIGURE 6-1

Analysis of amniotic fluid.

A second procedure commonly used in fetal assessment is amniocentesis. In this procedure a needle is inserted through the abdominal and uterine walls and into the amniotic sac where approximately 1 ounce of amniotic fluid is withdrawn.[11] Analysis of the fluid and the discarded fetal cells contained in the fluid allows the detection of specific chromosomal abnormalities, inborn errors of metabolism, and fetal malformations (Figure 6-1).

For example, if a concentration of the compound alpha-fetoprotein (AFP) is found in the amniotic fluid, spina bifida may be present. Tay-Sachs disease, thalassemia, and Down's syndrome may also be detected by evaluating the fetal cells. As the gender or sex of the fetus may also be determined by amniocentesis, parents concerned with the possibility that their baby may be born with a sex-linked disorder, such as muscular dystrophy or hemophilia, may be helped in their difficult decision-making process.

The risks associated with amniocentesis are considered very small, although instances of miscarriages, infections in the mother, and needle punctures of the fetus have been reported.[99] While it would seem that the benefits of the procedure far outweigh the risks, only a small percentage of at-risk mothers take advantage of the procedure.[11] Reasons for this phenomenon have been the high cost, fear of the procedure, fear of the associated risks, lack of knowledge that the procedure exists, and inaccessibility to the procedure.[11]

Fetoscopy is another diagnostic procedure that is being used to a greater extent. In this procedure a small tube is inserted through the mother's abdominal wall and into the amniotic fluid. A fiberoptic light source on the end of the tube, or fetoscope, allows the physician to detect congenital malformations. In addition, a syringe may be used to take placental blood samples that can be used to detect such blood diseases as sickle-cell anemia.[105]

Many high-risk pregnancies require the continued monitoring of various biochemical and hormonal factors through the use of specific laboratory techniques. For example, during a diabetic pregnancy, blood glucose concentrations must be constantly monitored to ensure that they stay within acceptable ranges. Other laboratory tests may be used to determine fetal pulmonary maturity. This factor is important to the physician in determining the optimal time of delivery, because it is now known that the risk of intrauterine death often increases approaching term in the diabetic pregnancy.[128] These procedures are believed to have helped reduce perinatal mortality in the diabetic pregnancy.[98]

It is anticipated that in the next decade many of these techniques will be refined and many new procedures developed. As a result, even more conditions and risk factors will be diagnosed prenatally, thus making that wish for a healthy baby a reality for more prospective parents than ever before.

Treatment of the fetus

Although most of the techniques now being used in fetal treatment have been developed within the last decade, the risks, benefits, and long-term impact of these techniques on all aspects of development are still largely unknown. Some of the risks that have been identified include infections, premature rupture of membranes, premature labor, puncture of fetal organs and blood vessels, and damage to the fetus, risks that often do not become critical until later in the pregnancy.

One of the first successful intrauterine procedures was the blood transfusion. In this procedure blood is directly administered to the fetus in cases of severe anemia as a result of blood incompatibility. Another technique, now commonly used, is the infusion of various drugs directly into the amniotic fluid where the fetus later ingests the drug. This procedure has been used to correct vitamin deficiencies, thyroid malfunctions, and heart rate irregularities.[69]

A procedure that is still in the experimental stages is the draining of excess fluid from fetal structures into the amniotic fluid. For instance, the treatment of fetal hydrocephalus consists of inserting a prenatal brain shunt into the enlarged ventricle in the brain and draining the excess cerebral spinal fluid into the amniotic fluid. A similar procedure is used in cases of hydronephrosis, a condition that results in urine backing up into the abdomen because of a urinary blockage.

Perhaps the most sophisticated procedure attempted so far is extrauterine surgery. The uterus is opened, then the fetus is exposed for surgery and returned to the uterus for the remainder of the pregnancy. This procedure has been attempted only a few times to date and is still considered highly experimental.[69] While fetal surgery may eventually save hundreds of babies a year from lives of disability, in the near future many medical problems still must be solved.

Fetal treatment also presents many moral and ethical questions. For example, is the therapy warranted? Which fetuses should be treated? What is the optimal period of intervention? Should the multiply handicapped child be treated? Can an obstetrician be sued for not diagnosing a fetal problem? Is it the parent's decision to decide if a procedure can or cannot be used on their child? When and under what conditions are abortions to be performed? The answers to these and countless other questions will unfold as the state of the art and science of perinatology is refined and expanded and as its procedures and policies are scrutinized by society.

Implications for occupational therapy

The role of the occupational therapist in prenatal care is still emerging and therefore must be hypothesized to some extent. Obviously the occupational therapist will not be directly involved in the medical procedures themselves, but as the focus of intensive care nurseries expands to include prevention and parent education, the occupational therapist will have a great deal to offer.

In the area of prevention an occupational therapist might be involved with the community task force charged with establishing and monitoring the prenatal network that is so necessary for high-quality care for the mother and fetus. Also, an occupational therapist would be helpful in working with the handicapped population in attempts to reduce some of the high-risk factors associated with pregnancies among that population.

Another role of the occupational therapist could be to share information at prenatal classes for prospective parents. Topics that occupational therapists might be asked to present include early infant stimulation, selection of infant toys, prenatal sensory or motor development, and activities to foster bonding and attachment.

Finally, the occupational therapist may become involved with the prospective parents of a handicapped baby. Who better than an occupational therapist could answer questions about the possible effects of a particular disability on the child's development or on specific tasks of daily functioning? These and other roles will emerge as techniques advance and new needs are discovered in this exciting new arena of practice.

PERINATAL COMPLICATIONS

The period just before, during, and immediately after birth is known as the perinatal period. Many factors can affect the birth process and also that critical period immediately after birth when the neonate must make so many biophysical adjustments to extrauterine life.

This section discusses major problems found in the perinatal period, describes medical procedures used with neonates in distress, overviews some of the neonatal assessments, and discusses implications for occupational therapy.

Complications surrounding the birth process

Labor and delivery are a very critical time in the pregnancy. Some of the factors that negatively affect these processes are maternal in origin, while others are caused by infant complications.

Many of the maternal illnesses that were discussed as presenting high-risk factors during the prenatal period of the pregnancy may also lead to the development of problems at this time of the pregnancy. For example, the diabetic pregnancy not only presents the prenatal complications already discussed, but it also involves complications in this period, such as toxemia, large babies, and babies who may be hypoglycemic after birth because of the excess insulin their bodies have produced.[77] Another example is the mother with a bacterial or viral infection, such as syphilis or gonorrhea, at the time of birth. While these diseases will no longer produce malformations, they may be transmitted to an immune-deficient neonate and cause serious and sometimes fatal results.[11]

A potentially dangerous maternal illness is toxemia, or preeclampsia. This syndrome consists of high blood pressure and edema in the lower extremities, and protein may be detected in the urine. If untreated, the mother may progress to eclampsia, which is often characterized by seizures, severe headaches, nausea, elevated pulse rate and temperature, and coma. Premature births, low birth weight babies, and even death have been attributed to these conditions.[68]

Other maternal complications may be related to placental problems or physical structural problems of the uterus or the pelvis. For example, placental problems can endanger the fetus by causing prematurity or by interfering with fetal blood circulation. Abruptio placentae is a condition in which the placenta prematurely separates from the uterine wall. In placenta previa the placenta lies over the cervical opening, and when labor begins, the cervix dilates and the placenta tears. Physical problems include uterine fibroid tumors that may hinder fetal growth, problems with premature dilation of the cervix, or a pelvis too small to allow passage of the fetal head.

The two most common infant factors affecting labor and delivery are birth defects and multiple pregnancies. Malformations of critical body organs are present in some birth defects. These may cause serious medical problems, some of which are incompatible with survival. Other birth defects may cause problems because of their unique characteristics. For example, babies born with hydrocephalus, or spina bifida myelomeningocele, or osteogenesis imperfecta may each have unique problems during the birth process.

Multiple births also have the potential to pose complications during this process. These complications include premature births, prolapsed cord, toxemia in the mother, and difficult deliveries as a result of unusual positioning of one or more of the fetuses.[11,127]

Medical management during labor and delivery

Many of these maternal and infant factors affect the oxygen supply to the fetus. Because there is a direct correlation between fetal oxygen level and fetal heart rate, heart rate is carefully monitored throughout the labor and delivery process. For instance, the normal range of fetal heart beats is 120 to 160 per minute. If this drops to below 100 beats per minute, it could indicate that the fetus is not getting enough oxygen and that immediate emergency medical care is required.[127]

Fetal heart rate may be monitored externally or internally. External monitoring is done by holding a stethoscope against the mother's abdomen and counting the number of beats per minute. Another method consists of strapping an electronic microphone to the mother's abdomen that continually monitors fetal heart rate and uterine contractions. Internal monitoring may be accomplished by inserting an electrode into the vagina and attaching it directly to the presenting part of the fetus.

The cesarean section may be performed as a lifesaving technique in many of the situations mentioned. This procedure consists of administering a general anesthetic to the mother and surgically removing the baby through an incision in the mother's abdomen. While the cesarean section must be performed to save the lives of babies, it does create some potential risks to both the mother and the baby. As the procedure is considered to be major surgery, the mother is subjected to potential hazards from the general anesthetic, the possibility of infection, and postoperative pain and discomfort. Babies delivered by cesarean section are more likely to develop respiratory distress, because they are born with fluid in their lungs. Normally, this fluid is expelled from the lungs during the first stages of labor.[127] They are also often more lethargic because of the effect of the anesthetic.[56]

Complications in the first weeks

The first 28 days of life require major adjustments to life outside the womb. Occasionally complications arise that require the services of a neonatologist, a medical specialist familiar with the problems and intricacies of this period of the life span.

In the first minutes and hours of life, major physiological changes take place that allow the neonate to breathe, blood to circulate to all parts of the body, nutrition to be absorbed, and temperature to be regulated.

Respiratory changes begin with the expulsion of the amniotic fluid from the lungs. Next, the force of the neonate's first breathing and first cries expands the lungs and opens the alveoli in the lungs. The chemical *surfactant* keeps these alveoli open, thus allowing an effective exchange of oxygen and carbon dioxide. When the amount of surfactant is decreased, *respiratory distress syndrome* of the newborn (RDS) occurs. The more immature the neonate, the higher the incidence of respiratory distress syndrome, as less surfactant has been produced. One study revealed that 60% of the neonates born at less than 32 weeks of gestation developed respiratory distress syndrome, whereas only 10% of the neonates born between 34 and 36 weeks developed the disease.[124]

Babies with respiratory distress syndrome must have their lungs artificially ventilated often for long periods of time. During this time a condition called *retrolental fibroplasia* (RLF) can occur. High concentrations of oxygen destroy delicate blood vessels in the eyes. Later, when the neonate is removed from the oxygen, new blood vessels begin to grow back in a disorganized manner. Often scar tissue accompanies this growth and, if not removed by surgical or laser treatments, can cause the retina to pull away from the choroid and result in blindness.[11]

Today's artificial respirators are sophisticated and allow careful control of the oxygen mixtures. In addition, they are designed to maintain a constant pressure on the alveoli, thus keeping them open in the absence of surfactant. This is known as *positive end-expiratory pressure* (PEEP), which has significantly lowered the rate of fetal death and overall risk of severe developmental delays.[52,65]

Three major cardiovascular changes must take place at birth. The foramen ovale, the hole between the right and left atria, must close. Also the ductus arteriosus and ductus venosus must close to allow blood to flow to the lungs and to the liver, respectively. Many complications can arise when these changes do not happen. One of the most common conditions found in premature newborns with respiratory distress syndrome is *patent ductus arteriosus* (PDA). In this condition the ductus arteriosus does not constrict, and this can lead to eventual heart failure and inadequate oxygenation of the brain. Treatment includes the administration of the drug *indomethacin*, which often triggers closure of the arterial wall. Surgery follows if the drug does not work.[61,86]

Another cardiovascular complication that may occur during the perinatal period is intracranial hemorrhage. This may occur prenatally, during the birth process, or postnatally. The site and the extent of the bleeding affect the prognosis. For example, extracranial bleeding, or cephalohematomas, are usually considered minor and usually cause no permanent damage. On the other hand, subdural, subarachnoid, and intraventricular hemorrhages are much more serious and, depending on the extent of damage, may cause seizures, brain damage, cerebral palsy and even death.[145]

Biochemical complications affect the premature neonate as well as the full-term neonate. One of the most common biochemical problems is jaundice, or icterus. This condition is characterized by a yellow discoloration of the skin and eyes as a result of an increase in the bilirubin level. Bilirubin is a by-product of the normal process that discards dead blood cells. When the bilirubin level rises slightly—a relatively common event in neonates—treatment may consist of simply placing the neonate under fluorescent lights. This speeds up the elimination of the bilirubin.

Hyperbilirubinemia poses a serious threat to newborns. The most common cause of hyperbilirubinemia is Rh incompatibility. In the past this syndrome, called *kernicterus*, caused many fetuses to die in utero, and those who survived suffered brain damage, cerebral palsy, a high-frequency hearing loss, discoloration of the teeth, and sometimes paralysis of the upward gaze.[104]

Today the drug *RhoGAM*, which is a gamma globulin, is injected into Rh-negative women after the birth or miscarriage of each newborn. It blocks the formation of antibodies in the mother's circulation, and subsequent Rh-positive newborns will be born without problems. This treatment has resulted in the virtual disappearance of kernicterus.[11]

Two other biochemical complications are hypoglycemia and hypothermia. Hypoglycemia, or low blood glucose level, can cause the newborn to be jittery, appear lethargic, vomit, and have seizures or apnea spells. Giving the newborn sugar intravenously usually prevents permanent damage. The premature newborn is very susceptible to loss of heat, or *hypothermia*. There are two major reasons for this: (1) an inability to regulate temperature and (2) a reduced amount of fatty tissue to act as insulation.

Immaturity of the central nervous system may also cause complications. For example, some neonates have spells in which they stop breathing. This is called *apnea*. If the apnea is persistent, it may be a precursor of *sudden infant death* syndome (SIDS).[11] While the exact cause and site of involvement are not as yet confirmed, the brain stem is believed to be involved, and sensory processing has been found to be slower in some infants. Equipment such as rocker beds have proved helpful to stimulate some infants to breathe, as have certain medications such as caffeine and aminophylline.[79] If the spells continue, it may be helpful to have an apnea monitor that sounds an alarm if the infant stops breathing. In addition, many physicians are recommending that the parents of infants with histories of apnea participate in cardiopulmonary resuscitation (CPR) courses.

In addition to apnea and sudden infant death syndrome, an immature central nervous system may cause sucking and swallowing problems that hinder nutritional intake. Some newborns may have to be fed intravenously by a gastrostomy tube, which is inserted through the abdomen into the stomach, or by a nasogastric tube, which is inserted up the nose and down the esophagus to the stomach. *Hyperalimentation* is the term used for the administration of intravenous solution that contains sufficient glucose, vitamins, amino acids, and electrolytes to meet the nutritional needs of these neonates.[139]

Generalized bacterial infection, or *sepsis*, is a serious concern in all nurseries. Neonates are susceptible to infection because of their incomplete defense or immune systems. Newborns can contract infections through the placenta, from the maternal vagina, from contamination of the amniotic fluid during delivery, from other newborns in the nursery, or from medical procedures such as blood transfusions. Early diagnosis is essential, because the infection can spread rapidly through the newborn's body. Blood cultures are taken to identify the specific organism, and antibodies are given intravenously. Usually the newborn's condition improves within 2 or 3 days with this treatment.[11]

Problems of neonates who are small or large for gestational age

The small for gestational age (SGA) neonate is defined as a newborn whose birth weight is below the 10th percentile for gestational age as measured by standardized growth charts.[84] The majority of small for gestational age newborns are born at or near term but are small for their age. These newborns may suffer from a number of medical problems, including congenital anomalies; difficulty with thermal regulation, polycythemia, or hypoglycemia; and pulmonary problems such as aspiration syndrome, pneumomediastinum, and pneumothorax.[136]

The growth of small for gestational age infants varies, depending on the duration of the intrauterine problems that caused the stunting.[136] Some studies indicate that if the child's growth and development have not caught up to normal curves by 3 years of age, the child will remain smaller than normal throughout life.[57] It has been stated that the small for gestational age infant has a higher incidence of developmental disabilities when compared to average infants.[57,127]

The large for gestational age (LGA) neonate is defined as the neonate whose birth weight is above the 90th percentile on the growth charts. Medical problems of these neonates include hypoglycemia; birth injuries resulting from prolonged or difficult labor or birth; and orthopedic problems resulting from the restricted room in utero.[138]

Problems of premature and postmature neonates

The premature neonate is defined as a baby born anytime before the 36th week of gestation or, in other words, more than 1 month before the anticipated due date. Because of aggressive obstetrical management and advances in techniques and equipment, more and more of these premature babies are surviving. Today neonates who weigh as little as 750 grams (1.6 pounds) and who are as young as 24 to 27 weeks of gestational age are surviving.

These preemies do not look like small babies but like fetuses. Specific characteristics vary with gestational age, but these newborns often have paper-thin skin that is brittle and red in color, and they may lack skin creases if they are younger than 32 weeks of gestational age. They may also have decreased tone and joint mobility. If they are younger than 34 weeks of gestational age, they may lack ear cartilage and breast buds.

In addition to the respiratory, cardiovascular, and biochemical complications already mentioned, these neonates may develop a disorder called *necrotizing enterocolitis* (NEC). The cause of this disorder is unknown, but it strikes at about 2 weeks of age. It is a serious intestinal disorder in which the bowel stops functioning and may rupture. Antibiotics may help, but in some instances a colostomy may have to be per-

formed. Unlike in adults, regeneration of the colon is often seen in these neonates.

Premature neonates often suffer problems that are a result of the techniques used to save their lives. These are known as iatrogenic disorders, and Table 6-2 lists some of the common ones.

The postmature, or post-term, neonate is defined as a baby born after 42 weeks of gestation. These neonates may possess the following physical characteristics: a long, thin body; thick scalp hair; and dry, cracked skin resulting from the loss of the vernix caseosa. In addition, they may show signs of recent weight loss if the placenta was no longer able to provide all the nutrition needed and stored fat was used as a food source. Two of the most common problems of the postmature neonate are hypoglycemia and respiratory distress resulting from meconium aspiration.[138]

Assessment of the neonate

At birth a neonate's neuromuscular, cardiovascular, and respiratory systems must be appraised to determine how well the neonate has responded to the birth process and extrauterine life. The Apgar scoring system provides this information by rating the neonate's color, heart rate, reflex irritability, muscle tone, and respiratory effort[5] (p. 151).

Assessment of a neonate's gestational age is very important, especially in planning for the needs of the premature neonate. Clinical assessment of gestational age is based on the knowledge of various postures, reflexes, and external body characteristics at specific fetal ages.[4,6,12,147]

The three most commonly used clinical assessments for determining gestational age are (1) the Dubowitz and Dubowitz Clinical Assessment of Gestational Age,[46] (2) the Lubchenco Clinical Estimate of Gestational Age,[84] and (3) the Newborn Maturity Rating and Classification. One of these assessments is usually given at birth and again during the first few days of life if low scores were noted in specific areas or if variations occurred between the results and other approaches to determine gestational age. All the assessments are used to evaluate neuromuscular signs as well as condition of

TABLE 6-2	Examples of iatrogenic conditions and disorders commonly found in premature neonates
Intervention or procedure	*Resulting disease or complication*
High concentrations of oxygen	Retrolental fibroplasia
Blood transfusions and intravenous procedures	Infections
Prolonged intravenous feeding	Liver damage or clots in the kidneys
Prolonged artificial ventilation	Bronchopulmonary dysplasia

skin, lanugo, breasts, plantar creases, ears, and genitalia.

A thorough physical examination is usually done after the newborn is 24 hours old, because it is after that time that problems such as seizures, intestinal obstructions, jaundice, apnea, hematomas, and other conditions become identifiable.[118] The physical condition and appearance of the following body structures are part of the examination: skin, head, eyes, nose, mouth, neck, thorax, lungs, heart, abdomen, genitalia, anus, trunk and spine, and extremities. In addition, general appearance, reflex presence and integration, tone, and quality of movement are observed.[118]

Many examinations also assess the social and interactive abilities of the neonate. The abilities to locate and orient to sensory stimuli, to react to environmental conditions, and to interact with caregivers are known to be important factors in growth and development and in the bonding and attachment process.

The Brazelton Neonatal Behavioral Assessment Scale (BNBAS) is one of the most commonly used measures of social-interactive responses in the neonate.[19] This scale is designed to look at both the neurological and interactional functioning of a neonate during the first month of life (pp. 191-192).

Other assessments that explore various aspects of the caretaker-child interactional processes are the Mother-Infant Play Interaction Scale[140]; the Maternal Attachment Assessment[8]; and the Neonatal Perception Inventories.[22] Assessments that specifically look at child abuse factors include the Perinatal Screening for Child Abuse Potential[64]; the Index of Suspicion[101]; and the Child Abuse Potential Inventory.[93]

Follow-up testing

Professionals in most health settings agree that the biophysical, cognitive, and psychosocial progress of the types of neonates discussed should be monitored throughout the infant and preschool years to detect any developmental delays. A variety of intelligence and general developmental tests have been designed to accomplish this goal, but the two most often used tests are the Denver Developmental Screening Test (DDST)[59] (Chapter 9) and the Bayley Scales of Infant Development (BSID)[12] (Chapter 11).

Implications for occupational therapy

The first goal of the neonatal intensive care nursery is to ensure the physical survival of the neonate. But once the medical problems have been overcome or at least stabilized, it is time to address other equally important factors that relate to the quality of life of both the neonate and the parents. For example, the environmental stimulation must be examined, caregiver-infant interaction must be nurtured, and the sensorimotor abilities, psychosocial skills, and functional skills of the neonate must be assessed.

An occupational therapist who is knowledgeable in the assessment and treatment of these factors can be a tremendous asset to the interdisciplinary team used in most neonatal units. In addition, occupational therapists have much to offer during follow-up evaluations geared toward monitoring the growth, development, and functional skills of high-risk neonates and neonates with diagnosed problems (Chapter 15).

MUSCULOSKELETAL PROBLEMS

This section will discuss the components of the musculoskeletal system, their reactions to disorders and injuries, and selected musculoskeletal problems of particular interest to occupational therapists.

Components and functions of the musculoskeletal system

The musculoskeletal system consists of the following six major components[121]:

1. Bones that provide a framework for the body; serve as levers for the skeletal muscles; protect body organs; produce platelets, erythrocytes, and leukocytes; and store calcium, magnesium, phosphorus, and sodium
2. Joints that allow for segmentation of the skeletal system and help facilitate movement
3. Articular cartilage that provides a cushioning effect and allows free movement
4. Skeletal muscles that provide active motion and the maintenance of posture
5. Ligaments that facilitate or limit motion and provide support
6. Tendons that also facilitate or limit motion and provide support

Musculoskeletal reactions to disorders and injuries

When subjected to abnormal conditions, bone tissue will either die or continue to live by making some type of adaptation. An increase or decrease in the amount of bone tissue deposited may take place; there may be an increase or decrease in bone resorption; or a combination of these two circumstances may occur.[123] If these reactions occur in just one bone, it is called a *localized reaction*; but if many bones are affected, it is referred to as a *generalized reaction*.

The epiphyseal plates are particularly susceptible to change as a result of abnormal conditions, such as decreased blood supply, pressure from fluid or tissue

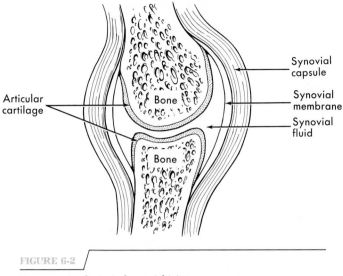

Articular cartilage

Bone

Bone

Synovial capsule

Synovial membrane

Synovial fluid

FIGURE 6-2

Components of a typical synovial joint.

buildup, and injury to the plate itself. As a result of these abnormal conditions, growth may be stopped entirely or restricted to one part of the plate and not another. The result of pressure and abnormal twisting forces can be the rotation of the bone toward the source of the pressure.

The various components of a synovial joint are shown in Figure 6-2. These parts may also react to abnormal conditions. For instance, articular cartilage has little power to regenerate itself; therefore, under abnormal conditions it often degenerates and the peripheral edges begin to thicken and eventually ossify.[121] Often the synovial membrane reacts by producing an excessive amount of fluid, by thickening, or by forming adhesions to the articular cartilage. The joint capsule and surrounding ligaments react by either stretching, which causes joint instability, or becoming tighter, which can impair the range of motion of the joint.

Finally, adverse conditions can affect any or all of the components of the skeletal muscle motor unit. When this occurs, the skeletal muscle may react by degenerating, contracting or shortening, becoming weaker and smaller (atrophy), becoming larger (hypertrophy), or regenerating.[121]

Selected musculoskeletal disorders and conditions

EPIPHYSEAL PLATE DISORDERS

Marfan's syndrome, also called arachnodactyly or hyperchondroplasia, is a disorder that causes excessive growth in all the epiphyseal plates. It is considered to be a hereditary condition with an unknown cause. Symptoms include increased height and decreased weight for chronological age, excessive length of the ex-

tremities, scoliosis, depressed sternum, stooped shoulders, flat feet, and excessive joint flexibility. Additional problems may occur, such as dislocation of the optic lens[121,139] and heart disease that includes dilation of the aorta. Medical treatment includes surgical intervention for any skeletal deformities that interfere with function.

Chondrodystrophia, also called chondrodystrophy or achondroplasia, has the opposite effect of Marfan's syndrome by stunting epiphyseal plate growth and causing dwarfism. This disorder is transmitted by an autosomal dominant gene and is characterized by very short limbs, a small face (head size is average because of normal growth of the cranial bones), and decreased height that seldom exceeds 4 feet. Skeletal abnormalities such as lumbar lordosis, coxa vara, and cubitus varus may also be present. To improve both function and appearance, orthopedic surgery is often performed.[121]

As mentioned earlier, twisting forces may cause changes in epiphyseal plate growth, causing the long bones to twist in the direction of the abnormal force. These are known as *internal, external,* or *combinational torsional deformities.* For example, "toeing out" is very common in young children. This deformity is characterized by externally rotated feet and knees and by limited internal rotation of the femur. It is often seen in infants who habitually sleep in the prone position with their legs externally rotated, and this causes external femoral torsion. Conversely, children who spend a great deal of time sitting on the floor with knees in front, feet out to the side, and femora internally rotated (the "television position" or "W-sitting"), may begin to "toe in," resulting from the internal femoral torsion.

Bow legs, or genu varum, is an example of a deformity caused by combinational torsional forces, that is, prolonged internal torsion to the tibia and external torsion to the femur. This deformity is often present at birth because of prenatal posturing, but it usually corrects itself unless compounded by specific neuromuscular problems or unusual sleeping and sitting postures that continue to apply the abnormal torsions.

DISORDERS CAUSED BY DEPOSITION OR RESORPTION IMBALANCES

Osteogenesis imperfecta, also called brittle bones or fragilitas ossium, offers an example of a disorder characterized by decreased bone deposition. It is a congenital type of osteoporosis that is transmitted by an autosomal dominant gene. The result is a serious disorder in which fractures can result from very minor traumatic situations. The severity of the disorder varies greatly depending on the time of onset (Table 6-3). Multiple fractures or repeated fractures to the same bone may cause a limb to become misshapen and eventually muscularly underdeveloped because of the long periods of immobilization and disuse. Prevention must be attempted through, at least, the use of padded arm and leg protec-

TABLE 6-3	Effect of onset of osteogenesis imperfecta	
Fetal type	Most severe	Fractures occur in utero and during birth. Mortality is high.
Infantile type	Moderately severe	Many fractures occur in early childhood. Severe limb deformities and growth disturbances occur also.
Juvenile type	Least severe	Fractures begin in late childhood. By puberty bones often begin to harden and fewer fractures occur.

tors and, in severe cases, long leg braces and crutches.[121] To provide internal support and to correct deformities that may develop, surgical procedures using metal rods and segmental osteotomies may be helpful.

Osteopetrosis, or marble bones or Albers-Schönberg's disease, is an autosomal recessive disorder that is characterized by a great increase in the amount of bone that results from defective resorption.[121] Gradually the bones become dense and the hemopoietic marrow spaces are infiltrated with bony deposits, causing aplastic anemia. Other local complications may include pathological fractures of the neck of the femur, nerve deafness or blindness as the nerve foramina begin to close because of bony encroachment, and enlargement of the liver and spleen. In severe cases hydrocephalus and mental retardation may be present. Prognosis is poor, and many children die in childhood. Treatment includes the administration of steroids and aggressive treatment of the anemia.

DISORDERS CAUSED BY INFECTION

Osteomyelitis is an inflammation of the bone marrow that may be caused by puncture wounds, infection adjacent to the bone, or microorganisms that travel in the blood.[115] Initially the organisms settle in the distal end of the metaphysis, and as the disease progresses the infection spreads throughout the bone and outward to the periosteum. Initial symptoms include pain, tenderness, and unwillingness to use or bear weight on the involved limb. These symptoms are followed by a fever, soft tissue swelling, and often anorexia.[150]

Treatment must be initiated as soon as possible, because prolonged infection may cause bone destruction, pathological fractures, septic arthritis, and eventually growth disturbances.[121] Diagnosis is usually made based on clinical signs, and confirmation is made from speci-

men aspiration test results, blood cell counts, and positive radiographic evidence.[115,121] Initial treatment usually consists of oral or intravenous antibiotic therapy for at least 3 weeks with bed rest and immobility of the affected body part. If improvement is not seen, surgery is done, which includes drilling into the bone to remove the pus and damaged tissue and putting in place drainage tubes and intravenous tubes that are used to infuse the site with a saline and antibiotic solution.[121] Following these procedures, splinting of the extremity or traction helps to prevent the spread of infection, reduces pain, and prevents contractures.[1] Relapses can lead to chronic osteomyelitis that may involve continued discharge of pus from a sinus over the infected area, pain, or the formation of an abscess cavity in the bone itself. Bed rest and antibiotics may clear the problem, or surgical procedures may have to be repeated. Chronic untreated osteomyelitis presents serious medical problems that can be minimized by early detection and prolonged antibiotic therapy.[1,115,121]

Another disorder that is spread by infection is *tuberculosis*. On occasion tuberculosis of the bone (tuberculous osteomyelitis) occurs as an isolated lesion, but it usually forms from infection at a primary lesion in another part of the body or from an adjoining joint.[1] The most common sites for tuberculosis of the bone are the long bones, synovial joints, and vertebrae.

The joints most often affected are the hip and the knee. Symptoms include pain, muscle spasm, reduced joint motion, and muscle atrophy. Initially swelling of the soft tissue around the joint is noted. Then the synovial membrane changes, and articular cartilage necrosis occurs. Finally the adjacent bones may begin to collapse.[121]

Tuberculosis of the spine, or Pott's disease, usually begins with pain, tenderness, and muscle spasms in the back. As the disease progresses, the anterior sections of the vertebral bodies begin to collapse, causing the spine to tilt anteriorly.[1] Infection may spread to adjacent disks and vertebrae or to the spinal cord. Pott's paraplegia may be a direct result of spinal cord involvement or a result of pressure on the cord.

The treatment for bone tuberculosis includes the use of antituberculous drugs, rest, a nutritious diet, immobilization of the infected joint or limb, surgical drainage, and, on occasion, arthrodesis or bony fusion.[1,115]

DISORDERS OF THE JOINTS

A major cause of physical disability in children under the age of 16 is *juvenile rheumatoid arthritis* (JRA). It is estimated that approximately 250,000 children in the United States suffer from some form of this disease.[1] This disease usually begins between the ages of 2 and 4 years of age and is more common in girls.[121]

The exact cause of juvenile rheumatoid arthritis is

unknown, but the following factors are believed to play undefined roles in its cause: genetics, emotional trauma, histocompatibility antigens, viruses, and antigen-antibody immune complexes.[1]

Juvenile rheumatoid arthritis is usually described as taking three different forms: (1) pauciarticular, (2) polyarticular, and (3) systemic, or Still's disease. The pauciarticular form usually affects only a few joints. Involvement is often asymmetrical, and there are few or no systemic manifestations. The joints most often affected are the knee, hip, ankle, and elbow. Many times overgrowth in the long bones surrounding the inflamed joint causes gait problems and flexion contractures. Many children suffering from pauciarticular juvenile rheumatoid arthritis develop iridocyclitis, an inflamed condition of the iris and ciliary body of the eye that can lead to blindness if early treatment is not begun.[1,121]

In the polyarticular form, onset is often abrupt and painful with symmetrical involvement of the wrist, hands, feet, knees, ankles, and sometimes the cervical area of the spine. Other symptoms include a low-grade fever, malaise, anorexia, listlessness, and irritability.[121]

Systemic juvenile rheumatoid arthritis, or Still's disease, consists of polyarticular symptomatology plus involvement in other organs such as the spleen and lymph nodes.[1] Signs and symptoms include a high fever, rash, anorexia, enlargement of the liver and spleen, and an elevated white blood cell count.[121] Epiphyseal plates adjacent to an affected joint may initially show an acceleration of growth but later may be destroyed, causing local growth retardation.

The prognosis for juvenile rheumatoid arthritis varies, depending on a number of factors, but it is important to remember that the largest percentage of children (the pauciarticular type) often recover completely within 1 to 2 years. Only about 15% of all children with the disease will have permanent disabilities.[121]

Medical management primarily centers on the use of the following therapeutic drugs (in order of preference): salicylates; nonsteroid, antiinflammatory analgesic drugs; gold salt injections; and adrenocorticosteroids.[121] Surgical repair and reconstruction are seldom recommended for children. Other forms of treatment may include splinting, active and passive range of motion of the joints, and monitoring each joint to maintain maximal function and prevent deformity.[115,121]

A disease that is a form of polyarthritis is *ankylosing spondylitis*, or Strümpell-Marie disease. The time of onset is usually 18 to 30 years of age, and it occurs predominately in young men.[1] This disease is characterized by a progressive bony ankylosing of the spine, beginning in the sacroiliac region and progressing upward to the cervical region. Eventually the spine becomes one rigid mass of bone. The proximal joints of the extremities are also often affected.

Treatment methods for this disease include the administration of salicylates or phenylbutazone, activity to maintain function, radiation therapy for relief of pain, and surgical procedures such as spinal osteotomy, interposition arthroplasty, and resection arthroplasty.[1,121] It should be remembered that no treatment halts the disease, but all methods must be used to limit immobility and prevent flexion of the spine.[1]

A severe orthopedic problem that is seen at birth is *arthrogryposis multiplex congenita*, or amyoplasia congenita. It is characterized by stiff, spindly, deformed joints in the extremities that are caused by either defectively formed (hypoplasia) or absent (aplasia) muscle groups or, on occasion, secondary to a defect in the anterior horn cells of the spinal cord.[121] Common clinical deformities include clubfoot, hip dislocation, flexion or extension deformity of the knee, flexion deformities of fingers and wrists, extension deformities of the elbows, and adduction deformities of the shoulder.[55]

Treatment presents an orthopedic challenge that may include casting, splinting, surgery on bones and soft tissue, and daily passive stretching of the joints.[121]

DISORDERS OF THE SPINE

The most common congenital abnormality of the spine is *spina bifida*, in which the laminae of one or more of the vertebrae are incompletely closed during the fourth week of prenatal development. This defect may be seen at any spinal level but most often occurs in the lumbosacral region.

The degree of impairment depends on the level and degree of spinal cord involvement. This continuum of impairment ranges from no functional impairment, to mild muscle imbalances and sensory losses, to paraplegia, and even to death in severe cases.[121]

The three types of spina bifida are illustrated in Figure 6-3. The mildest form is spina bifida occulta. Many times in this form of spina bifida there are no external manifestations visable, or the skin overlying the defect may be dimpled, pigmented, or covered with hair. Internally the spinal cord may be divided by a bony spur or congenital neoplasm, or there may simply be a slight bony malformation of one or more vertebrae.[89]

Spina bifida with meningocele is characterized by a sac, or meningocele, visible above the bony defect. This sac is covered with skin and subcutaneous tissue, contains cerebral spinal fluid, and while the meninges extend into the sac, the spinal cord remains confined to the spinal canal.

Spina bifida with meningomyelocele is the most severe form of the disorder. In this form the sac may be covered with only a thin layer of skin or the meninges, and the spinal cord or nerve roots protrude into the meningocele.

Complications with this form of spina bifida include meningitis and hydrocephalus. Infection is easily contracted because of environmental exposure of the

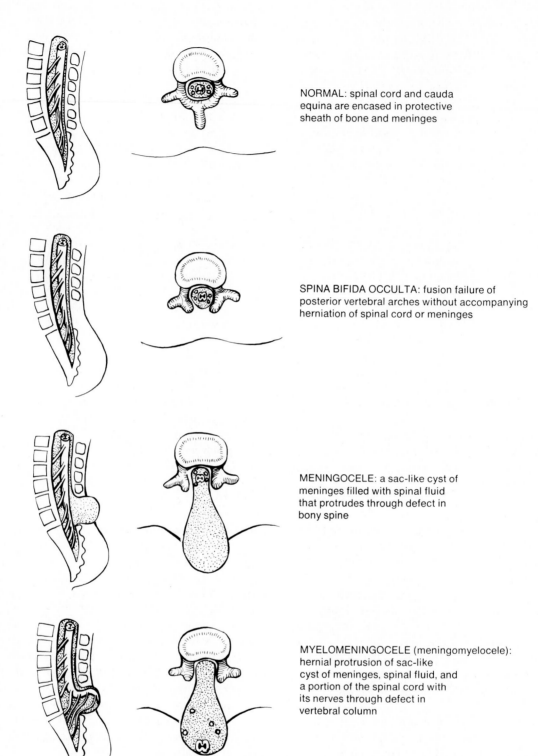

NORMAL: spinal cord and cauda equina are encased in protective sheath of bone and meninges

SPINA BIFIDA OCCULTA: fusion failure of posterior vertebral arches without accompanying herniation of spinal cord or meninges

MENINGOCELE: a sac-like cyst of meninges filled with spinal fluid that protrudes through defect in bony spine

MYELOMENINGOCELE (meningomyelocele): hernial protrusion of sac-like cyst of meninges, spinal fluid, and a portion of the spinal cord with its nerves through defect in vertebral column

FIGURE 6-3

Three forms of spina bifida.

From Whaley, L., and Wong, D.: Nursing care of infants and children, ed. 2, St. Louis, 1983, The C.V. Mosby Co.

meninges and spinal cord. Hydrocephalus is a common secondary complication that may be caused by either a developmental defect in the brain, such as aqueduct stenosis, or by the lower portion of the brain (and part of the cerebellum) slipping through the foramen ovale, a condition known as *Arnold-Chiari syndrome*.[11,121]

The medical management of the spina bifida child depends on the degree of involvement, but ideally the sac should be removed as soon as possible. Additional surgery may include the implantation of a shunt to relieve excessive ventricular pressure. Orthopedic intervention may include bracing, crutches, casting, and orthopedic shoes.[115,121] Other medical procedures may involve controlling urinary and bowel continence and infections and preventing renal deterioration.[115,129]

The rehabilitation goals for these children include the attainment of the highest level of physical functioning possible and the achievement of maximal independence in all areas of daily functioning. Counseling; the long-term monitoring of physical, cognitive, and psychosocial functioning; special education; and vocational training may be implemented to achieve these goals.

Congenital scoliosis is another relatively common spinal abnormality. The condition is usually characterized by two lateral spinal curves, the severity of which is variable. In mild cases the curvature may be inconspicuous to external observation, and if a healthy spine exists above and below the curvature, further progression is unlikely.[121] If the curvature is more severe or if the condition exists with other abnormalities such as absent or fused ribs or multiple hemivertebrae, early surgical treatment must be done to prevent permanent deformities and subsequent growth complications.[121]

DISORDERS OF THE UPPER EXTREMITIES

The most common congenital abnormalities of the hands are (1) excess number of fingers (polydactyly) and (2) webbing of the fingers (syndactyly). In *polydactyly* a variety of things may occur: the existence of one or more complete extra digits, or the duplication of just a portion of a finger or thumb. The decision to surgically remove a digit or portion of a digit is based on radiographic information, functional assessment, and cosmetic considerations.[121]

Webbing of the fingers may exist between two adjacent fingers or may involve three or four fingers. Usually the webbing extends along the proximal portion of the fingers, but occasionally it may extend the length of the fingers. Bones and joints may be involved in addition to the soft tissue. Typical reconstructive surgery involves surgical separation of the digits and skin grafts.[121]

Relatively rare abnormalities of the upper extremities include hypoplasia or aplasia of the radius; dislocation of the head of the radius; hypoplasia of the clavicles; and a congenital high scapula (Sprengel's deformity). In each of these problems surgical interventions will be attempted if function and cosmetic appearance can be improved.

Congenital amputations of the upper extremities may be as minor as a missing finger or part of a hand, or as major as the absence of one or both of the extremities. During the prenatal period, for varying reasons, the soft tissue and overlying skin in a small area of the limb fail to grow in circumference, thus forming what are called *congenital annular constricting bands*.[121] If the constriction is shallow, no deformity may occur, or the distal portion of the extremity may enlarge because of edema. But if the constriction is severe, the extremity may be amputated below the constriction.[121]

Types of limb deficiencies include *amelia*, which is the absence of an arm; *phocomelia*, which refers to a limb that is missing the proximal part; *paraxial deficiency*, which consists of a normal upper part of the limb with either the radial part of the arm and attached fingers undeveloped or the ulnar part of the arm and attached fingers undeveloped; and *transverse hemimelia*, in which a part of a forearm or hand or part or all of the fingers are missing.[116]

Treatment of children with severe congenital amputations consists of fitting them with prostheses as early as 6 months of age. This helps to prevent the formation of habits that might interfere with adapting to the prostheses and also allows the child to interact with the environment through age-appropriate bimanual activities.[121,133] Treatment may also include early referral to an amputee clinic. An interdisciplinary team can work with the child on preprosthetic activities as well as help the family adjust to the child's deficiency.

DISORDERS OF THE LOWER EXTREMITY

Congenital abnormalities of the feet include polydactyly, syndactyly, and assorted adduction (varus) and abduction (valgus) deformities of one or more toes. The treatment of these conditions is very similar to that described for the hands.

The most important abnormality of the foot is *clubfoot*, or talipes equinovarus. The incidence of clubfoot is high (2 per 1,000 live births), with boys being affected twice as often as girls.[1,121] The condition is often bilateral with major clinical features that include forefoot adduction and supination, heel varus, equinus through the ankle, and medial deviation of the foot in relationship to the knee.[1,121] Underdevelopment of the muscles in the lower legs may also be noted.

The exact cause or causes of clubfoot are unclear, but during fetal development something adversely affects the development of the muscles on the medial and posterior aspects of the legs, causing them to be shorter than normal.[1,121] These contractions in turn lead to the bone and joint problems.

Complete correction of clubfoot is very difficult to attain. Many times the deformity will be corrected in infancy only to recur during periods of rapid growth.[121] Initial treatment consists of manually correcting the deformity with gentle pressure and then using one of the following methods for holding the foot in the correct position: casting, metal splints of the Denis Browne type, adhesive strapping, and special boots.[1] Gradually the amount of time the child spends in the piece of equipment is decreased until the child is only in it at night. If progress has not been noted in 2 to 3 months, soft tissue operations such as tendon lengthenings, tendon transfers, and capsulotomies may be performed. Salter[121] states that these early operations can greatly decrease recurrence of the problem.

In older children and in neglected cases or recurrent cases, treatment may have to be geared toward the creation of a plantigrade foot so that the child can walk on the sole of his foot.[1] The soft tissue surgeries mentioned earlier may be used, as well as bony operations such as arthrodesis of joints, osteotomies, and the insertion of a bone wedge on the medial side of the calcaneus to correct the line of weight bearing.[1]

Hypoplasias of the fibula, tibia, and femur are rare but serious congenital abnormalities. Often when the fibula is affected, a built-up foot and brace may help to compensate for the leg length discrepancy. Hypoplasia of the tibia is often unsuccessfully resolved by reconstructive surgery; therefore, amputation is performed at the knee, and the child is subsequently fitted with a prosthesis.

Congenital problems of the knee include hyperextension of the knee, called genu recurvatum, and dislocation of the patella. Genu recurvatum is usually corrected with plaster casts, and dislocation of the patella may require reconstructive soft tissue operations.[121]

Congenital dislocation of the hip is almost as common as clubfoot (1.5 per 1,000 live births) and is also often bilateral, but, unlike clubfoot, many more girls than boys are affected.[121] The causes of congenital hip dislocation (head out of socket) and subluxation (head partially out of socket) are both genetic and environmental. For example, hip laxity may be genetically inherited or may be a result of a hormonal secretion of the uterus.[1] Environmental factors include birth complications from uterine pressure or poor presenting positions. Also, the unstable hip may be dislocated or subluxed by sudden, passive extension or by positioning that maintains the legs extended and adducted.[1,121]

Early diagnosis of this abnormality is critical, because delay can cause serious and permanent disabilities. Three clinical observations that may be used in diagnosing congenital hip dislocation are the Ortolani test, Galeazzi's sign, and Trendelenburg's sign.

The Ortolani test consists of flexing the infant's knees and hips and then alternately adducting and pressing the femur downward and then abducting and lifting the femur. If the hip is unstable, it will dislocate when it is adducted and reduced (back in the socket) as it is abducted.[121] The evaluator will feel and often hear a "click" as this happens. Galeazzi's sign consists of one knee being lower than the other when the child is placed in the supine position on a table with knees flexed to 90 degrees. This results from the dislocated femur lying posteriorly to the acetabulum.[121] Trendelenburg's sign consists of the hips dropping to the opposite side of the dislocation and the trunk shifting toward the dislocated hip when the child is asked to stand on the foot on the affected side.

If treatment is begun within the first few weeks of life, normal development of the hip can nearly always be assured. The longer it goes unresolved, the poorer the prognosis.[1] Specific treatment techniques vary according to the age of the patient when treatment is initiated, but generally the techniques, ranging from those used on the younger child to those used on the older child, include stabilizing the hip in an abducted and flexed position to facilitate femoral and acetabular development. This may be accomplished with splints, traction, the hip spica plaster cast, or the pillow splint.[1,121] If these methods do not correct the problem, a number of surgical procedures may be used to correct bony and soft tissue problems.[1] In severe cases arthrodesis or total replacement arthroplasty may be performed.[1] Again, it should be emphasized that every infant should be examined for this deformity in the first weeks of life to prevent the complications this defect can cause.

Congenital amputations of the lower extremities are not as prevalent as those in the upper extremities.[1,121] They are just as serious when they do occur. Terminology and management strategies are the same as described with the upper extremity amputee.

Implications for occupational therapy

Occupational therapists have worked with children with assorted musculoskeletal problems for many years. Specific treatment goals will vary, depending on the condition and the needs of each child. In general, occupational therapy goals will include assisting with the physical habilitation or rehabilitation of the child; monitoring and fostering development; and working on various self-care, play and leisure, and work skills that the child needs to perform his roles at home, in school, and in the community (Chapter 20).

NEUROMUSCULAR CONDITIONS

This section discusses various diseases and conditions that are of interest to occupational therapists because they primarily interfere with the ability of children to engage in motor interactions with their environment. The site of the damage may be the brain, the anterior horn cells, the peripheral nerves, the neuromuscular junction, or the muscle itself. These diagnostic problems are collectively referred to as neuromuscular conditions.

Selected neuromuscular diseases and conditions

THE MUSCLES

The muscle cells are thought to be the primary site of disease in the muscular dystrophies. All forms of muscular dystrophy are the result of specific genetic defects that cause biochemical and structural changes in the surface and internal membranes of the muscle cells. These changes cause a progressive degeneration and weakness of various muscle groups.[96]

A somewhat debated type of muscular dystrophy is *congenital muscular dystrophy* (CMD). While the literature dates back to the mid-1960s, it does not appear to provide definitive data on incidence, essential features, or long-term follow-up.[80]

It is known that the disease is transmitted by autosomal recessive inheritance. Essential features that have been reported in various studies include hypotonia and multiple joint contractures from birth, general muscle weakness and atrophy, and normal intelligence.[80] Associated problems include clubfoot, torticollis, diaphragmatic involvement, congenital heart defects, and spinal defects.[41,80] Often little to no progression of the disease is seen after childhood, and some functional improvement may be seen around this time.[80]

Diagnosis is made from the presence of high serum levels of the muscle enzyme creatine kinase; by electromyography analysis; and by examination of muscle tissue taken during biopsy. Clinical examination often reveals a "floppy" child with muscle weakness in the face, neck, trunk, and limbs; decreased muscle mass; and absent deep tendon reflexes.[80]

Two other forms of muscular dystrophy are *limb-girdle* and *facioscapulohumeral*. In *limb-girdle muscular dystrophy* the initial muscles affected are the proximal muscles of the pelvic and shoulder girdles. Onset may begin anywhere from the first to the third decade of life, with progression being either slow or moderately rapid. Its hereditary pattern is autosomal recessive like the congenital form.

Facioscapulohumeral muscular dystrophy is autosomal dominant, and onset usually occurs in early adolescence. Although severity varies greatly from patient to patient, involvement is primarily in the face, upper arms, and scapular region, as the name implies. Clinical manifestations include a slope to the shoulders, decreased ability to raise arms above shoulder height, and

decreased mobility in the facial muscles that gives a "masked" appearance.[96]

The most common and the most severe form of muscular dystrophy is called *Duchenne's dystrophy*, which is inherited in a sex-linked recessive manner, affects males, and has an incidence of 0.2 per 1,000 live births.[11]

Symptoms usually begin between the second and sixth years of life. Parents describe their child as having difficulty climbing stairs and rising from a sitting or lying position. The child stumbles and falls excessively and tires easily.[96] A distinctive characteristic of this form is the enlargement of calf muscles and sometimes of forearm and thigh muscles, giving the appearance of strong, healthy muscles. However, this enlargement is caused by extensive fibrosis and proliferation of adipose tissue, which, when combined with the other pathological changes in the muscle tissue, actually causes muscle weakness. This phenomenon is referred to as pseudohypertrophy of muscles.

Involvement begins in the proximal musculature of the pelvic girdle, proceeds to the shoulder girdle, and finally affects all muscle groups. As leg and pelvic muscles weaken, the child will often use his arms to "crawl" up his thighs into a standing position from a kneeling position. This is known as Gower's sign and is diagnostically very significant. Mobility is one of the first functions to be lost, and wheelchair dependence is common by 9 years of age. Gradually the simplest activities of daily living become difficult and then impossible. In the advanced stages of the disease, lordosis and kyphosis are common, as are contractures at various joints. Death, usually as a result of infection, respiratory problems, or cardiovascular complications, often occurs before the early twenties.[96]

At this time there is no treatment that will arrest or reverse the dystrophic process, but antibiotic therapy and other advances in dealing with pulmonary complications have helped to extend life expectancy.[96] Also, the use of orthopedic devices and adaptive equipment and activity can increase mobility, minimize contractures, delay spinal curvatures, and maximize independence in daily activities and thus in role functioning.

THE NEUROMUSCULAR JUNCTION

An example of a disease that affects the neuromuscular junction occasionally in children is *myasthenia gravis*.[92] When this disease enters the body, antibodies are produced that block or greatly reduce the neurotransmitter acetylcholine from being released into the synaptic gap, thus impairing nerve impulses and causing impairment of movement.[11]

Symptoms include drooping of the eyelids, and general muscle weakness that usually worsens as the day progresses.[11] Treatment includes a medication called

TABLE 6-4	Motor types of cerebral palsy and their suspected lesions

Motor types	Suspected site of lesion
Spasticity	Motor portion of cerebral cortex or pyramidal tract
Athetosis	Basal ganglia
Rigidity	Severe decerebrate lesion
Ataxia	Cerebellar lesion
Tremor	Basal ganglia
Atonia	Basal ganglia
Mixed	Many areas of the brain
Unclassified	Varies with combination

Adapted from Batshaw, M.L., and Perret, Y.M.: Children with handicaps: a medical primer, Baltimore, 1981, Paul H. Brookes Publishing Co.; Minear, W.: Pediatrics **18:**841, 1956; and Scherzer, A.L., and Tscharnuter, I.: Early diagnosis and treatment in cerebral palsy: a primer on infant developmental problems, New York, 1982, Marcel Dekker, Inc.

neostigmine that prevents the breakdown of acetylcholine. With medication and proper rest, these children can lead relatively normal lives.

THE PERIPHERAL NERVES

Guillain-Barré syndrome, or acute polyneuropathy, is caused by a virus that infects the peripheral nerve roots. For some reason the body interprets these infected roots as foreign bodies and begins to destroy them: a phenomenon known as an autoimmune response. This disease is normally rare (1 per 100,000 live births), but in 1976 the incidence rose sharply as a complication of the swine flu vaccination program.[11]

Clinical symptoms usually begin with an upper respiratory infection, progress to muscle weakness and paralysis in the lower extremities, and then involve the upper extremities and diaphragm.[11] However, the nerve fibers often regenerate over a period of months, and normal functioning usually returns.[47]

THE ANTERIOR HORN CELLS

Poliomyelitis is a viral disease that affects the anterior horn cells of the spinal cord. In less severe forms of the disease, symptoms may last a few days or weeks and consist of flu-like symptoms with no clinically detectable neurological deficit.[11,115] The paralytic form of polio, on the other hand, progresses quickly to meningitis and muscle weakness, followed by some degree of paralysis.[11] Often, for example, the anterior horn cells of the cervical and lumbar regions are involved, causing quadriplegia and interfering with innervation to the diaphragm and intercostal muscles, thus hampering or completely eliminating the person's ability to breathe independently.[11]

Before 1955 thousands of infants and children con-

tracted poliomyelitis each year, but for the last decade less than 50 cases have been reported in the United States.[115] The reason for this is the highly successful oral polio immunization program recommended for infants between 2 and 4 months of age (Chapter 5).

THE BRAIN

Cerebral palsy is a nonprogressive disorder resulting from brain insults or injuries occurring in the prenatal, perinatal, or infant period of development. It is primarily characterized by aberrant motor control and posture, but sensory difficulties and other associated problems often coincide with the motor difficulties.

Many of the high-risk factors already discussed may cause the lesion or lesions leading to cerebral palsy, but the ones most often described are prematurity, intracranial hemorrhage, neonatal anoxia, poor maternal prenatal conditions, hyperbilirubinemia, multiple pregnancy, and malformations of the central nervous system.[26,125]

In addition, cases of genetically determined lesions that cause specific types of cerebral palsy have been reported. These cases have been attributed to an autosomal dominant pattern of inheritance and have been traced through several generations of the families.[35]

Lesions that develop in the infant period are often caused by trauma, neoplastic factors, intracranial hemorrhages, central nervous system infections, toxicity, or complications surrounding conditions and diseases such as uncontrolled hydrocephalus or sickle-cell anemia.[71,102]

The incidence of cerebral palsy was reported to be 7 per 1,000 live births in 1956,[106] but a survey of more recent studies indicates a range of 0.6 to 2.4 per 1,000 live births.[66] Reasons for this apparent reduction in the overall number of cases include improved obstetrical care, technological advances in prenatal and neonatal care, and improved management of maternal infections and diseases such as rubella, diabetes, and Rh incompatibility.[58,66] For example, the incidence of athetosis has dropped because of improved treatment and prevention of hyperbilirubinemia,[58] and spastic diplegia has been reported to be declining in incidence because of advances in neonatal care.[66]

Injury to the brain often results in various disorders other than motor problems. Depending on the location of the damage, severity of the damage, and time of onset, the associated conditions that are commonly seen are visual and auditory impairments, dental problems, speech problems, sensory integration deficits, seizure disorders, mental retardation, perceptual motor deficits, and emotional problems.[48,71,115]

Since the late 1800s various authors have attempted to classify various types of cerebral palsy. In 1956 Minear[94] developed classifications for the American Academy for Cerebral Palsy (Table 6-4). Scherzer and

TABLE 6-5	Topographic patterns of cerebral palsy

Term	Description of location
Diplegia	Quadriplegia with mild involvement in upper extremities
Hemiplegia	Upper extremity and lower extremity on the same side of the body
Monoplegia	One extremity
Paraplegia	Lower extremities
Quadriplegia	Equal involvement in upper and lower extremities

Adapted from Roberts, K.B.: Manual of clinical problems in pediatrics, Boston, 1979, Little, Brown & Co.; and Scherzer, A.L., and Tscharnuter, I.: Early diagnosis and treatment in cerebral palsy: a primer on infant development problems, New York, 1982, Marcel Dekker, Inc.

Tscharnuter[125] questioned the use of such a fixed classification system today in which referral is made for younger and younger children who demonstrate changes in the manifestations of their lesions as their central nervous systems mature. These authors have suggested classifying the younger children as being developmentally delayed or as having developmental abnormalities in specific areas such as oral, motor, and psychological functioning; then at a later point in their maturation they suggest reevaluating them for classification into the more traditionally used categories.[125]

Cerebral palsy is also classified according to severity and distribution. The terms *mild*, *moderate*, and *severe* are used to describe the degree of involvement. The terms used to describe the topographical patterns of cerebral palsy are in Table 6-5.

The spastic type of cerebral palsy is characterized by abnormally high tone, which makes voluntary movement difficult and limited in range. The tone is often described as being very resistive when an extremity is initially moved, and then it suddenly releases later in the movement pattern. Because this is similar to the movement of a knife blade being closed, it is referred to as the "clasped knife" quality.[11] This form of cerebral palsy may be mild, moderate, or severe, and distribution may be quadriplegic, diplegic, hemiplegic, or sometimes paraplegic.

Symptoms generally associated with spastic cerebral palsy are absent righting reactions, protective extension, and equilibrium reactions; pathological tonic neck and tonic labyrinthine reflexes; and positive supporting reaction. In addition, deformities such as kyphosis, lordosis, heel cord shortening, and flexion contractions often develop as a result of the associated reactions and the abnormal postures and motor patterns.[71]

The symptomatology of pure athetosis is characterized by muscle tone that alternates from being low to being normal, and sometimes to being high.[71] This results in an inability to cocontract and stabilize a joint, which contributes to joint subluxation. Also characteristic of athetosis are slow, writhing involuntary movements that are more distal than proximal. Visible muscle twitches may be present.

Pure athetosis is rare and is more often combined with spasticity, tonic spasms, or chorea, resulting in combinations of symptoms from different types. For example, the athetoid child with spasticity often displays spasticity in proximal areas and athetosis in distal areas[71] and muscle tone fluctuates between normal and high. There may be some control in midranges and some cocontraction may be present in proximal joints, but they often lack selective movement and grading of muscle action.[70] Because of the spasticity, deformities may be present that are not seen in pure athetosis.

The child with athetosis and tonic spasms is faced with muscle tone that changes from low to high. The child has either a tonic spasm or has such low muscle tone that movement is severely hampered. In addition, righting, equilibrium, and protective extension reactions are absent; deformities may develop; and pathological symmetrical and asymmetrical tonic neck reflexes may be present.[71]

Finally, the child with choreoathetosis suffers from muscle tone that fluctuates from low to normal and from low to high. In addition, the chorea movements are jerky, involuntary, and proximally oriented. Hands are weak, and fingers and shoulders are often partially dislocated (subluxation).

Ataxia is characterized by muscle tone that fluctuates from normal to below normal. As with athetosis, it is rare to see this form of cerebral palsy in a pure form. But generally speaking, children with ataxia lack a stable base of support, which limits them to gross, total movement patterns. They appear uncoordinated and clumsy, have poorly timed motor patterns, and have difficulty maintaining or regaining balance. In an attempt to gain stability, these children compensate by adopting primitive or "fixing" patterns.

When infants and young children are flaccid they are often referred to as "floppy." Low muscle tone, lack of flexion, and little to no sensory or stretch feedback create a listless baby who is capable of very little voluntary movement.[71] The low tone also affects respiratory functions, making the child vulnerable to serious respiratory infections. As the child gets older more manifestations of the lesion become apparent, and the child can eventually be placed in the traditional categories that have been mentioned.

These forms of cerebral palsy have been presented in isolation for educational reasons, but it should be remembered that many children with cerebral palsy demonstrate symptoms from one or more of the individual types. This is known as "mixed type" cerebral palsy, and use of this category appears to be on the increase.[125]

A comprehensive medical assessment is necessary with cerebral palsy because of its multiple problems. The physician usually bases the diagnosis on abnormal delays in development that have been observed during physical examinations and on what the parents have reported over a period of months or years. Types of problems that should alert the physician that something may be wrong include: the retention of primitive reflexes, variable tone, hyperresponsive tendon reflexes, asymmetry in the use of extremities, clonus, poor sucking or tongue control, and involuntary movements.[11,115] Another clue might be a large discrepancy between motor and intellectual areas of development.[11]

Medical management of cerebral palsy may encompass pharmacological, orthopedic, and neurosurgical approaches. Many medications have been used in an attempt to help alleviate the motor problems associated with cerebral palsy. For example, dantrolene (Dantrium) and diazepam (Valium), have been reported to reduce spasticity and tone in some children.[11,115] Another medication, levodopa, is believed to have possible benefits with athetoid children.[115]

Orthopedic procedures range from bracing and splinting to orthopedic surgery. Batshaw[11] states that bracing and splinting may be used to maintain range of motion, prevent contractures, improve functioning, and prevent or delay orthopedic surgery. Bracing and splinting may also be used as an integral part of postoperative treatment.

Various surgical procedures may be employed with these children. Some of these procedures are designed to increase range of motion through the release, lengthening, or transfer of affected muscles.[11] For example, a hamstring release might benefit walking, or a transfer of hip adductors might help the child to sit. Surgery may also be needed to correct hip dislocation by releasing the hip adductors and severing their nerve connections.

Although prognosis varies for each type of cerebral palsy, most children with cerebral palsy will live to adulthood, but their life expectancy is less than that of the normal population.[11] Functional prognosis varies greatly from type to type, with hemiplegia and spastic diplegia having a better prognosis than the more severe, rigid types.

Seizures are another example of a group of neuromuscular conditions whose center of dysfunction is in the brain. Seizures are described as periodic stereotyped motor activities associated with impaired consciousness and perception.[115] These characteristics result when abnormal brain cells in the cortex begin to discharge excessive amounts of electricity because of nerve cell de-

polarization.[11] This activity spreads to adjoining cells, causing a seizure.

Some seizures may be directly attributed to the factor or factors that trigger the seizure. For example, acute factors often described are hypoglycemia, fever, trauma, hemorrhages, tumors, infections, and anoxia.[11,115] Other seizures may be attributed to previous scarring and structural damage or to hormonal changes.[115] Many seizures, especially in children, have no discernible underlying disease and are therefore idiopathic in nature.

Many authors classify seizures by their clinical characteristics or symptoms. With this form of categorization there are four major types of seizures: (1) grand mal seizures that account for 40% to 50% of the total incidence, (2) petit mal seizures that occur 12% to 15% of the time, (3) focal or psychomotor seizures that occur 5% of the time, and (4) mixed-type seizures that account for the remainder.[115]

A child having a grand mal seizure may have an aura, or sensation that the seizure is about to begin. This is usually followed by a loss of consciousness during which the body becomes rigid or tonic, and then rhythmical clonic contractions of all the extremities occur. Incontinence is frequent. The seizure may last for 5 minutes followed by a postictal period that may last from 1 to 2 hours in which the child is drowsy or in a deep sleep.[11,115]

Petit mal seizures are characterized by a momentary loss of awareness and no motor activity except eye blinking or rolling. There is no aura, the seizures usually last only 5 to 10 seconds, and there is no postictal period. One important factor to remember with this type of seizure is that they are frequently mistaken for "daydreaming." Petit mal seizures are common in children and in early adolescents, but they are seldom seen after the age of 15.[115]

Psychosocial seizures, or temporal lobe seizures, may consist of tonic-clonic movements, but they also show automatic reactions such as lip smacking, chewing, and buttoning and unbuttoning clothing. In addition, the individual may appear to be confused and disorganized, and he may have sensory experiences such as smelling and tasting items not in the environment and hearing sounds of various types.[11,115]

Minor motor seizures include those found in infancy.[90] The most common type of seizure in infancy is the febrile seizure. This is often a single, brief episode that is precipitated by fever and usually is unassociated with either prior or residual neurological signs or with an abnormal electroencephalogram (EEG).[115]

Two other mild forms of seizures are (1) myoclonic seizures that consist of contractions by single or small groups of muscles and (2) akinetic seizures in which the primary problem is a loss of muscle tone.[11]

A child who has a seizure must undergo a thorough

evaluation so that the factors causing the seizure can be determined. A family history, medical history, and developmental history must be completed, as well as an electroencephalogram to help determine the type of seizure.

Anticonvulsive medications are administered in an attempt to control the seizures. In theory these medications increase the intensity required to trigger the seizure or eliminate the recruitment of surrounding cells. Batshaw[11] and Roberts[115] have described the commonly administered anticonvulsive medications and their most common side effects, which include cataracts, weight gain, high blood pressure, pathological fractures, drowsiness, hair loss or gain, nausea, liver damage, vomiting, gum enlargement, hyperactivity, anorexia, and lymphoma-like syndrome. These various side effects are specific to the various medications prescribed, such as adrenocorticotropic hormone (ACTH), valproic acid (Depakene), phenytoin (Dilantin), phenobarbital, and ethosuximide (Zarontin).

Implications for occupational therapy

The services provided by occupational therapists to children with neuromuscular problems are steeped in years of tradition. Roles are well established and usually understood and accepted by parents and other professionals. With some of these children the first concern is to provide them with normal sensory and motor experiences. Another important goal is to position and support them so that they may begin to develop specific skills. In other children the focus may be on other aspects of daily functioning, such as selecting leisure activities or learning to drive or selecting activities that will foster vocational development (Chapters 16, 19, and 24).

DEVELOPMENTAL DISABILITIES

This section addresses other developmental disabilities found in childhood, namely, autism, learning disabilities, and mental retardation. In general, the developmental disabilities are characterized by prenatal, perinatal, or early childhood onset, and each disability has the potential to affect all areas of the child's development and to impair the child's performance of many functional tasks and skills.

Autism

Autism is one of the most devastating of the chronic developmental disabilities because of the unusual combinations of sensorimotor and behavioral characteristics displayed by these children.

The National Society for Autistic Children estimates that approximately 5 autistic children are born per 10,000 live births and that four times as many boys as girls are afflicted with the disorder.[7] Autistic children are found in families of all racial, ethnic, intellectual, and socioeconomic backgrounds.[103]

The disorder is complicated by the fact that it often coexists with other problems such as mental retardation, seizure disorders, and a number of diseases associated with organic brain damage. The fact that a large percentage of autistic children also suffer from cognitive deficiencies has been a controversial but relatively accepted issue. For example, Ornitz[103] explains that the cognitive deficiencies exhibited by autistic children are just as real as in mentally retarded children and that 75% of the autistic children can be expected to perform at a retarded level throughout their lives. DeMyer and others[39] state that 70% of these children have IQ scores lower than 35. The National Society for Autistic Children estimates that 60% of all autistic children have IQ scores below 50; 20% have IQ scores between 50 and 70; and 20% have scores of 70 or more.[7]

As mentioned earlier, autism is often seen in conjunction with conditions that are associated with brain damage, including phenylketonuria, congenital rubella, Addison's disease, celiac disease, retrolental fibroplasia, cerebral lipidosis, and infantile spasms.[36,78,113] Seizure disorders also occur in high incidence in autistic children. Both psychomotor and grand mal seizures have been reported in the autistic population.[36,78]

In the almost 40 years since Leo Kanner[74] first identified 11 children as having "extreme autistic aloneness," many theories have been suggested for autism. At first it was hypothesized that the parents' inability to provide appropriate nurture because of their extreme personality types and traits or because of their psychopathies caused the child to withdraw socially and become autistic.[14,30] Next came the theorists who proposed that various hereditary and biological factors were present but that the parents were still at least partially responsible for causing the syndrome.[109] These theorists were followed by ones who focused on the "psychological" problem of the child. During this period autistic children were described under the term *childhood schizophrenia*.[13,67] Today there is general agreement among most researchers that the syndrome of autism is caused by organic brain pathology. However, at this time the location of the exact affected site or sites in the central nervous system is not certain, nor are the factors that cause this organic pathology known.

The behavioral characteristics of autism are usually manifested before 30 months of age and may be categorized into five subclusters.[103] Disturbances in relating to persons and things affect the autistic child's ability to establish meaningful relationships with people and inanimate objects. While abnormalities in this area vary with age and degree of severity, they directly involve interactions that require initiative or reciprocal behavior from the child. Specific behaviors that are observed are poor or deviant eye contact, delayed or total lack of a social smile, apparent aversion to physical contact, delayed or absent anticipatory response to being picked up, and an apparent preference for being alone.[88,103] Disturbances in relating to inanimate objects are often observed during the play of autistic children. Many times a toy or an object is not used in the manner that it was intended but instead is twirled, spun, flicked, tapped, or in other ways manipulated, arranged or rearranged. In addition, the autistic child's use of play materials is often rigid and inflexible; these children seldom demonstrate cooperative and imaginative play.[153]

Disturbances in communication may be thought of as being on a continuum from severe to mild. At the severe end of the continuum appears a complete lack of speech, or mutism. At the other end of the continuum normal language accompanied by only slight articulation or tonal deficits may be seen. Many other communication problems have been described at points along the continuum. For instance, much of the speech of autistic children is repetitive, or echolalic, in nature. Classic echolalia consists of parrotlike repetitions of phrases immediately after the child has been exposed to them, while delayed or deferred echolalia consists of the repetition of phrases at a later time. Echolalic speech occurs out of social context and appears to have little or no communicative value. Other types of speech and language problems include syntax problems, atonal and arrhythmic speech, pronoun reversals, and a lack of inflection and emotion during communication.[111]

Onset can occur at either of two times, as described in the literature: at birth and anytime up to the age of 30 months. But regardless of the time of onset, most autistic children display disturbances of their developmental rate. Specifically, they will show deviations and discontinuities in the normal sequence of motor, language, and social milestones.[53,54] For example, an autistic child may demonstrate the ability to perform one task precociously, such as sitting up, but another motor task, such as pulling to the standing position, may be delayed well past the normal time. Or the child may walk on time but not learn to run until many years later.

Disturbances of motility are considered to be indicative of central nervous system dysfunction in autistic children.[38,112] Deviant motility may involve the arms, hands, trunk, lower extremities, or entire body. Motor patterns in the upper extremities are very common and include wiggling and flicking of fingers, alternating flexion and extension of the fingers, and alternating pronation and supination of the forearm.[112] Other motility patterns often seen include head rolling and banging, body rocking and swaying, lunging and darting movements, toe walking, dystonia of the extremities, invol-

untary synergies of the head and proximal segments of the limbs, and an inability to perform two motor acts at the same time.[31,38]

Disturbances of sensory processing and perception have been reported in autistic children for almost 20 years. Eric Schopler[126] in 1965 first described the abnormal responses of autistic children to various visual, vestibular, and auditory stimuli. Since then many research studies have attempted to unearth and describe these various dysfunctions by using techniques such as film microanalysis, electronystagmography, sensory-evoked potentials, and many less technical methods.[28]

A. Jean Ayres[9] describes two types of sensory processing problems in autistic children. The first deals with the registration of, or orientation to, sensory input. It appears that in autistic children the neurophysiological processes that decide what sensory stimuli will be brought to their attention are working correctly sometimes but not at others.[9] Therefore they react normally to sensory stimuli one minute, and the next minute (hour or day) they may overreact or underreact to the same stimuli.

The second sensory processing disturbance described by Ayres involves the control or modulation of a stimulus once it has entered the system.[9] Again, the autistic child is believed to be capable of exerting control at times but not at other times, resulting in a child who processes tactile information normally at times and who at other times appears to be the victim of uncontrolled overstimulation—the tactiley defensive child.

While most autistic children have normal life expectancies, the functional prognosis has not been good to date. In 1967 Rutter and Lockyer[120] reported in follow-up studies of autistic children that fewer than 2% were functioning effectively and holding a job in the community; 50% were institutionalized; and the remainder were at home functioning at various levels but needing considerable help from the family. Cerreto[24] predicted that about 20% of the autistic children should be capable of making a good social adjustment and able to lead an independent life and work; another 20% will need help in adjusting to life and work; and 60% will remain severely handicapped and be unable to live independently. These prognostic figures may be accurate indicators of the overall potential of these children, or they may simply reflect the state of the art today in diagnosing and treating these children's special problems.

As no one method of treatment has yet proved to be totally effective in treating autism, an interdisciplinary approach is usually selected. The role of the physician on the interdisciplinary team is to make appropriate referrals, offer support to the parents, monitor the child's progress, and often prescribe medications. The medications used with these children are varied: sedatives, stimulants, major and minor tranquilizers, antihistamines, antidepressants, and psychotomimetics.[103]

It is felt that these medications work best when used in conjunction with attempts at corrective socialization and special education.[103]

Learning disabilities

Many different labels are used synonymously with the term *learning disabilities*. Some of the more common labels that have been applied are the following:

Minimal brain dysfunction (MBD)

Minimal brain injured (MBI)

Minimal cerebral dysfunction (MCD)

Slow learner

Educationally handicapped

Educationally maladjusted

Special learning disorder

Neurologically handicapped

Neurologically impaired

Perceptually handicapped

Specific language disorder

Dyslexia

Hyperactive child

Attention deficit

Why so many labels? First of all, these terms reflect the jargon of the large number of professionals from both the educational and health fields who have become involved with these children. Also reflected in these terms are the demands, preferences, and restrictions of parental and political groups and agencies.

Defining learning disabilities has been as difficult as labeling the condition. Many "official" definitions are available, but the following definition taken from Public Law 94-142, the Education for All Handicapped Children Act,[146] has been the most influential:

> A disorder in one or more of the basic psychological processes involved in understanding or in using language, spoken or written, which may manifest itself in an imperfect ability to listen, think, speak, read, write or do mathematical calculations.

The learning disabled child has average or above average intelligence, has adequate sensory acuity (is not blind or deaf), and has been provided with appropriate learning opportunities. In spite of all these positive features, there is a significant discrepancy between the child's academic potential and the child's educational performance.

While different studies and agencies report varying incidence figures, the figure most often given is approximately 10% of the school population. As with autism, more boys than girls are affected, in this instance a 4:1 ratio.[11]

A child with learning disabilities may display any number of the behaviors listed under the following eight categories[29]:

Disorders of motor function include both motor skills and motor activity level. Motor skills dysfunctions may range from clumsiness, to poor performance in gross or fine motor skills, to problems planning new tasks (dyspraxia), to reflex and equilibrium problems, to sensorimotor problems in a number of areas. Occasionally tics, grimaces, and choreoathetoid movements in the hands may be seen. The child may be described as always being in motion (hyperactive) or being slow and lethargic (hypoactive).

Educational disorders can occur in one or more academic subjects. Related educational skills that are often described as being dysfunctional in a learning disabled child are copying from the blackboard, printing and cursive writing, the organization of time and materials, understanding written and oral directions, symbolic confusion (reversals of letters, and so on), cutting, coloring and pasting, and keeping place on the page.

Disorders of attention and concentration include short attention span and other attentional deficits, restlessness, impulsivity, and motor and verbal perseveration.

Characteristics included under *disorders of thinking and memory* are poor ability for abstract reasoning, difficulty with concept formation, and poor short- and long-term memory.

Difficulties with speech and communication may include difficulty shifting topics of conversation and difficulty with "small talk," the sequencing of words, sentences or sounds, slurred words, and articulation errors.

Auditory difficulties usually associated with learning disabled children often stem from auditory perceptual problems and not acuity (hearing) problems. Examples of various auditory perception problems are the child who cannot remember the oral directions just given to him or who cannot benefit from sounding words out and blending them or who cannot learn the different vowel sounds. The high incidence of allergies and ear infections in learning disabled children puts them at risk for auditory perceptual problems.

Learning disabled children often have various *sensory integrative and perceptual disorders*. Because the base of support (good tone and cocontraction, integrated reflexes, functional postural and equilibrium reactions, and adequate processing and modulation of sensory input) is weak in many of these children, they are not adequately prepared for various laterality and directionality concepts and tasks that require visual perception skills. Their specific sensory integration problems will be discussed in Chapter 19.

Last but not least, learning disabled children may demonstrate *psychosocial problems* such as throwing temper tantrums or demonstrating antisocial behavior. Their social competencies may be delayed based not only on their ages but also on their intelligence. Many of these children are sensitive and decidedly at risk for poor self-esteem and self-concept problems, because they have the intelligence to know when they are being teased and to know the frustration of being good at some things and not at others.

It appears that a number of factors can cause learning disabilities. In some cases, heredity appears to be a possibility, allergies are another factor, sensory integrative dysfunctions have been found in others, and all the prenatal, perinatal, and early childhood factors that have been mentioned earlier are potential contributors.

The role of the physician in the management of learning disabilities is similar to that with autistic children: referrals are made when special evaluations and services are needed, the child's progress is monitored, parental support and guidance are provided, and, on occasion medications are prescribed to control agitation and hyperactivity.

The prognosis for learning disabled children is the best of all the developmental disabilities. Although most will retain some degree of learning disability as adults, the vast majority will be contributing members of society.[72] As with all disorders, prognosis will be affected by the severity of the disability. Therefore the milder learning disabled persons should not be limited in their life and career skills. But those with severe learning disabilities may need vocational planning and counseling and minor adaptations to ensure as high a level of social, emotional, and vocational functioning as possible.

Mental retardation

The following definition for mental retardation is from Public Law 94-142, the Education for All Handicapped Children Act[146]:

> . . . significant subaverage general intellectual functioning existing concurrently with deficits in adaptive behavior and manifested during the developmental period, which adversely affects a child's educational performance.

This means that to be labeled mentally retarded an individual must score 2 or more standard deviations below the mean on a standardized IQ test, the individual must be impaired in the ability to adapt to the environment, and the cause of the mental retardation must have occurred prenatally to age 18 years.

Four degrees of severity are usually given: *mild, moderate, severe,* and *profound.* Figure 6-4 shows the bimodal distribution of intelligence. It also shows the levels of severity as they relate to this distribution. Mildly, or educable, mentally retarded children have an IQ range of 55 to 69. Characteristics include the ability to learn academic skills at the third to seventh grade level and the usual achievement of social and vocational skills adequate to minimal self-support (67% are employed and 80% are married[115]).

Moderately, or trainable, mentally retarded children have an IQ range of 40 to 54. This group is unlikely to progress past the second grade level in academics; they can usually handle routine daily functions and do unskilled or semiskilled work in sheltered workshop conditions. Some type of group home or supervised housing situation is usually the best placement for these individuals.

Severely retarded children have an IQ range of 25 to 39. These individuals can usually learn to communicate, they can be trained in elemental health habits, and they require supervision to accomplish most tasks.

Profoundly retarded children have IQs below 25. These children need nursing care for basic survival skills. Usually they have minimal capacity for sensorimotor or self-care functioning.

It has been estimated that there are over 300 causes of mental retardation.[51] These causes are usually categorized under the following headings: acquired conditions (toxins, trauma, infection, prematurity); chromosomal problems; multiple congenital anomaly syndromes; central nervous system malformations; neuro-

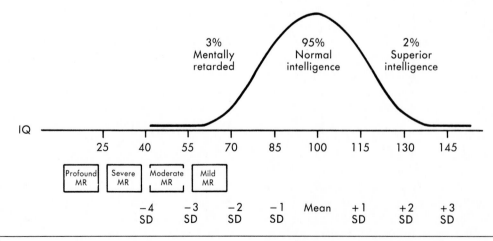

FIGURE 6-4

Criteria for determining the four degrees of severity in mental retardation.

cutaneous syndromes; and metabolic and endocrine disorders.

Approximately 80% of retarded children have additional problems.[115] For example, it is estimated that approximately 50% have speech problems, 50% have ambulation problems, 20% have seizures, 25% have visual problems, and 40% have chronic conditions such as heart disease, diabetes, anemia, obesity, and dental problems.[115]

The physician's role begins with a history that focuses on gestation, neonatal events, illnesses, and developmental progress.[115] During the physical examination all major and minor abnormalities must be identified to detect the possibility of a syndrome.[115] In addition, laboratory tests such as chromosomal analysis, metabolic tests, and EEGs may be ordered. Referrals for psychological, educational, developmental, and speech and hearing evaluations may be made and then interpreted for the parents. Services must be determined, and parents, siblings, and other family members must be given support and advice.

Today the emphasis in the field of mental retardation is toward deinstitutionalization, normalization, and providing mentally retarded individuals with every opportunity to be able to reach their maximal level of functioning in the least restrictive environment. Now more than ever the community is an integral component of the treatment process.

Implications for occupational therapy

Occupational therapists have been working with mentally retarded and autistic children for many years. What has changed is the expanded number of settings for therapy. Not long ago, mentally retarded children, no matter what their level of functioning, were institutionalized because that is where the services were offered. The same situation was true for autistic children. Today there is a varied continuum of program options available to these children. These options are offered not only by institutions but also by private developmental centers, public and private schools, governmental agencies, and parent and professional groups.

The most recent developmental disability to be of concern to occupational therapists is learning disabilities. Today a substantial percentage of occupational therapists work with learning disabled children in school-based practice (Chapters 17, 19, and 24).

RESPIRATORY PROBLEMS

This section discusses three major chronic respiratory conditions found in children. In addition, it discusses otitis media, which, while located in the ear, often accompanies upper respiratory infections, colds, and allergic conditions.

Selected diseases and conditions

CYSTIC FIBROSIS

Cystic fibrosis (CF) is an autosomal recessive inherited disorder in which the mucus secreted by various exocrine glands becomes abnormally thick and sticky.[115] Exactly what causes these changes is unknown. Cystic fibrosis is found almost exclusively in Caucasians and has an incidence of approximately 1 in 2,000 live births.[11]

Chronic pulmonary disease is the most serious complication of cystic fibrosis.[115] A chronic cough, wheezing, lower respiratory infections, abscesses and cysts, hemoptysis, and recurrent pneumothorax are all examples of the serious pulmonary complications that develop in cystic fibrosis. Other complications often related to cystic fibrosis are: clubbing of the fingers resulting from hypoxemia, nasal polyps, and enlargement of the right side of the heart (right ventricular hypertrophy), which may eventually cause heart failure.[40]

Pancreatic insufficiency causes characteristic foul smelling and greasy stools. Associated problems include malabsorption; clinical diabetes; deficiencies of vitamins A, E, and K; and gastrointestinal obstruction.[115]

In the liver, bile ducts often become blocked, resulting in destruction of cells behind the blocked ducts. While this is a serious problem, a positive point is that children's livers are often capable of regeneration.

In the female reproductive system the ovaries are not affected, and the child does not become infertile, but problems are commonly found with the cervical mucous glands. In the male the testes are not affected, but sterility does occur often because of the fact that sperm cannot travel through the vas deferens.

Also in cystic fibrosis the sodium absorption inhibiting factor is affected, which causes excessive amounts of sodium chloride to be secreted from the sweat glands onto the skin. This phenomenon provides important diagnostic information that is often gathered in two vastly different but important ways. First, mothers often detect that their children taste salty when they kiss them. This alerts the physician who will perform the simple diagnostic test known as the "sweat test." In this test an electrode is placed on the skin, causing the child to sweat at the contact site. A sample of the sweat is taken. If excessive levels of sodium chloride are detected, the diagnosis is made.[115]

Medical management consists of vigorous antibiotic, enzyme, and vitamin therapy and sound nutritional counseling. In an effort to keep the lungs as free as possible, the following physical or respiratory therapy techniques may be employed: mist tent therapy, intermittent positive pressure breathing, aerosol therapy, and postural drainage techniques.[115]

The prognosis for cystic fibrosis is not good. Some

of these children die in infancy, while others may do relatively well until adolescence, when there is some evidence that girls do more poorly than boys.[85,134] The life spans of children with cystic fibrosis are slowly lengthening as a result of improved maintenance techniques, but many still die before they are 20 years old.

OTITIS MEDIA

Otitis media is one of the most common infections in children. The eustachian tube becomes blocked, and fluid forms in the middle ear. *Pneumococcus, Hemophilus influenzae,* and *Streptococcus* are the usual pathogens found. Symptoms may include pain, a sense of fullness in the ear, irritability, and rhinorrhea.[115]

Three types of otitis media are described: (1) serous, (2) suppurative, and (3) chronic serous otitis media (CSOM), the chronic form often found in children with allergies.

The goal of treatment is to eradicate the organisms, clear the fluids, and prevent chronic serous otitis media.[16] This is accomplished by the administration of antibiotics such as penicillin, ampicillin, amoxicillin, or sulfonamides.[16] The insertion of tympanostomy tubes may be necessary in more chronic cases. Children with histories of otitis media should have their hearing acuity and auditory perceptual skills evaluated, because disuse of the auditory system as a result of the presence of the fluid can cause specific perceptual problems.

ASTHMA

Asthma is characterized by bronchial hyperreactivity that causes airway constriction in the lower respiratory tract and reported bouts of wheezing. Roberts[115] reported that approximately 5% of the boys and 3% of the girls under 15 years of age suffer from hay fever or asthma.

Many factors can cause the wheezing. If it is evoked by external factors, such as dust, it is called *extrinsic asthma,* and if it is evoked by internal stimuli, such as infection, it is called *intrinsic asthma.* In many instances a multifactorial etiology exists, which consists of environmental sensitivity and familial predisposition.

Status asthmaticus is a serious asthmatic condition in which normal outpatient assistance does not improve the condition and emergency medical intervention is needed.

Treatment for asthma may include environmental control measures, skin testing, immunotherapy for allergies, emotional support, and usually a combination of two classes of pharmacological agents: methylxanthine and beta-adrenergic agonists.[25]

TUBERCULOSIS OF THE LUNGS

Tuberculosis of the lungs is one of the oldest diseases reported to be found in humans. It is an infectious disease caused when the tubercle bacillus is inhaled into the lungs. Symptoms include fatigue, a persistent cough, hemoptysis, and chest pain.[139] Lesions occur in one or more lobes of the lungs. It is not uncommon for individual lesions to heal by calcification, thus allowing the disease to go into an inactive or arrested stage.[139]

A number of different tuberculin tests may be performed that indicate whether an individual has ever been infected or exposed to tubercle bacillus. However, these tests do not reveal whether the infection is currently active or inactive. These tests consist of applying tuberculin to the skin directly or intradermally and then watching for a local inflammatory reaction within 48 to 72 hours or 48 to 96 hours, depending on the test administered. Diagnosis may also be done through the examination of sputum samples and through chest x-ray films.

Treatment consists of chemotherapy using medications such as ethambutol, isoniazid (INH), para-aminosalicylic acid (PAS), or streptomycin.[115] Bed rest and nutritional counseling may also be recommended. In advanced cases various surgical procedures may be required.

While tuberculosis is not as prevalent as it was 20 years ago, it is still found in certain parts of the country and is more prevalent among certain populations, such as American Indians.

Implications for occupational therapy

Occupational therapy involvement with children with respiratory problems may occur at two different levels. At the secondary level the occupational therapist must be aware of complications, signs, and symptoms and possibly adjust some treatment methods. This situation would occur in those cases where the respiratory situation was secondary and probably an acute problem to the patient's major handicapped condition. Many days of treatment are missed because of respiratory illnesses.

On a primary level of involvement the occupational therapist might be directly involved in the treatment of the respiratory condition or disease. This might involve the implementation of activities to improve respiratory output, help with energy conservation, or direct concern with deficit self-care, play, and leisure activities or work tasks.

CONGENITAL CARDIAC DEFECTS

This section discusses the major cardiovascular conditions found in the neonatal and early childhood periods of life. Congenital heart defects are second only to problems concerned with prematurity when the leading causes of death in pediatric hospitals are determined.[76]

Patent ductus arteriosus (PDA) was discussed earlier in the perinatal section of this chapter. The other major types of congenital heart conditions will be described here. They are atrial septal defects, ventricular septal defects, tetralogy of Fallot, and transposition of the great vessels. In addition, rheumatic fever will be discussed, because it is one of the most serious cardiac illnesses found in children.

Atrial septal defects

When an opening in the septum between the right and left atrial chambers occurs, it is called an atrial septal defect (ASD). This opening may be of any size and can occur anywhere along the septum. As a result, when the left atrium contracts, blood is sent into the right atrium. This is called a left-to-right shunt and causes more blood than normal to be sent to the lungs, resulting in "wet lungs," a condition that makes the lungs more susceptible to upper respiratory infections. This also causes the right atrium, and especially the right ventricle, to work much harder, and it can eventually cause heart failure in the older child. Other symptoms include poor exercise tolerance and the appearance of being thin and small for age. Information for diagnosis is gathered from listening to the characteristics of the murmur, evaluating chest x-ray films and electrocardiograms, and administering heart catheterization.

Surgical procedures are not routinely done until the child is 4 or 5 years of age. Until that time, the child is closely watched for complications, especially signs of heart failure.

Ventricular septal defects

Ventricular septal defects (VSD) are the most common type of congenital cardiac malformations and are often more serious than atrial septal defects.[115] This type of defect consists of a hole or opening in the muscular or membranous portions of the ventricular septum.

Etiological factors are often idiopathic, but congenital infections, various teratogenic agents, and genetic predisposition may also contribute to the cause.[49]

In these defects the blood flows from the left ventricle to the right ventricle, a left-to-right shunt, and as in an atrial septal defect, an increased amount of blood is pumped to the lungs. The defect is considered more serious if the opening is in the membranous section of the septum, because the size of the hole is not, at least somewhat, diminished during contraction as happens in openings in the muscular part of the septum.

Symptoms associated with this defect include feeding problems, shortness of breath and increased perspiration, fatigue during physical activity, increased incidences of respiratory infections, and delayed growth.

As in atrial septal defects, the diagnosis is based on the murmur, chest x-ray film results, electrocardiograms, and heart catheterization. In these defects improvement often occurs after 6 months of age, and over 50% of the cases correct themselves by the age of 5 years.[33] However, if the extent of damage is great, or if the hole does not repair itself, surgical procedures to close the defect may need to be undertaken early in the child's life.

Careful monitoring of these children must occur to prevent the life-threatening situation known as Eisenmenger's complex. In this situation pulmonary vascular obstruction has occurred as a result of prolonged exposure to increased blood flow and high pressure. Eventually the heart is no longer capable of pumping against the increased pulmonary pressure, and blood pools in the right ventricle. This poses a medical emergency, requiring immediate surgical intervention.

The prognosis for infants with ventricular septal defects continues to improve as both surgical techniques and management of heart failure progress.[115]

Tetralogy of Fallot

As the name implies, there are four different problems associated with tetralogy of Fallot: (1) pulmonary valve or artery stenosis plus (2) ventricular septal defect present prenatally causing (3) a right ventricular hypertrophy, and (4) overriding of the ventricular septum by the aorta.[115]

The etiological factors are probably similar to those described under ventricular septal defects, but it is felt that they must occur in the early weeks of fetal development when the right ventricle is at a critical stage.[75]

Physiologically the unoxygenated blood that is returning from the body cannot easily exit to the lungs because of the pulmonary stenosis. Instead, it takes two paths of least resistance: the defect, creating a right-to-left shunt, and the aorta.

Symptoms include central cyanosis, coagulation defects, clubbing of fingers and toes, feeding difficulties, failure to thrive, dyspnea, and "tet" spells during which the child suddenly squats to his knees. It is believed that this squatting action raises systemic vascular resistance and decreases the shunting.[75]

Diagnosis is usually based on cyanosis; analysis of the heart murmur; right ventricular hypertrophy and right axis deviation demonstrated on the electrocardiogram; a chest x-ray film revealing the characteristic "boot-shaped heart"; and echocardiography demonstrating the overriding aorta.[75,115]

Management consists of medication to reduce the

frequency and severity of the "tet" spells.[115] Surgery is ideally delayed as long as possible. In severe cases a temporary shunt may be put in to bypass the stenosis. Later, "total correction" surgery is done in which the pulmonary outflow obstruction is removed, the VSD is closed, and the aorta may be enlarged.

As with VSD, prognosis is improving as techniques and maintenance improve. Operative mortality has been reduced to 20%,[115] but surgery is still a dangerous and complicated procedure.

Transposition of the great vessels

Transposition of the great vessels involves the anatomical transfer of the great arteries. Severity depends on the amount of mixing between the two sides of circulation.[76] This can be accomplished by coexisting congenital cardiac defects, such as a VSD, or a pulmonary stenosis, or congenital transposition of the ventricles, called *corrected transposition*.[115] The severity of the symptoms varies, but cyanosis, congestive heart failure, and respiratory distress are common.

Diagnosis may be helped by the use of echocardiography, which can help identify the transposition, and by heart catheterization.

Treatment techniques include enlarging the foramen ovale by inserting a catheter with a balloon tip through the foramen ovale and into the left atrium. Next the catheter is pulled back through the foramen ovale to enlarge it, thus increasing the flow of oxygenated blood to the right atrium.[115] Another procedure involves excising the atrial septum and inserting a patch that redirects the blood flow. A third technique that is very new involves severing the great vessels at their bases and reattaching them to the proper ventricles.[115]

Rheumatic fever

Acute rheumatic fever occurs from 2 to 4 weeks after an acute infection of streptococcal pharyngitis. The incidence of rheumatic fever has geen greatly reduced in the past century but should still be considered a potentially dangerous condition.

School-aged children are most frequently affected, especially following a streptococcal pharyngitis epidemic. Rheumatic fever usually begins with one of the following serious symptoms: carditis, polyarthritis, or chorea.[115]

As there is no laboratory test specific for diagnosing rheumatic fever, a combination of factors from the following diagnostic criteria must be substantiated[46]:

Minor criteria	Major criteria
Clinical	Carditis
Arthralgia	Polyarthritis
Fever	Erythema
History of infection in recent weeks	marginatum
	Chorea
	Subcutaneous nodules
Lab	
Increased erthrocyte sedimentation rate	
Presence of C-reactive protein (CRP)	

Treatment consists of prescribing bed rest plus administering antibodies (usually penicillin) and antiinflammatory agents. Most patients will take penicillin from the time of diagnosis until approximately 15 to 20 years of age as a preventive measure to prevent recurrence. It appears that a high percentage of children who experienced carditis during the first phase of rheumatic fever will experience future heart problems.[115]

Implications for occupational therapy

As in the case of respiratory conditions, the involvement of occupational therapy in congenital cardiac defects may be direct or indirect. For example, congenital heart defects are often found as secondary diagnoses in handicapped children. Children with Down's syndrome or other types of mental retardation and multiply handicapped children may have histories of congenital heart problems. In these cases occupational therapists must be aware of the associated signs, symptoms, treatment procedures, and medications to watch for complications and for the effect of these conditions on the child's functioning.

Direct involvement might include participation on a pediatric rehabilitation team. In this instance the occupational therapist would be concerned with physical restoration as well as the monitoring of various developmental and functional skills.

HEMATOLOGICAL PROBLEMS
Selected diseases and disorders

The following selected blood diseases and disorders found in children are reviewed in this section: sickle-cell anemia, hemophilia, and idiopathic thrombocytopenic purpura.

SICKLE-CELL ANEMIA

Sickle-cell anemia is a hereditary, chronic form of anemia in which abnormal sickle, or cresent-shaped, erythrocytes are present that contain an abnormal type of hemoglobin called Hemoglobin S.[130] In the United States most cases occur in black Americans, of whom 1 in 10 are carriers of the trait, and 1 in every 400 to 600 black neonates have the disease.[114]

The clinical course of children with sickle-cell anemia is interspersed with episodes of severe worsening called *sickle-cell crises* that can be grouped into four types.[130] *Aplastic* and *hyperhemolytic crises* are characterized by imbalances in the production and premature destruction of red blood cells, which may cause the hemoglobin to decrease by 50%, necessitating immediate transfusions. *Sequestrian crises* consist of the sudden and rapid enlargement of the spleen. This type of sickle-cell anemia traps much of the blood volume and can possibly cause shock or death. Painful, or *vaso-occlusive crises* are characterized by pain in the hands, feet, toes, and abdomen.

Sickle-cell anemia affects other organs as well. Lungs may become infected, and hypoxemia is common; liver and kidney involvement causes urine problems and hematuria; cerebrovascular accidents may occur; the legs develop ulcers; and spleen damage can leave the child defenseless against major infections.[130]

Medical management is limited to the treatment of symptoms: transfusions, antibiotic therapy, and making the child comfortable. Prognosis is poor, since this is a disease that is both physically painful and potentially emotionally crippling as well.[115] A prenatal determining procedure is currently being developed that offers new hope for this disease.[3]

HEMOPHILIA

The hemophilias are characterized by greatly prolonged coagulation time (clotting) that results in abnormal bleeding. They are sex-linked hereditary disorders and occur almost exclusively in males.[130]

There are two major types. Hemophilia A, or classic hemophilia, is caused by a deficiency of a factor in plasma necessary for blood coagulation. This factor has been called factor VIII, antihemophilic globulin, and antihemophilic factor.[139] Hemophilia B (Christmas disease) results from a deficiency of clotting factor IX.

Symptoms are not usually noticeable or bothersome until near the end of the first year of life, then soft tissue hemorrhages begin to occur. The intracranial hemorrhage is one of the most dreaded and serious complications of hemophilia. Bleeding into joints (hemarthrosis) can cause severe musculoskeletal problems that can lead to joint deterioration if untreated. The following procedures can be used to protect the joints: blood can be drained from a joint; chemical agents can be injected into the joint; and a specific preventive range of motion activities can be initiated. Surgical procedures, such as joint replacements or synovectomies contain some element of risk for hemophiliac patients.[114]

Soft tissue hemorrhages and hemarthroses are treated at home by replacing the missing factor to a level that will again control the bleeding. This is called *replacement therapy*, and most children can be trained to administer their own infusions.

The prognosis is steadily improving for this disease. The average age of death is 52 years.[83]

IDIOPATHIC THROMBOCYTOPENIC PURPURA

The central problem in idiopathic thrombocytopenic purpura (ITP) is the fact that the blood platelets are being destroyed faster than they can be produced. Simply stated, patients with this disease develop antibodies that destroy their own platelets.

About one half of the children with idiopathic thrombocytopenic purpura have had an infectious illness within 6 weeks of the diagnosis. These cases have a better prognosis, with 90% recovering.[139] Symptoms include bleeding from the mouth and skin when injured, intracranial hemorrhage, increased clotting time, and hemorrhages in internal organs.[87] Treatment with corticosteroids may help, but these agents have longrange side effects. Platelet transfusions and splenectomy are used as emergency procedures.

While most patients recover to the point that they may not demonstrate symptoms, their bodies often continue to destroy platelets but at a level that is matched by increased bone marrow production.[115]

TAY-SACHS DISEASE

Tay-Sachs disease is a degenerative nervous system disorder caused by the absence of an enzyme usually found in the blood called hexosaminidase A. This enzyme converts GM_2 ganglioside, a product of nerve cell metabolism, into a nontoxic substance. As this is not happening in Tay-Sachs disease, the toxic substance builds up in the brain and other body organs and leads to brain damage.

This disorder is common in Jewish persons whose ancestry can be traced to the Mediterranean region.[11] Today nearly 1 out of every 10 American Jews carry the Tay-Sachs gene.[11] As Tay-Sachs is an autosomal recessive trait, both parents must be carriers of the abnormal gene.

These children appear healthy at birth and seem to develop normally until about 6 months of age at which time they begin to deteriorate.[11] Within the next 3 to 5 years the children lose motor functioning, become profoundly mentally retarded, become blind and deaf, and often suffer seizures.[11] Death occurs usually no later than 5 years of age.

Carriers of Tay-Sachs disease can be detected by a simple blood test. In addition, through amniocentesis, the disease can be detected in the fetus by examining the amniotic fluid for the presence of hexosaminidase A. These tests, in addition to the relatively small and well-defined population in which the disease is primarily found, make Tay-Sachs disease hypothetically a preventable condition.[115]

Prevention becomes even more important when it is remembered that there is no cure. Treatment procedures can only make the child as comfortable as possible until death occurs. Research efforts are focusing on a number of treatment approaches that may someday offer help for these children. For example, the search continues for a substance that could substitute for the hexosaminidase A or for a procedure to graft healthy cells into Tay-Sachs patients so that the transplanted cells could produce hexosaminidase A. Research is also progressing on gene transplantation from normal into defective cells. Until an effective treatment is found, the best strategy is prevention through genetic counseling.

THALASSEMIA

Thalassemia is one of the most common inherited hematological diseases. It is an autosomal recessive trait affecting primarily those of Greek or Italian descent.[11]

In this disease the red blood cells are characteristically misshapen and lack normal amounts of hemoglobin. A blood test can determine if an individual carries the abnormal gene. In addition, this condition can also be detected prenatally through the use of amniocentesis.

This disease has a mild to severe continuum. As in Tay-Sachs disease, the children appear healthy at birth but during the first year or two they become pale and listless, develop poor appetites, and have frequent infections; their bones become thin and brittle; and facial bones take on a characteristic look.[11] As the condition worsens, the spleen, liver, and other organs enlarge. Many children require surgery to remove the spleen, and they require many blood transfusions. There is no cure for the disease at this time. As with Tay-Sachs disease, the hope lies in prevention and research.

Implications for occupational therapy

Advances in the medical treatment of hematological diseases, conditions, and disorders have helped to reduce the long-term biological effects. This fact has changed the overall role of occupational therapy with this population.

Fewer of the children require orthopedic equipment such as splints and adaptive equipment. Careful monitoring can be done of the child's biophysical development in general; in particular, the range of motion in joints, strength, asymmetrical changes, and pain can be monitored. Families may need help in selecting appropriate play and leisure activities that facilitate maximal activity levels in the child.

NEOPLASTIC DISORDERS

Cancer, somehow, seems even more insidious when it attacks children. This section will discuss some of the major cancers of children and young adults.

Acute lymphoblastic leukemia

Leukemia is the most common neoplastic disease of childhood, occurring in 3 to 4 children per 100,000, with a peak incidence between 2 to 6 years. The cause is unknown, but changes in gene structure, viruses, and various environmental teratogens are all being studied as possible etiological factors.

Acute lymphoblastic leukemia (ALL) is characterized by the uncontrolled multiplication of immature white blood cells, which prevents the bone marrow from producing normal blood cells.[115] Symptoms include loss of weight; night sweats; chronic fatigue; paleness; a high fever; repeated infections; purpura; and enlarged lymph nodes, spleen, and liver. Diagnosis is usually made by examining a specimen of bone marrow for lymphoblasts. Blood counts are also taken.

The goal of medical management is the achievement of complete "cure" by inducing remission, eliminating cells in "sanctuaries" like the central nervous system, and maintaining the remission.[115] Specifically, treatment is conducted in three phases. The first phase is called *induction therapy* and is designed to rid the bone marrow and the rest of the body of the leukemia cells. The second phase is called *central nervous system prophylaxis* and is aimed at killing cells in the brain and spinal cord. The third phase of treatment is called *maintenance therapy* in which chemotherapy is administered to treat small deposits of cells that remain after remission.[107]

Prognosis is much improved over previous years, with the majority of patients going into remission for at least 5 years. Many go long periods of time with no recurrent signs.[115]

Wilms' tumor

Wilms' tumor is the most common abdominal neoplasm in children, with an incidence of 1 in 10,000 to 15,000 live births. Peak incidence is at 3¼ years.[115]

Sonography may help to distinguish a tumor from a fluid-filled cyst. If a tumor is found to exist, surgery should be performed as soon as possible. This is followed by radiation and a chemotherapeutic regimen.[115]

Prognosis is now favorable for recovery, with even the most involved level of cases having a 50% cure rate.[115]

Hodgkin's disease in children

The highest peak of incidence of Hodgkin's disease in children is between 5 and 8 years, with a second peak in the mid-teens. Cause is unknown, but a viral agent is suspected.

The presenting problem is often an enlarged but painless cervical node. Other symptoms include fever, chills, night sweats, and weight loss.[139]

A histological examination of the node reveals the presence of Reed-Sternberg cells if Hodgkin's disease is present. A clinical examination may detect an enlarged liver and spleen. Diagnosis is based on the extent of the disease, as is prognosis. Treatment consists of radiotherapy and chemotherapy.

Implications for occupational therapy

While the prognosis for many childhood cancers is good, even the most hopeful situation is a crisis for the child and the family. Many times the diagnostic and treatment procedures have side effects that are physically and psychologically devastating.

If the child's condition is terminal, the situation is even more difficult. In our culture death is not only unexpected in childhood but it is also considered an unnatural event. Occupational therapy has a significant role to play with a child who is dying, the family, and significant others in the child's life (Chapter 25).

ENDOCRINE DISORDERS AND CONDITIONS

The hormones secreted by the endocrine glands enter the bloodstream and travel to a second site where they have a specific effect on a body organ or another gland. In children the endocrine glands have an effect on metabolism, growth, sexual maturity, and stress control. This section provides an overview of the endocrine conditions and disorders commonly seen in children.

Type I diabetes

Type I diabetes* (juvenile diabetes, growth onset diabetes mellitus, or insulin-dependent diabetes) is a chronic metabolic disorder resulting from an extremely low level of insulin production or no production at all. This type of diabetes is found in children and young adults. A large number of children seem to develop the disorder at 10 or 11 years of age.

*This type is insulin-dependent diabetes, which differs from Type II diabetes, or non-insulin-dependent diabetes.

The exact cause of Type I diabetes is unknown. It appears, however, that genetic predisposition plays a role, as does infection. One hypothesis is that the beta cells of the pancreas are damaged as a result of virus infections. It has been noted that newly diagnosed cases of Type I diabetes rise as the number of cases of viral infections rise at various times of the year.

Early symptoms include increased voiding, increased thirst, and dehydration. Later symptoms include acidosis, vomiting, hyperventilation, and eventually coma.

The general goals of treatment are to ensure satisfactory growth, ensure emotional development, help the child acquire some degree of normal life, resolve the symptoms, prevent ketoacidosis, and prevent long-term sequelae, such as renal and cardiac damage and eye disease.[44,142] The achievement of these goals is very difficult because it depends on maintaining a delicate balance between so many factors: exercise, nutritional intake, hormones, emotions, and many other internal and external influences on blood sugar levels.

Effect on growth and metabolism

Following stimulation by the hypothalamus, the pituitary gland secretes the thyroid-stimulating hormone (TSH) into the bloodstream. This hormone stimulates the thyroid gland to produce thyroxine, a hormone that is known to affect body growth, metabolism, and brain growth. If the thyroid gland secretes too little thyroxine, brain development may be hampered during the critical prenatal and infant periods of life. Later in development body growth may decrease or stop, and the child may develop dry skin, become constipated, and show a decreased heart rate.

To prevent, or at least minimize, the effects of thyroid deficiency, early diagnosis is critical. Today many states have mandated screening for this deficiency during the first few days of life. Once the deficiency is found, the children are given daily dosages of thyroxine for as long as they continue to show a deficiency.

On the other hand, an overproduction of thyroxine can cause sleeplessness, diarrhea, and a slight tremor in the upper extremities and increase in appetite with no weight gain. Growth is usually not affected in this condition. Treatment consists of the administration of a medication that blocks the production of thyroxine. In extreme cases surgery may be used to remove part or all of the thyroid gland, thus reducing the production of thyroxine. The child can then be given correct dosages of thyroxine on a daily basis.

Also influencing the growth of the child is a growth hormone that is produced in the pituitary gland. If this hormone is deficient or absent, growth is slowed or stopped and deviations appear on growth charts. Treatment consists of injections of a similar hormone taken directly from human cadavers or from pigs, as the hormone cannot yet be synthesized. In fact, this hormone is in such scarcity that dissemination is controlled by the National Pituitary Center, and children who qualify for the program are treated only until they reach a height of 5 feet, 6 inches.

Effect on sexual maturity

The hypothalamus stimulates the pituitary gland, which in turn stimulates the testes to produce testosterone and the ovaries to produce estrogen. Both these hormones accelerate growth of the bones, assist in the fusion of the growth plate, and contribute to the development of secondary sex characteristics. These hormones can be deficient or excessive. A balance can be achieved through medication and hormone administration.

Reaction to stress

Another example of an endocrine gland is the adrenal gland. The same cycle begins with the hypothalomus stimulating the pituitary gland, which in turn stimulates the adrenal gland to secrete dopamine, norepinephrine, and epinephrine.[115] These agents affect other organs as well by providing negative feedback to the pituitary gland to stop the secretion of the adrenocorticotropic hormone. The purpose of this particular cycle is to help the body deal with stressful situations.

Implications for occupational therapy

Advances in medical treatment have reduced the need for most of these children to receive occupational therapy. But therapists must be familiar with signs and symptoms, treatment techniques, and possible side effects of these techniques in case a child has or develops any conditions as secondary problems during therapy for other problems.

GASTROINTESTINAL AND RENAL CONDITIONS

This section discusses disorders of the gastrointestinal and renal systems in children.

Crohn's disease

Crohn's disease is a chronic, inflammatory disorder of the intestinal tract that is accompanied by the formation of granulomas, fistulas, abscesses, and perianal disease. Pain and bloody diarrhea are also present. The cause is unknown.[115]

Treatment consists of anti-inflammatory agents, steroids, a bowel management program, and psychological support.[115] Surgery does not reverse the damage, but 80% of all patients face surgery at one time or other. Recurrence is virtually assured.[34]

Renal failure

Acute renal failure (ARF) of the kidney may be a result of trauma, toxins, temporary obstruction, or decreased blood flow to the kidney. Treatment for the underlying cause and temporary dialysis should eliminate the problem.

Chronic renal failure (CRF) is a permanent, progressive reduction in renal function. Renal diseases, such as focal glomerular sclerosis and membranoproliferative nephritis, or systemic disorders, such as systemic lupus erythematosus and vasculitis, may cause chronic renal failure.[115]

The uremic syndrome refers to the group of symptoms caused by reduced renal functioning and compensatory behaviors. It includes acidosis, dermatological changes, gastrointestinal problems, changes in the eyes, cardiac problems, neurological changes, and bleeding.[2]

Treatment centers on dialysis and transplantation. The much publicized problem with transplantation is finding a donor in time. The irony is that the technique has been perfected to the point that 75% of the kidneys transplanted into children function well for at least 3 to 5 years.[115]

Implications for occupational therapy

The occupational therapist must know the signs and symptoms of gastrointestinal and renal conditions in case a child undergoing therapy develops any of these conditions. The occupational therapist must also know the side effects and precautions.

TRAUMATIC INJURIES

Hundreds of thousands of children are seriously injured and thousands more die each year as a result of accidents. The four leading types of fatal accidents are motor vehicle accidents, drownings, burns, and poisonings.[115] Other accidents, while not fatal, cause injuries that may leave the children with life-long physical or emotional scars. This section discusses three specific types of traumatic injuries that often require the evaluation and treatment services of occupational therapists.

Head trauma

Head injuries during childhood constitute a major medical and public health problem. Approximately

4,000 children per year die from head injuries in the United States. Three to four times that number are seriously injured and must endure prolonged hospitalizations and life-long complications of some degree.

The vast majority of these cases are caused by motor vehicle accidents involving cars, bicycles, or motorcycles. Other cases are caused by self-inflicted injuries such as falls, and still others are caused by assault or penetrating wounds, such as gunshots.

Head traumas are often classified as closed or open. A closed head trauma indicates a blow to the head that has not caused an open or penetrating wound. An open head trauma denotes a penetration or laceration. Open wounds often require additional treatment, such as debridement, removal of bone fragments or other foreign bodies, surgical repair of blood vessels, closure of the wound, and tetanus prophylaxis.

Damage to nervous system tissue may occur at the time of impact or penetration. However, secondary damage may occur resulting from brain swelling, intracranial pressure, hematomas, emboli, and hypoxic brain conditions.[73,110] It is these secondary causes of nervous system damage that must be prevented or at least minimized through early medical intervention.

Two distinct clinical patterns in unconscious children with head injuries are described.[110] In the first type the child goes into unconsciousness or coma immediately after the trauma. In the second type, known as the pediatric concussion syndrome, the child may become unconscious right after the injury but then become lucid before showing further signs of involvement. These may include drowsiness, vomiting, loss of consciousness, and even more serious indicators such as Babinsky's sign, decerebrate posturing, and even brain death.[110] The pediatric concussion syndrome may resolve at any stage of its continuum or complete its full course.

Once the child's condition is stabilized, his level of consciousness is determined. One scale that is often used is the Glasgow Coma Scale.[73] This system ranks children according to their ability to elicit sounds or words; their responses to tendon reflex testing and motor responsiveness in general; and their ability to voluntarily or involuntarily open their eyes.[110] Next, a neurological assessment of brain stem reflexes is conducted. Additional diagnostic procedures may involve computerized tomography (CT scan), electroencephalography (EEG), angiography, and radiography to determine the extent and location of fractures.

Treatment includes the close monitoring and control of cerebral circulation and of intracranial pressure through the use of sophisticated devices and control systems. When intracranial pressure cannot be controlled by use of traditional means, a large dose of barbiturate, such as phenobarbital, may be administered. If this attempt fails to control the pressure, lowering of the body temperature may help. Withdrawal from the latter two forms of treatment is difficult and may cause sleep disturbances, behavioral problems, apnea and some decreased intellectual functioning.

The prognosis for children who receive the type of treatment described is good. The majority of children with head trauma make a good recovery or are only moderately handicapped and are able to return to a regular school setting.[110] The milder effects include auditory and visual perceptual deficits, body image problems, difficulties with some minor gross and fine motor skills, and a slowing of response.[11,110]

Children who have shown decerebrate posturing, flaccidity, scores of less than 5 on the Glasgow Coma Scale, or prolonged coma are considered to have a guarded prognosis.[110] These children often require rehabilitation for ambulation, motor skills, and self-help skills.[21] In addition, some children will demonstrate severe emotional disturbances that will require professional help.[21]

Burns

Every year burn accidents cause the death of approximately 1,800 children and result in serious medical conditions in 1,500 other children.[115] Smoke inhalation, respiratory failure, hypovolemic shock, renal failure, and posttraumatic infection are the major factors associated with death from burns.[115] The severity of the burn injury is determined by the depth, exact location, and extent of body surface affected.

Clark[27] described the aims of burn treatment: prevention of infection and burn shock, early skin coverage, correction of cosmetic damage, restoration of function, and integration back into the environment. As burned tissue provides a fertile bed for infection, many types of intervention procedures must be used to minimize the possibility of sepsis. Environmental bacteria must be minimized. Surface bacteria must be reduced by using medicated ointments, administering antibiotics, removing dead tissue early, and covering the areas with skin grafts.[27] Burn shock is prevented by administering various intravenous solutions that help replace lost body fluids. Nutrition may be maintained through tube feedings, oral feedings, and intravenous feedings if indicated.[144]

Deformities, contractures, and loss of motion must be prevented by early intervention. Exercise programs, splinting, proper positioning, pressure garments, and reconstructive surgery are all methods used to limit the long-term effects of burn injuries. A child who faces a long hospital stay will need to have academic assistance to prevent any educational delays. The family and the child may need counseling in adjusting to any disfigurements or any limiting physical conditions. Without this help the emotional handicap may be as great as the physical one.

Musculoskeletal injuries resulting from trauma

Fractures are extremely common in children. While dislocations and soft tissue injuries are less common in children than adults, they are serious and painful when they do occur.[122]

Fractures may be classified in many ways. An open fracture refers to the fact that there is an open wound or penetration caused by an object outside the body or caused by the bone penetrating from within the body. A closed fracture indicates that no penetration has occurred. Open fractures present added complications because the wound must be closed in addition to treating the fracture. The risks of infection and healing complications are higher with the open fracture.

Fractures may also be described by the type of forces or trauma that causes them. An angulation or bending force may cause the bone to snap crosswise (transverse fracture), a condition called a greenstick fracture in children. If the two fracture surfaces separate and misalign, it is known as an oblique fracture. When there is a tension failure of bone resulting from stress applied by an attached ligament or muscle, it is called an avulsion fracture. When one bone wedges into another, it is called a compression fracture. A bulge in the cortex surrounding the bone causes bubble or buckle fractures. A hairline crack fracture consists of a slight crack in the bone with no displacement.[122]

Birth fractures and special congenital fractures are discussed in the musculoskeletal section of this chapter. A specific fracture of potential seriousness in children is that which involves the epiphyseal plates. This type of fracture has the potential to interrupt bone growth by causing bone deformities. Epiphyseal fractures account for about 15% of all childhood fractures.[122]

The Salter-Harris classification of epiphyseal fractures consists of descriptions of five types of injuries. Each type is described, possible causes and prognosis are listed, and general treatment techniques are described. Salter[122] states that 85% of epiphyseal plate injuries are uncomplicated by growth disturbances.

Children's ligaments are stronger than the associated epiphyseal plates. Therefore, when stress is applied, it is more common to find a fracture than a damaged ligament. Severe tension applied to muscles, nerves, and tendons, often results in damage. Treatment is usually aimed at protecting the damaged part from stretching during the healing process.[122] The child must begin to exercise as soon as possible to prevent decreased joint motion and muscle power loss. Surgical repair may also be needed.

Implications for occupational therapy

Occupational therapy treatment for acute musculoskeletal problems is limited to cases in which complications have occurred, such as growth deformities or severe damage requiring rehabilitation (Chapter 20). Serious head trauma cases often require occupational therapy services for evaluation and symptomatic treatment. Burn injuries require occupational therapy services if long-term hospitalization or residual problems are anticipated (Chapter 21).

SUMMARY

An overview of the major diagnostic categories of interest to occupational therapists has been presented. Many times therapists do not need to have full knowledge of disease processes to treat a child effectively. However, it is most important to have sufficient knowledge to recognize side effects and potential hazards in treatment. References cited throughout this chapter should be consulted for a more detailed discussion of each diagnosis.

REFERENCES AND SELECTED READINGS

1. Adams, J.C.: Outline of orthopaedics, ed. 9, New York, 1981, Churchill Livingstone, Inc.
2. Alfrey, A.: Chronic renal failure: manifestations and pathogenesis. In Schrier, R.W., editor: Renal and electrolyte disorders, Boston, 1976, Little, Brown & Co.
3. Alter, B., and others: Prenatal diagnosis of hemoglobinopathies, N. Engl. J. Med. **295:**1437, 1976.
4. Amiel-Tison, C.: Neurological evaluation of the maturity of newborn infants, Arch. Dis. Child. **43:**89, 1968.
5. Apgar, V.: A proposal for a new method of evaluation of the newborn infant, Curr. Res. Anesth. Analg. **32:**260, 1953.
6. Apgar, V., and James, L.S.: Further observations on the newborn scoring system, Am. J. Dis. Child. **104:**419, 1962.
7. Autism fact sheet, Washington, D.C., 1980, The National Society for Autistic Children.
8. Avant, K.: A maternal attachment strategy. In Humenick, S.S., editor: Assessment strategies in the health care of young children and childbearing families, Norwalk, Conn., 1982, Appleton-Century-Crofts.
9. Ayres, A.J.: Sensory integration and the child, Los Angeles, 1980, Western Psychological Services.
10. Ballard, J.L., Kazmaier, K., and Driver, M.A.: Simplified assessment of gestational age, Pediatr. Res. **11:**374, 1973.
11. Batshaw, M.L., and Perret, Y.M.: Children with handicaps: a medical primer, Baltimore, 1981, Paul. H. Brookes Publishing Co.
12. Bayley, N.: The Bayley Scales of Infant Development, New York, 1969, The Psychological Corp.
13. Bender L.: Schizophrenia in childhood: its recognition, description and treatment, Am. J. Orthopsychiatry **26:**499, 1956.
14. Bettelheim, B.J.: A mechanical boy, Sci. Am. **200:**117, 1959.
15. Birth defects: tragedy and hope, White Plains, N.Y., 1981, The National Foundation—March of Dimes.

16. Bluestone, C.D., and Shurin, P.A.: Middle ear disease in children: pathogenesis, diagnosis, and management, Pediatr. Clin. North Am. **21:**379, 1974.

17. Bradshaw, M.M.: Denver Developmental Screening Test. In Humenick, S.S., editor: Analysis of current assessment strategies in the health care of young children and childbearing families, Norwalk, Conn., 1982, Appleton-Century-Crofts.

18. Brashear, H.R., Jr., and Raney, R.B.: Shands' handbook of orthopaedic surgery, ed. 9, St. Louis, 1978, The C.V. Mosby Co.

19. Brazelton, T.B.: Neonatal behavioral assessment scale, Philadelphia, 1973, J.B. Lippincott Co.

20. Brazie, J.V., and Lubcheno, O.: Clinical estimation of gestational age: an approximation based on published data. In Kempe, C.H., Silver, H.K., and O'Brien, C., editors: Current pediatric diagnosis and treatment, ed. 3, Los Altos, Calif., 1974, Lange Medical Publications.

21. Brink, J.D., and Woo-Sam J.: Physical recovery after severe closed head trauma in children and adolescents, J. Pediatr. **97**(5):721, 1980.

22. Broussard, E.R.: Psychosocial disorders in children: early assessment of infants at risk, Contin. Educ. Fam. Physician **44:**42, 1978.

23. Campbell, S.: Fetal growth. In Beard, R., and Nathaniels, P., editors: Fetal physiology and medicine: the basis of perinatology, Philadelphia, 1976, W.B. Saunders Co.

24. Cerreto, M.: The diagnosis of childhood autism, Galveston, Spring 1980, The School Health Newsletter, The University of Texas Medical Branch.

25. Chai, H., and Newcomb, R.: Pharmacologic management of childhood asthma, Am. J. Dis. Child. **125:**757, 1973.

26. Churchill, J., and others: The etiology of cerebral palsy in premature infants, New York, 1971, American Academy for Cerebral Palsy.

27. Clark, A.M.: Burns in childhood, World J. Surg. **2:**175, 1978.

28. Clark, F.: Research on the neuropathophysiology of autism and its implications for OT, Occup. Ther. J. Res. **30:**3, 1983.

29. Clements, S.D.: Minimal brain dysfunction in children: terminology and identification, NINDB Monograph No. 3, Washington, D.C., 1966, U.S. Department of Health, Education and Welfare.

30. Clerk, G.: Reflections on the role of mother in the development of language in the schizophrenic child, Can. Psychiatr. Assoc. J. **6:**252, 1961.

31. Colbert, E.C., and Koegel, R.R.: Toe walking in childhood schizophrenia, J. Pediatr. **53:**219, 1958.

32. Collard, R.R.: Bayley scales of infant development. In Buros, O.K., editor: The eighth mental measurement yearbook, vol. 1, Highland Park, N.J., 1978, Gryphon Press.

33. Collins, G., and others: Ventricular septal defect: clinical and hemodynamic changes in the first five years of life, Am. Heart J. **84:**695, 1972.

34. Cooke, W.: Survey of results of treatment of Crohn's disease, Clin. Gastroenterol. **1:**521, 1972.

35. Cooper, W., German, J., and Lame, E.: Genetic implications of cerebral palsy, J. Bone Joint Surg. **47:**1673, 1965.

36. Creak, E.M.: Childhood psychosis: a review of 100 cases, Br. J. Psychiatry **109:**84, 1963.

37. Cruickshank, W.: Cerebral palsy: a developmental disability, ed. 3, Syracuse, 1976, Syracuse University Press.

38. Damasio, A.R., and Maurer, R.G.: A neurological model for childhood autism, Arch. Gen. Psychiatry **35:**777, 1978.

39. DeMyer, M., and others: Prognosis in autism: a follow-up study, J. Autism Child. Schizophr. **3:**199, 1973.

40. di Sant' Agnese, P.A., and Davis, P.B.: Research in cystic fibrosis, J. Pediatr. **8:**711, 1976.

41. Donner, M., Rapola, J., and Somer, H.: Congenital muscular dystrophy: a clinico-pathological and follow-up study of 15 patients, Neuropaediatrie **6:**239, 1975.

42. Drage, J.S., Berender, H., and Fisher, P.D.: The Apgar score at four years: psychological examination performance. Perinatal factor affecting human development, Scientific Pub. No. 185, 222-226, 1969, Pan-American Health Organization, World Health Organization.

43. Drage, J.S., and others: The Apgar score as an index of infant morbidity, Dev. Med. Child Neurol. **8:**141, 1966.

44. Drash, A.: The control of diabetes mellitus. Is it achievable? Is it desirable? J. Pediatr. **88:**1074, 1976.

45. Drillien, C.: The small-for-dates infant: etiology and prognosis, Pediatr. Clin. North Am. **17:**9, 1970.

46. Dubowitz, L.M.S., and Dubowitz, V.: Gestational age of the newborn; a clinical manual, Reading, Mass., 1977, Addison-Wesley Publishing Co., Inc.

47. Eisen, A., and Humphreys, P.: The Guillian-Barré syndrome, Arch. Neurol. **30:**438, 1974.

48. Ellenberg, J.H., and Nelson, K.B. Early recognition of infants at high risk for cerebral palsy: examination at age four months, Dev. Med. Child Neurol. **23:**6, 1981.

49. Engle, M.A.: Ventricular septal defects: status report for the seventies, Cardiovasc. Clin. **4**(3):282, 1972.

50. Fandal, Q.W., Kemper, M.B., and Frankenburg, W.K.: Needed: routine developmental screening for all children, Pediatric Basics, No. 24, Freemont, Mich., Gerber Products Co.

51. Fils, D.H.: The developmental disabilities handbook, Los Angeles, 1978, Western Psychological Services.

52. Fisch, R.D., and others: Physical and mental status at 4 years of age of survivors of the respiratory distress syndrome, J. Pediatr. **86:**497, 1975.

53. Fish, B.: Involvement of the CNS in infants with schizophrenia, Arch. Neurol. **2:**115, 1960.

54. Fish, B.: Longitudinal observations of biological deviations in a schizophrenic infant, Am. J. Psychiatry **116:**25, 1959.

55. Fishbein, J.: Birth defects, Philadelphia, 1963, J.B. Lippincott Co.

56. Fisher, D., and Paton, J.: The effect of maternal anesthetic and analgesic drugs on the fetus and newborn, Clin. Obstet. Gynecol. **17:**275, 1974.

57. Fitzhardinge, P., and Steven, E.: The small-for-date infant. I. Later growth patterns, Pediatrics **49:**671, 1972.

58. Franco, S., and Andrews, B.: Reduction of cerebral palsy by neonatal intensive care, Pediatr. Clin. North Am. **24:**639, 1977.

59. Frankenburg, W.K., and Dodds, J.: Manual: Denver Developmental Screening Test, Denver, University of Colorado Medical Center.

60. Frankenburg, W.K., and others: Reliability and stability of the Denver Developmental Screening Test, Child Dev. **42:**1315, 1971.

61. Friedman, W.F.: Medical management of ductus arteriosus, Prenatal care **77:**18, 1977.

62. Goodwin, J., Dunne, J., and Thomas, B.: Antepartum identification of the fetus at risk, Can. Med. J. **101:**458, 1969.

63. Gottfried, A.W., and Brody, N.: Interrelationships between and correlates of psychometric and Piagetian scales of sensorimotor intelligence, Dev. Psychol. **11**(3):379, 1975.

64. Gray, J.D., and others: Prediction and prevention of child abuse and neglect. Child Abuse Neglect Int. J. **1:**45, 1977.

65. Gregory, G.A. and others: Treatment of the idiopathic respiratory distress syndrome with continuous positive airway pressure, N. Engl. J. Med. **284:**1333, 1971.

66. Hagberg, B., Hagberg, G., and Olow, I.: The changing panorama of cerebral palsy in Sweden 1954-1970. I. Analysis of general changes, Acta Paediatr. Scand. **64:**187, 1975.

67. Havelkova, M.: Follow-up study of seventy-one children diagnosed as psychotic in preschool age, Am. J. Orthopsychiatry **38:**846, 1968.

68. Hellman, L., and Pritchard, J., editors: Williams' obstetrics, New York, 1975, Appleton-Century-Crofts.

69. Henig, R.M.: Saving babies before birth, The New York Times Magazine, vol. 18, Feb. 1982.

70. Hobel, C., and others: Prenatal and intrapartum high risk screening: prediction of the high risk neonate, Am. J. Obstet. Gynecol. **117:**1, 1973.

71. Hopkins, H.L., and Smith, H.D.: Willard and Spackman's occupational therapy, ed. 6, Philadelphia, 1983, J.B. Lippincott Co.

72. Ingram, T.S., Mason A.W., and Blackburn, I.: A retrospective study of 82 children with reading disability, Dev. Med. Child Neurol. **12:**271, 1970.

73. Jennett, B., and Teasdale, G.: Management of head injuries, Philadelphia, 1981, F.A. Davis Co.

74. Kanner, L.: Autistic disturbances in affective contact, Nervous Child **2:**217, 1943.

75. Karp, R., and Kirklin, J.: Tetrology of Fallot, Ann. Thorac. Surg. **10:**370, 1970.

76. Klaus, M.H., and Fanaroff, A.A.: Care of the high-risk neonate, Philadelphia, 1979, W.B. Saunders Co.

77. Koivisto, M., Blanco-Sequeiros, M., and Krause V.: Neonatal symptomatic and asymptomatic hypoglycaemia: a follow-up study of 151 children, Dev. Med. Child Neurol. **14:**603, 1972.

78. Kolvin, J.: Psychoses in childhood: a comparative study. In Rutter, M., editor: Infantile autism: concepts, characteristics and treatment, London, 1971, Churchill Livingstone.

78. Korner, A.F., and others: Reduction of sleep apnea and bradycardia in preterm infants on oscillating water beds: a controlled polygraphic study, Pediatrics **61:**528, 1978.

80. Lazaro, R.P., Fenichel, G.M., and Kilroy, A.W.: Congenital muscular dystrophy: case reports and reappraisal, Muscle Nerve **2:**349, 1979.

81. Leukemia: the nature of the disease, New York, 1981, The Medical and Scientific Advisory Committee of the Leukemia Society of America, Inc.

82. Lewis, A.J., and Besant, D.F.: Muscular dystrophy in infancy, J. Pediatr. **60:**376, 1962.

83. Lewis, J., Spero, J., and Hasiba, V.: Death in hemophiliacs, JAMA **236:**1238, 1976.

84. Lubchenco, L.O.: Assessment of gestational age and development at birth, Pediatr. Clin. North Am. **17**(1):125, 1970.

85. Mangos, J., and Talamo, R., editors: Cystic fibrosis: projections into the future, New York, 1976, Grune & Stratton, Inc.

86. McCarthy, J.S., Zies, L.G., and Gelband, H.: Age-dependent closure of the patent ductus arteriosus by indomethacin, Pediatrics **62:**706, 1978.

87. McClure, P.: Idiopathic thrombocytopenic purpura in children: diagnosis and management, Pediatr. Clin. North Am. **55:**68, 1975.

88. McConnell, O.L.: Control of eye contact in an autistic child, J. Child Psychiatry **8:**249, 1967.

89. Menelaus, M.B.: The orthopaedic management of spina bifida cystica, London, 1971, E. & S. Livingstone.

90. Menkes, J.H.: Diagnosis and treatment of minor motor seizures, Pediatr. Clin. North Am. **23:**435, 1976.

91. Merkatz, I.R., and Fanaroff, A.A.: Antenatal and intrapartum care of the high-risk infant. In Klaus, M.H., and Fanaroff, A.A., editors: Care of the high-risk neonate, Philadelphia, 1979, W.B. Saunders Co.

92. Millichap, J.G., and Dodge, R.R.: Diagnosis and treatment of myasthenia gravis in infancy, childhood, and adolescence, Neurology **10:**1009, 1960.

93. Milner, J.S., and Wimberly, R.C.: An inventory for the identification of child abusers, J. Clin. Psychol. **25**(1):95, 1975.

94. Minear, W.: Classification of cerebral palsy, Pediatrics **18:**841, 1956.

95. Moriarity, A.: Review: the Denver Developmental Screening Test. In Buros, O., editor: The seventh mental measurement yearbook, Highland Park, N.J., 1972, Gryphon Press.

96. Muscular dystrophy fact sheet, New York, 1980, Muscular Dystrophy Association.

97. Nesbitt, R., and Aubry, R.: High-risk obstetrics. II. Value of semi-objective grading system in identifying the vulnerable group, Am. J. Obstet. Gynecol. **103:**972, 1969.

98. New, M., and Fiser, R., editors: Diabetes and other endocrine disorders during pregnancy and in the newborn, Prog. Clin. Biol. Res. **10:**13, 1976.

99. NICHD National Registry: Midtrimester amniocentesis for prenatal diagnosis: safety and accuracy, JAMA **236:**1471, 1976.

100. Norris, D., and others: Hodgkin's disease in childhood, Cancer **36:**2109, 1973.

101. Olsen, R.J.: Index of suspicion: screening for child abusers, Am. J. Nurs. **1:**108, 1976.

102. O'Reilly, D., and Walentynowicz, J.: Etiological factors in cerebral palsy: an historical review, Dev. Med. Child Neurol. **23:**8, 1981.

103. Ornitz, E.: Childhood autism: a review of the clinical and experimental literature, Calif. Med. **118:**21, 1973.

104. Oski, F.A., and Naiman, J.L.: Hematologic problems in the newborn, Philadelphia, 1972, W.B. Saunders Co.

105. Patrick, J.E., Perry, T.B., and Kinch, R.A.: Fetoscopy and fetal blood sampling: a percutaneous approach, Am. J. Obstet. Gynecol. **119:**539, 1974.

106. Perlstein, M., and Barnett, H.: Nature and recognition of cerebral palsy in infancy, JAMA **148:**1389, 1952.

107. Pinkel, D.: Treatment of acute leukemia, Pediatr. Clin. North Am. **23:**117, 1976.

108. Ramey, C.T., Campbell, F.A., and Nicholson, J.E.: The predictive power of the Bayley Scales of Infant Development and the Stanford-Binet Intelligence Test in a relatively constant environment, Child Dev. **44**(4):709, 1973.

109. Rank, B.: Intensive study and treatment of preschool children who show marked personality deviations or "atypical development" and their parents. In Caplan, G., editor: Emotional problems in early childhood, New York, 1955, Basic Books, Inc., Publishers.

110. Raphaely, R.C., and others: Management of severe pediatric head trauma, Pediatr. Clin. North Am. **27**(3):715, 1980.

111. Ricks, D.M., and Wing, L.: Language, Communication and the use of symbols in normal and autistic children, J. Autism Child. Schizophr. **5:**215, 1975.

112. Ritvo, E., Ornitz, E., and LaFranchi, S.: Frequency of repetitive behavior in early infantile autism and its variants, Arch. Gen. Psychiatry **19:**341, 1968.

113. Ritvo, E., and others: Correlation of psychiatric diagnoses and EEG findings, Am. J. Psychiatry **126:**37, 1970.

114. Rizza, C.R., and Mathews, J.M.: Management of the haemophilic child, Arch. Dis. Child. **47:**451, 1972.

115. Roberts, K.B.: Manual of clinical problems in pediatrics, Boston, 1979, Little, Brown & Co.

116. Robertson, E.: Rehabilitation of arm amputees and limb-deficient children, London, 1978, Cassell, Ltd.

117. Robinson, R.J.: Assessment of gestational age by neurological examination, Arch. Dis. Child. **41:**437, 1966.

118. Rudolph, A.J., and Kenny, J.D.: Anticipation, recognition, and transitional care of the high-risk infant. In Klaus, M.H., and Fanaroff, A.A., editors: Care of the high-risk neonate, Philadelphia, 1979, W.B. Saunders Co.

119. Rugh, R., and Shettles, L.B.: From conception to birth: the drama of life's beginnings, New York, 1971, Harper & Row, Publishers, Inc.

120. Rutter, M., and Lockyer, L.: A five to 15 year follow-up study of infantile psychosis. II. Social and behavioral outcome, Br. J. Psychiatry **113:**1183, 1967.

121. Salter, R.B.: Textbook of disorders and injuries of the musculoskeletal system, Baltimore, 1970, Williams & Wilkins.

122. Salter, R.B.: Textbook of disorders and injuries of the musculoskeletal system, ed. 2, Baltimore, 1983, Williams & Wilkins.

123. Salter, R.B., and Field, P.: The effects of continuous compression on living articular cartilage: an experimental investigation, J. Bone Joint Surg. **42A:**31, 1960

124. Schaffer, A.J., and Avery, M.E.: Diseases of the newborn, Philadelphia, 1971, W.B. Saunders Co.

125. Scherzer, A.L., and Tscharnuter, I.: Early Diagnosis and treatment in cerebral palsy: a primer on infant developmental problems, New York, 1982, Marcel Dekker, Inc.

126. Schopler, E.: Early infantile autism and receptive processes, Arch. Gen. Psychiatry **113:**1183, 1965.

127. Schuster, C.S., and Ashburn, S.S.: The process of human development: a holistic approach, Boston, 1980, Little, Brown & Co.

128. Schwartz, R., Field, G., and Kyle, G.: Timing of delivery in the pregnant diabetic patient, Obstet. Gynecol. **34:**787, 1969.

129. Sharrard, W.J., and Zachary, R.B.: A controlled trial of immediate and delayed closure of spina bifida cystica, Arch. Dis. Child. **38:**18, Feb. 1963.

130. Sickle-cell anemia fact sheet, White Plains, N.Y., 1981, The National Foundation–March of Dimes.

131. Smith, C.A.: Effects of maternal undernutrition upon the newborn infant in Holland (1944-1945), J. Pediatr. **30:**229, 1947.

132. Synder, C., Eyres, S.J., and Barnard, E.: New findings about mothers' antenatal expectations and their relationship to infant development, Am. J. Matern. Child Nurs. **4:**354, 1979.

133. Spencer, E.A., Functional restoration—amputations and prosthetic replacement. In Hopkins, H.L., and Smith, H.D., editors: Occupational therapy, ed. 6, Philadelphia, 1983, J.B. Lippincott Co.

134. Stern, R., and others: Course of cystic fibrosis in 95 patients, J. Pediatr. **89:**406, 1976.

135. Stott, D.H.: The child's hazards in utero. In Howells, J.G., editor: Modern perspectives in international child psychiatry, New York, 1971, Brunner/Mazel, Inc.

136. Sweet, A.Y.: Classification of the low-birth-weight infant. In Klaus, M.H., and Fanaroff, A.A., editors: Care of the high-risk neonate, Philadelphia, 1979, W.B. Saunders Co.

137. Taylor, K.M.: The Apgar scoring system. In Humenick, S.S., editor: Analysis of current assessment strategies in the health care of young children and childbearing families, Norwalk, Conn., 1982, Appleton-Century-Crofts.

138. Taylor, K.M.: Gestational age assessment. In Humenick, S.S., editor: Analysis of current assessment strategies in the health care of young children and childbearing families, Norwalk, Conn., 1982, Appleton-Century-Crofts.

139. Thomas, C.L.: Taber's cyclopedic medical dictionary, ed. 14, Philadelphia, 1981, F.A. Davis Co.

140. Thompson, E., and others: The mother-infant play interaction scale, Austin, Tex., 1980, The University of Texas School of Nursing.

141. Thompson, H.: Evaluation of the obstetric and gynecologic patient by the use of diagnostic ultrasound, Clin. Obstet. Gynecol. **17:**1, 1974.

142. Thompson, R.: Juvenile onset diabetes, Can. Med. Assoc. J. **114:**783, 1976.

143. Tronick, E., and Brazelton, T.B.: Clinical uses of the Brazelton Behavioral Assessment. In Friedlander, B., Sterrit, G., and Kirk, B., editors: Exceptional infants, assessment and intervention, vol. 3, New York, 1975, Brunner/Mazel, Inc.

144. Trunkey, D., and Parks, S.: Burns in children, Curr. Probl. Pediatr. **6**(3):3, 1976.

145. Tsiantos, A., and others: Intracranial hemorrhage in the prematurely born infant, J. Pediatr. **85:**854, 1974.

146. U.S. Office of Education: Education for all Handicapped Children Act, Public Law 94-142, Fed. Reg. **42:**42478, 1977.

147. Usher, R., McLean, F., and Scott, K.E.: Judgment of fetal age: clinical significance of gestational age and an objective method for its assessment, Pediatr. Clin. North Am. **13:**835, 1966.

148. Walker, L.O.: The Brazelton Neonatal Behavioral Assessment Scale. In Humenick, S.S., editor: Analysis of current assessment strategies in the health care of young children and childbearing families, Norwalk, Conn., 1982, Appleton-Century-Crofts.

149. Waters, E., Vaughn, B.E., and Egeland, B.R.: Individual differences in infant-mother attachment relationships at age one: antecedents in neonatal behavior in an urban economically disadvantaged sample, Child Dev. **51:**208, 1980.

150. Weldvogel, F., Medoff, C., and Swartz, M.: Osteomyelitis: a review of clinical features, therapeutic considerations and unusual aspects, N. Engl. J. Med. **282:**198, 1970.

151. Werner, E.: Review: the Denver Developmental Screening Test. In Buros, O., editor: Seventh mental measurement yearbook, vol. 1, Highland Park, N.J., 1972, Gryphon Press, p. 734.

152. Widmayer, S.M., and Field, T.M.: Effects of Brazelton demonstrations on early interactions of preterm infants and their teenage mothers, Infant Behav. Dev. **3:**79, 1980.

153. Wing, L., and others: Symbolic play in the severely mentally retarded and in autistic children, J. Child. Psychol. Psychiatry **18:**167, 1977.

PART

III

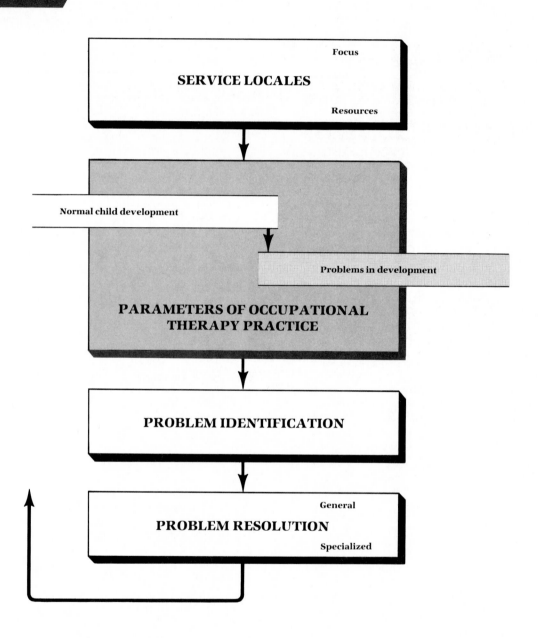

SERVICE LOCALES

Focus

Resources

Normal child development

Problems in development

PARAMETERS OF OCCUPATIONAL THERAPY PRACTICE

PROBLEM IDENTIFICATION

PROBLEM RESOLUTION

General

Specialized

Basic principles of occupational therapy intervention

PAT NUSE CLARK

Occupational therapy in pediatrics

The four theoretical approaches to pediatric occupational therapy reviewed in Chapter 3 share a humanistic view of the child (and the species) as an adaptive creator. An integration of the constructs of these and other theories and models of occupational therapy proposes an approach to practice that has been called "human development through occupation."[3,4] This chapter presents the philosophy of practice developed for this approach and discusses generic processes and modalities of occupational therapy. These concepts have been expanded and modified somewhat from their original presentation so that their ideas can be applied more directly to pediatric practice. In addition, a description of the sequence and basic components of occupational therapy in pediatrics is presented.

A PHILOSOPHY OF PRACTICE
View of man

Human adaptation is distinguishd by the child's capacity to purposefully affect his own world of self, culture, and environment. The unique richness of this creative function is the product of two biological characteristics: (1) the ability of the human brain to formulate and symbolize concepts and (2) the ability of the human hands to translate concepts into action. The child's awareness of these abilities, through successive and successful interactions with the environment, promotes the will for purposeful activities.[7,8]

Purposeful activities are broadly defined as the goal-directed use of a person's body systems, time, energy, interests, and attention in environmental interactions.[9,17,24] The child spends most of his time occupied in certain types of purposeful activities that support performance of chosen personal, social, and occupa-

tional roles.[1] Occupational roles and the supportive *occupational activities* are distinguished from other kinds of purposeful activities by two characteristics: (1) the use of hands and tools to explore and manipulate the environment and (2) the direct or indirect relationship of occupational activities to cultural continuity. There is a recognized sequence to the emergence and primary engagement of the human in such occupational activities.[19] This includes the development and use of

1. *Self-maintenance*, including self-care, sleep, rest, recreation, and other activities directed toward the preservation of the self and the species and preparation for work and play.[20,25]
2. *Play* as the anticipator and facilitator of subsequent goal-directed activities. Play includes sensorimotor exploration; symbolic activities such as art and drama; crafts; and games. The behaviors and skills acquired through playful exploration of the self, culture, and environment serve as the learning bridge to adult competence and creative achievement.[26]
3. *Work* as the economic function of humans in their world and the healthy state of man the achiever.[25,26] Work includes the educational and prevocational activities of the child in addition to the vocational and home management activities of the adult (Figure 7-1).

View of health

The child's maturing ability to direct and affect his or her purpose in life may be seen as a primary indication of general well-being, or health. Humans maintain health through engagement in a flexible balance of work, play, and self-maintenance activities, which develop and change throughout the life span.[7,20,25] The infant's work of learning is blended into playful sensorimotor exploration of the environment. As the child ages, the structure of his learning becomes more formalized through school, family, peer group, and community activities. The infant's involvement in self-maintenance activities is superficially passive until one considers the role of his crying behaviors in his daily routine. Again, with maturation the child gradually assumes more direct responsibilities for various self-care tasks.

In a healthy state the individual is able to adapt and achieve a satisfying life and is able to function adequately in chosen personal, social, and occupational roles.[23] *Role performance* involves the use of pertinent purposeful activities, including the various skills, habits, rules, tasks, and relationships acquired through the acculturation of the individual.[7,12,17]

The healthy performance of an individual is influenced by four major factors. First, the child's basic *biological endowment*, which includes the various body systems, functions, and genetic capacities, provides her with the potential to develop and learn a variety of skilled activities. Second, there is a hierarchical *maturation* of these basic endowments as the child grows and accommodates to changing environments, assimilating new experiences and learning. Together these two physiological processes provide a foundation of sensory, integrative, motor, and cognitive functions that permit the development of adaptive skills. The interaction between the individual and culture, physical space, and other environmental elements becomes increasingly complex throughout the life span. Therefore human performance must change and adapt as it is influenced by the third factor of *cultural, spatial, and temporal requirements*. The child must learn to effect a satisfying balance between meeting internal needs and adapting his behavior to external influences. The emergent, socialized *personal needs* change in concert with the three other performance factors, becoming the fourth determinant of one's "normal" performance. The human capacities that develop through the interaction between these internal and external forces provides a foundation of emotional and social functions (Figure 7-2).

Throughout life the individual encounters physiological, social, and psychological problems that may or may not impede performance of various roles and role activities. Analysis of the effect of such problems on socially adequate, personally satisfying performance and critical elements of development is both qualitative and quantitative.[16] Several questions arise. Is the individual capable of resolving the problem, adapting to it, or coping with it independently? With children in particular one needs to consider whether the coping process in itself is a hazard to the developmental progression. Is the nature of the problem such that it threatens to delay, disrupt, or impair functions, life role skills, or both? If the problem is sufficient to cause a dysfunction in the individual's performance and balance of daily tasks and roles, what resources are available, acceptable, and accessible to the child and family (Figure 7-2)? For example, a learning disabled child might have parents who both work, and therefore he needs to receive occupational therapy services through the school. However, he may not meet the eligibility requirements for that school's therapy services if his schoolwork is not 2 years below age level. If he lives in a county where there are no clinical occupational therapy services for children, and his parents cannot change their work schedules, life-style, and standard of living, he will probably go without occupational therapy treatment.

View of the profession

It is the heritage and concern of occupational therapy that awareness of the child's special needs for both

---

FIGURE 7-1

Conceptual model for the philosphy of practice: occupational activities and occupational therapy.

From Clark, P.N.: Am. J. Occup. Ther. **33:**578, Sept. 1979.

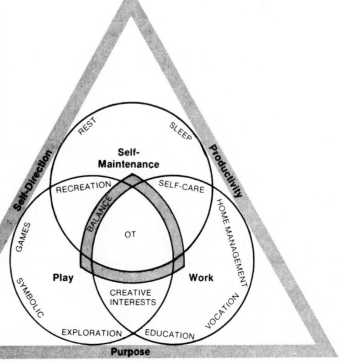

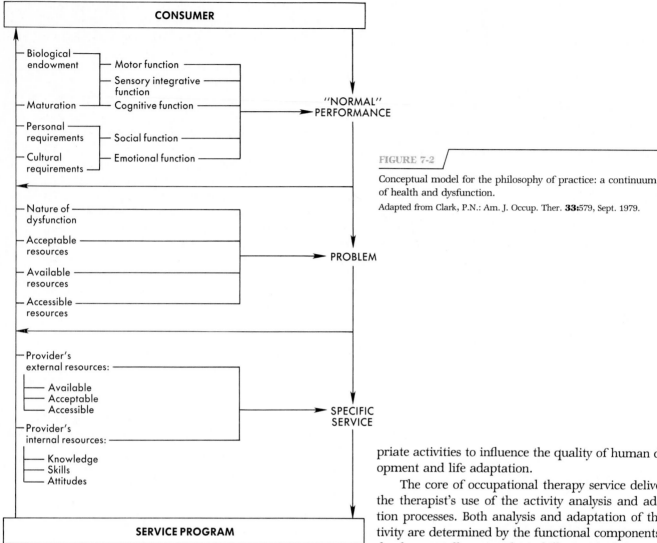

CONSUMER

Biological endowment ─── Motor function
Sensory integrative function
Maturation ─── Cognitive function
Personal requirements ─── Social function
Cultural requirements ─── Emotional function

"NORMAL" PERFORMANCE

Nature of dysfunction
Acceptable resources
Available resources
Accessible resources

PROBLEM

Provider's external resources:
Available
Acceptable
Accessible
Provider's internal resources:
Knowledge
Skills
Attitudes

SPECIFIC SERVICE

SERVICE PROGRAM

FIGURE 7-2

Conceptual model for the philosophy of practice: a continuum of health and dysfunction.

Adapted from Clark, P.N.: Am. J. Occup. Ther. **33:**579, Sept. 1979.

purpose and balance in life activities be applied to health service delivery.[7,25] Occupational therapy is viewed as an applied health service that is concerned with the quality and satisfaction of daily living from birth to death, as evidenced through occupational role performance.[16] The scope and delivery of such a service may be as complex and varied as the nature of human occupation.

It is the belief of the discipline that "man, through use of his hands, as they are energized by mind and will, can influence the state of his own health" (p. 2).[24] It is the mandate of occupational therapists to provide services that support the child's achievement of health through engagement in purposeful activities. Inherent in this mandate is a second: that occupational therapy services must be relevant to the time, cultures, and environments that are meaningful to the child. Accordingly, service programs must be designed and carried out that use goal-directed, meaningful, and age-appro-

priate activities to influence the quality of human development and life adaptation.

The core of occupational therapy service delivery is the therapist's use of the activity analysis and adaptation processes. Both analysis and adaptation of the activity are determined by the functional components and developmentally antecedent skills required to perform it. The intervention process will require attention to the enhancement and integration of sensory-integrative, motor, cognitive, emotional, and social functions *as these relate to* performance of daily occupational activities. The outcome of occupational therapy service delivery is always determined by the child's mastery of tasks and relationships necessary to actively engage in play, self-maintenance, school, and prevocational activities.[16] Regardless of the complexity of services to enhance functional components of behavior, if the program does not follow through to ensure an optimal level of performance in required everyday activities, it is not occupational therapy.

The occupational therapist may work with children of varied age and diagnostic groups in a broad spectrum of health care, educational, and social service settings. Services provided include assessment of the child's performance of play, self-maintenance, educational, and prevocational tasks and the design, execution, and evaluation of individualized, goal-directed programs.

The goals of occupational therapy intervention are always related to the following:[15]

1. The *development and maintenance* of functions and skills necessary for performance of the desired or required occupational activities
2. *Prevention* of inadequate development, deterioration, or loss of those functions necessary to engage in play, educational, prevocational, and the various self-maintenance activities
3. *Remediation*, or rehabilitation, of dysfunction that impairs acceptable performance of daily occupational activities
4. *Facilitation* of the child's adaptive capacity to influence his or her own life and health status
5. *Collaboration*, communication, and cooperation in the planning and achievement of goals with the child and significant others in the child's life, including family and other service providers.

BASIC PRINCIPLES OF PRACTICE

In essence, the practice of occupational therapy must be directly related to each child's overall mastery of age-appropriate occupational role requirements (that is, player or student) and must also support the achievement of goals and balance in the broader scope of personal and social roles (that is, son-daughter or boy-girl). Therefore the therapist must be familiar with the human development process, its functional and skill components, and its sequence, and the therapist must relate these to the needs of the child within a continuum of health and dysfunction.

The constructs of "human development through occupation" suggest that there are processes and modalities that are generic to occupational therapy services. The processes are activity analysis and activity adaptation. The modalities include occupational activities, relationships, special activity adaptation techniques, and the tools, materials, and equipment of the activity process.

Analysis and adaptation of generic modalities

Occupational activities are selected from the age-appropriate play, work, and self-maintenance categories described earlier. The therapist analyzes the activity by considering the functional content and quality required to perform the activity and the antecedent developmental skills that are needed. The activity is also analyzed to determine if it is meaningful to the age-related role requirements of the child. For example, if the child will be attending school, will the activity be required of the child there, or will it at least promote the child's performance of similar activities in the school setting?

Once the activity is selected, the therapist can structure it and make use of the other generic modalities. From the study of Freud, Piaget, and Erikson the therapist is aware of the motivational utility of the child's *relationships* with human and nonhuman objects. This characteristic of human behavior can be used to stimulate the child to active participation in the activity process. For example, a favorite toy can be used to stimulate the infant toward achievement of a new motor function. Or the therapist can urge the child to complete a craft project as a gift for a parent or favorite relative. When working with young children (Chapter 8), it has proven to be most effective to make direct use of infants' relationships with their mothers by training the mothers to carry out treatment programs.

The activity itself can be modified by use of special *adaptation techniques* that can include such a method as changing the position of the child's body or working surface. The therapist may use some special physical techniques, such as direct sensory stimulation, to enable the child to perform better in the chosen activity. The activity process itself may be modified by breaking tasks down into components by use of a simple-to-complex, step-by-step progression of skill development. Another method is to alter expectations for independent performance of the activity in view of the functional limitations of the child. For example, the therapist may scoop food onto a spoon for the child but expect the child to bring the spoon to his mouth independently.

The therapist may also teach the child to use compensatory methods. In essence, this means teaching the child to substitute the use of a well-developed function for a function that is either temporarily inadequate or poorly developed. For example, if a child has broken an arm but wants to stay independent in self-care, the therapist can teach the child to use one-handed techniques in the varied activities.

The *tools*, *materials*, and *equipment* of the activity are in themselves important modalities and are often the easiest part of the process to adapt. Adaptations can be made according to the developmental sequence of activity performance. Typically, small children can control a ball better with both hands before they can throw with one hand. Therefore the person helping the child learn to do this activity might start out with bilateral throwing of a large ball and progress to a smaller ball as the child gains control of the movement.

There is also a large variety of tools and materials that are collectively known as *adaptive equipment*. This equipment runs the gamut from bent-handle spoons to electronic door openers (and beyond) and often opens up a new world of independent performance for the child. However, adaptation of materials does not necessarily require special devices. Often a simple substi-

EXHIBIT 7-1

Model for activity analysis in pediatric occupational therapy

1. Description of the activity.

2. Properties of the activity.
   a. Tools, materials, techniques, and equipment used in the activity.

   b. Steps in the activity process.

   c. Relationship to occupational role development and performance.

   d. Human and object relationships inherent in the activity process.

3. Performance requirements of the activity.
   a. Developmentally antecedent skills.

   b. Component functions used in the activity process.

Function	*Essentials*	*Variables-adaptables*
Sensory integrative		
Motor		
Cognitive		
Emotional		
Social		

tution, such as Play-doh for plastic clay, may make the activity more achievable for a child. It is clear that in addition to having a good knowledge of developmentally appropriate activities, the therapist must also be able to approach activity performance in a flexible way.

The process of breaking an activity into steps to facilitate performance of the necessary skills is also used to enable the child to learn what to do. The teaching skills of the therapist are important, and the therapist must learn a variety of teaching techniques to deal with a varied pediatric population.[3,4,6,13,21]

This preliminary discussion of activity analysis and adaptation may be clarified further by Exhibit 7-1. This form allows the therapist to analyze the activity according to the components stressed earlier, and it provides information that can be used to adapt the activity to the needs of a child. For example, if the therapist finds that a child lacks the developmentally antecedent skills to perform an activity independently, then a program of the earlier occurring activities would be in order first. Analysis of essential and variable functions permits the therapist to identify activity adaptations that can be tailored to a specific child's functional capacity.

A SEQUENTIAL MODEL OF THE OCCUPATIONAL THERAPY PROCESS

As was previously mentioned, activity analysis and adaptation are generic processes of occupational therapy. A number of categories of occupational therapy modalities were introduced and briefly discussed in relation to the generic processes. These modalities may be used both to assess and to enhance the development and skill performance of the child throughout the occupational therapy intervention process. Figure 7-2, which demonstrates the continuum of normal performance and dysfunction, also represents the sequence of events that leads the child to occupational therapy services.

The two major components of the service process are (1) assessment and (2) program development and evaluation. The latter may be considered *treatment*, and the terms are often used interchangeably. However, this book will use program development and evaluation more frequently for several reasons. First, this terminology is more widely accepted in the educational and social service agencies that are the major employers of pediatric occupational therapists. In addition, it will serve as a reminder of the program evaluation requisite. Together the two components form a continuum of problem identification and problem resolution. Assessment is the problem identification component of practice, whereas program development and evaluation are concerned with problem resolution. These two components

are not mutually exclusive. Much valuable information for assessment purposes is evidenced during programming, and often assessment activities become the foundation of the child's program. In addition, each component has several distinct phases, which are shown in Figure 7-3 and will be discussed in detail here.

Assessment

Assessment is an evaluative process that is based on facts (data collected through different formal and informal objective measures of children's functions and performance) and sound clinical judgment. The latter is the subjective and interpretive component of assessment, and it is the product of the individual therapist's experience that includes training, practice, and theoretical frame of reference. The importance of clinical judgment should not be underestimated. It is the critical difference between a collection of data and meaningful assessment.[16]

Assessment is a continuing process as the therapist constantly thinks through interactions and activity experiences with the child. However, at initial contact and at designated intervals throughout intervention, assessment becomes more structured in formal reports. This allows the therapist to

1. Identify present performance
2. Define problems
3. Identify potential performance
4. Develop program objectives and modalities
5. Record and report progress to document change

The initial contact between the therapist and the child serves as a general performance *screening*. It is necessary to determine whether the child appears to have problems in play, self-maintenance, educational or prevocational activity performance. Also, at this time it may be useful to refer the child to other disciplines and resources for more effective problem identification. The therapist must determine if occupational therapy will help or hinder. Sometimes it may be more efficient to delay the start of occupational therapy until after another service provider has worked with the child. Or the problem may be minor or situational and merely require some timely discussion with the parents and available follow-up as needed.

BASIC METHODS OF ASSESSMENT

Decisions regarding intervention are usually based on data from a variety of resources and the therapist's general problem analysis. Several basic methods are used to collect pertinent information about a child. First, the therapist will *observe* the child, preferably within an uncontrived activity performance situation. For example, the child might be seen in a hospital playroom or in a classroom. Skilled observation requires that the therapist carefully use all senses and record

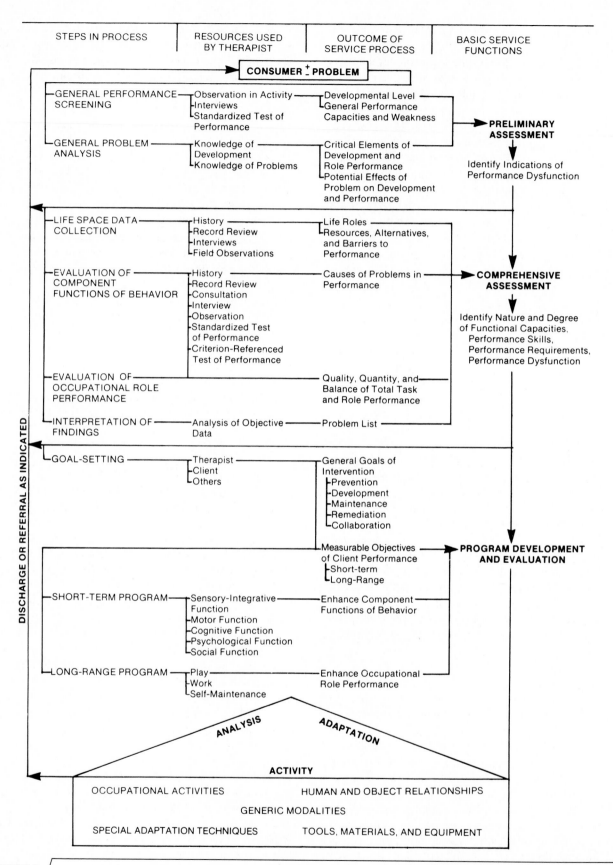

FIGURE 7-3

Sequential model of the occupational therapy process.

From Clark, P.N.: Am. J. Occup. Ther. **33:**583, Sept. 1979.

data objectively. An increasingly popular method of observation is to record the child's activity on videotape, which can then be analyzed later with less loss of information.

Whenever possible, the therapist will conduct short *interviews* with the child, significant others (family and associates), and other members of the service delivery team. The components of a good interview were described by Gillette[10] as being carefully structured, open-ended questions; unbiased observing, listening, and feedback; and objective recording of data.

Next, a *performance-based screening test* may be administered to the child to identify his developmental level, as well as his general performance capacities and weaknesses. The use of a standardized developmental evaluation is highly recommended, because it will provide a normative baseline for continued assessment and descriptive information for program planning.

Standardized tests are recommended for this part of screening because of the way they are constructed, administered, scored, and interpreted. A standarized test is constructed for use with a specific population of people who share some common characteristics. The population could be as specific as a group of multiply handicapped preschool children or as broad a population as 8-year-old children. When the test is constructed, it is repeatedly administered to a sample of this population until it is refined enough to make predictions about that population.

There is a prescribed way to administer a standardized test that is to be followed by anyone who uses the test. There are also prescribed ways to score the test and to interpret the scores. Usually raw scores are obtained from the number of test items passed by the child. These raw scores may be transformed into meaningful data through the use of tables that accompany a test kit. With use of the tables, raw scores are interpreted as developmental age levels, skill quotients, or standard scores. Standard scores are derived through analysis of the raw scores of the population of subjects who were tested during the test construction phase. These calculated scores indicate an individual's relative standing within the performance variations for that population. If the test has been administered and scored properly, and if the test has been found to be valid and reliable, then these interpretive scores (age levels, quotients, or standard scores) may be assumed to indicate the individual's capacities or weaknesses.

Before a standardized test is released for public use, it will be subjected to analysis for validity and reliability. The *validity* of a test indicates whether it measures the skill or function it was designed to meausre. There are several kinds of validity. Logical validity is demonstrated when the test items are directly and obviously examples of the process to be measured. Content validity refers to the relative weighting of test items as they are used to measure a quality. For example, when predicting motor ability, is the value given for raising one's head while in the prone position equal to the value of rolling from the supine position to the side? How many items would be needed to adequately assess the motor skills of an infant? The third, most important type of validity is called construct validity. Through correlations of scores obtained by the sample population on the new test and other recognized tests of the same phenomena, the test developer can determine if the test has predictive value.

The *reliability* data for a standardized test indicate the strength of its predictive value. Normally there are two measures of reliability, each having a different function. Test-retest reliability (also called stability) is determined by administering the test two or more times to each child in the sample within a fairly short time period. The objective is for the children's individual scores to remain fairly consistent in each administration. In addition, the test should be measured for interrater reliability. Typically, two or more testers will administer the test to each child in a sample. The goal here is to have score consistency regardless of who administers the test. If either reliability measure is weak, the test developer must reexamine the standardized administration and scoring methods and refine the test until more consistent (stable) findings are obtained.[11]

GENERAL PROBLEM ANALYSIS

General problem analysis is a thought process (adapted from Llorens[16]) that is used by the therapist to guide initial planning for individuals and groups. The process is based on the therapist's knowledge of child development and pathological processes. First, the therapist will identify the critical elements of development and role performance for the age of a given child. Next, the problem is defined and described. This would include prediction of the course and outcome of the problem, other service providers and procedures that are commonly associated with that problem, and special considerations and precautions involved in management of the problem by the therapist and others.

Next, the therapist will consider what the effects of the problem, as described, might be on attaining and maintaining the critical developmental task and performance requirements of that age. This estimation is a global process, but it requires the use of activity analysis and the consideration of how the component functions of behavior might be affected. The result of this analysis is the identification of potential areas of performance dysfunction that need to be assessed by the therapist and that later will serve as the focus of program development. The occupational therapist then evaluates data collected during screening in relation to the potential effects on occupation role performance predicted by the general problem analysis.

It should be reinforced here that general problem analysis is a thought process, a way of approaching *planning* for a new client or developing a service program for a group who share similar presenting problems. It is useful for occupational therapy students to practice using this method in written form until they become attuned to using the thought process. In addition, a written version of general problem analysis is valuable as a prospectus for a new service program. It will indicate the rationale for occupational therapy intervention, specific foci of the service programs, and space, staff, material, and equipment needs. A sample of a general problem analysis is shown in Exhibit 7-2. Although the information about general problem analysis is presented here after screening, this thought process begins as soon as the therapist is notified of a new referral.

COMPREHENSIVE ASSESSMENT

The preliminary part of the assessment process, or screening, can help the therapist begin to determine what the child needs to be able to do that he or she cannot do to satisfy self, family, and society. Results of general performance screening guide the design of further evaluation as the therapist seeks to identify more precisely the nature and degree of a child's functional capacities and skills, as well as program goals. Comprehensive assessment includes the following:

1. *Life space data collection.*[5] Through history-taking, interviews, and field observations the therapist defines the child's life roles and environmental and cultural performance requirements. External resources, alternatives, and barriers to performance are clarified.

2. *Evaluation of component functions of behavior.* Formal and informal measures of functional capacity are used to determine why a child has problems doing every day activities. The therapist, guided by general problem analysis and screening results, assesses sensory-integrative, cognitive, social, motor, and emotional functions. Specific evaluation of one functional area may be more indepth than others, depending on the presenting problems.

Information about functional capacities may be collected by the therapist through observation, interviews, and administration of standardized and criterion-referenced tests. Standardized tests were discussed in detail in the section on screening. *Criterion-referenced* tests are nonquantifiable measures of performance. They may be commericially produced or therapist made. Behavioral statements about functions or descriptions of a skill are collected from various legitimate resources and listed. For example, if a therapist wanted to evaluate a young child's emotional functions and used Erikson as a reference, a criterion-referenced test might include "Does not cry when mother leaves room." Typically performance is judged by arbitrary ratings that vary in precision. More precise ratings can sometimes be determined by frequency of behavioral occurrence, such as "never," "1 to 3 times out of 10," "4 to 7 times out of 10," and so on. However, a frequency rating may not always be useful for program planning; therefore, descriptive terms are often used. For the example given, there might be such descriptors as "in presence of therapist," "in presence of other children," or "in any situation." Both sets of descriptors are examples of quasi-ordinal scales, which use ranked levels of performance that have no weighted equivalence. Although not often subjected to the rigors of standardized test construction and lacking in reliability data, criterion-referenced tests usually have sufficient logical validity to provide useful information. An example of a well-constructed criterion-referenced test is the Early Intervention Developmental Profile (Chapter 11).

Data may also be collected from other service providers through the use of record review and consultation. Information is taken from charts, reports, team meetings, and individual discussions. The use of assessment findings from other sources helps to limit duplication of services to a child who may already be overwhelmed by professional attention. Interpretation of the assembled data will provide a picture of the child's capacities and deficits in the five component functions (Figure 7-3).

3. *Evaluation of occupational role and activity performance.* Concurrently, the therapist also measures the child's ability to perform specific activities required in daily self-maintenance, play, educational, and prevocational roles. The variety of assessment methods used remains the same but with focus on total task performance. Evaluations of performance in these activities will be both qualitative and quantitative and will also identify the appropriateness of balance between the different categories of occupational activities. For example, does the child take so long to put on a shirt independently that he frequently misses the bus for school? Would it be feasible to use some adaptive equipment or limited assistance from the mother so that he can benefit from school opportunities and still maintain a sense of independence? Considerations of this type guide the transition from assessment to program planning.

Program development and evaluation

Through the assessment process the therapist has identified child-specific performance dysfunctions and problems, that is, what areas and types of activity performance require occupational therapy intervention and why. Often a prioritized list of problems is constructed, either individually by the therapist or jointly with team members.

Program goals and objectives can be developed with the child and family through the consideration of the assembled data and the availability of occupational therapy and other services. *Program goals* describe long-term expectations of treatment and will be consistent with the general goals of occupational therapy, as described earlier and shown in Figure 7-2. *Objectives* can be conceptualized as the short-term accomplishments that will enable the child to achieve long-term goals. Objectives are written in terms of behaviors that will be demonstrated by the child or the therapist. It is usually preferable to write objectives about the child's behaviors because this gives more clues for program planning and regulatory bodies favor this approach. Sometimes, how-

---

EXHIBIT 7-2

General problem analysis
Client: Johnnie Jones
Age: 6
Sex: Male
Life and occupational roles: Boy, son, playmate, brother, student
Problem: Juvenile rheumatoid arthritis
Meaningful others: Parents, siblings, peers, teachers, other relatives, adults in the neighborhood.
Critical elements of development and role performance at this period of life: Learning academic skills; improving motor and perceptual skills; learning to get along with peers; learning social and sexual roles; developing an independent self-concept; moving into the community; developing concrete operations.
Common definition and description of presenting problem: A systemic disease with inflammation of the joint capsule; involves one or more joints; intermittent low-grade fever; pain, swelling, redness, and stiffness. Requires rest, periods of immobilization, medical and nursing care, laboratory procedures, chemotherapy.
Potential disruptions to performance:
  Sensory-integrative: General decrease in sensory stimulation, especially tactile and kinesthetic; vision may be impaired by fever and medications.
  Motor: Decreased muscle strength, speed, flexibility, precision, and impulsion. Decreased practice and refinement of motor patterns.
  Cognitive: Delay of academic learning; interference and effect on perceptual-motor experiences; possible delay on transition to concrete operations because of diminished activities.
  Emotional: Less opportunity for reaching out; forced into dependency; regression may occur; sexual identity could be disrupted.
  Social: Separated from meaningful others, especially peer group; decreased competitive and cooperative interaction experiences; decreased social language development.
  Developmental tasks: All tasks are affected by decreased opportunity, especially physical, academic, and peer group skills.
  Occupational role performance: Limited mobility affects skill development and maintenance in all areas. Subject to dependence in self-care and in initiating activities in other realms.
Areas indicated for occupational therapy assessment: Age-related task performance; evaluation of sensory, motor, and emotional functions. Information on other functions could be obtained from teachers, physician, nurses, parents, social worker, or psychologist.
Suggested procedures: Observation, standardized developmental evaluation for age, interviews with child and parents regarding occupational role and activity history; assessment of play and self-maintenance skills; range of motion and functional muscle strength tests; tests of visual perception and sensory awareness; possibly a projective activity battery. Check on family and developmental history; intellectual assessment and school performance; peer interaction if in a children's unit.
Possible goals for occupational therapy intervention:
  Direct: Maintain developmental-performance skills, especially play, self-care, and socialization; maintain healthy self-concept; prevent loss of joint motion; prevent excessive dependency.
  Indirect: Support bedside academic program; facilitate home management, including parent-child relationships; support medical regimen through the monitoring of performance response to medications and through the use of graded activity program and adherence to medical precautions.
Possible program modalities: Board games at bedside with two or three children; resting splints as necessary to protect joints and maintain range of motion; gross motor play on inflatables; adapted diet to facilitate self-care in feeding; adapted dressing techniques as necessary; reading, story-telling, and dramatic play.

Adapted from Llorens, L.A.: Application of a developmental theory for health and rehabilitation, Rockville, Md., 1976, American Occupational Therapy Association, Inc.

ever, objectives related to therapist behaviors are un-avoidable. An example of this would be when further evaluation or work with parents is indicated. Llorens and Schuster[18] have suggested that these objectives should be measurable and specify what tasks the child will be able to perform to demonstrate goal achievement.

The use of broad goals in combination with specific measureable objectives of task performance is now generally required by regulatory bodies involved with occupational therapy services. Goals will be short and clear, for example, "Johnny will develop age-appropriate feeding skills." This is adequate, but it would be clearer to say, "Johnny will self-feed at the 2-year-old age level."

In contrast, measurable objectives are more elaborate. Each contains three components. First, a *behavioral statement* specifies what the child will do that can be observed. If working on a behavior that cannot be observed, such as a "healthy self-concept," the therapist must specify an observable behavior that gives an indication of the desired phenomenon. For example, the objective might read, "Sally will smile at herself in the mirror." In addition, each objective will include a *condition statement* (descriptively, how the child will do it). The third component is a *performance criterion*, which denotes how acceptable performance will be measured.[27] For example: "Johnny will feed himself [behavioral statement] using a spoon [condition statement] without spilling [performance criterion]."

However, this is not descriptive enough to be useful for program planning or for parents or supervisors who are reviewing a program plan. So it is more likely that a typical objective will include more than one condition statement and often more than one performance criterion. Therefore the objective becomes: "Johnny will feed himself [behavioral statement] solid foods [condition statement] using a spoon or fork [another condition statement] at lunch in the cafeteria [still another condition statement] without spilling [a performance criterion] in 20 minutes [a second performance criterion]." This gives a more precise description of what is expected of the child, as well as how and where he will do it.

Next, a therapy program is designed to meet those objectives, based on the therapist's use of the activity analysis process with generic modalities. Fidler[7a] stated that occupational therapists select activities that duplicate, simulate, or represent the natural activities of the child's required repertoire. As discussed earlier, program activities may be adapted to facilitate independent activity performance. If this is done, the objective would be written to reflect this. The example mentioned earlier might be changed to "Johnny will feed himself solid foods, using a spoon or fork *with built-up handles,* at lunch in the cafeteria, without spilling, *for 10 bites each meal.*"

SHORT-TERM PROGRAM

Most frequently the initial, short-term goals and program will be directed toward improving basic capacities in the five component functions. This practice is supported by the theoretical frameworks presented in Chapter 3. It is proposed that most programs should begin with attention to the physiological components (sensory-integrative, motor, and cognitive functions.) Research reports support the effectiveness of this approach in early programming.[2,14,22] In pediatric occupational therapy, play activities provide the most appropriate modalities for development of component functions. The use of play as a therapeutic modality will be discussed in detail in Chapter 13.

LONG-TERM PROGRAM

The long-term objectives and program are concerned with promoting acceptable performance in required occupational role activities. Therefore the therapist works with the child to develop skills in specific play, self-maintenance, and academic and work readiness activities.

At different intervals throughout the process of intervention, the therapist will retest and reassess the performance status of the child to determine program effectiveness. Goals and objectives must maintain relevance to the changing needs of the child. It is particularly important for the therapist to keep in touch with the family and significant others to ensure continuity and consistency of the program with environmental demands. Moving to a new house or entering a new school can have profound implications for program changes. A two-dimensional review of the intervention process (Figure 7-3) may be used to check relationships between and within components of assessment data, program goals and objectives and program modalities.

DISCHARGE, REFERRAL, AND FOLLOW-UP

It should be remembered that at any time through the sequence of occupational therapy intervention, services may be discontinued. Occasionally this is because of circumstances beyond the therapist's control, such as acute illness or family relocation. However, termination is generally subject to tacit agreement by all parties involved. Because of growth patterns, children tend to reach plateaus of performance, and continued therapy during these times often becomes unproductive. In such instances it is useful to institute "vacation from therapy" periods. This pattern of discharge should be accompanied by a specific follow-up date as well as an open door for parents' contacts before that.

At other times therapy may be discontinued because of a life change of the child that necessitates delivery of occupational therapy through another agency. An example of this is when a child enters a school system that provides direct therapy services. In this case contacts need to be made early with the accepting agency therapist to ensure program continuity and to prepare the child for the changes. Very often children do become attached to their therapists, but they seem to respond nicely when changes are explained in terms of "growing up." Again, an open-door policy with the family should exist, but with the understanding that future contacts will be handled cooperatively with the new therapist.

The preceding cases relate to children whose problems require long-term occupational therapy services. The therapist will also see a number of children whose problems require only short periods of intervention. In this instance therapy is terminated with the expectation that the child can accomplish necessary tasks of the moment and should have little or no difficulty with future developmental requirements. Any problems that are foreseen are carefully discussed with the parents, and the child, if possible. Referrals to other agencies or services are made to ensure adequate supports for remaining or unforeseen problems. As usual, there exists an open-door policy, and the therapist will usually schedule a follow-up appointment within the next 6 months.

STANDARDS OF PRACTICE

In the 1970s the American Occupational Therapy Association (AOTA), through its Commission on Practice, developed standards of practice in different specialty areas. Included among these are standards for developmental disabilities and school system services. These standards are in Appendix A and should be reviewed and updated reularly. The sequential model of practice presented in this section is in accord with AOTA recommendations, and each may help clarify the other.

SUMMARY

The developmental theories used by occupational therapists and the "human development through occupation" model suggest that the therapist is concerned with development, integration, adaptation, competence, and initiative in task performance. Therefore therapy is directed toward providing opportunities to enhance the child's preparedness to deal with the activity performance requirements of daily living. The tools of the occupational therapist are the activities of daily living in the broadest sense.[15] The processes of activity analysis and adaptation are the core functions of the occupational therapist. These functions are used throughout an intervention process that identifies and resolves children's problems through assessment, program development, and evaluation.

REFERENCES

1. Bertrand, A.L.: Social organization: a general systems and role theory perspective, Philadelphia, 1972, F.A. Davis Co.
2. Carlsen, P.N.: Comparison of two ccupational therapy approaches for treating the young cerebral-palsied child, Am. J. Occup. Ther. **29:**267, 1975.
3. Clark, P.N.: Human development through occupation: theoretical frameworks in contemporary occupational therapy practice, part 1, Am. J. Occup. Ther. **33:**505, 1979.
4. Clark, P.N.: Human development through occupation: a philosophy and conceptual model for practice, part 2, Am. J. Occup. Ther. **33:**577, 1979.
5. A curriculum guide for occupational therapy educators, Rockville, Md., 1974, American Occupational Therapy Association, Inc.
6. Cynkin, S.: Toward health through activities, Boston, 1979, Little, Brown & Co.
7. Fidler, G.S., and Fidler, J.W.: Doing and becoming: purposeful action and self-actualization, Am. J. Occup. Ther. **32:**305, 1978.
7a. Fidler, G.S.: Personal communication, 1975.
8. Florey, L.L.: Intrinsic motivation: the dynamics of occupational therapy theory, Am. J. Occup. Ther. **25:**319, 1971.
9. Gilfoyle, E.M., Grady, A.P., and Moore, J.C.: Children adapt, Thorofare, N.J., 1981, Charles B. Slack, Inc.
10. Gillette, N.P.: Occupational therapy and mental health. In Willard, H.S., and Spackman, C.S., editors: Occupational therapy, ed. 4, Philadelphia, 1971, J.B. Lippincott Co.
11. Hasselkus, B.R., and Safrit, M.J.: Measurement in occupational therapy, Am. J. Occup. Ther. **30:**429, 1976.
12. Heard, C.: Occupational role acquisition: a perspective on the chronically disabled, Am. J. Occup. Ther. **31:**243, 1977.
13. Hopkins, H.L., and Smith, H.D.: Willard and Spackman's occupational therapy, ed. 5, Philadelphia, 1978, J.B. Lippincott Co.
14. King, L.J.: A sensory-integrative approach to schizophrenia, Am. J. Occup. Ther. **28:**529, 1974.
15. Lansing, S.G., and Carlsen, P.N.: Occupational therapy. In Valletutti, P., and Christoplos, F., editors: Interdisciplinary approaches to human service delivery, Baltimore, 1977, University Park Press.
16. Llorens, L.A.: Application of a developmental theory for health and rehabilitation, Rockville, Md., 1976, American Occupational Therapy Association, Inc.
17. Llorens, L.A.: 1969 Eleanor Clark Slagle Lecture: Facilitating growth and development: the promise of occupational therapy, Am. J. Occup. Ther. **24:**93, 1970.
18. Llorens, L.A., and Schuster, J.A.: Occupational therapy sequential client care recording system: a comparative study, Am. J. Occup. Ther. **31:**367, 1977.
19. Matsusuyu, J.: Occupational behavior: a perspective on work and play, Am. J. Occup. Ther. **25:**291, 1971.
20. Meyer, A.: The philosophy of occupational therapy, Am. J. Occup. Ther. **31:**639, 1977.
21. Mosey, A.C.: Occupational therapy: configuration of a profession, New York, 1981, Raven Press.
22. Norton, Y.: Neurodevelopmental and sensory integration for the profoundly retarded multiply-handicapped child, Am. J. Occup. Ther. **29:**93, 1975.
23. Pelligrino, E.: Preventive health care and the allied health professions. In Hamburg, J., editor: Review of allied health education, Lexington, 1973, University of Kentucky Press.
24. Reilly, M.: 1961 Eleanor Clark Slagle Lecture: Occupational therapy can be one of the great ideas in 20th century medicine, Am. J. Occup. Ther. **16:**1, 1962.
25. Reilly, M.: A psychiatric occupational therapy program as a teaching model, Am. J. Occup. Ther. **20:**61, 1966.
26. Reilly, M.: Play as exploratory learning: studies in curiosity behavior, Los Angeles, 1974, Sage Publications, Inc.
27. Sprinthall, R.C., and Sprinthall, N.A.: Educational psychology: a developmental approach, ed. 3, Reading, Mass., 1981, Addison-Wesley Publishing Co., Inc.

8

MARTHA S. MOERSCH

Parent involvement

The origin of the term *parent involvement* is unknown, but one can speculate that it must have been selected intentionally for its double meaning. Involve can mean to "occupy (oneself) absorbingly or engrossingly" and to "draw (one) into an entanglement"; the noun involvement can mean both the "action of involving" and the "fact or state of being involved." Parent involvement then becomes a relationship in which each person—the parent and the occupational therapist—assumes responsibility for entering the relationship and for drawing the other person into the relationship.

OCCUPATIONAL THERAPY LITERATURE ON PARENT INVOLVEMENT

Occupational therapists have always been aware of the important role that parents play in helping to carry out treatment plans for children, but the occupational therapy literature has not reflected this awareness to the extent that literature of other disciplines has.

Differences between the first and fifth editions of Willard and Spackman's traditional textbook of occupational therapy[79] indicate that therapists are increasing the documentation of their involvement with parents. In their 1947 edition, Willard and Spackman[79] mentioned parents three times. By 1978, in the fifth edition, Tiffany[69] noted that it was highly desirable that the occupational therapist be involved in parent counseling or family treatment. It was also noted that therapists in acute pediatric settings could expect to spend "50 percent of their time working with adults under stress—the patients' families" (p. 428)[33] and that the entire family of the child with cerebral palsy should be

active members of the treatment team.[40] Parents were discussed at length in the chapter on blindness and deafness: Wade[76] showed empathy for parents and recognized that good relationships with them were necessary to ensure maximal benefits to the blind or deaf child.

If the early occupational therapy literature made only casual mention of parents, it did give considerable coverage of therapist-child interactions. One explanation for this is that therapists of that time often worked with children who lived in residential medical facilities or received long-term care in hospitals. The most obvious explanation is that then, as now, the nature of pediatric occupational therapy, based on active involvement with adaptive response by the child, placed first importance on a close primary relationship with the child.

As therapists began working with younger and more severely handicapped children, it became necessary to bring the parents into more active roles. At the same time the practice of placing children in residential hospital schools ended. Hospital stays became shorter or were often replaced by outpatient services, and many parents made use of hospital live-in privileges.

Knickerbocker,[43] writing in 1965, appears to be the first occupational therapist to write about the art and philosophy of involving parents. Many of her suggestions are almost identical to the current literature on appropriate ways to involve parents. These include the following: ask for suggestions from parents; recognize the value of parents' contributions; do not isolate the child from the parents when treating the child; build on parents' strengths; direct actions toward maintaining a cohesive family unit; make sure that parents know why as well as how to carry out their child's program; help parents develop appropriate perspectives of the capabilities and deficiencies of their child; and structure the therapy program with the goal of developing more effective parent-child relationships.

In 1969 Vulpe[74] reported a home program that tried to provide successful experiences for parents by teaching them to use concrete activities related to their child's developmental patterns. From the early seventies to the present, occupational therapists have published increasing amounts of material for or about parents.*

THERAPIST-FAMILY RELATIONSHIPS
The child

As the therapist develops and maintains a relationship with parents, the parents must sense that the therapist always has the child's welfare as top priority. Otherwise, there is no basis for a therapist-parent relationship. This concept may be difficult to keep in mind during the sometimes stressful process of developing a rapport with parents. The following are some examples of behaviors the therapist can incorporate in interactions with children and parents.

- If the child is physically present during discussions, the therapist should acknowledge the child as an active participant. No one questions the logic of asking an infant, "Show mommy how you can close your lips on the spoon." It may be harder to refrain from talking to parents of a 4- or 5-year-old as if the child were not present or could not understand what was being said.
- Children should be included in the decision-making process whenever possible. It is better for the child to hear what takes place in the parent-therapist conference than to develop anxiety, fear, and fantasy about what is being said.[9]
- Children should be given appropriate explanations of what occupational therapy will try to accomplish and the uncertainties of therapy outcomes. Parents should know what explanations have been given to the child.
- Child need role models to help them develop self-esteem, someone to note or foster their accomplishments, opportunities to take part in usual childhood experiences, and independence in controlling their environments.[9] Parents can observe therapists providing for some of these needs and can be alerted as to how families can contribute.
- Therapists should show respect for the child as a person. Featherstone,[22] both a professional educator and a parent of a handicapped child, notes that a professional "offers parents a chance to savor the ordinary but delicious pleasure of parental

pride and delight" (p. 183) when he treats the handicapped child as any other valuable, real-life child, calling him by name, playing with him, and enjoying him.

The parents

GENERAL CONSIDERATIONS

The therapist should see that at least part of the initial visit of the child and his parents is spent in discussion of what occupational therapy is and what it can be expected to do for children in general. It is important that both parents be present for as much of the initial evaluation and parent-informing and program-planning sessions as possible. The therapist should schedule these sessions with consideration for the family's responsibilities. Developmental programs for young children are time-consuming and require cooperation among all persons involved. If only one parent is present at the first sessions, it will be necessary for this parent to later explain findings and recommendations to the other parent and thereby risk being put in the position of having to defend the program. Even when both parents are present for the informing and decision-making sessions, they should also be given written reports to review as they wish.

Parents are consumers of the therapist's services. They will, and should, make judgments about the services. As knowledgeable and involved consumers, perhaps these parents can become lifetime advocates of their handicapped children.

GUIDELINES FOR HOME PROGRAMS

The nature of a child's growth and development and the occupational therapist's goal to help children attain their maximal potential levels of growth and development require home programs to be included in occupational therapy treatment. The following guidelines will assist therapists in developing home treatment programs to be carried out by parents and families.

- Develop the home program following the initial meetings with the child and parents. These meetings are for orientation, interview, comprehensive evaluation, parent informing, and treatment planning and for parents and therapist to enter into a relationship for providing treatment to the child.
- Visit the child's home for some of the initial meetings, if possible.
- Give parents written reports of all findings and plans as they are developed.
- Determine jointly with the parents the treatment objectives, as well as the appropriate activities to meet the objectives, and specify what portions of the treatment will take place at home.
- Write objectives in areas of the child's strengths

---

*References 1, 7, 11, 15, 17, 18, 21, 23, 24, 32, 37, 42-44, 46, 51, 54, 55, 57, 58, 61, 62, 73-76, 80.

and weaknesses. This encourages parents and assures them of some success.

- Demonstrate the treatment activities and explain their rationale; teach the parents to perform the activities, observe their practice, correct their mistakes, and make necessary adaptations; answer parents' questions you have answers for and be honest about questions you do not have answers for; and provide emotional support to the parents.
- Encourage parents to join you in frequent problem-solving sessions.
- Make sure that necessary supplies and equipment are available.
- Monitor parents' program implementation and make appropriate adaptations and changes in conjunction with the parents.
- Reevaluate and write new objectives at frequent intervals (3- to 6-month intervals recommended).
- Vary activities to maintain continued interest of both child and parents and for generalization of learning. Encourage parents to think of variations and try them.
- Work toward parents' assumption of responsibility for the treatment program.
- Be guided by the suggestion that the "development of realistic parental perceptions and expectations may be a major goal of treatment" (p. 39).[64]

Occupational therapists have discussed home programs in numerous publications.* Program suggestions appear throughout the discussions of practice in this text.

MOTIVATING PARENTS

Therapists often ask how to motivate parents to carry out treatment programs. Two ways are (1) be sure that the program works for the child and (2) be sure that the parent will achieve some success.

Parent motivation is usually increased by setting up treatment activities that can be carried out in the daily routine of the family, such as gross motor activities during bath and diapering times, rough and tumble play with a parent or sibling, or fine motor manipulation board games that other family members enjoy.

Parents are usually more motivated if they have had a part in planning the program. The therapist should make reasonable requests of the parents. It is not necessary that the treatment program be done in the same way or at the same time each day. However, for some parents a very structured program seems to be more motivating.[51] A parent who is overwhelmed by the constant problems brought on by a handicapped child and has experienced feelings of helplessness may welcome a home program that is written precisely and includes a

---

*References 1, 18, 37, 42-44, 46, 51, 54, 62, 74, 75.

section for recording treatment time and comments by the parent.

FOSTERING PARENT-THERAPIST INTERACTIONS

Therapists must be objective in evaluating their own actions as they try to work out positive relationships with parents. Knickerbocker[43] has suggested that therapists who assume major treatment responsibility for the child may "imply that the parents' responsibility ends at the clinic door" (p. 129). Therapists should guard against assuming authoritarian roles that seem to put them in superior positions because this can interfere with therapist-parent communication and make it more difficult for parents to assume their responsibilities. Therapists should be alert to possibilities that they may "mother" or "father" the child as a way of fulfilling their own needs for parental roles; in so doing they "may tend to usurp the rightful responsibilities of the child's own parents" (p. 130).[43]

The following suggestions, paraphrased from Roos[61] are ways of building productive work relationships between parents and professionals.

- Parents should be accepted as team members, considered as colleagues, and their contributions treated with respect.
- Parents and professionals should recognize and discuss their preconceived notions or negative expectations of each other.
- Professionals should accept parents "where they are."
- Professionals should be aware of and willing to listen to expression of existential anxieties of parents.
- Professionals should share relevant information with parents.
- Professionals should maintain good communication with a minimum of professional jargon.
- Professionals should select methods and techniques; parents, and children if appropriate, should make the final selection of goals and objectives.
- Parents and professionals need mutual support and encouragement from each other.
- Parents and professionals should never compete with each other or undermine each other's efforts with the child.

SPECIAL CIRCUMSTANCES OF PARENTS

The pediatric occupational therapist is likely to find that a variety of circumstances exist among parents. The circumstances become important to the therapist only if the welfare of the child is affected, but knowledge of them may be of help in working with parents.

Marital problems affect many parents of handicapped children because marital problems affect a high percentage of the population as a whole and because there is the added stress of caring for a disabled child.[22,78]

Single parents head many families with handicapped children. Problems that may arise are not necessarily related to singleness itself, but to the lack of another adult who can provide support.[4] Bronfenbrenner[6] noted that one of the five factors that determine the effectiveness of early intervention programs for children is the "presence in the home of another adult besides the principal caretaker" (p. 18).

Therapists will encounter *those other than biological parents in the parental role*, such as adoptive parents, stepparents, foster parents, guardians, grandparents, siblings, other relatives, agency representatives, and friends. The occupational therapist's relationship with surrogate parents will usually be the same as with biological parents, and the suggestions of Roos[61] will usually apply to anyone in the parental role. Exceptions could exist in those instances in which there are unusual circumstances. However, the person who is legally designated as responsible in the child's state of residence, including the handicapped or ill person, must sign all legal documents.

Mentally retarded parents are sometimes found among parents of handicapped children. Such parents can usually manage to maintain themselves and their families in at least a marginal manner, but they may need help in crises. Occupational therapists are well aware of the knowledge and skills required to help physically or mentally disabled parents to cope with management of their handicapped children.

Parents who abuse children are as likely to be found among parents of handicapped children as they are in the population as a whole.[12,21,78] Child abuse creates very difficult situations. It has received much concern and study, but it is far from being eradicated. There is speculation about the long-term effectiveness of mandatory reporting of suspected child abuse by persons providing care and education to children.[27]

Therapists should also be aware of possible problems among parents at low economic or educational levels who have other ill or dependent family members or who make frequent geographical moves and must therefore locate new community resources and emotional support.

Siblings

Through discussions with parents or through their own observations, therapists can determine the need of siblings to know and understand the handicapped child's condition, to know the implications of the handicapping condition as it relates to them, and to know the future expectations related to the handicapped child.[7,9,45] There are numerous publications explaining handicapping conditions in suitable terms for siblings of all ages. Many books on handicapped children and their families have sections on siblings and list resources for helping them.[7,78]

Grandparents

Parents may report that they have more difficulty coping with the concerns and questions of their parents than they do with those of their nonhandicapped children. This is not unexpected, since grandparents have concerns for both the beloved grandchild and their own beloved child. Parents may also report more difficulties with grandparents who live far away. Dickerson and Brown[19] noted, "It is a lot easier to maintain unreal expectations for a child over a period of time if you don't have any experiences living with the particular child" (p. 87).

However, parents usually report positive aspects of involvement of the grandparents in the care of a handicapped child. The grandparents provide emotional support, sitter or respite care, financial assistance, and attention to the other children in the family so that the parents are able to spend more time with the handicapped child.[19] Therapists are likely to have relationships with grandparents that can facilitate the child's therapy. Grandparents are good sources of information about the child, because many children willingly cooperate with grandparents. Grandparents often have more time than working parents to play with or teach the child, and they contribute in many ways to a normal family life for the child.

Grandparents can also contribute to friction within a family, as when a husband or wife may be forced to take sides for or against inlaws or each other.[9] Moersch[56] described some possible problems in households made up of children, parents, and grandparents. When fathers are too busy to accompany mothers to clinic visits of the child, the grandmother often goes along to help with the child. This may result in increasing the competency and effectiveness of the mother and grandmother and strengthening their alliance. By contrast, the father becomes less competent and effective. Extreme examples have shown that grandparents, especially the grandmother, assume the parental role in opposition to one or both parents and to the extent that the child is uncertain as to who the real mother or father is. In such families, children who are already prone to learning or emotional problems seem to suffer from living with too many adults who expose them to different and contradictory expectations of behavior. Other factors negatively affecting the child are parents and grandparents who act as individuals rather than family units in managing the children and the broken homes. Infantilization, a particularly undesirable trait in a handicapped child, may result.

Northcott,[59] who worked with young deaf children for many years, cautioned those professionals in programs for young handicapped children to be aware of the special situation of the single parent and the parent in a multigeneration family under one roof.

Others: relatives, neighbors, friends, the public

Therapists do not usually have active relationships beyond the immediate family of the child. However, the welfare of the child can be affected if the parents have difficulties maintaining a normally functioning environment. To educate relatives, neighbors, friends, or other persons who seem likely to interfere with family relationships, the therapist can make use of the ongoing efforts of schools, churches, the press, movies, television, the government, and others to influence attitudes toward people with handicapping conditions. These efforts can provide information and influence public policy. It is hoped they can also suggest positive alternative actions to family associates.[5,10,48,67,81]

THE THERAPIST'S PREPARATION TO RELATE TO FAMILY MEMBERS

Many persons who become certified as occupational therapists do so with minimal knowledge and experience in forming working relationships with parents and families of patients. If academic courses dealing with families are offered, they may not be useful. Turnbull[70] noted that many university courses on families give limited attention to helping parents solve their day-to-day problems. Instead, courses are likely to spend time on the "psychological insight approach to parental guilt." Such courses tend to "insure conflict and unsatisfactory relationships between parents and professionals. Extended practicum with families of handicapped children . . . should be standard requirement for courses which purport to prepare students for working with parents" (p. 138).[70]

Clinical placements may provide opportunities for some students to work with parents in pediatric acute care hospitals and other programs that emphasize parent involvement. But when and where do most occupational therapists get sufficient practice in working with parents to feel comfortable in doing so? Probably only when they begin working in a program in which parent involvement is an integral part of the structure. Early intervention programs for handicapped or high-risk infants have been good sources for learning to work with parents, especially those programs that include home visits. Home visits bring about intimate associations with families who have to add the care of a handicapped child to the normal responsibilities of the family. Here the occupational therapist becomes a "participant in both the joys and sorrows of the families, including critical illnesses and death as well as the successful attainment of program objectives" (p. 41).[56]

While reading should not be emphasized over active participation, there are many excellent publications on working with parents and families (see References). For example, therapists could learn a great deal from Roos's discussion[61] of the existential conflicts that most people have at times but that parents of handicapped children are especially likely to have. Roos[61] noted that he and his wife found that "professionals seemed strangely disinclined to listen to our concerns. . . ." He lists the critical conflict areas most likely to be reactivated by the realization of having a retarded child as disillusionment, aloneness, vulnerability, inequity, insignificance, past orientation, and loss of immortality (p. 20).[61]

As therapists increase their awareness of all the facets of coping with the presence of a handicapped child in the family, they will also increase their own creative skills and sensitivity in developing and maintaining interactions with parents and other family members.[34,71]

NATURE OF PARENT INVOLVEMENT
Infant and preschool years

Literature on parent involvement since the mid-1960s pertains overwhelmingly to the infant and preschool years. This is explained in part by the focus of medical and educational research on young children, belief in the importance of the family setting for early learning, availability of funds, expectations of parents to care for their young children, and recognition by professionals of the personal satisfaction and career opportunities in working with preschool children.

The majority of early preschool programs[30,31,35,77] were for disadvantaged children and were aimed at improving cognitive and social levels of the children. Handicapped children were added as the result of the movement toward guaranteeing the rights of all people and because of the influence of parent groups. Medical advances in prenatal and perinatal care, studies of parent-infant bonding, and general feelings of "the earlier the better" reduced the age level of special programs to birth, and the parent involvement literature increased even more.

Childhood years

State and national mandatory special education laws were enacted and reflected the concept of parents' rights in legislative and educational practices. The numbers of children placed in residential institutions were greatly reduced, and education was broadened to include individualized training appropriate to the child.

Literature on parent involvement in programs for school-aged children has focused mainly on the decision-making mechanism for individualized programs.

Adolescent years

The nature of parent involvement in the lives of all children changes drastically when the children reach adolescence. It appears that adolescence is such a critical time that whether the child is ill or handicapped seems secondary in importance. At the same time, the presence of a handicapping condition increases the possibility that the child will not acquire the basic survival skills so important in adult life.[13]

Parents of children with all levels of handicapping conditions are well aware of the changes that occur when the children reach adolescence. Parents of a severely retarded son were surprised at the abrupt changes that came with puberty after they had assumed that a mentally slow child would also show slow physical development. They found instead that there was a difference between having a retarded child and having a retarded teenager. In another case, parents of a child with the hidden disorder of bronchial asthma (which resulted in acute crises that periodically disrupted an otherwise normal development) described the difficult decision they had to make to send their son to a residential treatment center where "the psychological atmosphere . . . was one of freedom and independence in which the youngsters controlled much of their own life situation . . . [and could] be as physical and active as they wished to be" (p. 207).[25] One intellectually bright but severely physically handicapped person considered that the success of her life was a result of her parents' repetitions throughout her early years that she could be anything she wanted to be.[8] It is especially hard for parents of mildly handicapped children of adolescent age to strike a balance between their love and concern for their children and their children's need to acquire the "skills and competencies necessary to function independently of parents, to become gainfully employed, and to assume adult responsibilities" (p. 1).[50]

Some special educators believe that both parents and professionals should have a thorough understanding of all that adolescence implies,[13] that "emotional development and the self-concept of a mildly handicapped adolescent may be of paramount importance" (p. 52),[50] and that the period of secondary education often brings about increased family stress, socialization problems, and interpersonal conflict.[50] Most of the interactions of professionals and parents of mildly handicapped adolescents will take place in the secondary educational environment, and the parent involvement will of necessity be less visible and less active. Professionals must realize how important it is that there be candid discussion between themselves and parents with under-standing on the part of both.[50] Persons filling parent counseling roles must be aware of the special problems of the secondary school because of the number of personnel involved and the "impersonal structure of the school" (p. 124).[50]

The *Exceptional Education Quarterly* devoted an entire issue to the subject of mildly handicapped adolescents. Entitled "Special Education for Adolescents and Young Adults,"[16] it presented such topics as educational options, career preparations, work-oriented curriculums versus academic education, and the similarities between learning disabled and low-achieving secondary school students. It also dealt with emotional factors, such as the depression and suicide potential and the vulnerability of partially blind and hard-of-hearing adolescents to psychiatric disturbance, and the need for sex education for handicapped persons. The importance of social skills, the impact of mandatory minimal competency testing, and the greater prevalence of learning disabled persons among officially delinquent youth were discussed. This issue is an exceptionally informative resource for both professionals and parents.

Mental retardation

The literature on parent involvement has been greatly influenced by the problems associated with mental retardation. Both early and contemporary programs for high-risk children have had prevention of mental retardation as a major purpose. As preschool programs for handicapped children became widespread, many of the children served were mentally retarded, such as those with Down's syndrome or those who were multiply handicapped with various degrees of mental retardation as one of the handicaps, or were severely handicapped by blindness, deafness, cerebral palsy, emotional disturbance, or unusual medical conditions. For this last group of children there was a need to provide them with appropriate stimulation and adaptations for cognitive learning so that they would not be restricted in their learning. Since all children have the same growth, development, and learning needs, the literature on mental retardation is appropriate for all children and parents at some stages of the children's lives. It is also appropriate for professionals.

Other disability areas

The literature on parent involvement with learning disabilities,* chronic medical conditions,[25,45] physical disabilities,† sensory deficits,‡ or emotional problems§

---

*References 1, 13, 16, 24, 44, 65.
†References 10, 18, 32, 38, 43, 52, 62.
‡References 18, 37, 54, 62, 76.
§References 1, 18, 21, 23, 52, 63.

is available but in lesser degree than that which is related to mental retardation. One area that needs to be covered in parent involvement literature is that of severe traumatic head injuries that result in brain damage. Such injuries are becoming more common among children of childhood and adolescent years. Thoms Rehabilitation Hospital[52] has published an informative handbook for families. It is fortunate that the fostering of self-esteem, play skills, social competence, and emotional development is usually stressed in most parent involvement literature.

Children at risk

As occupational therapists expand their practice areas to include facilitation of growth and development in well children who are at risk for developmental problems, they see parent involvement as a major vehicle for implementation of their programs.

Finn[23] described a community intervention and prevention model for children, parents, and school personnel in an inner-city area. Parents were helped to learn about mothering skills, elements of children's developmental processes, toy construction from household items, and other positive parent-child interactions in both group and home visit situations. The program emphasized the parents as decision makers regarding their children, the provision of basic emotional support for parents, and preserving and respecting the values and life-styles of the parents.

Gillette[26] set up an art workshop for the mothers of preschool children who were identified by the school as exhibiting less than optimal mothering behaviors toward their children. The mothers who were selected had difficulties in one or more of the areas of "discipline; intimacy; giving (in other than material ways); allowing freedom of expression, especially when it was 'messy'; permitting the development of autonomy in the child; and denying the existence of certain personal needs which resulted in a sense of depletion and frustration in the mother herself" (p. 128).[26] The preschool children themselves were "considered to be poor educational, emotional, or behavioral risks for the community" (p. 127).[26] Results of the program led to the assumption "that an increase in [the mother's] own sense of personal value can lead to more mature behavior in regard to other persons" (p. 129).[26] It was not possible to identify specific changes in the mothering behavior at the time of reporting. The program itself is an example of how occupational therapists can take part in parent involvement with the intent of benefiting children.

Llorens[46] included a brief description of a program for teenage mothers as one example of her use of objective setting to establish an occupational therapy pro-

gram with an inner-city community. The mothers were helped through an education-consultation process to increase their own interpersonal growth and development as one means of preventing interpersonal difficulties within the mother-infant relationship.

In 1978 Morris[58] suggested parent education in well baby care as a new role for the occupational therapist. She reported that pediatric clinics were ideal locations for parent education programs for teaching mothers the mental health aspects of child care, how to support their child's cognitive development, and alternative ways of interacting with their child.

Ellsworth[21] described a parent education program that was designed to counteract the increasing incidence and severity of child abuse and neglect among children of Army families, as well as the alarming prevalence of parents ill prepared to rear socially and emotionally healthy children. The program, developed and directed by an occupational therapist and an Army health nurse, followed a 10-week seminar and group counseling format for parents, accompanied by developmental assessment and play therapy sessions for their children. Provisions were made for appropriate follow-up treatment for the children and counseling for the parents.

ISSUES OF PARENT INVOLVEMENT
Play and parent-family involvement

It is appropriate to link play and parent involvement in a book on how occupational therapy can help children play, grow, learn, and develop skills that will enable them to enjoy satisfying adult lives. Various types of play, from infant stimulation to educational games for teenagers, take place within the family environment.

During the past decade much attention has been paid to infant sensory stimulation, which was said by White[77] to be "an extension of the love of two caring people for their child" (p. 64). Occupational therapists have used the normal day-to-day interactions of mothers and children to determine how mothers can provide sensory stimulation to their infants,[15] how mothers can be helped to understand sensory integrative problems of their children,[1] and how mothers can make their children's everyday environments more positive.[24] Day[15] found that in a 4- to 6-week-old infant, playing was second only to feeding in providing the greatest amount of stimulation. On a per minute basis, playing provided more stimulation than any other activity, and playing was an important provider of all types of stimulation. Ayres[1] described how parents can involve their children in sensory integrative activities in the form of play to encourage adaptive responses and to enhance the children's self-esteem. Gordon and Lalley[30] used play activities in their research studies of disadvantaged mothers and their children. Later, the play activities were published for the use of other parents.[28,29]

Many of the intervention programs[30,31,77] in the 1960s and early 1970s for high-risk children made extensive use of home visitors. One of the major duties of the home visitor was to demonstrate play activities to the parents and to encourage parents to play with their children. There are many books on play, crafts, and games for children of all ages. Parents should be warned to inspect them carefully before purchasing to be sure that they will be useful.

Parent as teacher or therapist

The topic of parents as teachers or therapists arises often in descriptions of programs for individuals or groups of children with handicaps. For the most part, the situation is either casually accepted or upheld as being desirable, beneficial, and expedient.*

Positive reports of parents acting as teachers come from persons well known in early programs for children at risk, such as Gray,[31] Weikart,[77] and Gordon and Lally.[30] Subsequently, others such as Shearer and Shearer,[66] Vulpe,[74,75] and Baker[3] developed programs in which parents were teachers for retarded children and others. Morris[58] wrote that "The parent can serve as an effective teacher when given training and experience in learning alternative ways of interacting with the child" (p. 75).

Shapero and Forbes[65] reviewed parent involvement in programs for learning disabled children and reported that a hands-off policy for parents as teachers was evident throughout the 1960s, but the policy changed completely by the early 1970s. In a study of more than 100 college and university teacher training programs in special education, 65% of the respondents had developed at least one course on training teachers to work with parents from 1973 to 1978. They concluded from their review that although the available research in nonclinical settings was inconclusive, it appeared that parents as teachers could positively affect the academic performance of learning disabled children. California allows parents to go beyond being teachers or therapists and serve as program coordinators[60] for their developmentally disabled children. Formal and structured training programs have been set up to assist parents to assume this role.

Another term to describe parents in the teaching role is *cotherapist*, which was used by Schopler[63] in a statewide program for autistic children in North Carolina. Parents carry out individualized home programs and also help out in the classrooms. *Provider of infor-*

mal therapy is the term used to describe "the introduction of therapeutically useful actions into the daily care and handling program" (p. 383),[38] especially for children with cerebral palsy.

In 1970 Moersch established the major feature of an early intervention program that was incorporated into the Early Intervention Project for Handicapped Infants and Young Children[57] in 1973: parents were to be supported as the major treatment providers for their handicapped children. *Major treatment provider* could be looked on as a general term, since staff members were from various disciplines. The term was selected after thoughtful consideration of the intended philosophy of the program, namely, that such young handicapped children need as much care as possible throughout their waking hours. Specialized therapy programs two or three times a week were not sufficient.

The term *treatment* was selected because of its current usage by interdisciplinary teams to denote purposefully and thoughtfully planned management. The parents' treatment would include what all parents do to care for their babies. Tasks that were easy with normal babies would be harder and take more time with handicapped babies, but they would be parent oriented instead of teacher-therapist oriented.

With the terminology established, it then became the responsibility of the project staff to develop treatment plans to fit into routine child care. The physical therapist determined what the child needed under the rubric of physical therapy, what part of the physical therapy could be done as exercises by the parents, and how the parents could incorporate the exercises into diapering, dressing, bathing, and playing with the child. The occupational therapist, speech therapist, psychologist, and special educator made similar discipline-related decisions. Parents became aware of the importance of establishing communication, naming items around the house, or singing to the child but would never stop everything to have a period of speech therapy.

The Early Invervention Project made a point of not calling the parents "teachers" or "therapists." The outcome was that many of the activities of occupational, physical, and speech therapists; special educators; and psychologists were translated into normal child care activities and carried out by people called "parents."[57]

There are those who oppose putting parents in the position of teachers or therapists on the grounds that this practice can diminish their roles as mothers or fathers. Tyler and Kogan[73] reviewed findings from studies reported in 1972 and 1974 of parent-child interactions with young children with cerebral palsy. They found that both mother and child showed more negative behaviors when the mother was performing therapy than when mother and child were playing. There was pro-

---

*References 2, 3, 31, 39, 66, 74, 75, 77.

gressive reduction of warm and positive behaviors in both mother and child over a 2-year period. They suggested that teaching mothers to be therapists could be an intrusion into the parent role, and they recommended that parents be guided toward healthy interactions with their children. A subsequent study was undertaken in which mothers were provided behavioral instruction to help them develop warm and positive behaviors toward their children. The positive effect of mothers in the second study emphasized that the "mother's role as an attentive audience and in enjoying the child's play can be important components" (p. 155)[73] in mother-child interactions.

Turnbull and Turnbull,[72] both professionals and parents of a handicapped child, urge that more study be done on parents as teachers and on the consequences of this practice for the parent-child relationship and for the child's self-image. They caution about the "possible implicit message to the child: 'You need to get well—you are unacceptable as you are' " (p. 120).

Whether one speaks of the parent as teacher, therapist, cotherapist, or treatment provider, the important point is whether the professional feels comfortable helping the parent to assume the role and whether the parent feels comfortable in doing so. In *Helping Your Exceptional Baby*, Cunningham and Sloper[14] used the following low-key way of introducing the helping process to parents:

> Teaching is the art of getting someone to learn. Learning has taken place when someone can do something [he] could not do before. So anything that helps someone learn something new can be called teaching. Seen like this, we are all teachers. We all help each other and our children to learn (p. 101).

Parent as advocate

The establishment in 1950 of the Association for Retarded Children (later changed to the Association for Retarded Citizens) and other parent groups is generally noted as the beginning of parent advocacy. Parent involvement does not necessarily have an active connotation, but parent advocacy requires the watchful and active participation of parents in securing services for their children.[47,50]

Staff members of the Early Intervention Project worked to help parents become advocates for their own and for all handicapped children.[7,57] Two of the parents described a successful parent advocate situation in their own words[41]:

> We have found it necessary to advocate for Laura with regard to the school bus. We needed to be sure that a seat appropriate to her size and type of handicap was provided for her. Since she was not sitting independently when she first began to ride the bus, we had to request an infant safety seat. As she has grown and developed,

we've made sure that the appropriate safety changes have been made. . . . We feel that advocating in school for our child is not just a privilege but a responsibility that we are obligated to fulfill in order to ensure the best possible education for our daughter (p. 28, 29).

Markel and Greenbaum[49] saw the need for parents to take more assertive roles, including advocacy, and compiled in workbook format *Parents Are to be Seen and Heard: Assertiveness in Educational Planning for Handicapped Children*. This book used actual situations reported by parents and is helpful for parent group meetings, workshops, and individual parents.

Parent counseling

When a telephone caller asks, "Will you talk with a mother about feeding her cerebral palsied child?" what pediatric occupational therapist would say no? If the same therapist was asked whether he or she is qualified as a counselor, what would the answer be?

What qualifies someone for counseling? Buscaglia[8] said that it depends on the questioner's definition of counseling and that "there appears to be little agreement concerning what counseling really is or should be. What is viewed as a *given assumption* or *common sense* to a traditional psychotherapist may be seen as a vague, meaningless opinion to a behaviorist" (p. 43). Buscaglia challenged

> Medical doctors, psychologists, counselors, educators, physical and occupational therapists, social workers, psychiatrists, and all those in the helping professions, to become more cognizant of the desperate need the disabled person and the family have for good, sound, reality-based guidance (p. 5).

It appears that many occupational therapists are reluctant to call themselves counselors. However, in reality they often find themselves in counseling roles with patients, clients, students, and others. As is true with counselors from any discipline, occupational therapists must be aware of the limitations of their knowledge and expertise and must decide when the needs of the person being counseled go beyond their expertise. At this point the occupational therapist has the same professional obligation as does any other counselor: to refer the person to a counselor with the appropriate expertise. Within these constraints, occupational therapists can still provide a great deal of beneficial counseling to the parents of handicapped, ill, and at-risk children.

The reading parent

Reading materials should be made available to parents who wish to use them. Therapists should be sensitive to the reluctance of parents of young handicapped children to read technical books that discuss disabilities in great detail and that are accompanied by photographs of persons of all ages and in all stages of the disability.

Many books on handicapped children[7,20,50,68] have lists of resources and readings for parents. From such lists, parents and therapists can identify books and articles on play and stimulation activities, sex education, growth and development, adaptive equipment, child abuse, attitudes toward people with handicaps, terminal illness and death, managing behavior problems, baby sitting and respite care, sibling reactions, the future of the handicapped child, and many types of handicapping conditions.

REACTIONS AGAINST PARENT INVOLVEMENT

It would be dishonest to imply that all parents are totally in favor of being involved in training and educating their handicapped children. Parent involvement appears to develop more naturally among parents of infants, since parents naturally assume that they will provide care for their infants. Such assumptions do not necessarily apply to older children.

Meyer,[53] in describing the life of her 18-year-old severely retarded son, said that she "would have been very grateful for any therapeutic help when he was an infant, but there was none available at that time" (p. 110). When her child was finally accepted into a program, she was grateful that the program "did not encourage parental involvement in other than typical school functions. I had spent twenty-four hours a day for six years with my child . . .; relief from constant child management allowed me the luxury of contributing [as a volunteer in community social and health agencies] and increased my own feelings of worth" (p. 110).

Turnbull and Turnbull[72] commented on the amount of time involved in educational matters. They feel that parent involvement and advocacy keep some parents so busy that they are thereby excluded from their own mainstream experiences with parents of nonhandicapped children. They question the emphasis on benefit to the child and suggest that parent involvement should also benefit the parents by "reducing stress, increasing family coping, and improving relationships within the family (parent and sibling) and with the handicapped child" (p. 116).[72]

Turnbull and Turnbull[72] felt strongly about the current emphasis on parents under Public Law 94-142, in which the "concept of parent participation pervades the requirements [of the law and] extends the right and arguably the duty to parents of handicapped children to assume the role of educational decision maker" (p. 115).[72] Some parents have neither the desire nor the capabilities to assume this responsibility; furthermore, opportunities for actual decision making are much more limited than the law implies. Turnbull and Turnbull suggested that programs "tolerate a range of parent involvement choices and options, matched to the needs and interests of the parents" (p. 120).[72]

It is also important that the nature of parent involvement in occupational therapy programs consider the need to establish independence in the growing child.

SUMMARY

As occupational therapists become more active in programming for infants and for children whose disabilities require long-term or lifetime attention of parents or other adults, the topic of parent involvement in therapy programs becomes increasingly important. Since the beginning of the 1970s, public opinion and philosophy, legislation, and governmental regulations have created a climate of child care that makes it necessary for individual or agency service providers to be sure to involve parents or to state their reasons for not doing so.

It may be useful for therapists to keep in mind that the new directions for the future that were identified in the eleventh annual report of the President's Committee on Mental Retardation[60] in 1978 included parent participation options in which

> Parents have a wide range of talents and temperaments. The best way to utilize parents is to recognize these differences and provide them with options which they can choose on the basis of their individuality. The worst: to involve them in narrow, heavily structured activities which do not fit their best capabilities (p. 73).

REFERENCES

1. Ayres, A.J.: Sensory integration and the child, Los Angeles, 1979, Western Psychological Services.
2. Badger, E.: The infant stimulation/mother training project. In Caldwell, B.M., and Stedman, D.J., editors: Infant education: a guide for helping handicapped children in the first three years, New York, 1977, Walker & Co.
3. Baker, B.L.: Support systems for the parent as therapist. In Mittler, P., editor: Research to practice in mental retardation: care and intervention, vol. 1, Baltimore, 1977, University Park Press.
4. Baker, B.L., Clark, D.B., and Yasuda, P.M.: Predictors of success in parent training. In Mittler, P., editor: Frontiers of knowledge in mental retardation: social, educational, and behavioral aspects, vol. 1, Baltimore, 1981, University Park Press.
5. Baskin, B.H., and Harris, K.: Notes from a different drummer: a guide to juvenile fiction portraying the handicapped, New York, 1977, R.R. Bowker Co.
6. Bronfenbrenner, U.: Who needs parent education? Position paper prepared for the Working Conference on Parent Education, Flint, Mich., 1977, sponsored by the Charles Stewart Mott Foundation.

7. Brown, S.L., and Moersch, M.S., editors: Parents on the team, Ann Arbor, 1978, The University of Michigan Press.

8. Buscaglia, L.: The disabled and their parents: a counseling challenge, Thorofare, N.J., 1975, Charles B. Slack, Inc.

9. Chinn, P.C., Winn, J., and Walters, R.H.: Two-way talking with parents of special children, St. Louis, 1978, The C.V. Mosby Co.

10. Clearly, M.: Please know me as I am: a guide to helping children understand the child with special needs, Sudbury, Pa., 1975, Jerry Clearly.

11. Cohn, M.S., and Caffey, K.J.: Handi-sitters: how to sit for the handicapped, 1812 Mapleleaf Boulevard, Oldsmar, Fla., 1979, Handi-Sitters.

12. Colman, W.: Occupational therapy and child abuse, Am. J. Occup. Ther. **29:**412, 1975.

13. Cruickshank, W.M., Morse, W.C., and Johns, J.S.: Learning disabilities: the struggle from adolescence toward adulthood, Syracuse, N.Y., 1980, Syracuse University Press.

14. Cunningham, C., and Sloper, P.: Helping your exceptional baby, New York, 1980, Pantheon Books, Inc.

15. Day, S.: Mother-infant activities as providers of sensory stimulation, Am. J. Occup. Ther. **36:**579, 1982.

16. Deshler, D.D., editor: Special education for adolescents and young adults, Except. Educ. Q. **1**(2):entire issue, 1980.

17. D'Eugenio, D.B.: But he doesn't fit in the car seat anymore. In Brown, S.L., and Moersch, M.S., editors: Parents on the team, Ann Arbor, 1978, The University of Michigan Press.

18. D'Eugenio, D.B., and Moersch, M.S., editors: Developmental programming for infants and young children, vol. 4, 5, Ann Arbor, 1981, The University of Michigan Press.

19. Dickerson, M.U., and Brown, S.L.: A search for a family. In Brown, S.L., and Moersch, M.S., editors: Parents on the team, Ann Arbor, 1978, The University of Michigan Press.

20. Ellis, N.E., and Cross, L., editors: Planning programs for early education of the handicapped, New York, 1977, Walker & Co.

21. Ellsworth, P.D.: Parent education: a definitive approach to the problem of child abuse and neglect. In U.S. Army Health Services Command Publication: Current trends in ambulatory patient care, Fort Sam Houston, Texas, Washington, D.C., 1978, U.S. Government Printing Office.

22. Featherstone, H.: A difference in the family: life with a disabled child, New York, 1980, Basic Books, Inc., Publishers.

23. Finn, J.L.: The children's developmental workshop. In Llorens, L.A., editor: Consultation in the community, Dubuque, Iowa, 1973, Kendall/Hunt Publishing Co.

24. Friedman, B.: A program for parents of children with sensory integrative dysfunction, Am. J. Occup. Ther. **36:**586, 1982.

25. Gallagher, J.J., and Gallagher, G.C.: Family adaptation to a handicapped child and assorted professionals. In Turnbull, A.P., and Turnbull, H.R., III, editors: Parents speak out: views from the other side of the two-way mirror, Columbus, Ohio, 1978, Charles E. Merrill Publishing Co.

26. Gillette, N.P.: Occupational therapy belongs to the community. In Llorens, L.A., editor: Consultation in the community, Dubuque, Iowa, 1973, Kendall/Hunt Publishing Co.

27. Goldstein, J., Freud, A., and Solnit, A.J.: Before the best interests of the child, New York, 1979, The Free Press.

28. Gordon, I.J.: Baby learning through baby play: a parent's guide for the first two years, New York, 1970, St. Martin's Press, Inc.

29. Gordon, I.J., Guinagh, B., and Jester, R.E.: Child learning through child play: learning activities for two and three year olds, New York, 1972, St. Martin's Press, Inc.

30. Gordon, I.J., and Lally, J.R.: Intellectual stimulation for infants and toddlers, Gainesville, Fla., 1967, Institute for Development of Human Resources.

31. Gray, S.W.: Home-based programs for mothers of young children. In Mittler, P., editor: Research to practice in mental retardation: care and intervention, vol. 1, Baltimore, 1977, University Park Press.

32. Griswold, P.A.: Play together, parents and babies, New York, 1972, United Cerebral Palsy, Inc.

33. Hamant, C.: Pediatrics. In Hopkins, H.L., and Smith, H.D., editors: Willard and Spackman's occupational therapy, ed. 5, Philadelphia, 1978, J.B. Lippincott Co.

34. Hanson, M.J.: Teaching your Down's syndrome infant: a guide for parents, Baltimore, 1977, University Park Press.

35. Heber, R., and Garber, H.: The Milwaukee project: a study of the use of family intervention to prevent cultural-familial mental retardation. In Friedlander, B., and Sterritt, G., editors: Exceptional infant. Vol. 3: assessment and intervention, New York, 1975, Brunner/Mazel, Inc.

36. Heward, W.L., Dardig, J.C., and Rossett, A.: Working with parents of handicapped children, Columbus, Ohio, 1979, Charles E. Merrill Publishing Co.

37. Hill, L.: Working with blind pre-schoolers, Am. J. Occup. Ther. **31:**417, 1977.

38. Holt, K.S.: Neurological and neuromuscular disorders. In Gabel, S., and Erickson, M.T., editors: Child development and developmental disabilities, Boston, 1980, Little, Brown & Co.

39. Honig, A.S.: The children's center and the family development research program. In Caldwell, B.M., and Stedman, D.J., editors: Infant education: a guide for helping handicapped children in the first three years, New York, 1977, Walker & Co.

40. Howison, M.V., Perella, J.A., and Gordon, D.: Cerebral palsy. In Hopkins, H.L., and Smith, H.D., editors: Willard and Spackman's occupational therapy, ed. 5, Philadelphia, 1978, J.B. Lippincott Co.

41. Jaworowski, S., and Jaworowski, R.: A baby goes to "school." In Brown, S.L., and Moersch, M.S., editors: Parents on the team, Ann Arbor, 1978, The University of Michigan Press.

42. Kinnealey, M.: Service programs in the university affiliated programs. In Llorens, L.A., editor: Consultation in the community, Dubuque, Iowa, 1973, Kendall/Hunt Publishing Co.

43. Knickerbocker, B.M.: A parent-oriented occupational therapy program for the multiply handicapped child. In West, W.L., editor: Occupational therapy for the multiply handicapped child, Chicago, 1965, Board of Trustees of the University of Illinois.

44. Knickerbocker, B.M.: A holistic approach to treatment of learning disorders, Thorofare, N.J., 1980, Charles B. Slack, Inc.

45. Kramer, R.F.: Living with childhood cancer: healthy siblings' perspective, Comp. Pediatr. Nurs. **5:**155, 1981.

46. Llorens, L.A.: Problem-solving the role of occupational therapy in a new environment. In Llorens, L.A., editor: Consultation in the community, Dubuque, Iowa, 1973, Kendall/Hunt Publishing Co.

47. Magrab, P.R., and Johnson, R.B.: Mental retardation. In Gabel, S., and Erickson, M.T., editors: Child development and developmental disabilities, Boston, 1980, Little, Brown & Co.

48. Mancini, P.N., editor: Friday's child, New York, 1977, The New American Library, Inc.

49. Markel, G.P., and Greenbaum, J.: Parents are to be seen and heard: assertiveness in educational planning for handicapped children, San Luis Obispo, Calif., 1979, Impact Publishers.

50. Marsh, G.E. II, and Price, B.J.: Methods for teaching the mildly handicapped adolescent, St. Louis, 1980, The C.V. Mosby Co.

51. McKibbin, E.H.: An interdisciplinary program for retarded children and their families, Am. J. Occup. Ther. **26:**125, 1972.

52. Mebane, W.M., editor: Getting our heads together: a helpful handbook for families of head-injured people, One Rotary Drive, Asheville, N.C., undated (approx, 1982), Thoms Rehabilitation Hospital, Inc.

53. Meyer, J.Y.: One of the family. In Brown, S.L., and Moersch, M.S., editors: Parents on the team, Ann Arbor, 1978, The University of Michigan Press.

54. Moersch, M.S.: Training the deaf-blind child, Am. J. Occup. Ther. **31:**425, 1977.

55. Moersch, M.S.: History and rationale for parent involvement. In Brown, S.L., and Moersch, M.S., editors: Parents on the team, Ann Arbor, 1978, The University of Michigan Press.

56. Moersch, M.S.: The handicapped child in a trigenerational family, Paper presented at American Occupational Therapy Association Conference, Detroit, April 25, 1979.

57. Moersch, M.S., and Wilson, T.Y., editors: Early intervention project for handicapped infants and young children, final report, Ann Arbor, Mich., 1976, Institute for the Study of Mental Retardation and Related Disabilities (ERIC Document #ED 132804).

58. Morris, A.G.: Parent education in well-baby care: a new role for the occupational therapist, Am. J. Occup. Ther. **32:**75, 1978.

59. Northcott, W.L.: Developing parent participation. In Lillie, D.L., editor: Parent programs in child development centers, Chapel Hill, 1972, The University of North Carolina Press.

60. President's Committee on Mental Retardation: Mental retardation: the leading edge, service programs that work, Washington, D.C., 1978, U.S. Government Printing Office.

61. Roos, P.: Parents of mentally retarded children—misunderstood and mistreated. In Turnbull, A.P., and Turnbull, H.R. III, editors: Parents speak out: views from the other side of the two-way mirror, Columbus, Ohio, 1978, Charles E. Merrill Publishing Co.

62. Schafer, D.S., and Moersch, M.S., editors: Developmental programming for infants and young children, vol. 1, 2, 3, rev. ed., Ann Arbor, 1981, The University of Michigan Press.

63. Schopler, E.: Treatment of autistic children: historical perspective. In Mittler, P., editor: Research to practice in mental retardation: care and intervention, vol. 1, Baltimore, 1977, University Park Press.

64. Serbin, L.A., Steer, J., and Lyons, J.A.: Mothers' perceptions of the behavior and problem-solving skills of their developmentally delayed sons, Am. J. Ment. Defic. **88:**86, 1983.

65. Shapero, S., and Forbes, C.R.: A review of involvement programs for parents of learning disabled children, J. Learn. Disabil. **14:**499, 1981.

66. Shearer, M.S., and Shearer, D.E.: Parent involvement. In Jordan, J.B., and others, editors: Early childhood education for exceptional children, Reston, Va., 1977, Council on Exceptional Children.

67. Stein, D.B.: About handicaps, New York, 1974, Walker & Co.

68. Thain, W.S., Casto, G., and Peterson, A.: Normal and handicapped children: a growth and development primer for parents and professionals, Littleton, Mass., 1980, PSG Publishing Company, Inc.

69. Tiffany, E.G., Psychiatry and mental health. In Hopkins, H.L., and Smith, H.D., editors: Willard and Spackman's occupational therapy, ed. 5, Philadelphia, 1978, J.B. Lippincott Co.

70. Turnbull, A.P.: Moving from being a professional to being a parent: a startling experience. In Turnbull, A.P., and Turnbull, H.R., editors: Parents speak out: views from the other side of the two-way mirror, Columbus, Ohio, 1978, Charles E. Merrill Publishing Co.

71. Turnbull, A.P., and Turnbull, H.R. III, editors: Parents speak out: views from the other side of the two-way mirror, Columbus, Ohio, 1978, Charles E. Merrill Publishing Co.

72. Turnbull, A.P., and Turnbull, H.R. III: Parent involvement in the education of handicapped children: a critique, Ment. Retard. **20:**115, 1982.

73. Tyler, N.B., and Kogan, K.L.: Reduction of stress between mothers and their handicapped children, Am. J. Occup. Ther. **31:**151, 1977.

74. Vulpe, S.G.: Home care and management of the mentally retarded child, Toronto, 1969, National Institute on Mental Retardation.

75. Vulpe, S.G.: Vulpe Assessment Battery: developmental assessment, performance analysis, individualized programming for the atypical child, ed. 2, Toronto, 1977, National Institute on Mental Retardation.

76. Wade, A.S.: Occupational therapy for problems with special senses: blindness and deafness. In Hopkins, H.L., and Smith, H.D., editors: Willard and Spackman's occupational therapy, ed. 5, Philadelphia, 1978, J.B. Lippincott Co.

77. Weikart, D.P.: Designing parenting education programs, Paper presented at the Working Conference on Parent Education, Flint, Mich., 1977, Charles Stewart Mott Foundation.

78. White, R.: The special child: a parents' guide to mental disabilities, Boston, 1978, Little, Brown & Co.

79. Willard, H.S., and Spackman, C.S.: Occupational therapy, Philadelphia, 1947, J.B. Lippincott Co.

80. Zissermann, L.: Sex of a parent and knowledge about cerebral palsy, Am. J. Occup. Ther. **32:**500, 1978.

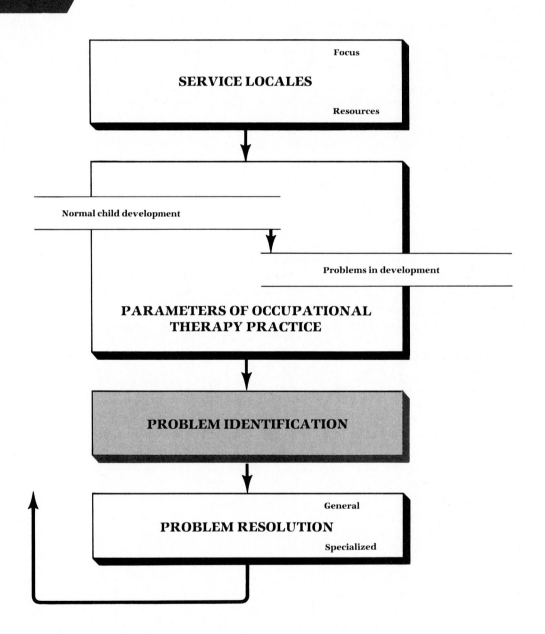

SERVICE LOCALES

Focus

Resources

Normal child development

Problems in development

PARAMETERS OF OCCUPATIONAL
THERAPY PRACTICE

PROBLEM IDENTIFICATION

PROBLEM RESOLUTION

General

Specialized

Principles and techniques of occupational therapy assessment in pediatrics

PAT NUSE CLARK
IDA LOU COLEY
ANNE STEVENS ALLEN
KAREN E. SCHANZENBACHER

Basic methods of assessment and screening

BASIC METHODS

This chapter stresses the importance of a questioning mind in evaluating function. It is an asset to know what questions to ask of oneself and others. Questions are formulated and answers often found through the study of normal development, principles of structure and function, and the behavioral sciences.

This chapter focuses on the use of a variety of basic methods to screen children to determine the need for occupational therapy services. Guiding questions for clinical observation of the child will provide a foundation for any other screening or formal evaluation. In addition, this chapter discusses a number of commonly used standardized and criterion-referenced screening instruments that are often used by occupational therapists in pediatric settings. Information on basic methods used for assessment was presented in Chapter 7. It might be useful to review that section before proceeding further.

Among the most valuable skills a therapist can possess are the abilities to observe, to be flexible and spontaneous, and to be creative with play and other activities that foster intrinsic motivation in children. Supporting these clinical attributes are foundation skills that are solidly grounded: a sense of organization and problem-solving strategies for developing the child's potential in daily life activities.

To begin, the importance of taking a broad view is emphasized. The therapist must look at the total child interacting within multiple environments. The child should not be considered merely in terms of an "oral-motor problem" or a "dressing problem." Life systems

are too closely intertwined. The task of the therapist is to make a thorough search: unravel and discover *why* the child can do some things and not others in his daily life routine.

Looking at the total child: clinical observations of basic skills

The following information will provide a foundation for and direction to the therapist's search for what a child can or cannot do.[5] Assessment begins by focusing attention on the child at rest in supine and prone positions. Movement is minimal, but signs of head control and the child's use of his head for orientation may be noted. The broad task is to view postural tone throughout the body and to survey structural components, carefully considering the inhibitors of activity performance. These may include stress, static postures, contractures of muscle tissue, tightening of skin, fusion of joints, structural deformities, and atrophy of muscles. Conditions that contribute to discomfort and pain, such as swelling, inflammation, and tenderness, can also affect mobility. Observations of the child at rest permit the therapist to develop a baseline picture from which to evaluate subsequent movement and its quality. Philosophically, and in practice, movement and independence in activity performance are linked together, each contributing to the other.

THE CHILD AT REST: SUPINE POSITION

Postural components. The therapist should ask the following. What is the child's prevailing posture?

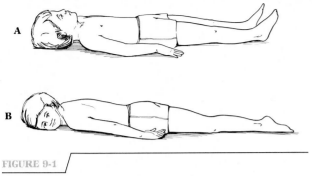

FIGURE 9-1

Normal resting postures. **A,** Supine. **B,** Prone.

Does flexion or extension predominate, or is his body position asymmetrical? Is the child bound by prevailing postures, or can he easily initiate volitional movement? What is the quality and type of postural tone: hypertonic, hypotonic, fluctuating, or appropriate to the age of the child? Does the child appear to rest comfortably in this position (Figure 9-1, *A*)?

Stabilization and control of the head. Can the child turn his head to the side without moving his arms or legs? Can he follow an object visually without head movement? Is the child's head in midline? Does he demonstrate neck extension or shoulder retraction?

Structural components of body systems. Are the child's shoulders level? Is his rib cage symmetrical? What is its shape? Is the pelvis level? Are there discrepancies in arm or leg length? Are there obvious joint contractures in the elbows, wrists, fingers, hips, knees, or ankles? Are there deformities or joint subluxation at the shoulder, wrist, metacarpophalangeal joints of the fingers, hips, or knees? Are the joints enlarged or reddened? Are there nodules around the child's joints? What is the appearance of muscle tissue: tense, flaccid, atrophied, or hypertrophied? What is the appearance of the child's skin: dry, moist, tight, loose, warm, or cold? What is its color?

THE CHILD AT REST: PRONE POSITION

Stabilization and control of the head, trunk, and shoulders. Postural components of the prone position are examined as with the supine position. In addition, the therapist will consider any changes in the child's head control in the prone position. Can the child extend his neck so that his head is free in space? Can neck extension be maintained without bobbing his head? Are the child's arms caught under his body or are they used appropriately to support upper body weight on his elbows or in an extended position? Where are the child's elbows in relation to his shoulders, and are his hands open or fisted? Is the child's head in a normal position in space (Figure 9-1, *B*)?

Structural components of body systems. Are the child's scapulae symmetrical? Is the child's spine relatively straight, or is there evidence of lordosis, kyphosis,

or scoliosis? Are the buttocks elevated by tightness at the hips or spinal deformity? Are there obvious joint contractures at the elbows, hips, knees, or ankles?

ROLLING

The body is engineered for flexibility so that individuals can move freely, easily, and in most instances without conscious effort. However, patterns of movement are learned through practice and repetition and are gradually refined. During observation, note the child's use of his head, shoulders, and hips, as well as his ability to rotate along the body axes. Abnormal patterns and asymmetry may interfere with mobility. Factors related to body structure may require adaptation.

Where does the child initiate movement for the roll: from the head, shoulder and arm, trunk, hip and leg, or combinations of these? Does the child use head movements appropriately? Does he become asymmetrical and lose control? Is rolling accomplished more readily to the right or left side? Are movements exaggerated with head thrust backwards or back extended? Does the child demonstrate log or segmental rolling, or has the child developed an adaptive pattern to accomplish this activity?

ACHIEVING THE SITTING POSITION

As infants gain stability of the neck and shoulders, acquire increased extensor tone for trunk stability, and are able to break through mass patterns of flexion and extension, they develop the ability to flex at the hips and elevate the upper body in space. They come to grips with the forces of gravity and are helped to maintain sitting position by postural reactions, guided by visual and vestibular processes, that keep the body upright in space. Can the child bring his head forward and lift it from a resting surface? How does the child "come to" sitting: with ventral push-off, dorsal push and partial rotation, or symmetrical push-off from the supine position (Figure 9-2)? Does the child roll to the side and push up sideways? Do the hips and knees flex when sitting is achieved? Do the child's legs need to be stabilized before sitting can be achieved? If the child cannot come to the sitting position alone, what is the position of his head when he is pulled to sitting? Is there head lag? Is the back rounded? Is there resistance at the hips?

SITTING

Sitting is normally an effortless task. The individual is not aware of the mechanisms at work that orient his head in space nor the work of his extensor muscles to keep his head erect. Trunk stability, or the balance of the vertebral column, depends largely on the posterior trunk musculature, the abdominal and intercostal muscles. As one sits, the trunk balances on the pelvis, which is a narrow sitting base unless the legs are extended and spread. The body, with its numerous movable parts, is

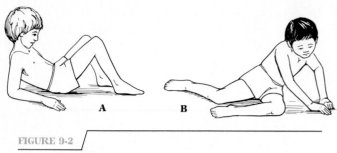

FIGURE 9-2

Coming to sit. **A,** Symmetrical. **B,** Ventral push.

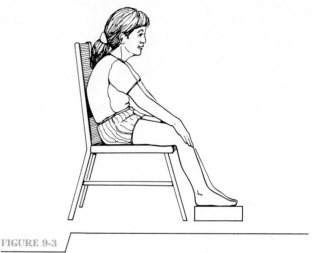

FIGURE 9-3

Insufficient hip flexion in sitting results in rounded spine and forward thrust of head.

able parts, is a series of structural segments, one placed on top of the other. Maximal stability is assured when the centers of gravity of the segments lie in a vertical line centered over the base of support. In the body structure, when one segment is unaligned, there is usually a compensatory disalignment of another segment to maintain a balanced position of the body as a whole (Figure 9-3).

The important functional areas to observe as the child sits are head and trunk alignment, the sitting base, and the amount of support required and provided by the arms. What is the position of the child's head? Is control maintained effortlessly in a stationary position or during free rotation? What does the child's back look like: is it rounded, symmetrical, or asymmetrical? What is the position of the hips? Are they extended or comfortably flexed? Is the child's weight distributed evenly over a narrow or wide sitting base? Can the child sit with her legs extended for a reasonable period of time? Is the child comfortable in the sitting position, or is he insecure?

Where are the child's arms, and does she use her hands as props? If so, how is her weight-bearing on the arms achieved: forward, right or left side, or backward propping? Is protective extension active and functional with elbows extended, or does the child tend to flop over on bent elbows? Are her hands open or fisted?

If a child can sit unsupported, can she lean forward and then recover balance? Can the child pivot her trunk while sitting to reach for objects that are not at midline? Are her hands free for manipulative play, or are they held insecurely close to the body? Is the child's head up with her eyes alert? Is the child comfortable in this position, or is there evidence of postural insecurity?

REACHING

Reaching multiplies the demands for postural security. Observe that as the child extends his arms outward from his body the center of gravity rises and his balance is less stable. Movement of the arms requires the child to make quick shifts in position to maintain balance. The maturation of postural stability to the point of maintained upright positioning permits development of the amazing process of human hand use.

Obviously, this cannot occur while the child must use all of his energy to maintain body position against the forces of gravity.

If the arms and hands are to do something, cocontraction is required at the proximal joints and at the midline to stabilize and maximize the forces exerted by the moving muscles. To reach all body parts, including those at the periphery, the child must actively move his scapulae and shoulders in all planes. The elbow joint calibrates the reaching parameters toward the head and feet. Combinations of range at the shoulder, elbow, and wrist bring the child's hand, with its valuable prehensile qualities, in contact with superior body surfaces. Flexibility of the spine and range of motion at the hips and knees permit the child to reach all the way to his toes.

Can the child bring her hands together at midline? Can she bring one or both hands to her mouth, behind her head, and to the small of her back; pronate and supinate her hand and forearm; reach straight overhead and out to the side without loss of trunk stability; and bend over at the waist, touch her toes, and return to an upright sitting position without loss of control and balance? Are her arm movements smooth, circumductive, or awkward? Does the child reach equally well with each side and with both arms together? What seems to interfere with her function?

HAND USE

As the child performs fine motor tasks with his hands, the rest of his body tends to be quiet, as if providing a silent framework for intricate movement. This is an important message from nature that should be recalled by the therapist when working with the child on eating skills or the fine manipulations required for fastening clothing. Postural stability is a critical prerequisite to human hand use.

Grasping involves complex movements. The long

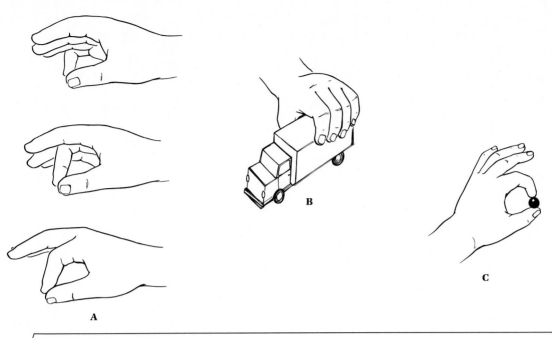

FIGURE 9-4

Normal prehension pattern. **A,** Checking opposition, thumb to fingers. **B,** Gross grasp with wrist extended. **C,** Pincer grasp, tip prehension.

flexors and extensors of the hand pass over several joints, potentially affecting movement in multiple locations. The tenodesis action of the wrist is an example of such phenomena. Fine prehension includes rotation and abduction of the thumb for opposition to the volar finger pads. Similarly, slight flexion of the fingers at the metacarpophalangeal and interphalangeal joints is needed to position the fingertips for prehension. Various degrees of movement between pronation and supination place the hand in angular planes during performance of such manual skills as writing, eating, playing, and cleansing after a bowel movement.

The therapist should observe to see if the child can oppose all fingers to the thumb (Figure 9-4, *A*). Are such movements awkward or fluid? Are they performed in digital sequence or arbitrarily? Can the child straighten his fingers with his wrist in a neutral position? Can his fingers be fully extended from a fisted position? Is extension of the child's fingers exaggerated when he reaches for an object?

What is the position of the child's wrist during grasping? (Figure 9-4, *B*). Is the child's grasp on objects forced? What is the position of the forearm during grasping: pronated, supinated, or in midposition? Is the thumb used in an immature scissors pattern, or is mature pincer function evident? (Figure 9-4, *C*). What is the quality of muscle tone, strength, and coordination? Are fine tremors noted in the hand? Does the child drop objects easily, or does she have difficulty releasing objects?

Clinical observations: the child interacting with the environment

The focus thus far has been on the components of motor function, such as balance, stability, muscle strength, synergy, coordination, and range of motion. These indispensable elements of movement and static postures are required for activity engagement. This view has been directed toward seeing the "entire body" in space. Now it is appropriate to look at the "whole child."

The questions to be asked are the following: How does the child respond to stimuli in the environment? What is the child's style of interaction with inanimate and animate objects? What attracts the child's attention and what intrigues, motivates, distracts, or disorganizes him? How does interaction with the environment affect the "doing" of the child? The search continues to find the child's unique combination of strengths that promote function and to sift out those elements that interfere with use of those strengths.

THE CHILD'S USE OF SENSORY MODALITIES

Does the child show preferential use of a sensory modality? For example, an individual may place his reliance on sight, hearing, or touch in his interactions with people and objects. Does the child look selectively and have visual interest in people, in people's activities and interactions, in objects, and in furnishings? Does the child attend to sound and explore objects that have a distinctive smell? Are heights and balancing activities avoided or approached eagerly? Does the child tend to touch and manipulate objects before proceeding with a task?

THE CHILD'S MOTOR RESPONSES

Does the child organize and carry out motor tasks in logical sequence, or does his motor planning appear impaired? Is it necessary to demonstrate a task or put a child passively though task patterns, or does the child initiate a new activity independently? Are the child's movements impulsive, controlled, or restrained?

COGNITIVE STYLE

The therapist will need to analyze problems of task performance in light of all observed characteristics. Sometimes motor ability is adequate to the task, but performance may be immature or impaired because of cognitive factors. How does the child approach a task: impulsively, automatically, analytically, or by using trial-and-error methods? How does the child respond to verbal direction? How many steps of a task can the child remember and process at a time? Is thinking concrete or abstract, and does the child show any awareness of and judgment related to safety factors?

SOCIAL RESPONSES AND COMMUNICATION

Intricately interwoven with engagement in activity is the child's participation in the larger activity of a social world. As skill in object manipulation increases, the activity itself requires less concentration, and the child looks out to compare his performance against that of others. Or, the child recognizes that other people around him are doing things that may or may not relate to him. The child's social interaction is commensurate with his ability to communicate by using verbal and nonverbal processes.

Does the child demonstrate eye contact during interactions with other people? How much does she pay attention to others, whether engaged in an activity or not? Does the child seem to prefer to play alone, alongside others, or in cooperative interaction? Does the child appear to perceive social feedback related to herself or others?

Does the child rely predominantly on speech to express himself, or does he use manual and facial expressions as well? Does he use automatic phrases? Does the child show indications of perseveration of ideas, word searching, or blocking? Does the child initiate conversation with elaboration of ideas, or does he merely answer questions with brief phrases?

Although specific behaviors can be observed, the reality is that behaviors occur within the context of the total environment. Therapists are also processing global interactions and integrating all that is seen into composite impressions of function. It is advisable to care-fully consider the setting within which one gathers those impressions. The clinical setting is always artificial and therefore limits the scope of evaluation and problem-solving. It does not represent the natural arenas of the child. In a sense, one is seeing the child in isolation, removed from the familiar surroundings of daily life: home, school, and playground.

THE CHILD AT HOME

At the child's home the therapist has the opportunity to view the child's characteristic adaptation in its fullest dimension. This is the most significant environment, because it contains those persons who can contribute most to the quality of the child's life.

There are many things to consider in this environment that directly or indirectly affect the child's development of function. These include the type of neighborhood; rural, urban, or suburban location; the terrain; and climatic factors. The therapist should explore the house and yard, noting the presence of stairs and other barriers to mobility. The interior of the house is important, including space for mobility aids and other adaptive equipment, storage areas, and how the family feels about changing the home environment to make it easier for the child to function. The therapist needs to know how busy the family life is and how the family manages daily schedules. The primary caregiver's skills and attitudes must be assessed to identify how much assistance is given to the child, how it is given, how responsibility is shared by other family members, and what the stresses of caretaking are. The availability of extended family help and respite care should be explored. Therapists need to determine how well the family will be able to follow through with therapy goals, including what realistic expectations can be established. The family's understanding of their child's potential and limitations, and their attitudes toward fostering maximal independence will be important to the outcome of occupational therapy intervention. The therapist needs to clearly identify what help the family is seeking, what they want to change, and where they want to begin.

THE CHILD AT SCHOOL

Success in school depends in large part on how comfortable the child feels in the environment and how well the environment is structured to permit the child to use her strengths, gain satisfaction, and receive recognition. Teachers, bus drivers, classmates, and other persons with whom the child comes in contact and who understand the disability can give valuable support for increasing independence by encouraging efforts. School represents a major part of the child's life and is critical to preparation for adulthood.

When therapists observe a school environment, they are bound by tradition and tend to look at practicalities to begin identifying and then solving problems. They will want to know if the child can sit at a desk or if some other arrangement will be necessary. Will the teacher's body and voice, as well as the blackboard, be readily accessible to the child? Will the child be able to reach for and put away books without assistance? How will toileting and eating be managed, as well as mobility within the school classroom, hallways, and grounds? What are the time constraints for mobility? What arrangements are needed regarding use and maintenance of wheelchairs and other adaptive equipment? Where will these items be stored? Who will assist the child with these? Do school personnel understand when to assist and when to insist on independent performance? These are important considerations that require the collective help of the child, parents, school staff, classmates, and therapists.

There are other issues to consider as well that are related to peer acceptance and the child's integration into the social fabric of the school. Factors to note include whether the child stands out as being different from peers in the classroom. For example, is the child dressed like the others in the class? Does the child's disability affect others in the room to the point of overt or covert reactions? Are the students and teacher comfortable with a child who may be different? How well does the child communicate with others? Since gaining acceptance from peers is a gradual process in all situations and for all human beings, the child may require help in relating, in making appropriate social overtures, and in being able to help others become at ease in his presence.

Through the basic process of clinical observation of the child at rest, in a variety of functional postures, at play, and in familiar environments, the therapist records impressions and evolving questions. One of the recurring questions should be: Does this child already have the resources to achieve a satisfying level of independence, or will occupational therapy services make a critical difference in the quality of this child's life? As the therapist reviews his or her notes of observation, the need for more information generates the need for other forms of screening.

Interviewing

Various types of interview formats are used to obtain information about children. Interviews are often conducted by the therapist with both parents, sometimes supplemented with data obtained through questionnaires.

There are several basic forms of interviewing. The most structured type is guided by an outline of questions. The interviewer asks the questions as specified on the outline, and the respondent provides answers that are linked by the constraints of the outline. The interviewer discourages discussion of extraneous material. This is called the *limited or structured response interview*.

A *semistructured interview* uses a basic outline of questions that have been developed to elicit thoughtful responses from the person. Although the interviewer will be careful to ensure collection of basic data, the questions have an open-ended quality that allows additional useful information to be obtained. In other words, the therapist who uses a semistructured format does so to prevent overlooking important information about a child that might not fit into frequently used categories. For example, a question might be worded, "How does your child play with brothers and sisters?" Clearly, such questions are designed to elicit descriptive information rather than yes-no responses.

A third type of interview is designed to obtain *free responses*. Open-ended questions are used to help the respondent examine and report on the meaning of experiences and perceptions. This method is frequently used in nondirective therapy as well as in assessment for mental health programs. The free response method differs from the semistructured interview in that the interviewer has fewer preconceived expectations about the nature of the information to be revealed.

INTERVIEWING SKILLS

To obtain useful information through an interview, the therapist must have command of the subject matter to be discussed. When an interview elicits information that is outside the therapist's expertise, appropriate referral for problem resolution is indicated. The therapist must have the ability to analyze and conceptualize content obtained through interviews into a meaningful whole (gestalt). Simple completion of interview forms without this follow-up step of integrating details into the overall assessment of the child is a waste of everyone's time.

It may be noted that the expertise of the professional level occupational therapist (OTR) is rarely needed for the administration of the limited response interview. Instead, the skills of the therapist are better used in semistructured and free response formats. Within these formats the therapist's knowledge is used to develop and explore new ideas that surface during an interview. Responses to one question may be seized on to develop new questions or to obtain more considered information.

The skilled therapist becomes expert in gaining the participation of the respondent. This may be done in a number of ways. First, the purpose and focus of the interview are clearly explained. The therapist develops a comfortable atmosphere that permits the respondent to reply openly. The therapist frequently reviews assembled information with the respondent to ensure accurate understanding of what has been said. The therapist listens attentively and without bias, making a conscious effort to allow for feedback. The therapist is aware of shifts in conversation, recurrent references, and inconsistencies and gaps and explores concealed meanings. Finally, the occupational therapist considers the effect of the physical setting, hour of the day, and other external influences on the interview process.

USE OF HISTORIES FOR SCREENING

Many occupational therapists have developed interview formats to obtain histories of skill development, activity participation, and life-space data. Two are included here. The *developmental history* (Exhibit 9-1) was constructed to obtain initial intake information as well as background data on developmental milestones and parental expectations of occupational therapy. It serves as a representative semistructured interview and has been used in face-to-face discussion with parents. It can also be given in questionnaire form to parents to complete at home where they may have more complete records available.

Takata's play history was also developed for use with an interview or questionnaire. It examines previous play history by obtaining information about the child's preferred forms of play and play context. In addition, this form is used to obtain information about current

EXHIBIT 9-1

Developmental history

Child's name: _____ Birthdate: _____ Age: _____

Mother's name: _____ Father's name: _____

Home address: _____

Home phone no.: _____ Business phone no.: _____

Prenatal history: Please describe the pregnancy:

Birth: Weight: _____ Height: _____ Duration of pregnancy: _____

Type of delivery: _____

Complications at birth? _____

Treatment received by baby or mother? _____

Postnatal history: Please list and describe any important injuries or illnesses, including ear and chest infections. At what ages did these occur?

_____

_____

Milestones: At what age did your child:

Turn head side to side? _____ Sit alone? _____

Lift head while lying on tummy? _____ Crawl-creep? _____

Roll over? _____ Pull to standing? _____

Cruise, walk with support? _____ Walk alone? _____ Run? _____

Climb stairs? _____ Walk down stairs? _____ Swallow? _____

Chew? _____ Drink from cup? _____ Feed self with spoon? _____

Babble? _____ Say words? _____ Speak in phrases? _____

Speak in sentences? _____ Play with children? _____

Have you noticed any differences compared to your other children?

_____

_____

Do you have any family/living problems which you think might affect your child's development or therapy?

_____

_____

What does this child like?

_____

_____

Dislike?

_____

_____

play content and skills of the child. From the data collected the therapist develops a description of the child as a player and a prescription for necessary play experiences that will be provided through occupational therapy intervention[9] (Exhibit 9-2).

SCREENING INSTRUMENTS
Test development

A veritable supermarket of screening instruments is available commercially. Most screening tests are performance based and therefore examine the child's skills in activity situations. Screening tests may focus on self-care activities, object manipulation skills, social skill development, language and cognition, or a combination of these areas. Such combination tests are considered adaptive development tests.

As discussed previously, many screening tests are standardized. (By definition, screening tests are criterion referenced.) Some may be standardized for administrative procedure, while others are standardized for both administration and scoring.

The process of test development and its necessary constraints merit attention. It is generally agreed that the variability of human characteristics and behaviors makes the development of "the perfect test" an elusive dream. The standardization of a test requires the par-

---

Please describe your child's problems?
_____
_____

What would you like us to help you and your child do?
_____
_____

What other therapy and/or special education programs has your child had? Now receiving?
_____
_____

Please indicate with a plus (+) the items which you feel are strengths in this child and please use a minus (−) to identify those factors which you feel are weaknesses in this child.

_____ response to smells and tastes   _____ response to touch
_____ response to visual stimuli   _____ response to movement
_____ response to sounds   _____ response to eating
_____ ability to manage physical/motor requirements of play/school activities.
_____ ability to manage thinking requirements of play/school activities.
_____ self-feeding _____dressing _____ toileting
_____ grooming _____ gross-motor coordination
_____ fine-hand coordination _____ general activity level
_____attention span _____ social skills _____motivation
_____response to family _____ response to other children

Does your child use glasses, hearing aid, braces, wheelchair, or other special equipment for daily activities?
_____
_____

Are there any allergies, seizures, or other medical problems we should know about?
_____
_____

Is there anything else you would like us to know at this time that you feel can help us provide better services for your child?
_____
_____

Do we have your permission to take photographs of your child for evaluation and student training purposes?
_____ Yes _____ No

May we obtain copies of your child's records from your child's physician or other agencies? Please list:
_____
_____
_____

Signature: _____ Date: _____

ticipation of human subjects. Given people's commitment to freedom of choice, it is always difficult to find adequate samples of subjects to take a test in its development stage, especially when the sample aims to represent every conceivable segment of minorities and majorities of the total population distribution. When children are to be tested, this task is compounded because of parental considerations regarding the privacy of their own lives and sensitivity about the exploitation of their children. Therefore test developers who are able to obtain a sizable sample of children (N = >1,000) have accomplished an admirable feat. When they have been able to obtain a sample of subjects that somewhat approximates a regional population distribution according to age, race, sex, and socioeconomic factors, this is even more appreciable. Finally, in the rare cases when fairly representative samples are obtained in different regions of the country, there is evidence of herculean effort on the part of the test developers that may take a decade or more to achieve.

Therefore, although therapists are well advised to check out carefully the reliability, validity, and normative data of standardized tests, consideration of the constraints of test development should be weighed against negative criticism. Obviously some tests will be poorly constructed, standardized, and evaluated. However, many tests that have flaws in these areas may still be useful and represent application of the highest standards of test development within a constrained situation. As long as the therapist is aware of the limitations of a test, it may be used knowledgeably.

Still other tests that are neither standardized nor

EXHIBIT 9-2

Takata's play history

(1) *General information*
   Name: Birthdate: Sex:
   Date: Informant(s):
   Presenting problem:
(2) *Previous play experiences*
   A. Solitary play
   B. Play with others:
      mother father sisters brothers playmates
      other family members   pets
   C. Play with toys and materials (earliest preferences)
   D. Gross physical play
   E. Pretend and make-believe play
   F. Sports and games: group collaboration
      group competition
   G. Creative interests: arts   crafts
   H. Hobbies, collections, other leisure-time activities
   I. Recreation social activities
(3) *Actual play examination*
   A. With what does the child play?
      toys   materials   pets
   B. How does the child play with toys and other materials?
   C. What type of play is avoided or liked least?
   D. With whom does the child play?
      self parents brothers sisters peers others
   E. How does the child play with others?
   F. What body postures does the child use during play?
   G. How long does the child play with objects?   With people?
   H. Where does the child play?
      Home: indoors   outdoors
      Community: park school church other areas
   I. When does the child play?
      Daily schedule for weekday and weekend?
(4) *Play description*
(5) *Play prescription*

From Takata, N.: Play as a prescription. In Reilly, M., editor: Play as exploratory learning: studies of curiosity behavior, Beverly Hills, Calif., 1974, Sage Publications, Inc.

EXHIBIT 9-3

Test analysis format

Title and authors:

What the test proposes to measure:

Population for whom the test was developed:

Test format
A. Type of instrument
B. Test content
C. Administration
D. Scoring
E. Interpretation
Include information about the basic type of instrument that is being used, for example, interview, criterion-referenced, or standardized test. Then briefly discuss basic administration guidelines that pertain to the entire test. For example, is information obtained by report of parents, or by presenting tasks to children. How is the test set up? Are there time limits for items in general? Include basic information about scoring and interpretation procedures.

Advantages of the test:

Disadvantages of the test

Purchasing information:

References:

commercially available have been so well researched to develop items that they are equally, if not more, useful. A good example is the clinical observations format developed by Ayres[4] that will be presented later in this chapter. The key to working with such "therapist-made" tests is in the clarity of description for administration of test items. In addition, referencing of resources used to develop the test is important for future generations of therapists who adopt its use at the same or different facilities.

The remaining purpose of this chapter is to describe and discuss some representative screening instruments that can be used in a variety of occupational therapy settings for children. For purposes of organization, these are divided into commercial tests and therapist-made tests. A test analysis format has been developed (Exhibit 9-3). This chapter will present a completed analysis of the Denver Developmental Screening Test because it is the screening instrument most commonly used with children. Other screening methods that are discussed here or encountered in practice may be similarly analyzed. The model analysis provided here will organize additional study of tests through the primary test reference and evaluative information from other similar resources.

Commercial tests

APGAR SCORING SYSTEM

The technology of neonatology has grown tremendously (Chapter 16), and screening of the newborn is critical to timely application of life-sustaining and enhancing procedures. Cardiac, neurological, and respiratory systems must be appraised to determine how well a neonate has responded to the birth process and extrauterine life. The Apgar Scoring System provides this information by rating the baby's color, heart rate, reflex irritability, muscle tone, and respiratory effort.[1] This test is not given by occupational therapists. However, information from the test is frequently used by therapists and others who treat high-risk, developmentally disabled, and medically unstable infants.

Scores for each of the five factors are computed 1 minute and again 5 minutes after birth. Each factor is rated on a scale of 0 to 2, and the sum of individual scores is called the Apgar score. The closer the total is to 10, the better the condition of the neonate is considered to be. Scores equal to or less than 6 usually indicate the need for some type of intervention. Table 9-1 further details the Apgar Scoring System.

It is generally agreed that the Apgar score accomplishes its purpose: to provide delivery room personnel with important information that helps them to plan the management of the neonate immediately after birth.[10] Attempts have also been made to determine the ability of the Apgar score to predict survival potential and to see if there is a correlation between the Apgar score and long-range intellectual, neuromuscular, and other specific disorders. These studies have produced a variety of conclusions. For example, one study found that the Apgar score was satisfactory for the prediction of survival of infants whose birth weight was over 1,000 grams but had poor prognostic value for infants weighing less than that.[2] A study by Drage and others[7] found that low birth weight infants who had unsatisfactory 5-minute Apgar scores had an increased percentage of neurological abnormalities at 1 year of age. But these same subjects at 4 years of age showed almost no neurological abnormalities, indicating that limitations may be short-lived.[6] No follow-up study of the school performance of these children was reported, although such assessment seems warranted. These and other studies attempting to confirm or deny the predictive validity of the Apgar score are most interesting, but more research is needed.

TABLE 9-1	**Apgar scoring system**		
Sign	*Score 0*	*Score 1*	*Score 2*
Heart rate	Absent	Slow (below 100)	Over 100
Respiratory effort	Absent	Slow, irregular, hypoventilation	Good, crying lustily
Muscle tone	Flaccid	Some flexion of extremities	Active motion, well flexed
Reflex irritability	No response	Cry, some motion	Vigorous cry
Color	Blue, pale	Body pink, hands and feet blue	Completely pink

Total score	*Condition*
0 to 3	Severe distress
4 to 6	Moderate difficulty
7 to 10	Absence of stress

From Apgar, V.: Curr. Res. Anes. Analges. **32:** 260, 1953; and Apgar, V., and others: JAMA **168:**1985, 1958.

DENVER DEVELOPMENTAL SCREENING TEST (DDST)

The Denver Developmental Screening Test[8] is widely used by pediatricians, occupational therapists, nurses, physical therapists, and other child care personnel to screen for developmental delays. It was developed in 1967 by Frankenberg and Dodds of the University of Colorado Medical Center and has generally well-accepted normative data.

Because this test is simple to administer, actual test administration is easily performed by well-trained assistant-level personnel. Therapists are cautioned to remember that this is a screening instrument. Its developers did not intend that it be used to establish clear-cut developmental levels of performance or be used for diagnostic purposes. They recommend the administration of comprehensive developmental and neurological evaluations for such purposes. The test analysis for the Denver Developmental Screening Test is shown in Exhibit 9-4, and a sample score sheet is shown in Figure 9-5. Awareness of the types of items used in this test is

useful to the therapist because similar items are used on the more comprehensive developmental evaluations. Of course, many more items would be used in the administration process.

Therapist-made tests

CHECKLISTS

Very often therapists will develop checklists to assist with referrals and screening. Checklists are simple lists of factors or behaviors that the therapist considers important to note. For example, a checklist to guide one's clinical observations according to the process presented earlier in this chapter would be a useful tool. Checklists do not constitute comprehensive evaluations. They are merely reminders to guide the direction of the screening or assessment.

A one-page checklist for referral to occupational therapy was developed by Carol Leaman, Fulton County Schools, Atlanta, Georgia (Exhibit 9-5). To help determine the need for occupational therapy services of

---

EXHIBIT 9-4

Test analysis: Denver Developmental Screening Test

Test measures: Screening of developmental accomplishments in four areas
1. Personal-social: Ability to get along with people and care for self
2. Fine-motor adaptive: Ability to see and use hands
3. Language: Hearing, comprehension, vocabulary, verbal expression
4. Gross motor: Postural and locomotive patterns

Test identifies delays in development in these areas.

Population: Children from birth to 6 years.

Test format: This is a standardized test involving
1. Task performance of specific activities by child.
2. Parent interview using specific questions; pass by "Report" of "R." To be used only if child cannot be observed performing tasks.

A standard, purchased test kit, forms, and manual are used. The form can be reused at successive test periods, rather than a new one.

Administration:
1. Establish rapport with parent and child. Child may sit on parent's lap during testing time but should be able to reach test material easily.
2. Calculate child's age in years and months.
3. Draw age line on form, connecting child's age top to bottom: include subtractions of time if child was more than 2 weeks premature.

NOTE: *Steps two and three should be completed with care as correct interpretation of results depend on accuracy here.*

4. Although the order in which test items are given is flexible, the items must be administered in the manner specified in the manual. An easy procedure to follow is to give the child blocks to play with as questions regarding birthdate and prematurity are asked and the age line is drawn. Items in the personal-social sector that are not likely to be observed during the test and can be passed on parental report can then be asked while the child continues to explore the blocks and becomes comfortable with the examiner.

5. The number of items to be administered may vary with age of the child. The recommended procedure is to identify the first three items to the left of the age line in each of the four sectors and make sure that the child can pass at

classroom students, the teachers can review items on the checklist to see if problem students demonstrate one or more of the behaviors indicated. Leaman has divided checklist items into four categories to assist the therapist in determining primary problem areas. Although this checklist was developed for elementary school children under 9 years of age, similar behavioral items can be developed to assist with referrals for other age groups and problems. In Leaman's checklist, section I relates to terminal behaviors. Sections IA through IC are used to identify clusters of behaviors for diagnostic purposes.

Another type of checklist was developed by therapists at the Colerain Elementary School in Columbus, Ohio. This Student Checklist (Exhibit 9-6) is used by therapists to organize initial data collection from records and reports that is related to ambulation, self-care, and communication activities. Therapists can make note of reported independent and dependent performance, as well as assistive devices already in use by the student.

A developmental checklist (Exhibit 9-7) can be useful for screening large groups of children in an agency where therapist hours are limited. Three to five representative activities are given at each age level that generally indicate adequate performance of play, self-maintenance, and school-work tasks. Therapists might ask the referring individuals to use the checklist as a guide for identifying children who are unable to meet the performance criteria in two or more items at each age level.

PERFORMANCE TESTS

Therapists frequently develop screening tools that assess a child's performance in different representative activities. Such screening instruments may be considered criterion-referenced tests. For example, a fundamental component of Ayres' Southern California Sensory Integration Tests (SCSIT)[4] is the clinical observation of the child's performance in a group of neuromotor tests. Many of these clinical tests were drawn by Ayres from traditional neurological examination procedures. A

Text continued on p. 158.

least those 12 items. To complete a full Denver Developmental Screening Test, the examiner should offer all items that intersect the age line or fall to the right of the line until the child fails to perform at least three of these more difficult items in each sector.

6. Scoring: P = Pass; F = Failure; R = Refusal; NO = No opportunity.
7. Delays: Items to left of age line that are failed. These are colored in on ends of bars for easy identification. Percentages indicate number of children at each age who have passed item. R = Parent interview accepted performance by report if cannot be observed. 23 = Footnote number = Instructions given on back of test form.

25%	50%	75%	90%
R		/ / / / / / / / / / / / /	
23		/ / / / / / / / / / / / /	

8. Interpretation:
Abnormal = a. 2 or more sectors with 2+ delays, or
        b. 1 sector with 2+ delays and 1 sector with 1+ delay and no passes intersecting the age line
Questionable = a. 1 sector with 2+ delays, or
        b. 1 sector with 1+ delay and no passes intersecting the age line
Untestable = When refusals occur in numbers large enough to cause the test result to be questionable or abnormal
        if refusals were scored as failures.
Normal = Anything else.
Advantages of test:
1. Speedy administration and scoring
2. Can be done by support staff with training and supervision
3. Validated against Bayley and Stanford-Binet tests
4. Large and good socioeconomic and ethnic distribution of standardization sample (N = more than 1,000)
5. Test-retest reliability: 90%-100%
6. Interrater reliability: 80%-95%
7. Validity: Positive 0.73 agreement on passes
        Negative 0.22 agreement on failures
Disadvantages: Cannot get clear-cut developmental level without abusing test.

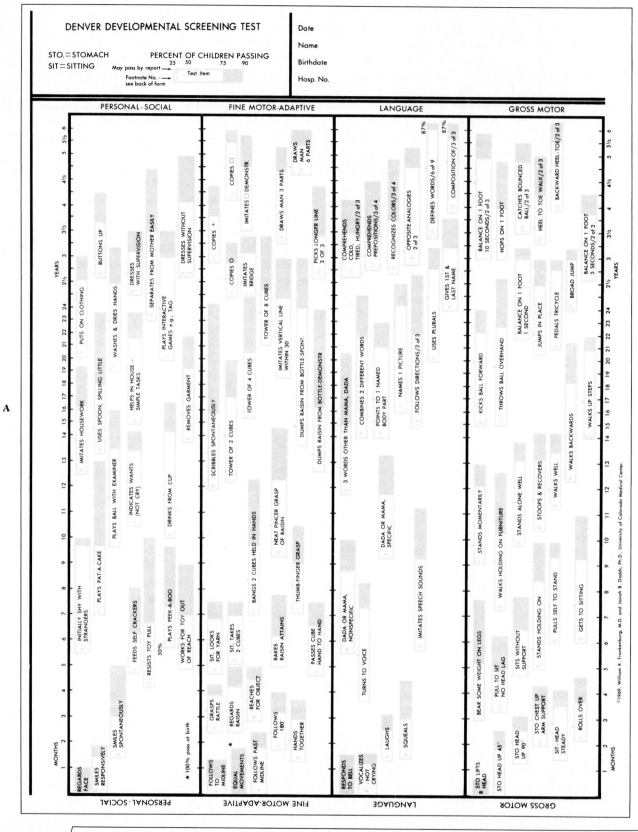

FIGURE 9-5

Denver Developmental Screening Test form. **A,** Front.

From Frankenburg, W.K., Dodds, J.B., and Fandel, A.W.: Denver Developmental Screening Test manual, ed. 2, Denver, 1970, LADOCA Project & Publishing Foundation, Inc. Available from LADOCA Project & Publishing Foundation, Inc., E. 51st St. & Lincoln St., Denver, Colo. 80216.

DATE

NAME

DIRECTIONS   BIRTHDATE

HOSP. NO.

1. Try to get child to smile by smiling, talking or waving to him. Do not touch him.
2. When child is playing with toy, pull it away from him. Pass if he resists.
3. Child does not have to be able to tie shoes or button in the back.
4. Move yarn slowly in an arc from one side to the other, about 6" above child's face. Pass if eyes follow 90° to midline. (Past midline; 180°)
5. Pass if child grasps rattle when it is touched to the backs or tips of fingers.
6. Pass if child continues to look where yarn disappeared or tries to see where it went. Yarn should be dropped quickly from sight from tester's hand without arm movement.
7. Pass if child picks up raisin with any part of thumb and a finger.
8. Pass if child picks up raisin with the ends of thumb and index finger using an over hand approach.

9. Pass any enclosed form. Fail continuous round motions.
10. Which line is longer? (Not bigger.) Turn paper upside down and repeat. (3/3 or 5/6)
11. Pass any crossing lines.
12. Have child copy first. If failed, demonstrate

When giving items 9, 11 and 12, do not name the forms. Do not demonstrate 9 and 11.

13. When scoring, each pair (2 arms, 2 legs, etc.) counts as one part.
14. Point to picture and have child name it. (No credit is given for sounds only.)

B

15. Tell child to: Give block to Mommie; put block on table; put block on floor. Pass 2 of 3. (Do not help child by pointing, moving head or eyes.)
16. Ask child: What do you do when you are cold? ..hungry? ..tired? Pass 2 of 3.
17. Tell child to: Put block on table; under table; in front of chair, behind chair. Pass 3 of 4. (Do not help child by pointing, moving head or eyes.)
18. Ask child: If fire is hot, ice is ?; Mother is a woman, Dad is a ?; a horse is big, a mouse is ?. Pass 2 of 3.
19. Ask child: What is a ball? ..lake? ..desk? ..house? ..banana? ..curtain? ..ceiling? ..hedge? ..pavement? Pass if defined in terms of use, shape, what it is made of or general category (such as banana is fruit, not just yellow). Pass 6 of 9.
20. Ask child: What is a spoon made of? ..a shoe made of? ..a door made of? (No other objects may be substituted.) Pass 3 of 3.
21. When placed on stomach, child lifts chest off table with support of forearms and/or hands.
22. When child is on back, grasp his hands and pull him to sitting. Pass if head does not hang back.
23. Child may use wall or rail only, not person. May not crawl.
24. Child must throw ball overhand 3 feet to within arm's reach of tester.
25. Child must perform standing broad jump over width of test sheet. (8-1/2 inches)
26. Tell child to walk forward, → heel within 1 inch of toe. Tester may demonstrate. Child must walk 4 consecutive steps, 2 out of 3 trials.
27. Bounce ball to child who should stand 3 feet away from tester. Child must catch ball with hands, not arms, 2 out of 3 trials.
28. Tell child to walk backward, ← toe within 1 inch of heel. Tester may demonstrate. Child must walk 4 consecutive steps, 2 out of 3 trials.

DATE AND BEHAVIORAL OBSERVATIONS (how child feels at time of test, relation to tester, attention span, verbal behavior, self-confidence, etc,):

FIGURE 9-5, cont'd

Denver Developmental Screening Test form. **B,** Back, with directions from numbered items on testing form.

EXHIBIT 9-5

Checklist of symptoms that may suggest a need for an occupational therapy referral

Guidelines:

1. Child is 9 years old or under
2. Child has many of the symptoms checked in Section I *plus* one of the other sections.

Section I

_____Has trouble with cutting, tracing activities

_____Has trouble pasting one piece of paper on another

_____Has difficulty reading the writing on the blackboard

_____Has difficulty copying from the blackboard

_____Has difficulty spacing his letters as he writes them

_____Reverses letters more often than his classmates

_____Sometimes reads words backwards

_____Does not have normal hand dominance; not skillful with either

_____Sometimes gets right and left confused

_____Hyperactive; distractible; poor attention span

Section IA (underreactive vestibular disorder)

_____Has trouble holding head up while sitting

_____Becomes tired easily

_____When shifting body in chair, sometimes falls out of seat

_____Stumbles and falls more frequently than others his age

_____Sometimes makes no attempt to catch himself when falling

_____Large movements are clumsy

_____Has a hard time keeping his balance in games, in P.E., on equipment

_____Is not really good at sports or does not enjoy them

_____Throwing or catching a ball may be difficult

_____Walks or runs into furniture, walls

_____Oversteps or understeps obstacles

_____Feels heavy or stiff when you try to help him position body

_____Runs in the wrong direction when playing a team sport

_____Often stands too close to other people

_____Often bumps into people

Section IB (overreactive vestibular disorder)

_____Does not stumble or fall, yet wants physical assistance

_____Becomes anxious when feet leave the ground

_____Has an unnatural fear of falling or of heights

_____Does not have fun on the playground equipment or with moving toys

_____Dislikes rough-housing, somersaults, rolling on the floor, jumping

_____May avoid climbing, walking on a raised surface, over bumpy ground

_____Is alarmed if suddenly pushed backward

_____Is threatened when other people move him

_____May not allow others to stand nearby when he is working

_____Uses the stair banister more than other children

Section IC (developmental dyspraxia: a motor planning problem)

_____Has not learned to do many self-help activities at age approp. level

_____Has trouble putting on clothes, using buttons and zippers, with laces

_____Does things in an inefficient way

_____Appears weak, has low muscle tone

_____Is accident-prone; has many little accidents (spilling milk)

_____Needs more protection than other children

_____Is more emotionally sensitive; feelings are easily hurt

_____Cannot tolerate upsets in plans and expectations

_____Complains more about minor physical injuries

_____Bruises, bumps, and cuts seem to hurt more than they do in other children

_____Is apt to be stubborn or uncooperative

_____Wants things his way

_____Has a shortage of skills; has to practice each skill over and over

_____Once a skill is learned, it is performed well

_____Has trouble with pencil control; is messy

_____Is slow to learn new games or new motor skills

From Carol Leaman, OTR, Fulton County Schools, Atlanta, Ga.

Adapted from text of Ayres, A.J.: Sensory integration and the child, Los Angeles, 1979, Western Psychological Services, Inc.

EXHIBIT 9-6

Student checklist

Name _____ Birthdate _____
Diagnosis:
Precautions:

Activities of daily living skills

Ambulation

Walks _____   Wheelchair _____
Independent _____ Walker _____   Independent _____ Dependent _____
Crutches _____ Cane _____   Assistance, long distances _____
Stairs: Independent _____ Dependent _____ Assistance _____
Comments: _____

Dressing

	Dependent	Needs some assistance	Independent
Coat	_____	_____	_____
Upper extremity	_____	_____	_____
Lower extremity	_____	_____	_____

Comments: _____

Feeding

Independent _____ Set up only _____ Minimal assistance _____ Dependent _____
Special utensils, equipment needed _____
Comments: _____

Toileting

	Yes	No
Bathroom independence	_____	_____
Urinary appliance _____	_____	_____
Diapers (independent) _____	_____	_____
Braces (independent) _____	_____	_____

Transfers: Independent _____
Assistance _____ Dependent _____

Comments: _____

Communication

Verbal _____   Nonverbal _____
Clear _____ Articulation problems _____   Bliss symbols _____
                                                   Other _____

Written communication	Legible	Illegible
Prints _____	_____	_____
Cursive _____	_____	_____
Types _____	_____	_____

Comments: _____

_____   _____
Therapist   Therapist

If you have any questions, concerns or problems please feel free to contact us.

Reprinted with permission of the Columbus Public Schools and Colerain Elementary School, Columbus, Ohio.

EXHIBIT 9-7

Developmental checklist

Neurological development to 5 years	1. Tonic neck reflex
	2. TLR
	3. Response to touch
	4. Protective extension
	5. Body righting

| 1 to 3 months | Lifts head |
| | Follows moving object |

| 4 to 7 months | Transfers toy hand to hand |
| | Approaches mirror |

| 8 to 12 months | Raises self to sitting position |
| | Finger-feeds self |

| 13 to 18 months | Makes pencil marks |
| | Cooperates in dressing |

19 to 24 months	Squats in play
	Identifies pictures by pointing
	Feeds self with spoon

25 to 36 months	Runs well
	Holds pencil with fingers
	Pulls on simple garment

37 to 48 months	Alternates feet going upstairs or rides tricycle
	Copies circle
	Feeds self well (spoon and fork)

49 to 60 months	Catches ball
	Copies crosses
	Distinguishes front, back of the clothes or *self*
	Acts out fantasies in play

5 to 7 years	Recites letters of alphabet
	Differentiates right from left
	Exhibits hand dominance
	Performs somersault
	Plays well with other children

7 to 10 years	Performs well in competition sports with other children
	Verbalizes plans for adult life
	Can read and write at grade level
	Can do math at grade level
	Independent in self-care

10 to 15 years	Prefers peer group activities
	Enjoys one hobby
	Travels independently
	Grade level academic performance (C − or better)
	Grade level athletic performance (C − or better)

15 to 20 years	Active interest in community-world affairs
	Preparation for adult occupational role
	Grade level academic performance
	Satisfactory peer relationships

basic format for content of clinical observation was described by Ayres[4] in 1976, based on procedures reported earlier.[3] Although a standard format for these procedures has not been published by Ayres, a number of interpretive forms have been developed by therapists who are certified in the administration of the SCSIT. The modification of one such form is shown in Exhibit 9-8. This clinical observation process incorporates some additional measures that have proved to be useful in practice.

MAKE YOUR OWN TESTS

All of the screening instruments presented here, including commercial tests, were at one time drafted together out of need by one or two individuals with knowledge and ingenuity. Some were developed to the point of usefulness in one facility, while others have been modified and subjected to extensive item analysis and standardization procedures. Within that one facility, the therapist-made test may be more reliable than other tests that have been developed further for commercial use.

This point is made to emphasize the importance of the therapist's grounding in developmental processes and problems, and the ability to formulate questions that will provide answers to guide effective treatment. Often the therapist may find that parts, but not the wholes, of different tests are useful with a particular population of children. Such a finding is common among therapists who work with developmentally disabled children because of children's variable age level development in different skill areas. Rather than subjecting a child to lengthy evaluation by using all tests, it may be more practical and sensitive to develop a therapist-made test that integrates the critical items from a variety of appropriate tests. It is important for the therapist who does this to retain information on the test form about the sources of items used, as well as any variations made in the items for the new test format. Clearly the usefulness of any instrument depends on the experience, perceptiveness, and knowledge of the test administrator. It is advisable for therapists to be familiar with correct administrative procedures for test items before adapting them.

SUMMARY

This chapter has presented basic methods of clinical evaluation, including observation, interviewing, and history taking, as well as a number of screening instruments for children. The test instruments discussed include both commercially available and therapist-made tests that are used to obtain information about developmental history and identify problems in functional status and general performance competencies. This ini-

EXHIBIT 9-8

Southern California Sensory Integration Tests: Clinical Observations

Student name: _____

School: _____ Class: _____

Date: _____ Examiner: _____

Date of birth: _____

Chronological age: _____

1. Eye preference for sighting: Offer spy holes at midline. Say, "Look at me through this with one of your eyes."
   a. Student's eye through ring of examiner's thumb and index finger.   R _____ L _____
   b. Student's eye through a paper cone to focus on examiner.   R _____ L _____
   c. Student's eye through a small hole in large cardboard.   R _____ L _____

   Score: 3 = Same as hand preference: R _____   L _____
          2 = Inconsistent
          1 = Opposite
   Comments: _____

2. Eye pursuits: Move pen back and forth, up and down, and diagonally, holding it about 10 to 12 inches from child's eyes at midline. Use child's shoulders, chin, and top of head as landmarks for ends of ranges. Instruct the child to follow the pen with his eyes without moving head. If necessary, examiner hold child's chin firmly to prevent head movements. To check convergence, begin with pencil at examiner's nose and move it slowly forward to student's nose and then back. Ask child to tell you when he sees "two pens."
   Score: General pursuits:
          3 = Basically smooth, coordinated movements. May show small jerks or hesitations.
          2 = Slight irregularities in most planes, even after child becomes accustomed to testing.
          1 = Unable to follow or loses target; unable to separate eye movements from head movements (normal to 6 years).
   Comments: _____
   Score: Across midline:
          1 = Basically smooth, coordinated movements as above.
          2 = Midline jerk, then refocuses.
          3 = Midline jerk, cannot refocus.
   Comments: _____
   Score: Convergence:
          3 = Basically smooth.
          2 = Movement jerky and unsure.
          1 = Eyes break apart or do not converge.
          0 = Unable to fixate.
          Check eyes together and then independently by first covering one eye, then the other. Observe and note right/left differences.
          L _____   R _____   Both _____
   Comments: _____

3. Forearm rotation: Test for adiadochokinesis, 10 seconds. Sit facing child, both with arms resting in laps. Demonstrate rapid supination and pronation, then ask child to imitate and say: "Do it fast." Count the number of times the palms slap thighs in 10 seconds. Observe for incoordination, and compare right and left scores.
   R _____ times   L _____ times
   Score: Bilateral coordination:
          3 = Normal
          2 = One arm slower than other throughout: R   L
          1 = Both arms deficient
   Comments: _____

4. Thumb-finger touching: Thumb touches each finger in sequence from index to little and then back in sequence to index finger, repeating several times. Observe speed, coordination, and right-left differences.
   Score: 3 = Performs easily   L _____ R _____ Both _____
          2 = Slight irregularities   L _____ R _____ Both _____
          1 = Awkard or unable   L _____ R _____ Both _____
   Comments: _____

Adapted from Ayres, A.J.: Sensory integration and learning disorders, Los Angeles, 1972, Western Psychological Services; and Ayres, A.J.: Interpreting the Southern California Sensory Integration Tests, Los Angeles, 1976, Western Psychological Services; and Adams, S., 1976.

Continued.

EXHIBIT 9-8, cont'd

Southern California Sensory Integration Tests: Clinical Observations—cont'd

5. Muscle tone: Examiner places student's shoulder, elbow, and hand flexor muscles on stretch. Note degree of hyperextension. Palpate muscles for tone.

    Score: 3 = Normal   R/L differences: _____

           2 = Slightly hypotonic

           1 = Definitely hypertonic

           0 = Hypertonic

    Comments: _____

6. Cocontraction: Examiner applies force against student's position. Sit facing child. Do not let him stabilize against back of chair. Ask child to "freeze like a statue" and not let you push or pull him. (This should be fully developed by 7 to 8 years of age.)

    Score: 3 = Can withstand moderate resistance.

           2 = Can withstand light resistance.

           1 = Unable to hold against resistance.

Arm: Student holds examiner's thumbs, with elbows flexed.	3 2 1
Shoulder: Examiner holds student's hands, elbows straight:	3 2 1
Neck: Examiner gives force against different planes:	3 2 1
(Do not expect as much strength as in arms.)	

    Comments: _____

7. Flexor postural pattern: Student assumes "curled up" position, arms crossed across chest, ankles crossed, knees and hips flexed, neck flexed forward. Do not allow child to clasp hands behind knees. Examiner applies resistive force at head and knees. Decrease force for children under 6 years.

    Score: 3 = Holds 20 seconds or more with moderate effort.

           2 = Holds 10 to 19 seconds with great exertion.

           1 = Holds less than 10 seconds against resistance.

           0 = Unable to hold against resistance.

    Comments: _____

8. Prone extension postural pattern: Student assumes pivot prone position with arms overhead, slightly abducted, and elbows slightly flexed. Legs should be straight together, fully extended. Have child lift head, arms, and legs off the floor (superman position).

    Score: Duration

           3 = Holds 20+ seconds with moderate effort.

           2 = Holds 10 to 19 seconds with great exertion.

           1 = Holds less than 10 seconds.

           0 = Unable to hold.

        Quality

           3 = Lifts four extremities simultaneously.

           2 = Lifts arms, then legs, or reverse.

           1 = Lifts one part at a time.

           0 = Unable to assume position.

    Comments: _____

9. Schilder's Arm Extension Test (AET)

    Part I: Student stands with feet together, arms stretched forward, fingers abducted, and eyes closed. Student counts aloud to 20.

        Check: _____Able to maintain posture with ease.

              _____Able to maintain posture but with effort.

              _____Postural change in arms during count (describe).

              _____

              _____Difficulty with assuming posture (describe).

              _____

              _____Unable to assume posture.

              _____Spooning of hands, hyperextension of elbows.

    Comments: _____

EXHIBIT 9-8, cont'd

Southern California Sensory Integration Tests: Clinical Observations—cont'd

Part II: Student assumes same position, without counting. Examiner turns student's head from side to side.

Check: _____Minimal or no rotation of shoulder following head.

_____Rotation of shoulder.

_____Rotation of shoulder and hips.

_____Equilibrium is disturbed.

_____Extreme exaggeration of asymmetrical tonic neck reflex attitude.

_____Resistance to head movement.

_____Facial or verbal manifestations of discomfort.

Comments: _____

Score: Arm position change:	Equilibrium:
3 = Normal	3 = Normal
2 = Slight Change	2 = Slight loss
1 = Marked change	1 = Marked loss
Head resistance:	Emotional response:
3 = Normal	3 = Stable
2 = Slight resistance	2 = Slight discomfort
1 = Marked resistance	1 = Marked discomfort
Arm raised: R _____ L _____	Elbow hyperextension: R _____ L _____

Comments: _____

10. Choreoathetoid movements: Observe movements of hands during pivot prone and Schilder's AET.

   3 = No movements

   2 = Slight jerking

   1 = Marked response

   Comments: _____

11. Asymmetrical tonic neck reflex (ATNR): Student assumes quadruped position, then places right hand on right hip and lifts left leg. Examiner turns student's chin to right shoulder. Reverse position for left side.

   Score: Right ATNR: Left ATNR

   4 = Assumes and holds for 10 seconds.   4

   3 = Slight wobbling but holds 10 seconds.   3

   2 = Difficulty assuming, holds less than 10 seconds.   2

   1 = needs assistance to assume, cannot maintain.   1

   0 = Unable to assume posture with assistance.   0

   Comments: _____

12. Space visualization contralateral use score (SVCU):

   FORMULA: $SVCU = 30 - I/C$, drop fraction

   Score: 3 = Score of 28 is normal.

          2 = Score of 29 indicates use of one side only; questionable deficit on opposite side.

          1 = Score of 27 or less suggests lack of adequate dominance for skilled motor tasks.

   Comments: _____

13. Postrotatory nystagmus test: Spin child 10 times in each direction, 2 seconds per revolution. Have child look up at ceiling at end of each spin. Estimate amount of excursion and duration. Repeat in other direction.

   Score: R _____ mm _____ _____ seconds

           L _____ mm _____ _____ seconds

Comments: _____

tial part of the occupational therapy assessment clarifies the need for more comprehensive evaluation and treatment. Considerable information can be obtained through careful observation of the child in relation to various activities and environments. This requires that the therapist use a questioning attitude based on and supported by knowledge of the human growth and development processes and human function.

REFERENCES

1. Apgar, V.: A proposal for a new method of evaluation of the newborn infant, Curr. Res. Anes. Analges. **32:**260, 1953.
2. Apgar, V., and James, L.S.: Further observations on the newborn scoring system, Am. J. Dis. Child. **104:**419, 1962.
3. Ayres, A.J.: Sensory integration and learning disorders, Los Angeles, 1972, Western Psychological Services.
4. Ayres, A.J.: Interpreting the Southern California Sensory Integration Tests, Los Angeles, 1976, Western Psychological Services.
5. Coley, I.L.: Pediatric assessment of self-care activities, St. Louis, 1976, The C.V. Mosby Co.
6. Drage, J.S., Berendes, H., and Fisher, P.D.: The Apgar score at four years: psychological examination of performance. In Pan American Health Organization: Perinatal factors affecting human development, World Health Organization Scientific Publications **185:**222, 1969.
7. Drage, J.S., and others: The Apgar score as an index of infant morbidity, Dev. Med. Child Neurol. **8:**141, 1966.
8. Frankenburg, W.K., Dodds, J.B., and Fandel, A.W.: Denver Developmental Screening Test manual, ed. 2, Denver, 1970, LADOCA Project & Publishing Foundation, Inc.
9. Takata, N.: Play as prescription. In Reilly, M., editor: Play as exploratory learning: studies in curiosity behavior, Beverly Hills, Calif., 1974, Sage Publications, Inc.
10. Taylor, K.M.: The Apgar scoring system. In Humenick, S.S., editor: Analysis of current assessment strategies in the health care of young children and child-bearing families, Norwalk, Conn., 1982, Appleton-Century-Crofts.

PAT NUSE CLARK
ANNE STEVENS ALLEN
FLORENCE CLARK
KAREN E. SCHANZENBACHER

Instruments to evaluate component functions of behavior

Through the screening process and general problem analysis (Chapters 7 and 9) the therapist is able to identify deficits in the child's performance that indicate the need for occupational therapy services. Screenings typically raise more questions in the therapist's mind than answers. These questions guide the selection of formal evaluation measures. The therapist will want to determine why the child has problems doing everyday activities. To begin to find the causes of these problems, the therapist will evaluate the status of sensory integrative, motor, cognitive, social, and emotional functions. Depending on the presenting problems, specific evaluation of one functional area may be done in more depth than others.

Evaluation procedures used to determine functional states include interviews, observation, administration of standardized and criterion-referenced tests, and manipulation and palpation of the child's body parts by the therapist. Again, the variety of tools available through commercial resources, the literature, and colleagues is virtually limitless. However, for this chapter a representative sample of some of the more widely known evaluative procedures is presented. Test analyses are included for the Frostig Developmental Test of Visual Perception, the Developmental Test of Visual-Motor Integration, the Purdue Perceptual Motor Survey, the Erhardt Developmental Prehension Assessment, and the Knox Play Scale. A number of other tests will also be discussed.

TESTING MOTOR FUNCTION

Because the occupational therapist is greatly concerned with the manifestations of motor behaviors in activity performance, considerable emphasis is often placed on motor function tests. Therefore the variety and specificity of tests for motor function that have been developed for and by occupational therapists are greater than for other functional areas. It would be difficult to familiarize oneself with every test available that measures motor function. However, selections from the group of tests presented here should permit the therapist to develop a comprehensive assessment of the motor functions of most children.

Tests for neurodevelopmental reactions and reflexes

A number of systems for testing the maturational patterns of the neuromotor system have been developed, including those by Fiorentino[14] and Milani-Comparetti.[29] To use any of these tests, an understanding of the general categories of neurodevelopmental reactions is necessary, along with an awareness of the principles of reflex maturation and testing. Exhibit 10-1 provides an overview of critical information. (Reference to relevant sections of Chapter 4 is also useful.)

Bearing the infant's state in mind, despite the fact that reflex evaluation may be the procedure used most often with younger children, it is generally best to perform these tests at the close of a testing session. The responses of infants and young children to the different tests range from slightly irritated to openly resistive, and the procedure does little to establish rapport between the child and the therapist. Therefore it is better to present the child with enjoyable play activities early in the therapeutic relationship and save the reflex testing until after a recognizable amount of positive responsiveness is shown by the child.

GENERAL PROCEDURES

In most neurodevelopmental tests the child is placed in a relatively static posture by the examiner. Postural tone and body symmetry are noted in the resting position. Then the examiner will touch or move the child, using a prescribed pattern of stimulus. The motor response that is elicited by the stimulus constitutes the reflex or reaction.

MILANI-COMPARETTI MOTOR DEVELOPMENT SCREENING TEST

The Milani-Comparetti Motor Development Screening Test[29] is a particularly useful system because the evaluation form clearly demonstrates time ranges for the emergence and disappearance of primitive and postural reactions. The reactions are tied to the develop-ment of locomotor patterns that begin in the supine position and progress to movement in upright walking. The instructions for test administration are clear, concise, and easy to follow. The protocol sheet provides a graphic record of the child's progress toward neuromotor maturity (Figure 10-1). Therapists are referred to the administration manual for more detailed information about the development and use of this test.[23]

FIORENTINO REFLEX DEVELOPMENT SYSTEM

The Fiorentino Reflex Development System is widely used. It was developed by Mary Fiorentino,[14] an occupational therapist. It is organized according to postural patterns of apedal, quadrupedal, and bipedal locomotion, and the level of central nervous system control of the reflexive pattern. There are subcategories of different types of reactions that occur and recur at each level. There is a maturational component through different forms of similar reactions as the child matures, and primitive subcortical reflexes are replaced by higher reactions with more cortical control. The Fiorentino system is well documented elsewhere.[14,19]

Motor performance tests

NORTON'S BASIC MOTOR EVALUATION

Norton's Basic Motor Evaluation was designed to assess the quality of sensorimotor performance and to identify the predominating inborn reactions that are related to a child's deficits in sensorimotor function. Therefore this test battery examines both reflex reactions and purposeful movement patterns. The original format of the test was developed by Semans in 1965 for assessment of children with cerebral palsy. In the Semans version the child was placed in a position and asked to hold it. In contrast, Norton's adaptation[30] was designed for the child with a less severe motor handicap, and it requires that the child assume and hold the position after a verbal command is given. Demonstration and physical assistance are given only if the child appears to have difficulty following directions.

The therapist observes the child according to a number of criteria. These include the quality of movement (such as smoothness and balance), motor planning and body scheme, flexibility and bilateral symmetry, and comprehension and memory for instruction. The therapist analyzes patterns of pathological movement to determine problems in balance, coordination, perception, or behavior. Because this evaluation includes interesting activities, children appear to enjoy participation. The test provides a useful measure of the movement criteria mentioned if the therapist closely observes the child's performance. Use of a videotape to record the child's performance can be particularly use-

EXHIBIT 10-1

Neurodevelopmental reactions and reflexes

Definitions
1. *Attitudinal (postural) reflexes:* Those reactions that automatically provide for maintenance of the body in an upright position through changes of muscle tone in response to the position of the body or its parts.
2. *Equilibrium reactions:* Responsible for body adaptation in response to a change in the center of gravity. Results in head and trunk righting toward vertical body alignment, changes in extremities to balance weight shifts through extension and abduction, and also protects body balance.
3. *Labyrinthine:* Refers to the inner ear that contains vestibular sensory organs that are sensitive to progressive movements, acceleration or deceleration forward, turning movements, and to changes of direction in relation to gravity.
4. *Phasic reactions:* Movement reflexes that coordinate muscles of the limbs in patterns of either total flexion or total extension.
5. *Righting reactions:* Function to keep the upper part of the body upright and to maintain the head and trunk in their proper relationship. Stimuli go through the labyrinths and to tactile receptors in the trunk, neck, and ears.
6. *Optical righting reactions:* Considered separately because these are dependent on the occipital cortex of the cerebral hemispheres.
7. *Static or tonic reactions:* Changes in distribution of muscle tone throughout the body, either in response to a change in position of the head and body in space (stimulus through labyrinths) or in the head in relation to the body (stimulus through proprioceptors in the neck muscles).

Principles of reflex maturation and testing
1. Maturation of central nervous system control results in the appearance of more adaptive and discriminative reactions rather than totally different, new reactions.
2. Neuromotor development is continuous, although not all areas mature simultaneously or at the same rate.
3. A child experiences both dormant and regressive periods of neuromotor maturation.
4. Flexor tone predominates in the limbs of the newborn. This decreases in the arms by 3 to 4 months and in the legs by 4 to 5 months.
5. There is an important interrelationship between muscle tone and reflex development. Reactions that include extension components do not appear until flexor tone begins to diminish.
6. It is important to differentiate the stimuli used to elicit a specific reflex (for example, noxious, tactile, proprioceptive).
7. Close observation is important as the infant moves constantly into and out of reflex patterns.
8. Some reflexes can be observed only through spontaneous behavior and cannot be elicited through testing.
9. Some reflexes are imposable (can be elicited by testing) at one age and not another.
10. Confusion exists because various authors label the same reflex with different names, label different reflexes with the same names, and test the same reflex with different stimuli. These practices lead to conflicting conclusions regarding ages of onset, disappearance, and so on.
11. The infant's state of being is important during testing:
    a. Wakefulness: During sleep there is complete hypotonia. The infant should be observed both during the resting state (awake, but not engaged in activity) and during spontaneous activity. Be alert to any signs of postural asymmetry between the two sides of the body.
    b. Mood: Crying increases muscular tension.
    c. Health: Pathology influences reflexive behaviors.
    d. Satiation: Hypotonia occurs after nursing when the infant is satiated, while increased muscular tension resulting from crying occurs shortly before feeding.
    e. Age: Specific age is determined by period of gestation.

Adapted from Carol Johnson, University of Florida, Gainesville, Fla., 1973.

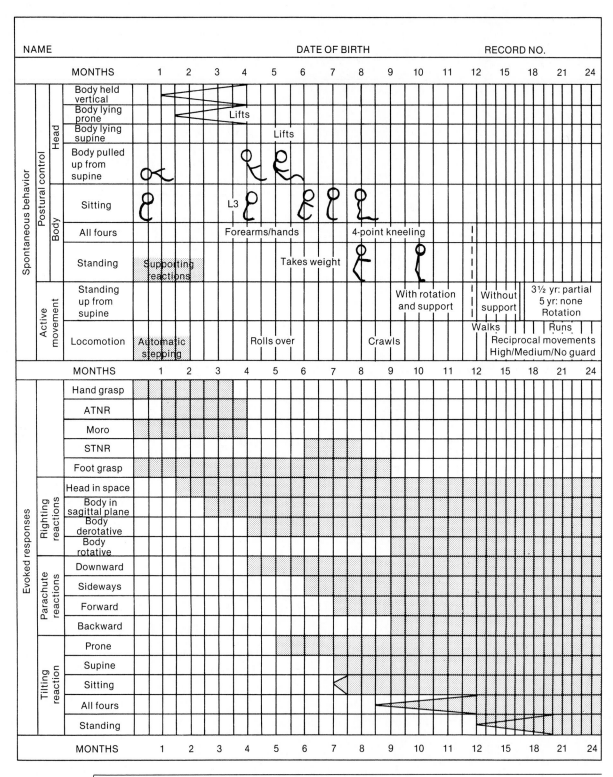

FIGURE 10-1

Milani-Comparetti Motor Development Screening Test.

From Milani-Comparetti, A., and Gidoni, E.: Dev. Med. Child Neurol. **9:**631, 766, 1967.

ful for analysis and follow-up. Although the test was designed for use with learning disabled children, it can readily be applied to other populations to obtain information about general motor function (Exhibit 10-2).

MOTOR EVALUATION OF HAND FUNCTION

A number of hand evaluations, both published and unpublished, have been developed for children. These are based on the maturational development of prehension patterns from gross "raking" movements of the whole arm to fine tip prehension. An illustration of these prehension patterns is found in Chapter 4. Through observation and activity analysis, any therapist can select representative developmental activities to assess the emergence and precision of hand use.

Two systems of prehension development testing are especially useful as models. Erhardt[13] has developed a research-based assessment that is commercially available and deserves special attention. A test analysis is shown in Exhibit 10-3.

In 1971 Skerik, Weiss, and Flatt[36] and then Weiss and Flatt[39] described a developmental test of prehension patterns. It was originally developed through their work with children who had congenital hand anomalies. However, because the test uses everyday children's activities to assess hand function, it can be used with other children as well. An adapted version of the Skerik, Weiss, and Flatt evaluation is shown in Exhibit 10-4.

BRUININKS-OSERETSKY MOTOR DEVELOPMENT SCALE

The Bruininks-Oseretsky Motor Development Scale is a standardized test of motor development that is administered individually to children 4½ to 14½ years of age. Gross and fine motor skills are evaluated according to performance on a group of 46 items that are divided into eight subtests. The fine motor subtests include upper limb coordination, response speed, visual-motor control, and upper limb speed and dexterity. Gross motor skills are measured on the running speed and agility, balance, bilateral coordination, and strength subtests. Activities include gross motor and paper-and-pencil tasks, such as walking a balance beam and drawing a straight line between two points.

The entire battery can be administered in under an hour, and requires a large room. Using the manual enables the tester to convert raw scores to standard scores and approximate age equivalents. Test development and evaluation of the Bruininks-Oseretsky scale has been extensive. The tests discriminate well between nonhandicapped populations and learning disabled and mentally retarded children. Interrater reliability is excellent, probably because of the well-written and amply illustrated administration and scoring procedures. Test-retest reliability is generally good for the entire battery. Individual subtest stability at the higher ages in the range shows more variability. In general this is an excellent evaluation instrument to use with school-aged children who demonstrate motor problems without obvious physical handicap, if adequate space is available.[8]

PURDUE PERCEPTUAL-MOTOR SURVEY

The Purdue Perceptual-Motor Survey is used to assess performance of a series of perceptual motor skills that are designed to detect errors in perceptual-motor development in children. Its purpose is to identify areas for remediation. The skills are grouped into five main areas: posture and balance, body image and differentiation, perceptual-motor match, ocular movements, and form perception. The test battery was designed by Roach and Kephart[34] at Purdue University in Indiana and was one of the earliest tests developed to evaluate this area of function. It is a performance-based test and is included in this section because clinical experience has shown that it is more useful to the occupational therapist for the assessment of motor functions than for sensory-integrative functions. The test analysis is found in Exhibit 10-5.

Evaluation of general motor function

Occupational therapists will also want to assess muscle strength, range of motion, and muscle tone of many children seen in practice. Methods for evaluation of these characteristics are well documented.[19,31] Assessment of muscle tone is discussed in Chapters 9 and 16. There are many other formats available through the sources mentioned. Exhibit 10-6 shows page one of a composite form that can be used to record this information. This format was developed as part of the initial evaluation process used by the occupational and physical therapy staff of Colerain Elementary School, Columbus, Ohio. The Colerain form is also used to record developmental locomotor skills, from head control to walking, as measured on the Milani-Comparetti Motor Development Screening Test, the Denver Developmental Screening Test, and other developmental evaluations.

It should be noted that data related to the areas of muscle strength and range of motion are generally not measured or recorded in as much detail as might be used for adult clients. This is in part because there are few normative data on strength in children and in part because of the limited usefulness of such data. With children the emphasis of assessment tends to focus more on the end performance of motor function than on isolated measures of musculoskeletal movement axes. The primary exception to this rule would be with those children who are seen before and after surgery for traumatic musculoskeletal injuries. In such cases therapists will perform detailed assessment of joint movement and muscle strength preoperatively and postoperatively. *Text continued on p. 175.*

EXHIBIT 10-2 **Norton's basic motor evaluation**

ASSESSMENT CHART: MINIMAL CEREBRAL DYSFUNCTION
Movement and posture with inborn reactions

Name _____ Bd. _____ Patient's clinic _____

0—Cannot assume test posture even after demonstration.
1—Can assume an approximate test posture after demonstration.
2—Can assume test posture in an awkward manner on command.
3—Can assume and sustain test posture in a near normal manner on command (note abnormal details).
4—Normal.

Examiner:

D.A.	Test movements and postures	
Supine 6-7 mo.	1. Rolls completely over: a. to right. b. to left.	
4-10 mo.	2. Pulls hips and knees to chest fully flexed, arms crossed, palms on shoulders, fingers extended.	
4 mo.	3. With hips, knees fully flexed: a. Extend right leg. b. Extend left leg.	
5-7 mo.	4. Head in midline, arms at side, raise head: a. Influence on arms. b. Influence on legs.	
36-60 mo. (3-5 yr.)	5. Pulls up to sit, support on forearms, then by extending elbows.	
Prone 4-6 mo. +24 mo.	6. Extends arms beside head, legs abducted. a. Raises head in midline. b. Supinates forearms (palms toward ceiling).	
+24 mo.	7. Brings arms down beside body, extends arms, palms down.	
3-6 mo. +36 mo.	8. a. Flex right knee, hips extend. b. Flex left knee, hips extend.	
3 mo.	9. a. Support trunk on forearms, upper trunk extended, face vertical. b. Flex knees.	
5 mo. 8 mo. 6 mo.	10. a. Supports trunk on hands with elbows and hips extended, face vertical. b. Flexes neck. c. Extends neck. d. Balance.	

From The American Occupational Therapy Association, Inc., Copyright 1972, Vol. 26, No. 4, pp. 193-198, *Minimal Cerebral Dysfunction*, Y Norton.

+ − = Present or absent inborn reactions.
I.R. = Inborn reactions.
* = Equilibrium reactions = learned reactions.
M.&P. = Movements and Posture.
( ) = Retarding influences.
S.T.N.R. = Symmetrical Tonic Neck Reflex.
D.A. = Age that normal responses, movement behavior develop in these positions due to presence or absence of certain basic reflexes and reactions.

Test				**Retest**			
Inborn reactions			**Date**	**Remarks: M.&P.**	**I.R.**		**Date**	**Remarks: M.&P.**
(Neck righting) Head on body	+	−			+	−		
(Body on body) Body on head			R				R	
Labyrinthine			L				L	
(Tonic neck) Associated reactions (Tonic labyrinthine)								
(Crossed extension) (Tonic labyrinthine)			R				R	
(Tonic neck)			L				L	
(Tonic) labyrinthine Associated reactions +			a				a	
S.T.N.R.			b				b	
(Tonic) labyrinthine Head on body								
Head on body (Tonic) labyrinthine			a				a	
Landau on floor (Tonic neck)			b				b	
(Neck righting) (Tonic neck) (Tonic labyrinthine)								
(Amphibian)			R				R	
			L				L	
Labyrinthine Optical righting			a				a	
Body on head			b				b	
Labyrinthine Optical			a				a	
(S.T.N.R.)			b				b	
Equilibrium			c				c	
			d				d	

Continued.

EXHIBIT 10-2, cont'd / **Norton's basic motor evaluation—cont'd**

8 mo.	11. Moves from prone to sit.
+9-11 mo.	a. All fours pushing back.
	b. Transitional between quadripedal and adult method: (1) side sit right.
	(2) side sit left.

Sitting erect

	12. Sits with soles of feet together, hips flexed and externally rotated to at least 45°.
8 mo.	a. Round sit.
10 mo.	b. Push laterally: (1) right.
	(2) left.
10 mo.	c. Balance-extended, flex legs.

	13. Extends knees, abducts legs: push forward, backward.
8 mo.	a. Hips 60°-70°.
10 mo.	b. Hips 90°-100°.
10 mo.	c. Hips 110°-120°.

	14. Hangs legs over edge of platform.
+15 mo.	a. Extends right knee.
	b. Extends left knee.

Kneeling and crawling

7 mo.	15. Gets into four point kneel and rocks (back straight).
	a. Weight on knees.
	b. Weight on hands.
	(1) Neck extended.
	(2) Neck flexed.
8 mo.	c. Crawl.

9 mo.	16. Moves to kneel stand, head in mid-position, arms at side. Hips fully extended.
36 mo.	a. Push: (1) Forward.
	(2) Backward.

10 mo.	17. Moves to half kneel:
	a. Weight on right knee.
	b. Weight on left knee.

Squat

21 mo.	18. Squats heels down, toes not clawed, knees pointing in same direction as toes, hips fully flexed, head in line with trunk. Arms forward.

Standing and components of walking

+15 mo.	19. Stands up. Correct alignment. Feet separated 6″.

36 mo.	20. Bear weight on one leg.
	a. Shift weight over right leg: _____ secs.
	b. Shift weight over left leg: _____ secs.

	21. Walks—Adult method.
+24 mo.	a. Forward.
	b. Backward.
36 mo.	c. Stairs: alternates feet.
	(1) Up.
	(2) Down.

Labyrinthine Optical Head on body Body on head (Amphibian) Equilibrium			a R L					a R L	
Labyrinthine Optical Protective extension of arms Equilibrium			a R L c					a R L c	
Labyrinthine Optical Protective extension of arms Equilibrium			a b c					a b c	
Labyrinthine (Adductor reflex)			R L					R L	
Labyrinthine Optical (S.T.N.R.) (Asymmetrical T.N.R.) Equilibrium			Rock Knees (1) (2) Crawl					Rock Knees (1) (2) Crawl	
Labyrinthine Optical Protective extension of arms Equilibrium			F B					F B	
Labyrinthine Optical Equilibrium			R L					R L	
Labyrinthine Equilibrium									
Labyrinthine Optical Equilibrium									
Labyrinthine Optical Equilibrium			R L					R L	
Positive Negative Support Equilibrium			a b c (1) (2)					a b c (1) (2)	

Continued.

EXHIBIT 10-2, cont'd

HEAD IN MIDLINE FOR POSITIONS

Tests: Supine

Test 1

Purpose: To test the level of and ability to roll completely over in both directions.

Instructions: "Roll to your tummy and keep rolling to your back again. Now do it on the other side. . . Lie on your back."

Note: Stiffness. Lack of trunk-pelvis separation (body on body righting). Hyperextended neck in backward roll. Rolls at angle. Normal: Head, hip, top knee slightly flexed in turning over to side.

Test 2 (From position of Test 1)

Purpose: To test for freedom from hypertonicity and lack of associated movement in the supine position.

Instructions: "Pull your knees close up to your chest. Bend your elbows and cross your arms. Put your hands on your shoulders. Raise up your elbows. . . Rest your arms."

Note: Fingers claw. Downward pull of scapular depressors preventing elbows from remaining away from the body. (Children with this difficulty seem to have trouble with writing.) Feet neither inverted nor dorsiflexed.

Test 3 (From position of Test 2)

Purpose: To test for lower extremity differentiation or identify hypertonicity preventing that differentiation.

Instructions: "Put your arms beside your body. Straighten that leg (right). Bend that same knee (right) and straighten the other leg (left). . . Relax!"

Note: Internal rotation of either leg. Adduction of either thigh. Feet inverted, plantar flexed. Extension of opposite leg when one extends. Back arched. Body asymmetry.

Test 4 (From position of Test 3)

Purpose: To test ability to raise head from the supporting surface and not affect the extremities.

Instructions: "Raise just your head. Put it back down . . . Now relax."

Note: Inability of head to differentiate from the rest of body. Symmetrical tonic neck reflex causing arms to flex and tone to increase in the legs. Feet inverted.

Test 5 (From position of Test 4)

Purpose: To test the ability and method of getting from supine to sit.

Instructions: "Sit up, please. . . Now lie down."

Note: Adult method, 5-year level: symmetry of movement, head forward, bilateral elbow flexion to extension, hips flexing; versus pathology of hypertonicity in back and lower extremities preventing hip flexion as back raises off support. Transitional method: +10-month level: from prone to side sit. Infant method, 8-month level: from quadripedal position to sit. (See illustration: Test 2)

Tests: Prone

Test 6

Purpose: To test freedom from hypertonicity in prone.

Instructions: "Get onto your tummy. Straighten your arms beside your head. Raise it. Turn the palms of your hands toward the ceiling. Straighten your fingers. . . Put your head down."

Note: Shoulders and hips: tightness in upper or lower extremities. Inversion of feet. Inability to supinate

(after +24 months). Inability to straighten fingers (asymmetry). Hypertonic upper extremity and trunk flexors, adductors, of upper extremity and trunk shoulder girdle depressors and pronators affect ability to do cursive writing. Heavy head: tonic labyrinthine abnormality. Lower extremity tightness can affect the degree of upper extremity freedom of movement.

Test 7 (From position of Test 6)

Purpose: To further test freedom of shoulders and arms from flexor hypertonus in prone.

Instructions: "Bring your arms down straight beside your body. Put the palms of your hands on the mat . . . Now relax."

Note: Freedom of head movement. Influence of head position on tone of extremities (asymmetrical tonic neck reflex), affecting ability in fine skill and possibly figure-ground. Balance, during movement and upright positions. Feet adducted, inverted.

Test 8 (From position of Test 7)

Purpose: To test selective control of hips and knees.

Instructions: "Bend your right knee. Put it down and bend your left knee. . . Now relax."

Note: 90-degree knee flexion with completely extended hips sometime after 36 months. Record hip raising, toppling of leg in inward or outward direction, foot inversion. Tightness at hips and knees affecting balance during movement and in upright positons. Amphibian reactions of forward flexion may be a retarding influence for hip extension, but a precursor for crawl.

Test 9 (From position of Test 8)

Purpose: To test postural control in spinal extension; and with knee flexion.

Instruction: "Pull up onto your elbows. Bend both knees . . . Now straighten your knees."

Note: Inability to place arms at a 90-degree flexion, with slight abduction, forearms straight, hands opened: hypertonicity of adductors, flexors of arms, forearms, and fingers. Toppling to either side. Hip flexion when knees flex. The control in this position is basic to crawl and the beginning use of hands with balance.

Test 10 (From position of Test 9)

Purpose: To test the ability to support weight on extended arms, regardless of the position of the head.

Instructions: "Straighten your elbows. Put your weight on your opened hands. Now bend your neck. Raise your head, (push laterally for balance). . . Now get onto your tummy."

Note: Inability to carry weight on extended elbows, finger extending with neck flexion, or to bend elbows with neck extension. Leg thrust with neck flexion, (due to symmetrical tonic neck reflex). Hip internal rotation and foot inversion. Lack of equilibrium reactions.

Test 11 (From position of Test 10)

Purpose: To test the ability and method of getting from prone to sit.

Instructions: "Sit up, please. . . Now bring your legs in front."

Note: Symmetry in getting up if the infant method in the quadrupedal position is used. The preferred side that the child turns toward if the transitional method is chosen, or whether the child pushes up to his knees, sits, swings his legs over and forward. (See illustration Test 5).

Tests: Sitting Erect

Test 12 (From position of Test 11)

Purpose: To test the ability to round sit and the development of lateral protective extension, balance reactions.

Instructions: "Sit up tall. Put the soles of your feet together. Relax your arms (push the child gently and laterally at each shoulder to observe balance and protective extension of the supporting arm with abduction of the opposite arm, and balance reactions as the therapist alternately flexes and extends the legs). . . Now put your legs out straight."

Note: Inability to balance. The presence or absence of protective extension of arms and the side of the absence. Straight (normal) back versus the need for head forward flexion compensation to prevent backward tipping. Lack of adequate hip flexion and external rotation of the legs.

Test 13 (From position of Test 12)

Purpose: To test balance reactions, protective extension of the arms in long sit.

Instructions: "Separate your legs. Sit up tall and let your arms go limp (push child forward then backward) . . . Now sit at the edge of the platform."

Note: Inability to balance or lack of protective extension of the limbs (elbows extended) when pushed forward, backward. Inadequate amount of hip flexion in forward, straight position. Internal rotation of thighs, foot inversion.

Test 14 (From position of Test 13)

Purpose: To test the ability to extend one leg without associated reactions in the other.

Instructions: "Sit up tall. Raise that (right) leg and straighten your knee. Relax, raise and straighten the other (left) knee. Rest. . . Now get onto your hands and knees."

Note: Any adduction or internal rotation of the other leg when either [first] leg extends. Foot inversions.

Tests: Kneeling and Crawling

Test 15 (From position of Test 14)

Purpose: To test weight bearing, balance and control in four-point position on open hands, regardless of the position of the head.

Instructions: "Rock backwards. Rock forwards (3 ×). Raise your head. Lower your head. Crawl. . . Now raise up onto your knees."

Note: Lordosis, flexion of elbows when the neck flexes with thrust of lower extremities (symmetrical tonic neck reflex); extension of the elbows only if the neck extends (symmetrical tonic neck reflex); extension of one arm only when the head turns toward that arm (asymmetrical tonic neck reflex); raising of knees off the supporting surface in moving onto extended elbows (symmetrical tonic neck reflex); inversion of feet and asymmetry in crawling.

Test 16 (From position on Test 15)

Purpose: To test for anterior-posterior control of pelvis, trunk and thighs during movement.

Instructions: "Straighten your trunk and hips (push forward, backwards). . . Remain in that position."

Note: Inability to regain balance without difficulty from forward, backward push. Lack of, or inadequate protective extension of arms. Feet inverted, hips flexed, back lordosed.

Test 17 (From position of Test 16)

Purpose: To test the control of hip rotation, and the effect on the lower extremities; balance.

Instructions: "Raise the left leg, bend the knee, and put your foot down flat. Change legs. . . Squat."

Note: Inadequate flexion of hip, knee, angle of forward leg (more than 90 degrees). Thigh adducted. Balance unstable. Toes constantly clawed. Heel off ground. Lower leg of supporting leg occasionally raised off support, that foot inverted and the hip of the supporting leg inadequately extended.

Tests: Squat

Test 18 (From position of Test 17)

Purpose: To test control of hypertonicity throughout the body.

Instructions: "Squat. Separate your knees. Put your heels down on the floor. Bring your arms forward. Shift weight sideways. . . Now stand up."

Note: Inability to put heels down on the floor. Constant clawing of toes. Tendency to topple backwards, or sideways in movement. Pain behind the knees or in the buttocks or calf of the leg.

Tests: Standing, Components of Walking

Test 19 (From position of Test 18)

Purpose: To test for normal distribution of tone in standing.

Instructions: "Stand up tall. Separate your feet so far (about 6″). . . Remain in that position."

Note: Inability to extend hips adequately. Excessive lordosis, geno recurvatum. Unequal weight distribution: shoulders of unequal height, spine curved laterally, feet inverted. Balance tenuous.

Test 20 (From position of Test 19)

Purpose: To test the time ability (in seconds) to support the body over one leg.

Instructions: "Shift your weight onto the (right) leg and hold it as long as you can. Do it on the other leg. . . Now stand on both legs."

Note: Time (recorded) in seconds that steady balance can be maintained on either leg. Flexed leg has inadequate hip extension; thigh is internally rotated and adducted; foot inverted. Difficulty in weight shift.

Test 21 (From position of Test 20)

Purpose: To test heel strike and dorsiflexion in forward movement; adult approach: hip extension in backward walk; freedom of upper extremity in stair climb.

Instructions: "Walk forward to that. . . and stop. Walk backwards to me and stop. . . Climb those stairs."

Note: Internal rotation of the thigh, hip-knee flexion, foot inversion; a lack of reciprocal arm movement with rigid spine. Forward walk: alignment of hips, knees, ankles. Dorsiflexion of forward foot on heel strike. Rear leg outwardly rotated at hip; roll off from head of first metatarsal. Slight rotation of trunk. Arms swing freely and alternate with leg movements (right arm with left leg in normal postural control). Backward walk: alignment of hip, knee, ankle or forward leg. Back leg extended, outwardly rotated at hip. Hip extended, knee flexes so that back foot touches first metatarsal, leg somewhat laterally for support. Feet *not* inverted in normal postural control. Climb stairs (without bannister): alternate flexed hip, knee, ankle dorsiflexion. Weight firmly on lower stair. Pulls up onto forward extending leg. Back leg flexed at knee, hip extended, and thigh abducted. Standing leg: leg, foot aligned, arms free in normal postural control. *Not* internally rotated thigh, adducted forward leg, nor inverted feet. (For children of at least four years of age.)

EXHIBIT 10-3

Erhardt Developmental Prehension Assessment

Test measures: Components and skills of hand function development. Test items were developed through extensive literature review. Three major sections, divided into 17 subsections, measure involuntary arm-hand patterns; the arms at rest; the asymmetrical tonic neck reflex; grasping reactions; placing responses; avoiding responses; voluntary movements; arm approach in prone and sitting positions; grasp and release of dowel, cube, and pellet; manipulation skills; crayon or pencil grasp; and drawing skills.

Population: Different sections of the test contain criterion-referenced behaviors that normally occur from birth to 6 years. Erhardt states that the 15-month level indicates prehensile maturity and would therefore be the baseline for measurement of older children.

Test format:

Content: This is a criterion-referenced test that uses a test booklet, the primary reference for scoring and interpretation, and a test kit of items specified by Erhardt but developed by the individual therapist.

Administration: Test items are presented in the sequence shown in the test booklet. Items are administered through observation of movement patterns and presentation of selected objects to the child. With older children, test administration may be expected to take up to 1 hour.

Scoring: As items are administered, the examiner makes notations in the test booklet according to prescribed symbols. Developmental age levels for each of the subtests are determined by the highest level pattern that is considered well integrated. Each of the subsections indicates which patterns should be considered permanent throughout life. Performance that indicates the need for intervention is also noted in scoring.

Interpretation: Approximate age levels for the three main areas of hand function (primarily involuntary hand-arm patterns, voluntary movements, and prewriting skills) are synthesized from av-

erage developmental levels in each pertinent subsection. Erhardt makes clear that the test is a clinical tool that is designed primarily to identify discrete areas for intervention. Therefore the derived developmental levels for each of the three areas would be considered less important than the descriptive information about hand function that is generated by the test.

Advantages: This test provides a detailed assessment of a broad range of motor skills and functions that contribute to the development of prehension. The gradings of the sequences of function are more highly developed than in any other test of prehension patterns available. It is therefore a highly useful tool to the occupational therapy clinician and researcher.

Disadvantages: The administration and scoring instructions for the test are in general poorly detailed. Use of the author's text assists the examiner to some extent with this problem through the detailed case examples that are given. More precise definitions for some of the objects to be used for test administration would be helpful. In the primary reference Erhardt discussed the interrater reliability study that was conducted. Two groups of eight therapists used the test booklet to score the videotaped performance of two handicapped children per group, and agreements were subjected to statistical analysis. Interrater correlations varied from fair to very good. Individual items were analyzed in light of the variable correlations, but the outcome of this process is not clear. It is unfortunate that interrater comparisons were not performed with the evaluations of normal children. Erhardt also stated that the test had been evaluated through clinical use by a number of therapists in several states. However, the results of this field testing have not been reported to date.

Purchasing information: From Erhardt, R.P.: Developmental hand dysfunction: theory assessment treatment, Laurel, Md., 1982, Ramsco Publishing Co.

EXHIBIT 10-4

Hand function evaluation

Score: 0 = Child cannot grasp object.
     1 = Child completes grasp in manner
          of his own adaptation.
     2 = Child uses mature grasp pattern.

Pattern-activity	*R-L*	*Comments*
Hook grip: MCP joints flexed. Carry a small suitcase.		
Hook grip: MCP joints extended. Carry a plastic pail with handle.		
Power grip: Thumb abducted. Use a toy hammer.		
Power grip: Thumb abducted. Hold a 1-inch dowel.		
Lateral pinch: Standard. Hold a key.		
Tip pinch: Standard. Insert tipped lace through 1-inch bead.		
Palmar pinch: Standard. Use a needle for sewing cards.		
Palmar pinch: Cylindrical. Hold an empty tin can.		
Palmar pinch: Spherical Hold a small rubber ball.		
Palmar pinch: Disk. Hold a plastic stacking ring.		

Pinch strength:
Differences between active and passive range of motion in hand:

Adapted from Skerik, S.K., Weiss, M.W., and Flatt, A.E.: J. Occup. Ther. **25**:98, 1971.

TESTING SENSORY INTEGRATIVE FUNCTIONS

What occupational therapists refer to as sensory integrative function has had numerous other labels. For the purposes of this book, the term *sensory integrative functions* will include the awareness, discrimination, and recognition of sensory stimuli from the environment and the central nervous system's use of this sensory information to direct motor behavior. The occupational therapist focuses on sensory integrative function as the individual's capacity to use his senses to guide movements in daily life activities. This is a broad concept, and it refers to thinking and planning as well as execution of the broad range of motor behaviors.

Many tests have been developed to assess visual perception (that is, visual sensory awareness, discrimination, recognition, and utilization). Fewer tests are available to assess sensory integrative processing of the other five senses. This has resulted in the occupational thera-

pist's heavy reliance on the Southern California Sensory Integration Tests (SCSIT) and on therapist-made tests of the other sensory modality functions.

Tests of visual perception

THE MOTOR-FREE VISUAL PERCEPTION TEST

The Motor-Free Visual Perception Test was developed by Calarusso and Hammill[9] to provide a rapid measure of visual sensory processing that does not require hand movements on the part of the child. Children are shown a series of test plates that measure simple visual discrimination, visual form constancy, gestalt perception, visual matching, and visual memory. The child can give a verbal response if he is unable to point to the correct item. Obviously the test is used with great difficulty with children whose severe motor handicap affects communicative ability.

The test is fairly well standardized with an ade-

EXHIBIT 10-5

Purdue Perceptual-Motor Survey

Test measures: The survey was designed to detect errors in perceptual motor development and to designate areas for remediation. It does not provide diagnostic information. It is a survey of perceptual motor skills that are grouped into five areas of posture and balance, body image and differentiation, perceptual-motor match, ocular pursuits, and form perception.

Population: It is recommended for children aged 6 to 10 years. The survey should not be used with children who have specific sensorimotor deficits such as blindness, paralysis, or known motor involvement. Results of tests administered to children with a measured IQ below 80 may be questionable.

Test format:

Content: This is a performance-based test that requires a manual, rating sheet, and the following equipment: balance beam, 4-foot-long pole, small pillow, mat, chalkboard, chalk, penlight, paper and pencil, and a table and chair appropriate to the child's size.

Administration: By use of the manual and equipment, 22 items plus 11 subitems are administered, and results are recorded in a scoring booklet. Common problems are listed for each task, and the examiner places a checkmark by each observed characteristic.

Scoring: Ratings from 1 to 4 are assigned for the child's performance on each item. A 4 indicates adequate performance, whereas a 1 indicates that the child had considerable difficulty with an item. Ratings for items are transferred to a summary sheet to allow for

score comparisons among the five areas. A composite score of 65 or higher indicates that the child is achieving within normal limits.

Interpretation: The lack of information concerning interpretation of ratings has been a source of criticism. The examiner is instructed to check the profile on the summary sheet to estimate major areas of difficulty that will require programming. Therefore the survey is most useful to experienced clinicians who are able to extract diagnostic information through observation of the child during test administration.

Advantages: Administration can be accomplished in about 30 minutes and is relatively simple. The survey can be used as a screening device and as a valid indicator of the need for diagnostic testing. Results are very useful for program planning. Reliability correlations for this test are generally good.

Disadvantages: Norms were obtained from 200 children in grades 1 through 4 at one school in Indiana only. A clinical sample of 97 "nonachievers" was matched to children in the normative group to establish validity estimates. Ratings were also correlated with teacher estimates of pupil performance, but the coefficient was not strong. Interpretations of findings are not well discussed in the manual. Standardization norms are not clearly presented for each age range.

Purchasing information: From Roach, E.G., and Kephart, N.C.: The Purdue Perceptual-Motor Survey, Columbus, Ohio, 1971, Charles E. Merrill Publishing Co.

---

quate normative sample, validity, and reliability data. The test can be administered in its entirety in less that 15 minutes. Scoring provides a perceptual age and perceptual quotient. Although such scores are useful for monitoring progress and communicating with other professionals, they should not be considered inviolate indications of the child's level of function. It is more pertinent to look at the child's performance in each of the five areas of the test to determine areas of weakness and the need for remedial activities.

DEVELOPMENTAL TEST OF VISUAL-MOTOR INTEGRATION (VMI)

The Developmental Test of Visual-Motor Integration was developed by Berry[5] to determine specific areas of difficulty in visual motor behavior, with an emphasis on visual perception and motor coordination during pencil reproduction of geometric forms. The test is widely used by educators and psychologists and has proved

useful to occupational therapists who want a quick measure of a child's eye-hand coordination in a pencil-and-paper task. A test analysis is shown in Exhibit 10-7.

FROSTIG DEVELOPMENTAL TEST OF VISUAL PERCEPTION

Frostig and others[16] first published the Frostig Developmental Test of Visual Perception in 1964, and it has been widely used since. The test represents one of the earliest and most durable tests of visual perception. The test seeks to measure five skill areas that Frostig defined as eye-motor coordination, figure-ground perception, shape constancy, position in space, and spatial relationships. These areas were chosen because of their importance to school readiness. The test can be administered to individuals or groups, and it is therefore useful for occupational therapists who need to screen large numbers of children. Exhibit 10-8 provides detailed information about the Frostig test in a test analysis.[15,16]

EXHIBIT 10-6

Colerain Elementary School Occupational and Physical Therapy Screening Evaluation

Child's name _____
Birthdate _____   Date of evaluation _____
1. Area of involvement/diagnosis:

2. General information—previous program, family, medical:

3. Development skills—motor skills, residual reflexes:

4. Muscle tone:

5. Muscle strength:

     Upper extremity   *Lower extremity*
     R   L   R   L

6. Limits in ROM:

     Upper extremity   *Lower extremity*
     R   L   R   L

7. Appliances:

8. Ambulation/mobility and transfers:

Reprinted with permission from Columbus Public Schools and Colerain Elementary School, Columbus, Ohio.

Tests of auditory perception

Whenever possible, tests of auditory perception are best administered and interpreted by speech pathologists or audiologists, who have greater expertise in these areas. Occupational therapists can readily obtain and discuss relevant information with these professionals in preparation for program planning. However, when speech or hearing services are not available, occupational therapists may need to obtain information about such areas as auditory discrimination and memory. In such instances the following tests are useful.

ILLINOIS TEST OF PSYCHOLINGUISTIC ABILITIES (ITPA)

The Illinois Test of Psycholinguistic Abilities is a widely accepted test battery that is used to delineate areas of difficulty related to communication skills. It is well standardized, and norms are available for children

EXHIBIT 10-7

Developmental Test of Visual-Motor Integration (VMI)

Test measures: The text is a measure of the child's ability in eye-hand coordination. The test correlates best with reading ability and is basically a tool for educational assessment.

Population: This test can be administered to children 2 to 15 years of age, but it was designed to be used primarily for children in preschool and in the early primary grades. The manual includes instructions for individual and group administration.

Test format:

    Content: This is a pencil-and-paper test that uses a test booklet with 24 geometric forms to be copied.

    Administration: The test may be administered to individuals or groups. Shapes are to be copied in the sequence presented in the booklet, without use of an eraser. It is best to provide the student with a pencil that has no eraser. Only one attempt is allowed for each form. The examiner begins by presenting the first form and, when certain that the child understands what is to be done, allows the child to proceed independently.

    Scoring: Raw scores are obtained by counting the total number of forms passed, up to three consecutive failures. The manual provides scoring criteria with extensive examples of correct and incorrect reproduction of forms.

    Interpretation: Raw scores are converted to perceptual age equivalents. Performance on items is to be used for program strategies. Beery presents a sequence of worksheet-type program recommendations that may be used to improve performance.

Advantages: The test can be administered quickly to groups and individuals and is best used as a screening device.

Disadvantages: The information obtained from test administration is limited by the nature of test items. Test development data are not contained in the administration manual for ready reference.

Purchasing information: From Beery, K.E.: Developmental test of visual-motor integration: administration and scoring manual, Chicago, 1967, Follet Publishing Co.

aged 2 to 10 years. Kirk, McCarthy, and Kirk[22] developed the test to measure components of communication according to a psycholinguistic model. This model states that the three major processes involved are decoding (stimuli reception), association, and encoding (expressive behavior). The test measures 12 areas of these processes, including grammatical closure and sound

EXHIBIT 10-8

Frostig Developmental Test of Visual Perception

Test measures: Frostig and associates postulated that what is usually referred to as visual perception actually consists of a number of different functions that develop relatively independently of each other. The test proposes to measure what the authors consider to be five fairly discrete areas that have particular relevance to school performance. These five abilities are:

1. Eye-hand coordination
2. Figure-ground perception
3. Perception of shape constancy
4. Perception of position in space
5. Perception of spatial relationships

Population: The Frostig test was developed for use as a screening device for preschool through first-grade children. Normative data for ages 4 to 8 are available. It is believed that any child over 10 years of age who does not score within the maximum age group for which any subtest is scaled may be presumed to have difficulty in the skill that subtest assesses.

Test format:

Content: This is a paper-and-pencil test that uses a protocol booklet, manual, and scoring materials. The booklet contains five subtests with several items in each test that are graded according to difficulty.

Administration: Normally individual administration should take no more than 45 minutes by following the manual, but there is great variability. Children who have learning disabilities frequently take longer or become too restless to complete the test at a single sitting. Group administration is possible if auxiliary personnel are available to monitor children and answer questions. Children with known problems should always be tested individually.

Scoring: Raw scores are determined for performance on each subtest. Scoring materials, such as overlays and lists of criteria, are included with test kits.

Interpretation: The raw scores are converted to perceptual age equivalents that serve as indicators of the age levels at which a child is believed to be functioning in abilities measured by each of the subtests. The perceptual age equivalents are then computed into scale scores that correlate the child's perceptual age to chronological age. In general, uniformly low scores suggest retardation rather than specific learning disability. A scatter of high and low scores suggests a disorder of visual perception. A perceptual quotient can be calculated in a manner similar to that for determining IQ. This may be converted to a percentile ranking by indicating how the child's performance compares to that achieved by the normative sample for his age group.

Advantages: The Frostig test is a good initial screening instrument, because it allows evaluation of a variety of behaviors in addition to evaluation of a variety of visual skills. These include test taking, following instructions, and the handling of the motor-planning tasks involved in writing. The test is simple to administer and grade because the manual has been written clearly. Adaptations of test administration are available for children who are deaf, do not speak English, are physically handicapped, and are emotionally disturbed.

Disadvantages: Standardization of the test was done with a somewhat small and primarily middle-income population. Therefore findings with children of different socioeconomic or ethnic backgrounds should be viewed accordingly. Some of the subtests become less valid for the older child because of worksheet experience in school and because the child can use cognitive skills to second guess the items in spite of genuine visual perception problems. This is particularly true of the position in space and spatial relationships items.

Purchasing information: From Frostig, M., and others: The Marianne Frostig Development Test of Visual Perception: 1963 standardization, Palo Alto, Calif., 1964, Consulting Psychologists Press.

References: Frostig, M., Lefever, D.W., and Whittlesey, J.R.B.: Administration and scoring manual for the Marianne Frostig Developmental Test of Visual Perception, Palo Alto, Calif., 1966, Consulting Psychologists Press and Frostig, M., and others: The Marianne Frostig Developmental Test of Visual Perception: 1963 Standardization, Palo Alto, Calif., 1966, Consulting Psychologist Press.

blending. Of particular interest to occupational therapists are its subtests that assess the following auditory perceptual functions: auditory reception, auditory association, verbal expression, auditory closure, and auditory sequential memory. The Illinois Test of Psycholinguistic Abilities measures visual areas as well: visual reception, visual association, visual closure, and visual sequential memory. The entire test battery frequently takes several hours to administer and requires careful preparation on the part of the administrator. As with the Southern California Sensory Integration Tests, it is recommended that therapists who plan to use this test practice its administration with a number of normal children before using it clinically.

In a review of literature related to the Illinois Test of Psycholinguistic Abilities, Clark[10] cautioned occupational therapists to be aware that its predictive validity is questionable for learning disabled students. Test stability has been found to vary from weak to good. Therefore researchers have recommended that the test not be used by itself but in conjunction with other standardized tests.

DICHOTIC LISTENING TESTS

FLORENCE CLARK

The dichotic listening test, which was developed by Broadbent[6,7] and later refined by Kimura,[20] is used by occupational therapists and audiologists to assess the status of speech lateralization in children. These tests provide an index believed to represent the relative efficiency of the right versus the left cerebral hemisphere functions that process auditory input of various types. It should be noted that the derived index is not considered to be a perfect indicator of speech lateralization.[20]

The procedure involves simultaneous presentation through headphones of a pair of auditory stimuli that have been stereophonically taped in a manner that administers one of the pair to each ear. Single sets of two digits, words, or nonsense syllables are used most frequently. Following the presentation of each stimulus pair, the subject is asked to indicate what was heard. Typically, right-handed individuals demonstrate greater accuracy in reporting what they heard through the right ear. When this result occurs, the computed index suggests a right over left ear advantage in accuracy of auditory processing.[4]

According to Kimura,[21] right ear advantage is interpreted to suggest lateralization of language processing in the left hemisphere of the brain. The basis for this inference resides in the arrangement of the neuroanatomical pathway from the ears to the regions of the cerebral cortex that are specialized for auditory processing.[35] Kimura[21] believed that impulses that travel via contralateral pathways from the ears to the hemispheres are processed more readily than stimuli that are conveyed over ipsilateral pathways.

Occupational therapists have used the dichotic listening tests as part of an overall assessment of sensory integrative function in which status of cerebral lateralization is one consideration (Chapter 19). Ayres[3,4] and Koomar and Cermak[25] are recommended reading.

Somatosensory tests

THE TEST OF SENSORY INTEGRATION

In 1979 DeGangi[11] of the Georgetown University Child Development Center published a performance-based test of sensory integrative function for children aged 3 to 5. The original test was made up of 21 items that assessed postural control, reflex integration, bilateral motor integration, oculomotor control, and vestibular function. Normative data were obtained from 113 children who represented a mix of racial and socioeconomic characteristics. Over the course of time, the test was developed to include 36 items.[12] Items related to vestibular and oculomotor functions were subsumed into the other three areas of measurement. Although a fairly small sample was used for standardization, item analysis and test validation procedures were generally rigorous, and the test is useful to occupational therapists.

Test administration is similar to Norton's Basic Motor Evaluation, but the emphasis is on relating scores to sensory integrative development. The manual provides comprehensive information on grading and interpretation of scores in each item and for clusters related to the three areas assessed. DeGangi noted variability of discriminative value of different test items in relation to different levels of dysfunction. The entire test can be administered to a preschool child in about half an hour, which is advantageous when considering the test tolerance of younger children.[11,12]

SOUTHERN CALIFORNIA SENSORY INTEGRATION TESTS (SCSIT)

As developed by Ayres,[1] formal assessment of sensory integrative functions is accomplished through the administration and interpretation of the Southern California Sensory Integration Tests, the Southern California Postrotary Nystagmus Test (PRNT),[2] and clinical observations[3] (Chapter 9) with additional information obtained from dichotic listening and academic tests. Ayres[3] described the Southern California Sensory Integration Tests as "tools (that may be used) to augment professional judgment in assessing patterns of neuropsychological disorder" (p. 1). She specified that the group of tests be used in their entirety, rather than selectively use individual tests. With the Southern California Postrotary Nystagmus Test, this means the administration of 18 tests, which usually requires 2 to 3 hours of formal testing.

The sequence of tests measures visual perceptual functions, somatosensory functions, and motor manifestations of postural and bilateral integration. Selection of test items was based on the use of similar items in other tests, logical validation by theory, and clinical experience. The tests must be presented in the order given in the manual, with no extraneous conversation. Talking should be limited to administrative procedures to control the amount and degree of environmental sensory stimulation to the child. Unnecessary conversation on the part of the tester simply generates additional sensory stimulation for the child that can confound test results. As a rule of thumb, it is helpful to tell the child in advance that you will not be talking much during the test but will have a long conversation afterward. The order of test administration is particularly vital with the somatosensory tests because these are sequenced to elicit tactile defensiveness. Experience suggests that test findings are most reliable if the entire group of tests is administered in one sitting. However, few children tolerate such a demand, so a recommended sequence is the following:

Session 1: Visual perception tests
Session 2: Somatosensory and motor tests
Session 3: Clinical observations and Southern California Postrotary Nystagmus Test

These are long, complex tests to administer and take, so it is useful to first screen the child with short tests such

as the Developmental Test of Visual-Motor Integration and Norton's Basic Motor Evaluation to determine the need for the Southern California Sensory Integration Tests.

Following test administration, raw scores are converted to standard scores, and these are in turn clustered in relation to Ayres' hypothesized syndromes (Chapter 19). Because each test must be considered by itself and in relation to score clusters and performance test results, interpretation is a complex process. Certification courses in administration and interpretation of the Southern California Sensory Integration Tests are offered by the Center for the Study of Sensory Integrative

---

EXHIBIT 10-9

Definitions and functional correlates of the Southern California Sensory Integration Tests

Visual perception tests

1. *Space visualization:* This test demonstrates the child's ability to discriminate spatial elements of objects (geometric forms) including, in the more advanced items, mental manipulations (movements) of objects in space. Formboard puzzles are presented to the child in different positions, with variable visual coordinates. Space visualization is critical to daily tasks that require object assembly-construction.

2. *Figure-ground discrimination:* This visual perceptual function allows the individual to concentrate on one stimulus against a field of many competing stimuli. The test items require the child to select a specific picture from a background of distracting pictures. Visual figure-ground discrimination enables the child to focus on words during reading.

3. *Position in space:* This test is designed to measure perception, recognition, and memory of the same form in different sequences. This visual function permits the child to discriminate numbers and letters in different words and math problems.

4. *Design copying:* This pencil-and-paper test measures a combination of visual perception of a geometric design and the capacity of the brain to direct the hand in duplicating that design. This combination allows the child to learn to write letters and numbers.

Somatosensory tests

5. *Kinesthesia:* Administration of this test can be used to assess the individual's capacity to perceive the position and movement of body parts.

The child is asked to duplicate movement patterns with vision occluded. Kinesthesia allows the individual to perform familiar motor activities, such as walking, with a sense of security and also helps guide the child as he tries out new movements and skilled activities, as in sports and crafts.

6. *Manual form perception:* This tests the complex of processes that allows people to use the sense of touch to identify forms and details of objects (stereognosis). The child is asked to identify the visual design that matches a plastic geometric form that is manipulated (unseen) in the hand. Again, this sense allows people to perform routine activities precisely and helps with the new activities such as buttoning and counting money.

7. *Finger identification:* This is a basic test of tactile sensory awareness. The student must identify which finger of either hand was touched by the examiner, while his vision was occluded. (NOTE: Vision is not occluded while identification is made, only when stimulus is given.) This basic sensory process is protective.

8. *Graphesthesia:* This tests intersensory integration of tactile discrimination, visual awareness, and fine motor planning. The child must recognize the form of, and then duplicate, a design drawn on the back of his hand. Vision is occluded when the tester draws designs on the back of the child's hand, but not when the child is duplicating the design. This complex sensory-motor process allows the child to become a proficient writer.

Adapted from Sandy Adams, University of Florida, Gainesville, Fla., 1977; Ayres, A.J.: Southern California Sensory Integration Tests: manual, Los Angeles, 1972, Western Psychological Services; Ayres, A.J.: Southern California Prostrotary Nystagmus Test: manual, Los Angeles, 1975, Western Psychological Services; Ayres, A.J.: Interpreting the Southern California Sensory Integration Tests, Los Angeles, 1976, Western Psychological Services.

Dysfunction at various locations across the United States each year. Therapists who intend to use the tests on a regular basis are well-advised to attend such a course. All therapists who use the tests are urged to heed Ayres' advice to practice administration with at least 20 normal children before clinical application.

The validity of the Southern California Sensory Integration Tests has not been conclusively established to date. Some parts of the test have been correlated to performance on the Gesell scales. All types of items on the test have been criterion referenced. Therefore it is critical that the test administrator have a strong background in relevant theory and science and in tests and measurements as well. The tests are valuable tools, but their value increases in concert with the academic and clinical expertise of the therapist who administers and interprets.

The Southern California Sensory Integration Tests have been analyzed only for test-retest stability, with ratings for individual tests varying from poor to acceptable. Ayres hypothesized that because the tests measure underlying, dynamic neurophysiological processes, they are likely to show lower test-retest stability than a test that measures end product behavior only. This concept is supported somewhat by the stronger reliability shown by the Motor Accuracy and Design Copying Tests, which

9. *Localization of tactile stimuli:* This is a test of tactile discriminative ability. The child must point to a spot on his arm that was touched by the examiner's pen, with vision occluded. This is a basic sensory process that helps individuals with such activities as self-dressing, washing, and hairbrushing.

10. *Double tactile stimuli:* This test measures the ability of the child to detect two touch stimuli that are applied at the same time to either or both the hand and the cheek. This test is administered with the child's back to the therapist and tends to elicit information about tactile defensiveness. Double tactile stimuli perception is a more advanced form of the sensory process described previously.

Motor tests
11. *Motor accuracy:* This test is designed to measure the degree of and changes in sensorimotor coordination in the arms and hands, guided by visual cues. This test emphasizes the motor aspect of tracing over a large pattern. The function relates to coordinated activities such as cutting, writing, and performing sports activities.

12. *Imitation of postures:* This test evaluates the coordinated use of information from visual and kinesthetic senses. The test requires the student to duplicate body postitions that are demonstrated by the examiner, a process that involves planning what to do with different body parts. This capacity enables people to learn new activities by imitation.

13. *Crossing midline of the body:* These items measure the tendency of an individual to avoid crossing the center of the body with a hand. The test requires pointing to the eye or ear with either hand. This function permits the child to perform activities that require coordinated use of both sides of the body.

14. *Bilateral motor coordination:* This test requires smoothly executed movements of, and interaction between, both arms as the student imitates rhythmic patterns demonstrated by the examiner. Both motor planning and coordination of the two body sides are demonstrated. Bilateral coordination is particularly important to smooth performance of gross motor activities such as riding a bicycle or dancing.

15. *Right-left discrimination:* This tests recognition of the right and left of the child, when looking at another person, and the right or left location of an object. The student points to or verbally identifies right or left according to different commands from the examiner. This function relates to the ability to plan body movements and to the sense of direction.

16. and 17. *Standing balance: eyes open and eyes closed:* These tests measure the ability of the child to maintain standing balance on one foot using visual cues (SBO) and using the vestibular sense of balance (SBC). These balance functions are critical to stable walking, running, stair climbing, and skilled motor activities.

18. *Postrotary Nystagmus Test:* This test measures the width (excursion) and duration of lateral, alternating eye movements after the child spins on a board a set number of times to each side. This test is considered pivotal to identification of the source of sensory integrative dysfunction in either cortical or vestibular structures.

do provide a concrete end product in addition to a sensorimotor pattern.

Normative data for the tests are provided in extensive tables in the administration manual. One of the major controversies about the Southern California Sensory Integration Tests has been their relatively small and localized normative sample. Although standard scores are printed for raw scores on all tests at all ages, many standard scores have been derived by extrapolation, and there is no way to differentiate those scores that were derived from subject performance from those that were extrapolated.

Therapists who plan to use the Southern California Sensory Integration Tests and the Southern California Postrotary Nystagmus Test need to be aware that these tests have been criticized by psychologists, neurologists, and professionals from other disciplines. Therapists must also recognize that much of the criticism is warranted because of the weak areas in test standardization discussed here. In addition, much of Ayres' neurobiological basis is admittedly hypothetical, and the validity of ideas has yet to be established. To use these tests intelligently, it is imperative that therapists be aware of these weaknesses and exercise sound clinical judgment in test interpretation. A defensive or aggressive posture in response to criticism from neurologists and psychologists is neither productive nor well considered. In most instances neurologists have better backgrounds in neurology and psychologists have better backgrounds in tests and measurements than do occupational therapists. The occupational therapist's strength is in the analysis of the relationship between activity and function. Perhaps this is why, in spite of weaknesses, the Southern California Sensory Integration Tests are such useful tools to occupational therapists. The clinical impressions of the child that are gained through test administration are rich in information that can be used for treatment planning and monitoring the child's progress through the treatment program. Again, therapists are advised to remember that sensory integrative function is a component of activity performance, not an end product in itself.

At the present time these two tests are being subjected to full-scale restandardization. A large sample of "normal" children, distributed across the country, will be used to refine test administration, scoring, and interpretation. It is hoped that this project will more conclusively demonstrate the strength of these tests for clinical use.

The point of this concern with validity, reliability, and normative data is that each user must consider carefully how much credence may be placed on the scores obtained. Ayres[3] stated that adequate interpretation of the Southern California Sensory Integration Tests is based on several factors:

1. Accuracy of test administration

2. Interpreter's knowledge of neurobiology, tests, and measurements

3. Interpreter's experiences with sensory integrative deficiency in practice

She stated further that there is no final, discrete interpretation of test scores because interpretation is based on what is known at any one time by the therapist who administers the test, and this knowledge is dynamic.

Because of the current restandardization project, it seems inappropriate to include a test analysis of the Southern California Sensory Integration Tests and the Southern California Postrotary Nystagmus Test here. Each test merits thorough scrutiny that is beyond the constraints of this chapter. However, Exhibit 10-9 provides an overview of the different tests related to the functions that each proposes to measure. This information is often helpful to parents of children who will be tested.[1-3]

EXHIBIT 10-10

Stereognostic test for preschool children

Child's name: _____ Date of birth: _____
Test date: _____

Object   *Right-left* *Comments*
1. Two-inch diameter rubber ball
2. Five-inch plastic spoon
3. Two-inch metal car with movable wheels
4. Three-inch plush stuffed dog
5. One-inch toy plastic chair
6. U.S. penny
7. One-inch plastic button, two times as thick as penny, with four holes*

TOTAL SCORE: _____ RIGHT: _____ LEFT: _____

Scoring: 2 = Identifies correctly when object is first presented.

    1 = Gives incorrect label on first presentation, but then self-corrects after additional manipulation.

    0 = Unable to give correct known label.

Note: Omit any items from the test that the child cannot label during the initial exploratory period.

*Correct identification of the button may be considered indicative of the development of finer discriminative abilities.

From the American Occupational Therapy Association, Inc., Copyright 1972, Vol. 26, No. 5, p. 256, A Stereognostic Test for Screening Tactile Sensation, NB Tyler.

SENSORY AWARENESS TESTING

Tests for sensory awareness, such as those of tactile recognition (stereognosis) and dermatomal patterns, are occasionally used with children who have lower motor neuron problems. Methods for these tests have been described.[19,31] However, the therapist needs to remember that sensory testing must be adapted to the experiential and cognitive levels of the children to be tested. For example, very young children cannot be expected to discriminate between pennies and dimes, for which their only concept may be "money."

Tyler[37] reported on a sensory test that was specifically designed for use with children aged 2 to 4 years. Seven common play and self-care items were chosen for manual identification by the child. Criteria for item selection included familiarity to children, small size, availability, texture variation, and presence of the items in the young child's language repertoire. Tyler encouraged children to manipulate and verbally label items before testing and eliminated items from individual test protocols if the child could not label them.

Tyler administered items as a "guessing game" to a normative sample of 98 children. Items were presented to seated children to feel with their hands behind their backs. Items were presented to the children in random order, first in one hand and then in another. If the child incorrectly labeled the object, the examiner encouraged the child to manipulate it, with his vision occluded, for additional time. Average time for test administration was 4 minutes.

An adapted format for Tyler's test is found in Exhibit 10-10. Tyler found the greatest variability of correct responses among the 2-year-olds, and hypothesized that the skills required for stereognosis develop during this period. The entire range of 2- to 4- year-olds had the most difficulty with identifying the button, possibly because of language inadequacy or because this item is similar to the penny.

Organizing results: the sensory integrative profile

Often therapists will find that they have obtained a multitude of potentially related scores after administering a number of sensory integrative and motor tests. In 1975 Llorens and Sieg[28] published a profile that can be used to organize data from many of the tests described earlier. Results can be charted on the profile to identify performance level in auditory discrimination, body awareness, orientation in space, integration of two sides of the body, fine motor control, gross motor control, ocular control, visual perception, and tactile and kinesthetic perception. Performance levels that are determined by conversion of raw and standard scores are classified as above age expectancy, appropriate for age, somewhat deficient, and markedly deficient.

TABLE 10-1 | **Conversion of test scores for Llorens-Sieg sensory integration profile**

Conversion of test scores

| Tests | Score conversion | | | |
	Above age expectancy	Appropriate for age	Somewhat deficient	Markedly deficient
Southern California Sensory Integration Tests	SD: +1.1 or more	SD: +1.0 to −1.0	SD: −1.1 to −2.0	SD: −2 or less
Purdue Perceptual Motor Survey		Score 4 or 3	Score 2	Score 1
Frostig Developmental Test of Visual Perception	Age equivalent above chronological age: 1 year	Age equivalent: ± 1 year	Age equivalent below chronological age: 1 year	Age equivalent below chronological age: −2 years
Goodenough-Harris Draw-A-Man Test	Mental age above chronological age: 1 year	Mental age: ± 1 year	Mental age below chronological age: −1 to −2 years	Mental age below chronological age: −2 years
Wepman Test of Auditory Discrimination (example for ages 8 years and older)		Error: 0-1	Errors: 2-3	Errors: more than 3
Clinical observation of primitive postural reflexes		Absence of reflexes	Presence of reflexes	

From The American Occupational Therapy Association, Inc., Copyright 1975, Vol. 29, No. 4, p. 208, A Profile for Managing Sensory Integrative Test Data, LA Llorens, KW Sieg.

EXHIBIT 10-11

Sensory integrative profile

Name: _____

Birthdate: _____ Age: _____

Sex: _____

School/unit: _____

Examiner: _____

Date: _____

			AB**	AP	SD	MD
Tactile kinesthetic perception		Kinesthesia (SC)*		▓		
		Manual Form Percep. (SC)				▓
		Finger Identification (SC)				▓
		Graphesthesia (SC)				▓
		Localization tact st (SC)	▓			
		Double tactile st (SC)			▓	
Visual perception	FG					
		Figure ground perception (SC)				▓
	FC	Figure ground (Fr)				▓
		Form construction (Fr)				▓
Ocular control		Ocular pursuit—both (P)	▓			
		Ocular pursuit—right (P)	▓			
		Ocular pursuit—left (P)	▓			
		Ocular pursuit—convergence (P)	▓			
Gross motor control		Walking board—forward (P)			▓	
		Walking board—backward (P)			▓	
		Walking board—sidewise (P)			▓	
		Obstacle course (P)		▓		
		Kraus-Weber (P)				
		Imitation of movement (P)		▓		
		Imitation of posture (SC)		▓		
		Tonic labyrinthine (Fi,B)				
		Asymmetrical TNR (B,A)				▓
		Symmetrical TNR (Fi,B,A)				▓
		Cocontraction (R,A)				▓

Category	Test	1	2	3	4
Fine motor control	Eye-motor (Fr)		▓		
	Rhythmic writing-rhy (P)			▓	
	Rhythmic writing-rep (P)			▓	
	Rhythmic Writing-orientation (P)		▓		
	Visual achievement forms (P)			▓	
	Visual achievement F-organization (P)			▓	
	Design copy (SC)				▓
Integration of two sides of body	Motor Acc-Acc (SC)	L R	L R	L R	L R
	Motor Acc-Adj (SC)	L R	L R	L R	L R
	Jumping (P)			▓	
	Perceptual motor mat cir (P)		▓		
	Perceptual motor mat DC (P)		▓		
	Perceptual motor mat lateral (P)		▓		
	Perceptual motor mat vertical (P)		▓		
	Cross midline (SC)		▓		
	Right-left discrimination (SC)			▓	
	Bilateral motor coordination (SC)				▓
Orientation in space	Spatial visualization (SC)				▓
	Position in space (SC)				
	Position in space (Fr)		▓		
	Spatial relationships (Fr)			▓	
	Angels-in-snow (P)			▓	
	Standing balance—open (SC)				
	Standing balance—closed (SC)		▓		
Body awareness					
	Draw man (G-H)			▓	
	Identify body parts (P)		▓		
Auditory discrimination					
	Auditory discrimination (W)				▓

*Key to tests and measures: SC, Southern California Sensory Integration Tests; FR, Frostig Developmental Test of Visual Perception; P, The Purdue Perceptual Motor Survey; Fi, Fiorentino Reflex Test; B, Bobath (literature); A, Ayres (literature); R, Rood (literature); G-H, Goodenough-Harris Draw-A-Man Test; W, Wepman Test of Auditory Discrimination.

†Key to performance designations: AB, above age expectancy, AP, appropriate for age; SD, somewhat deficient for age; MD, markedly deficient for age.

Llorens and Sieg stated that the integrated data on the profile can be used to design remedial programming that will facilitate development in areas determined to be somewhat and markedly deficient. In addition, program activities can be selected to maintain proficiency in areas that are deemed age appropriate or higher. This very useful profile is shown in Exhibit 10-11, and a conversion table for ranking of scores according to performance levels is presented in Table 10-1.

TESTING COGNITIVE FUNCTIONS

Superficially it may appear that there are fewer tests of cognitive, social, and emotional functions. However, it should be remembered that it is difficult to obtain physical measures of function in these areas. Instead these functions must be inferred through evaluation of the child's maturing performance in developmental tasks. The child's performance is reflected against the therapist's study of human development and the therapist's familiarity with the variations that normal children exhibit in manifestation of theoretical constructs. Therefore, although several tests that have been designed to measure cognitive levels and psychosocial functions are presented here, most assessment of these areas will be done during the therapist's administration of developmental and performance evaluations that will be discussed in Chapter 11.

Collaboration with psychologists and educators

Cognitive development and function are often tested by teachers and clinical psychologists who are well trained in the administration of intelligence tests. Specialized training and even certification are necessary to administer and interpret many such instruments. Therefore the occupational therapist should consult with these professionals to determine if reports are available about a child's performance on the Wechsler Intelligence Scale (WISC-R), the Stanford-Binet, the Bender-Gestalt, the Wide Range Achievement Test (WRAT), or other similar tests. Careful review of these reports should provide the therapist with substantial information about the child's intellectual capabilities, as well as offer clues to the child's thinking and learning styles.

However, if such information about cognitive function is not available from psychologists or teachers, there are several commercial tests that are fairly valid and reliable that can be easily administered by the occupational therapist without additional training. These include the Goodenough-Harris Drawing Test and the Wachs Analysis of Cognitive Structures.

Cognitive tests

GOODENOUGH-HARRIS DRAWING TEST

The Goodenough-Harris Drawing Test is relatively simple to administer, and because it uses drawing, children generally enjoy taking it. The test is based on the premise that children's drawings reflect the maturation of cognitive representations.[17]

The test may be administered on an individual basis or in groups. Normative information is provided for children ages 3 to 15 years, although Harris cautions that the sample of 3- and 4-year-olds was smaller, and therefore the test is less predictive for this age range. The child is asked to draw three pictures: a man, a woman, and a self-portrait. The test administrator will ask the child to explain each of the pictures, to clarify what each component of the drawings represents to the child. To score the test the therapist contrasts body part details included in the child's drawing with normative criteria. The test manual gives clear definitions and examples of scoring for the various body parts so that scoring is generally objective. Raw scores (for number of acceptable body parts) can be converted to standard scores, quality scores, and percentile rankings to yield an impression of the child's intellectual development.[18] It should be noted that the test manual does not contain information about test development. The user is referred to Harris' formal text[17] for more detailed information about theoretical framework and standardization.

WACHS ANALYSIS OF COGNITIVE STRUCTURES (WACS)

Wachs, an optometrist, became interested in cognitive development and learning problems through his work with children who had visual-motor and perceptual disorders. In collaboration with Hans Furth, Wachs studied Piagetian theory and research methodology extensively. With this background, Wachs and Vaughan[38] developed a test that uses typical Piagetian tasks to evaluate cognitive development of children in the preoperational age range (3 to 6 years). The Wachs Analysis of Cognitive Structures is more complex to administer than the Goodenough-Harris Drawing Test, but the information it provides can be helpful to occupational therapists. The test also serves as a model for the construction of Piagetian tasks for evaluative purposes.

The Wachs Analysis of Cognitive Structures is composed of 15 task clusters that relate to four cognitive abilities: manipulation of materials, visual representation, graphic representation, and manual identification. The test requires little verbal response from the child; instead it is a performance-based assessment of the child's use of body and sense thinking. The test demonstrates the development of cognitive schemes in each of the four areas. Raw scores are converted to standard scores and percentile rankings.

Internal consistency and interrater reliability of the test are excellent. The normative samples for this test were small. However, one of the special features of the test is that it was also administered experimentally to a number of "atypical" groups of children, including high-risk, Eskimo Indian, retarded, African, and deaf children. The test manual provides considerable data that can be used by the therapist for interpretation of test results, and it makes note of cultural implications for treatment planning.

As with other tests mentioned earlier, it is advisable for the interested therapist to practice administration of the Wachs Analysis of Cognitive Structures with normal children before clinical use. Naturally, one should study the manual carefully, as well as review pertinent information about Piagetian theory.

TESTING PSYCHOSOCIAL FUNCTIONS
Projective techniques

For many years occupational therapists have used projective techniques to assist in the assessment of emotional states of their patients. Unstructured art materials are presented to the clients with variable instructions from the therapist about how the media are to be used. The therapists record observations of the client with regard to task involvement, approach to the activity, attention span, motivation, and feelings expressed by the client during engagement in the activity. A number of projective batteries that are used with adult clients have been reported in the occupational therapy literature, but there is less information about the use of projective techniques with children. Typical activities that are used to elicit projective information include finger painting, drawing, clay sculpture, and mosaic tile arrangement. The most essential element to the process is the therapist's ability to encourage the client to discuss what he is thinking about and doing.

Llorens and Bernstein[26] reported on the use of finger painting as a projective medium for emotionally disturbed children. The unstructured and reversible nature of finger painting was found to allow one child to express a range of feelings about his family problems, as well as recognize changes in his own behavior through discussions with the therapist. In another publication related to programming for this population, Llorens and Rubin[27] suggested that behavioral observations during activity involvement be rated according to the adequacy of attention span, ability to concentrate, ability to follow verbal directions, degree of motor activity, relatedness to therapist, dependence-independence (of behavior), and affect and mood. Behavioral manifestations of these characteristics may be rated as inadequate, transitional, and adequate. It is recognized that assessment through projective techniques is more subjective and depends on the sound clinical expertise of the therapist. Essentially the use of projective techniques represents the use of activity analysis as an evaluation tool.

Data-based observation of behavior

One of the most frequently employed techniques for the identification and assessment of adaptive and maladaptive behaviors is the use of data-based observation. The occupational therapist or another professional begins the assessment with detailed note-taking on observed behaviors. *Target behaviors* that appear to interfere most with effective social adaptation and emotional adjustment are identified and ranked. From this list the therapist and program team can identify a few behaviors that are most suited to immediate intervention. It should be noted that the behaviors that are first targeted for change might not be the most maladaptive. Instead the behaviors chosen will generally be those that are believed to be most amenable to change within the current time frame.

The next step is for the therapist and other staff who will work to eliminate the target behaviors to obtain baseline *frequency rates* on the occurrence of said behaviors. Most facilities have a specific internal data collection sheet, or they use commercial forms for this purpose. Data are usually collected within fixed time intervals, such as 5-, 10-, or 30-minute periods. Often therapists will use a small mechanical counter so that they can "click off" behaviors as these occur without interrupting the task. At the end of the data base period the behavioral frequency is recorded. The staff members will review baseline data and establish objectives for behavior change. For example, if a child was observed pushing other children five times in a 10-minute period on the playground, the staff members might establish an immediate objective to reduce the frequency of pushing by 40%, that is, to three times in one 10-minute period in that location. A long-term goal might be to eliminate the behavior completely.

Thereafter at regular intervals the frequency of the behavior is measured and notes may be made by the therapist regarding any variations in the behaviors. One of the critical observational requirements throughout the process will be the therapist's identification of situations (*environmental contingencies*) that appear to stimulate or inhibit behavioral frequency. This type of assessment process is used throughout the course of treatment as data collection continues until there is closure on the target behaviors. It should be noted that the *treatment* itself will usually consist of a reward for performance of an adaptive behavior, such as asking another child to move out of the way. Or the child may be rewarded for not exhibiting the maladaptive behavior, that is, when he has not pushed. In this behavior modification approach it is considered inappropriate to punish the child for exhibiting the maladaptive behavior unless all other routes to behavior change have been exhausted without success.

Although the example just mentioned relates to psychosocial dysfunction, data-based observations can be used to record changes in all areas of concern to the occupational therapist. For example, the therapist might use this technique to record changes in standing tolerance, increased assistive use of a weak hand, or spontaneous interactions with other children. Data-based observation is a powerful tool for measurement of change. The most important elements are the identification of appropriate targets for observation and data collection, as well as recognition of environmental contingencies for behavior change. Again, the therapist's use of activity analysis is the key to successful application of this technique.

EXHIBIT 10-12

Knox Play Scale

Test measures: The scale is used to evaluate observed, spontaneous play behavior of a child and compare this behavior to age-level and age-appropriate behaviors. Expectations of play have been derived primarily through Erikson's theory of child development. Play is assessed through the following dimensions.

1. *Space management:* How the child manages his body and the surrounding space through use of postural mechanisms.
2. *Materials management:* How the child handles objects and materials and the purposes for the use of materials through sensation, process, and result.
3. *Imitation:* How the child understands the world and the child's ability to express feelings through observation and imitation of others.
4. *Participation:* The degree and manner by which the child participates with others in the environment, including cooperation, independence, and dependence.

The first two categories may be used to assess motor, cognitive, and sensory integrative development as well as play performance. The third and fourth categories are particularly useful to assess the psychosocial development of the child.

Population: This play scale was constructed to provide descriptions of normal play behavior for newborn to 6-year-old children. The only reported experimental use of the scale is with a small clinical sample of mentally retarded children.

Test format:

Content: This is a descriptive, performance-based test that requires no special materials other than notebook and pencil for recording.

Administration: Administration of the test is fairly simple but requires that the examiner take notes on the child's play for a specified time period. Videotape recording, if relatively unobtrusive, is highly recommended. The examiner should be familiar with Knox's material before observations.

Scoring: The test analysis format provided in the primary reference categorizes and describes behavior but provides no numerical shorthand for grading. A "+" is marked before those statements that best describe observed behavior, and a "−" is marked when the behavior is absent. "NA" and "NE" are used when opportunity for a behavior does not arise or when a behavior is not evident. Items of special interest are underlined, such as when a child engages in one type of behavior excessively.

Interpretation: Interpretations are determined by comparisons with age-level play expectations and are based on the sound clinical judgment of the therapist. The test is best used in conjunction with other instruments.

Advantages: The Knox Play Scale is a descriptive tool that may yield useful information that often cannot be obtained or analyzed through standardized tests. It provides a carefully constructed framework for analysis of situational play behavior. The lack of a numerical rating scale does not appear to reduce the value of the scale.

Disadvantages: Although the scale is based on a well-established theory of play development, the derived format has not been checked against the actual performance of a sample of "normal" children. Therefore findings of the test will need to be corroborated to some extent by results of other, more formal tests.

Purchasing information: From Knox, S.H.: A play scale. In Reilly, M., editor: Play as exploratory learning: studies of curiosity behavior, Beverly Hills, Calif., 1974, Sage Publications, Inc.

A revision of this instrument, called the Preschool Play Scale, was recently reported by Bledsoe and Shepherd.[5a] The derived scale was checked for interrater and test-retest reliability, as well as concurrent validity with several other measures of play behavior.

The Knox Play Scale

The Knox Play Scale, which is actually a framework for analysis of observed activities, was developed to assess the social-emotional maturation of newborn through 6-year-old children through their play behaviors. Knox's scale[24] is based primarily on Erikson's concepts of play and psychosocial development. Children are observed, preferably in a group situation, and their behavior is recorded by the therapist or on videotape. The latter method is believed to be more reliable because it preserves every nuance of the child's interactions with objects, environment, and people. An analysis of the Knox Play Scale is detailed in Exhibit 10-12. Descriptive information of expected behaviors at different age levels should be obtained from the primary source.[24]

Piers-Harris Children's Self-Concept Scale
KAREN E. SCHANZENBACHER

Subtitled "The Way I Feel about Myself," the Piers-Harris Children's Self-Concept Scale is a self-report instrument designed to look at correlates of the self-concept of children in grades 3 through 12. The scale consists of 80 questions that may be answered in 15 to 30 minutes, depending on whether it is administered individually or to a group. Results may be reported in stanines, percentiles, or individual scores for each of the six factors measured: behavior, intellectual and school status, physical appearance and attributes, anxiety, popularity, and happiness and satisfaction. While this test was designed primarily as a research tool to look at the development of a child's self-concept, it is also useful in clinical and counseling settings and as a screening instrument to identify children in need of intervention.

Studies measuring the internal consistency and stability reported coefficients ranging from .71 to .93. Concurrent validity studies comparing the Piers-Harris to other self-concept, peer, and teacher rating methods are inconclusive, with correlations ranging from − .64 to .68. Further information on reliability and validity studies are discussed in a research monograph.[33]

SUMMARY

This chapter has focused on the presentation of a selected group of tests, some more widely known than others. These tests are used to evaluate different component functions of behavior: the sensory integrative, motor, cognitive, psychological (emotional), and social processes that enable children to do the things they do. Assessment of these functions is critical to the therapist's understanding of why children have problems in everyday activities. Findings from these tests allow the therapist to develop treatment programs that will improve functional processes to improve the child's task performance. Testing in these functional components accompanies comprehensive evaluation of the child's performance skills in play, self-maintenance, school work, and prevocational activities (Chapter 11).

REFERENCES

1. Ayres, A.J.: Southern California Sensory Integration Tests: manual, Los Angeles, 1972, Western Psychological Services.
2. Ayres, A.J.: Southern California Postrotary Nystagmus Test: manual, Los Angeles, 1975, Western Psychological Services.
3. Ayres, A.J.: Interpreting the Southern California Sensory Integration Tests, Los Angeles, 1976, Western Psychological Services.
4. Ayres, A.J.: Dichotic listening performance in learning-disabled children, Am. J. Occup. Ther. **31:**441, 1977.
5. Beery, K.E.: Developmental test of visual-motor integration: administration and scoring manual, Chicago, 1967, Follett Publishing Co.
5a. Bledsoe, N.P., and Shepherd, J.T.: A study of reliability and validity of a preschool play scale, Am. J. Occup. Ther. **36:**783, 794, 1982.
6. Broadbent, D.E.: Listening to one of two synchronous messages, J. Exp. Psychol. **44:**51, 1952.
7. Broadbent, D.E.: Speaking and listening simultaneously, J. Exp. Psychol. **43:**267, 1952.
8. Bruininks, R.H.: Bruininks-Oseretsky Test of motor proficiency: examiner's manual, Circle Pines, Minn., 1978, American Guidance Service.
9. Calarusso, R.P., and Hammill, D.D.: Motor-Free Visual Perception Test, Novato, Calif., 1972, Academic Therapy Publications.
10. Clark, F.A.: The Illinois Test of Psycholinguistic Abilities: considerations of its use in occupational and physical therapy practice, Phys. Occup. Ther. Pediatr. **2:**29, 1982.
11. DeGangi, G.: Assessment of sensorimotor integration in preschool children, Washington, D.C., 1979, Georgetown University Child Development Center.
12. DeGangi, G.A., and Berk, R.A.: Psychometric analysis of the Test of Sensory Integration, Phys. Occup. Ther. Pediatr. **3:**43, 1983.
13. Erhardt, R.P.: Developmental hand dysfunction: theory assessment treatment, Laurel, Md., 1982, Ramsco Publishing Co.
14. Fiorentino, M.R.: Reflex testing methods for evaluating CNS dysfunction, Springfield, Ill., 1972, Charles C Thomas, Publisher.
15. Frostig, M., Lefever, D.W., and Whittlesey, J.R.B.: Administration and scoring manual for the Marianne Frostig Developmental Test of Visual Perception, Palo Alto, Calif., 1966, Consulting Psychologists Press.
16. Frostig, M., and others: The Marianne Frostig Developmental Test of Visual Perception: 1963 standardization, Palo Alto, Calif., 1964, Consulting Psychologists Press.
17. Harris, D.B.: Children's drawings as measures of intellectual maturity: a revision and extension of the Goodenough Draw-a-Man Test, New York, 1963, Harcourt, Brace, & World, Inc.
18. Harris, D.B.: Goodenough-Harris Drawing Test: manual, New York, 1963, Harcourt, Brace, & World, Inc.
19. Hopkins, H.L., and Smith, H.D.: Willard and Spackman's occupational therapy, ed. 6, Philadelphia, 1983, J.B. Lippincott Co.
20. Kimura, C.: Cerebral dominance and perception of verbal stimuli, Can. J. Psychol. **15:**166, 1961.
21. Kimura. D.: Some effects of temporal lobe damage on auditory perception, Can. J. Psychol. **15:**156, 1965.
22. Kirk, S.A., McCarthy, J.J., and Kirk, W.: Illinois Test of Psycholinguistic Abilities, Urbana, 1968, University of Illinois Press.
23. Kliewer, D., Bruce, W., and Trembath, J.: The Milani-Comparetti Motor Development Screening Test: administration manual, Omaha, Neb., 1977, Meyer Children's Rehabilitation Institute.

24. Knox, S.H.: A play scale. In Reilly, M., editor: Play as exploratory learning: studies of curiosity behavior, Beverly Hills, Calif., 1974, Sage Publications, Inc.

25. Koomar, J.A., and Cermak, S.A.: Reliability of dichotic listening using two stimulus formats with normal and learning disabled children, Am. J. Occup. Ther. **35:**456, 1981.

26. Llorens, L.L., and Bernstein, S.P.: Finger painting with an obsessive-compulsive organically-damaged child, Am. J. Occup. Ther. **17:**120, 1963.

27. Llorens, L.L., and Rubin, E.Z.: Developing ego functions in disturbed children: occupational therapy in milieu, Detroit, 1967, Wayne State University Press.

28. Llorens, L.L., and Sieg, K.W.: A profile for managing sensory integrative test data, Am. J. Occup. Ther. **29:**205, 1975.

29. Milani-Comparetti, A., and Gidoni, E.: Routine developmental examination in normal and retarded children, Dev. Med. Child Neurol. **9:**631, 766, 1967.

30. Norton, Y.: Minimal cerebral dysfunction. Part II: modified treatment and evaluation of movement, Am. J. Occup. Ther. **26:**186, 1972.

31. Pedretti, L.W.: Occupational therapy: practice skills for physical dysfunction, ed. 2, St. Louis, 1985, The C.V. Mosby Co.

32. Piers, E., and Harris, D.: Piers-Harris Children's Self Concept Scale, Nashville, Tenn., 1969, Counselor Recordings & Tests.

33. Piers, E., and Harris, D.: Children's self concept scale: research monograph #1, Nashville, Tenn., 1977, Counselor Recordings & Tests.

34. Roach, E.G., and Kephart, N.C.: The Purdue Perceptual-Motor Survey, Columbus, Ohio, 1971, Charles E. Merrill Publishing Co.

35. Rosenzweig, M.R.: Representations of two ears at the auditory cortex, Am. J. Physiol. **167:**147, 1951.

36. Skerik, S.K., Weiss, M.W., and Flatt, A.E.: Functional evaluation of congenital hand anomalies, part 1, Am. J. Occup. Ther. **25:**98, 1971.

37. Tyler, N.B.: A stereognostic test for screening tactile sensation, Am. J. Occup. Ther. **26:**256, 1972. (Abstract.)

38. Wachs, H., and Vaughan, L.J.: Wachs Analysis of Cognitive Structures, Los Angeles, 1977, Western Psychological Services.

39. Weiss, M.W., and Flatt, A.E.: Functional evaluation of the congenitally anomalous hand, part II, Am. J. Occup. Ther. **25:**139, 1971.

PAT NUSE CLARK
ANNE STEVENS ALLEN
IDA LOU COLEY
KAREN E. SCHANZENBACHER

Instruments to evaluate childhood performance skills

COMPREHENSIVE DEVELOPMENTAL SCALES
Scope of developmental evaluation

One of the basic components of any occupational therapy assessment for children is a developmental evaluation (Chapter 7). The most common practices are to use standardized tests or criterion-referenced, therapist-made tests that contain items drawn from a variety of standardized tests and from resources in the literature.

Developmental testing is usually thought to measure such early adaptive skills as controlling the head, building block towers, and recognizing pictures. In fact, developmental testing may be more broadly conceptualized as the evaluation of child and adolescent performance in any age-appropriate activity. Therefore a test could, and should, include such items as ordering a hamburger, making one's own bed, getting from class to class, and handing homework in on time. With this concept in mind, the occupational therapist may consider evaluations of schoolwork, prevocational preparation, self-care, and community living activities as logical extensions of the developmental assessment. For purposes of organization, this chapter will separate different types of evaluation. But the continuity between categories of performance evaluation cannot be overemphasized.

Brazelton Neonatal Behavioral Assessment Scale (BNBAS)
KAREN E. SCHANZENBACHER

The Brazelton Neonatal Behavioral Assessment Scale is included here because it most closely approximates a developmental evaluation of the neonate.[7] This text is one of the most commonly used measures of the newborn's socially interactive responses. The scale is designed to look at both the neurological and interactive functions of an infant during the first month of life.

To measure neurological function, the test includes 20 items that evaluate reflexes and other relevant responses:

Plantar grasp	Automatic walking	Tonic deviation of head	Rooting
Hand grasp	Placing	Tonic deviation of eyes	Sucking
Ankle clonus	Incurvation	Nystagmus	Passive movement of arms
Babinski reflex	Crawling	Tonic neck reflex	Passive movement of legs
Standing	Glabella	Moro reflex	

This portion of the scale has been found to be as successful for identification of neurological problems in the newborn as a pediatric neurological examination.[29]

The scale also includes 27 items that were designed to measure the neonate's capacity for interaction with the environment and caregivers:

Response decrements to light, rattle, bell, and pinprick.
Orientation: Inanimate visual, inanimate auditory, animate visual, animate auditory, animate visual and auditory.

Alertness	Irritability
General tonus	Activity
Motor maturity	Tremulousness
Pull-to-sit	Startle
Cuddliness	Lability of skin color
Defensive movements	Lability of states
Consolability	Self-quieting activity
Peak of excitement	Hand-mouth facility
Rapidity of build-up	Smiling

These items have been found to be especially useful for demonstration of neonatal behavioral capabilities to parents.[31] When parents understand what their babies are capable of doing through demonstration of the item skills, parental interaction skills may improve.[33] There may also be an increase in parental expectations, a phenomenon that over the long-term can foster the baby's development.[26]

Clinically the interactions portion of the scale has been used to monitor behaviors between mother and child if either demonstrated early inappropriate skills. Another use that has been explored is the capability of the scale to identify long-range infant temperament and interactive problems. While some preliminary studies have demonstrated potential value in this application, the results are not conclusive.[32]

In summary, Brazelton Neonatal Behavioral Assessment Scale has proved to be an effective predictor of neurological problems, a teaching tool for parents, and an indicator of interactional skills present in the neonate. The scale has also been used extensively in research.

Bayley Scales of Infant Development (BSID)

The Bayley Scales of Infant Development were developed as part of a large-scale longitudinal study of human development carried out by Bayley and associates at the University of California at Berkeley.[27] The scales[5] use typical developmental items to assess mental, motor, and behavior levels of infants and toddlers aged 2 to 30 months. This test battery is an excellent, comprehensive, and well-standardized instrument that requires some advance preparation by the therapist before clinical administration. As with most standardized tests, it tends to be most reliable for the middle of the age range represented. The test uses both performance and parental reports to obtain data and may take several hours to complete. (Any of the three different sec-

tions may be used by itself but with a substantial loss of information.) Therefore it is more appropriate to administer the scales to young children through several sessions. A complete test kit of materials and manual are commercially available. Review of the items found for this age range on the Denver Developmental Screening Text form (Chapter 9, Figure 9-5) should give a picture of the types of skills measured by the Bayley tests.

Gesell Developmental Scales

The Gesell Developmental Scales were developed by Arnold Gesell and his associates at the Yale University Institute for Child Study, beginning in the 1930s. The test items and procedures have been modified and updated through the years.[22] It is helpful to review some of Gesell's concepts (Chapter 3) in preparation for administration of the scales. Several forms are available according to the age level of children from early infancy through 10 years of age.

The test measures performance according to Gesell's behavior patterns: motor, adaptive, language, and personal-social. It also provides developmental levels by months for each of the areas tested. The test has been widely used for diagnostic purposes and is often given by pediatricians as a follow-up to developmental delays identified by the Denver Developmental Screening Test. The kit for this test is commercially available.

Interrater reliability and predictive validity for the Gesell scales are generally excellent. Normative samples for the early schedules (ages birth to 36 months) were large, but there is less information available about parts of the schedules that are used with older children. The user should remember that the tests should be used primarily to determine satisfactory or delayed development of neuromotor and cognitive skills.[22]

Vineland Social Maturity Scale

Although in many ways outdated, the Vineland Social Maturity Scale[14] is in a class by itself. Developed in the 1920s by Edgar Doll at the Vineland Training Center, Vineland, N.J., the Vineland Social Maturity Scale is the only durable standardized instrument that has attempted to measure development from infancy through adulthood. The scale measures performance in eight areas.

1. to 3. *Self-help skills* include eating, dressing, and general related activities.
4. *Locomotion* includes both basic movement patterns and the use of transportation resources as necessary to function as a productive member of society.
5. *Occupation* includes involvement in play, household tasks, creative pursuits, recreation, and employment.

6. *Self-direction* items assess personal independence and exercise of individual responsibility.
7. *Socialization*, in the sense of being socialized, assesses the individual's ability to live in a social culture and contribute to the general welfare of society.
8. *Communication* items are used to assess social use of different forms of communication.

The test is administered by interview with a protocol booklet and manual as guides. The examiner generally interviews the person who is the primary caretaker for the child or adult. (The test was originally developed to assess social maturity of individuals who are mentally retarded.)

The test administrator begins the session with a fairly open-ended question such as, "Tell me what your child does?" or "Describe a typical day." It is important to ask nonleading questions and to follow up on partial responses. At first this is difficult to do, but with experience the therapist can easily become proficient. The therapist should practice asking questions like, "Why do you do that?" "How is that accomplished?" The therapist should avoid questions that can be answered with "Yes," "No," or "I guess so." Generally, once the informant gets involved with information related to one of the categories, the therapist can continue with that category until the current level of function is identified. The test manual gives fairly good descriptors for what activities constitute performance of an item.

Scoring of the test is relatively simple once the notation has been mastered. Variations of 0 and 1 point are assigned for each item passed or failed. In some instances the examiner must make judgments about whether a child might be able to do an activity with which the child has had no experience, based on descriptions of the child's achieved performance in similar items. Raw scores are converted to provide a social age equivalent and a social quotient. Doll warns that the test is to be used for descriptive purposes, not as a rating scale.

Criticisms of the test address content, source of information, and variability of scoring. As might be expected, because the test was developed several generations ago, current expectations related to many items have changed. Some items are expected at an earlier age. For example, it is now anticipated that children will "follow current events" much earlier than age 15. Other items will need to be redefined by the examiner to match current practices more closely. For example, "goes about home town" freely may be appropriate to a small town but will need to be modified for the rural or urban youth of 9.

The test results can be questioned because information is typically obtained by parental report. Although Doll and associates recommended a number of ways, such as the questioning techniques described above to tease out truthful descriptions from parents, the methods are not always foolproof. To reiterate, whenever there is any doubt about whether a child can actually do something, it is best to ask the parent to explain in detail how the child does the activity.

Finally, scoring of specific items has an element of subjectivity when the examiner must decide whether to give credit for an item that the child has never attempted *because of lack of opportunity*. Again, careful questioning is the only method that can be used to make such determinations. The element of subjectivity remains, but it is hoped that decisions will be based on sound clinical judgment rather than on expediency. The test manual, protocols, and scoring forms are available commercially.[14]*

AAMD Adaptive Behavior Scales (ABS)

The AAMD Adaptive Behavior Scales[1,2] also provide comprehensive measures of behavior from infancy through adulthood, although the tests are of more recent origin. These scales are descriptive and also provide numerical ratings that may be used to chart progress. Age equivalents for behaviors are not provided. The AAMD Adaptive Behavior Scales are available in two versions. The original scale, the AAMD Adaptive Behavior Scales[1] was developed for use in institutional settings and day programs for mentally retarded individuals and therefore has a wide age range of behaviors. The public school version, the AAMD Adaptive Behavior Scales—Public School Version,[2] was developed later and measures a narrower age range of behaviors. Both scales are used to record adaptive and maladaptive behaviors.

Both tests have two parts. The first part measures adaptive behavior in the areas of independent functioning, physical development, economic activity, language development, domestic activity, vocational activity, self-direction, responsibility, and socialization. Items are broad and generally do not give the discrete, detailed information about components of activity performance usually preferred by occupational therapists. The second part of the tests identify an exhaustive array of maladaptive behaviors against which the individual's actual behaviors are compared according to duration, severity, and frequency.

The record review, data-based observation, and informant interview are used to obtain information. In general, reports of behaviors must be corroborated by more than one informant for documentation purposes. The AAMD Adaptive Behavior Scales contain many items and can consume a considerable amount of time to complete at the initial assessment. Space is provided

---

*A revised version of the Vineland Social Maturity Scale was in press and unavailable for preview prior to publication of this text.

in both versions of the protocol booklet for updated assessments (usually conducted annually). In most mental retardation programs the primary recorder for the test will be a psychologist or behavior specialist who obtains data from parents and other members of the team who work with the child. Consideration regarding application of findings is generally determined by the entire interdisciplinary team rather than by one individual. Because of the format of the items, behavioral objectives for program plans are easily generated.

Because of relatively recent origin and the increasingly sophisticated technology of test development the two scales do not manifest exactly the same problems of content, source of report, and subjective scoring that are of concern to users of the Vineland Social Maturity Scale. However, because of length and complexity of requirements regarding documentation of behaviors, these tests are not efficient instruments for use by the occupational therapist who works alone. Typically the therapist will use these tests only when working at a facility that has adopted them as its primary assessment instrument.

Early Intervention Developmental Profile (EIDP)

Under the direction of Schafer and Moersch, an interdisciplinary team at the University of Michigan university affiliated facility spent a number of years developing a comprehensive assessment and practice system for newborn to 3-year-old children. The developmental items for evaluation and early intervention broadly reflect the concerns of occupational, physical, and speech therapists as well as psychologists. The Early Intervention Developmental Profile is that part of *Developmental Programming for Infants and Young Children*[25] that is used to assess skill development over the course of time. The profile is designed to be administered by an interdisciplinary team.

The profile is divided into six sections: perceptual-fine motor, cognition, language, social-emotional, self-care, and gross motor development. The occupational therapist administers the perceptual-fine motor and self-care items. In addition, the therapist may assist with evaluation on the gross motor and cognitive sections. A speech therapist might be best to administer the language items, a physical therapist administers the gross motor section, and a psychologist usually has primary responsibility for the cognitive assessment.

Administration of test items is thoroughly explained in the evaluation manual. References for each item are well documented. Test items are administered to the child until he fails two consecutive items in each major portion of the profile. Basal and ceiling levels of performance determine the range of the child's transitional development at the time of the test. The total time required for test administration may vary from half an hour to several hours. No cumulative score is obtained. Age levels for each performance area are charted on a composite table to yield a profile. Each protocol booklet can be used for several subsequent evaluations, with the composite profile recorded with a different color or line notation each time to document progress.

The Early Intervention Developmental Profile was designed specifically to guide program planning. It is not to be used for diagnostic purposes. Nicely tied into the behavioral items on the profile is a series of intervention activities that can be used to help children achieve skilled performance in subsequent developmental tasks.

Interrater and test-retest reliability studies of the profile used small samples, but with generally excellent results. Significant correlations were found between children's scores on the Early Intervention Developmental Profile, the Bayley Scales of Infant Development, and the Vineland Social Maturity Scale, indicating strong content validity. The sample was small and the test was performed with a clinical population, so findings should be viewed accordingly. The Early Intervention Developmental Profile is best used as a clinical instrument for interdisciplinary team planning. The varied expertise of the team lends itself to more knowledgeable interpretation and application of test findings.[25]

Vulpe Assessment Battery

The Vulpe Assessment Battery was developed by Vulpe[30] under a grant from the Canadian National Institute of Mental Retardation. This test battery is a long and detailed assessment of children's competencies and developmental skills. The battery is used to assess performance in the following areas: basic senses and functions, gross motor behaviors, fine motor behaviors, language behaviors, cognitive processes and specific concepts, organizational behaviors, and activities of daily living. A final component of the battery is assessment of the child's environments. Skills are cross-referenced from one area to another.

Because of its length, administration of the Vulpe Assessment Battery on initial assessment can be time-consuming. However, reevaluation proceeds from the cut-off point fairly quickly, and therefore many therapists believe this justifies the time spent earlier. It may be helpful to administer the test in partnership with another therapist to alternate observation, item presentation, and recording duties. It becomes apparent that as our knowledge of child development and function increases, so does the complexity and length of developmental evaluations. Most comprehensive developmental scales are now best administered cooperatively with one or more professionals to support documentation, to provide expertise in the broad range of areas assessed, and to share the physical and time demands of test administration.

Like many other developmental assessments, the Vulpe Assessment Battery is not considered a true standardized test. Items have been carefully selected and are based on validation through the literature and clinical experience. Interrater reliability for the test is strong, probably because administrative procedures are explained in considerable detail. This latter characteristic of the battery makes it a useful tool for the development of program activities.[30]

Brigance Diagnostic Inventories

The Brigance Diagnostic Inventories use two elaborate test batteries to assess the functional and academic skill development of children aged newborn through 11 years. The Brigance Diagnostic Inventory of Early Development (IED)[9] is designed for children to 7 years of age and measures psychomotor skills, self-help skills, communication, general knowledge and comprehension, reading skills, printing skills, and math skills. The Brigance Diagnostic Inventory of Basic Skills[8] is administered to elementary school children to evaluate skill development in academic areas. The latter would be less useful to occupational therapists but may be encountered in practice in school systems.

The Brigance Diagnostic Inventory of Early Development has been adopted in many education-oriented early intervention programs. Test items are written in behavioral terms and are designed to tie in to programming. Brigance stated that all test items are "norm referenced" for expected age level through extensive review of the literature. Different items are administered through parental report, observation of spontaneous behavior, and specific performance. The packaging of the Brigance test is impressive, and its detail leaves little room for erroneous administration. Experimental editions of the tests were field tested at numerous facilities across the United States, with subsequent refinement of items. Because of its clear detail, including illustrations of appropriate patterns and self-contained instructions in the scoring records, the test is easy although time-consuming to administer.[9]

Other developmental evaluations

For every test that has been discussed here, there are a dozen available commercially and many times that number of therapist-made tests. Most tests draw on items and use formats in combinations that are based on or similar to tests described here. It is probably best for therapists to become skilled administrators of two or more standardized commercial tests to become familiar with typical and useful test items and response variance. However, with experience the therapist may wish to develop a personalized series of test items that have proved most useful with a given clinical population and age range. One such format was developed by Carol Leaman to assess preschool and primary elementary school children. Because Leaman had been unable to locate a satisfactory commercial test that included items for this entire age range, she was forced to use two separate standardized assessments. Very often, when testing an older preschool child or a younger primary grade child, she found that items from both tests were needed to accurately assess the developmental level of the individual. Therefore she developed a therapist-made test that spanned the entire age range of her student population, incorporating test items from standardized tests for both age groups. The resultant developmental checklist is shown in Table 11-1.

EVALUATION OF SPECIFIC PERFORMANCE SKILL CATEGORIES

This section presents measurements of selected tasks of performance in one or more of the occupational activity groups: play, self-maintenance, schoolwork, and prevocational activities.

Play assessments

KNOX PLAY SCALE

The *Knox Play Scale* was discussed in Chapter 10 with reference to its usefulness for assessment of psychosocial functions of children in a play situation. The therapist is reminded to consider use of the scale to examine play skills for their own sakes because much valuable information can be obtained. Within this context, the Knox Play Scale can also be used to identify play experiences that may be used in treatment to promote development.

CURRIE MOTOR EVALUATION

The Currie Motor Evaluation[12] uses a series of familiar play activities to assess developmental level and gross, fine, and perceptual motor skills. The test is designed for use with children aged 4½ to 8½ years. Administration requires a protocol sheet (Table 11-2), toys familiar to children, and a room conducive to play. This is a performance-based test. Performance levels are compared with standard scores, and decisions are based on clinical judgment. Currie's tests can identify deficiencies related to neuromuscular function, performance ability, perceptual-motor abilities, and laterality, and they may be used by the knowledgeable therapist to predict problems in everyday activities, based on the child's ability to perform related motor behaviors.

Standard scores for this test were derived from normative study of a small sample of children. Therefore

TABLE 11-1	Developmental checklist		Initial evaluation			Re-evaluation		
			+	+/−	−	+	+/−	−
Age	Activity							
2.0	Builds tower of 6 to 7 blocks							
2.0	Imitates building a 3-block train							
2.0	Strings 1 to 4 (1 inch) beads							
2.0	Cuts gashes in edge of paper							
2.0	Imitates circular strokes							
2.2	Imitates vertical line within 30 degrees							
2.5	Answers "What do you hear with?"							
2.6	Builds tower of 8 to 9 blocks							
2.6	Adds chimney to train							
2.6	Holds pencil in fingers							
2.6	Makes 2 or more strokes for cross							
2.6	Screws, unscrews top							
2.6	Formboard—3 forms; adapts in 4 trials							
2.6	Gives full name							
2.6	Names 1 to 2 colors							
2.10	Points to teeth and chin on request							
3.0	Builds tower of 9 to 10 blocks							
3.0	Imitates building a 3-block bridge							
3.0	Imitates drawing a horizontal line							
3.0	Imitates drawing a cross crudely							
3.0	Copies a circle							
3.0	Cuts paper in half							
3.0	Puts 10 pellets into bottle in 30 seconds							
3.0	Formboard—3 blocks; no error or correction							
3.0	Names 3 colors							
3.0	Puts together 2 piece puzzle of person							
3.0	Determines size constancy in 3 dimensions							
3.0	Unbuttons medium shirt buttons							
3.6	Copies a 3-block bridge							
3.6	Puts together 3-piece puzzle of person							
3.6	Puts together a 7-piece puzzle							
3.6	Comprehends 3 prepositions (in, on, under)							
3.6	Finds pictures of animals that are alike							
3.8	Points to tongue, neck, arm, knee, thumb							
4.0	Imitates building a 5-cube gate							
4.0	Attempts to cut a straight line							
4.0	Copies a cross							
4.0	Puts 10 pellets into bottle in 25 seconds							
4.0	Puts together a 4-piece puzzle of person							

Reproduced with permission of Carol Leaman, Atlanta, Ga., 1982.

the scores should be used only to represent a trend of performance, rather than serve as validated scores. Because of the clinical usefulness of the test, it merits additional refinement.

PLAY SKILLS INVENTORY

The Play Skills Inventory is a test battery developed by Hurff[20] at Children's Hospital in Los Angeles. It pro-
vides a description of development and play characteristics in four general areas, including sensation, motor function, perception, and intellect. The test has been reported through several sources.[20,21] Materials for the test are not commercially available but may be readily assembled by using instructions from the primary reference.[20] A test analysis is shown in Exhibit 11-1.

Age	Activity	Initial evaluation			Re-evaluation		
		+	+/−	−	+	+/−	−
4.0	Adds 3 parts to incomplete man						
4.0	Determines size constancy in 2 dimensions						
4.0	Knows front and back of clothes						
4.0	Buttons large buttons						
4.2	Imitates square						
4.3	Puts together a 7 piece puzzle in 150 seconds						
4.6	Copies a 5-cube gate						
4.6	Copies a square						
4.6	Prints a few capital letters						
4.6	Counts 4 objects and answers "how many?"						
4.6	Knows day and night						
4.6	Knows pictorial likes and differences						
4.6	Knows 4 prepositions						
4.8	Follows 3 commands in proper sequence						
4.8	Puts together a 5-piece puzzle of man						
5.0	Copies a 2-step block						
5.0	Cuts out simple shape with 1/8 inch outline						
5.0	Copies a triangle						
5.0	Prints first name						
5.0	Prints a few numbers						
5.0	Compares textures						
5.0	Buttons medium buttons on shirt						
5.0	Draws house with a door, windows, roof, chimney						
5.4	Judges weights						
5.4	Gives age						
5.6	Prints numbers 1 to 5						
5.6	Knows pictorial likes and differences (9 out of 12)						
5.6	Knows which is bigger, "cat or mouse?"						
5.8	Can form a rectangle of 2 triangular cards						
6.0	Builds 3-step block on demand						
6.0	Copies a diamond						
6.0	Prints most capital letters						
6.0	Prints first and last names						
6.0	Gives name and address						
6.0	Cuts out a simple design						
6.0	Ties shoelaces						
6.0	Buttons small buttons						
6.0	Knows right from left						
6.0	Differentiates morning and afternoon						
6.0	Understands numbers up to 10						

OTHER PLAY ASSESSMENTS

In 1981 Florey[16] published a review of literature related to occupational therapy evaluation of play behaviors and components. She included a table of clinical instruments that had been developed by students of Reilly's occupational behavior theory. Some of these instruments, such as Knox's Play Scale and Hurff's Play Skills Inventory, have been discussed in detail in these chapters. However, the other instruments discussed by Florey are noteworthy and are included in an adaptation of her table in Table 11-3.

Assessments of self-maintenance skills

Many of the developmental tests described earlier in this chapter provide a good range of self-help and other self-maintenance activities to be assessed by the therapist. However, occupational therapists frequently desire

TABLE 11-2	Currie evaluation of function	

Skill tested and age (years)	Level of difficulty	Score
Physical skills		
Test 1	Ball bounce and catch (no variations)	Highest number of successes in 3 tries
Test 2	Successive bouncing of ball (no variations)	Highest number of successes in 3 tries
Test 3	Target aim	Cumulative scores in 12 attempts
5½ to 6½	Target distance 3 feet	
6½ to 7½	Target distance 4 feet	
7½ to 8½	Target distance 5 feet	
Dexterity		
Test 4	Bead stringing	Time required to complete task
5½ to 6½	Large beads	
6½ to 8½	Small beads	
Test 5	Peg board—cross-diagonal design	Time required to complete task
5½ to 6½	Construct by imitation	
6½ to 7½	Construct by copying	
7½ to 8½	Construct by verbal instructions	
Perceptual motor		
Test 6	Relationship of form-space and parts-whole	Time to complete
5½ to 6½	9-piece puzzle	
6½ to 7½	13-piece puzzle	
7½ to 8½	21-piece puzzle	
Test 7	Motor planning—3-dimensional construction	Time to complete
5½ to 6½	10-block pyramid	
6½ to 7½	8-piece object	
7½ to 8½	15-piece object	
Test 8	Spatial relationships—parquetry block design layout	Time
5½ to 6½	Match blocks to design	
6½ to 7½	Build design within frame	
7½ to 8½	Build design, no boundaries	

From The American Occupational Therapy Association, Inc., Copyright 1969, Vol. 23, p. 35, Evaluating Function of Mentally Retarded Children Through the Use of Toys and Play Activities, C. Currie.

TABLE 11-3	Pilot instruments-guides for play assessment	

Name of instrument	Content area	Clinical yield
Guide to play observation Age range: not specified Author: Florey[15]	Rules and skills	Interpretation of current play in dimensions of generation of rules, achievement of objective, skilled acts with objects and people, and flexibility of skill
Guide to status of imitation Age range: not specified Author: deRenne-Stephan[13]	Imitation	Interpretation of current status of imitative processes in dimensions of child, role models, family organization, and physical environment
Specification for a play milieu Age range: not specified Author: Takata[28]	Play	Examination of balance of human, nonhuman, qualitative, and quantitative elements in play milieu
A play agenda Age range: birth to 12 years Author: Michelman[23]	Art-games	Specifications for environment, experiences, and activities that promote risk taking and decision making

From The American Occupational Therapy Association, Inc., Copyright 1981, Vol. 35, No. 8, p. 520, Studies of Play: Implications for Growth, Development, and for Clinical Practice, L. Florey.

EXHIBIT 11-1

Play skills inventory

Test measures: The Play Skills Inventory was designed to monitor status of skill development in middle childhood. Specifically, items are designed to elicit data about four areas. Hurff's definitions of these areas include the following:

1. *Sensation:* The ability to identify and detect stimulus change.
2. *Motor:* Includes physical strength, endurance, speed, flexibility, and motor accuracy.
3. *Perception:* The ability to attend selectively to a group of stimuli and to recognize patterns.
4. *Intellect:* The ability to pull past learnings from memory, to select the best solution for a task, to adapt actions to meet the task, and then to reflect on the outcome of the task.

Hurff proposed a model of skill development that used sensation and motor skills as the foundation for the development of, first, perceptual skills and, finally, intellectual skills.

Population: Hurff stated that the test may be administered to children in the range from 8 to 12 years of age. The children who made up her normative sample were all 10 years old.

Test format: This is a criterion-referenced, performance-based test that uses a variety of commercial and therapist-designed games and equipment. Indoor and outdoor activities are included in the 20 items that are specified. These include, among others, physical fitness test, walking on a balance beam, identification of objects hidden in a picture, size estimations, and building block construction. The entire test battery can be administered in 1 to 2 hours, depending on the capabilities of the child.

Administration and scoring information is detailed in the primary reference.[20] A point system and time limit are specified for each test and are used to classify performance as acceptable or unacceptable. Normative data from the sample of 21 subjects were used to determine classifications. A profile is included to record raw scores and interpretation. Interpretation of deficit areas is global, dependent on clusters of unacceptable scores in one or more of the four areas.

Advantages: Because familiar play activities are used, this test is appealing to the age group and tends to elicit optimal performance. Selection of test items by the age level appears well grounded. Although it will require some effort to obtain or construct the materials needed for the test, Hurff's descriptions of items are clear.

Disadvantages: The Play Skills Inventory has not been subjected to standard test development procedures. Although considerable literature review was used to determine test items, only 21 subjects were used to determine the final form of the test and provide normative data. Hurff stated that there was no intent to standardize the test. In view of its clinical usefulness, this is unfortunate.

Interpretation is limited and depends more on the therapist's knowledge of Hurff's model, occupational behavior, and child development theory. Therefore support from stronger standardized tests would be needed to supplement data and impressions obtained from administration of the Play Skills Inventory.

Purchasing information: From Hurff, J.M.: A play skills inventory. In Reilly, M., editor: Play as exploratory learning: studies of curiosity behavior, Beverly Hills, Calif. 1974, Sage Publications, Inc.

References: Hurff, J.M.: Am. J. Occup. Ther. **34:**651, 1980.

more detailed information about this area of performance than can be obtained from the multicategory tests. Therefore a number of self-care instruments have been developed, although not subjected to formal test development procedures and publication. Most activities of daily living tests are criterion referenced and use a graded rating of the individual's ability to perform each task according to the amount of independence demonstrated. For example, a test might use a quasi-ordinal scale and give differential, but arbitrarily defined, points for ability to perform a task (1) without demonstration, (2) after demonstration, (3) with verbal cuing, or (4) with physical assistance (Chapter 7). This method is demonstrated by the two self-care assessments that are shown in Exhibits 11-2 and 11-3 and discussed here.

ACTIVITIES OF DAILY LIVING ASSESSMENT: TIME-ORIENTED RECORD

The format for the Activities of Daily Living Assessment: Time-Oriented Record was developed by Coley[10] and associates at the Children's Hospital of Stanford University Medical Center and was reported in 1978. It is a comprehensive assessment of self-maintenance activities organized according to a developmental sequence, and it contains items related to home and hospital living. The test items can be administered and passed during a formal evaluation session or as achievement is observed by the therapist during treatment. Scoring of the test is explained on the forms in Appendix B. Again, a quasi-ordinal scale is used. The test record provides the opportunity to differentiate between the child's use of right and left body sides.

EXHIBIT 11-2

Activities of daily living

Name _____ Birthdate _____

Communication _____ Ambulation _____

Key: 0 = Totally dependent, cannot perform
    1 = Dependent, but can help
    2 = Assisted or supervised with fine and gross activities
    3 = Assisted or supervised with fine activities
    4 = Normal independence for chronological age

I. *Feeding activities*   Date

Eat finger food
Pick up and feed self sandwich
Eat with fork
Eat with spoon
Spoon liquids, such as soup
Drink through straw
Drink from cup
Spread butter with knife
Cut soft food
Cut meat
Can eat with standard service
Can eat in normal time

Comments (note special equipment, avoided or modified foods):

III. *Fastenings*   Date

Large buttons—open
Large buttons—close
Small buttons—open
Small buttons—close
Hooks and eyes—open
Hooks and eyes—close
Snaps—open
Snaps—close
Safety pins–open
Safety pins—close
Zippers—open
Zippers—close
Buckles–open
Buckles–close
Shoelaces–open
Shoelaces—close
Bows—open
Bows—close

Comments (note special equipment, etc.):

II. *Dressing activities*   Date

Remove socks
Remove shoes
Remove braces
Remove underpants
Remove bra
Remove trousers
Remove skirt
Remove slip-over garment
Remove cardigan garment
Remove hat
Remove gloves
Remove rubbers, boots
Put on socks
Put on shoes
Put on braces
Put on underpants
Put on bra
Put on trousers
Put on skirt
Put on slip-over garment
Put on cardigan garment
Put on hat
Put on gloves
Put on rubbers, boots

Comments (note special equipment, unusual position):

IV. *Hygienic activities*

Operate water faucet
Wring wash cloth
Wash hands
Get into tub
Bathe self in tub
Get out of tub
Apply toothpaste to brush
Brush teeth
Shampoo hair
Comb hair
Clean, trim nails
Use handkerchief
Adjust clothing for toileting
Get on toilet
Use toilet paper
Get off toilet
Flush toilet
Use urinal
Empty urinary appliance
Apply deodorant
Feminine hygiene

Comments (note special equipment, mobility):

Occupational therapist: _____

EXHIBIT 11-3

A reference form for eating function assessment

Identification of child _____

History: _____

_____

Body position: _____
Abnormal signs: _____
Primitive signs: _____
Normal signs: _____

Oral structures:

Lips: symmetry, retraction, pursing

Teeth: number, caries, abnormal formation, color, position, hygiene

Gingiva: tenderness, inflammation, bleeding, edema, hypertrophy

Tongue: size, position in mouth, deviation, tremors, length of frenulum, scars

Hard, soft palates: clefts, abnormally high arch, abnormal areas of hypertrophy

Uvula: mobility and length

Functional ability:

Suck: movement of tongue, lip prehension

Food: liquid, puree

Utensil: bottle, spoon

Swallow: coordination with respiration, position of lips, amount of drooling

Food: liquid, thickened liquid, puree, lumpy, solid

Drinking: stabilization on rim of cup, movement of jaw, stabilization of jaw, sealing lips

Food: liquid, thickened liquid

Utensil: cup, glass

Biting, chewing: stabilization of jaw, munching pattern

Chewing pattern: up-down, lateral, rotary

Tongue movement: lateral, midline

Food: crunchy, solid

Utensil: fingers, spoon, fork

Straw drinking: position of lips

Hand use:

Palmar grasp, pincer grasp, opposition finger/thumb, hand to mouth reach, hand to mouth control

Developmental level in eating:

Type of food

Skill in using utensils

Record:

Time required for feeding

Amount of food intake

Amount of fluid intake

Adaptive equipment: _____

Recommendations for intervention: _____

_____

Expected outcome of intervention: _____

_____

COLERAIN SCHOOL ACTIVITIES OF DAILY LIVING TEST

The Colerain School Activities of Daily Living Test is another useful therapist-made tool and is shown in Exhibit 11-2. This form is used to assess performance of specific activities that are common expectations of elementary school children. Because the therapists' concern was with performance rather than diagnosis, no developmental levels were assigned to the test items. It is assumed that the student who can pass every item would be independent in self-care within a school environment. Note the differences in the scoring criteria on this form in comparison to the previous test.

EATING FUNCTION ASSESSMENTS

A number of therapist-made eating assessments have been reported in the literature and at professional conferences. In recent years these assessments have become increasingly complex as the knowledge of oral-motor structure and function has expanded and the technology to develop eating and other prespeech mechanisms has expanded. The Eating Function Assessment form (Exhibit 11-3) is a composite of information sought by the occupational therapist who deals with children who have problems in eating. This instrument, developed by Coley, is not all-inclusive. However, it should provide a foundation to begin assessment of such children and may be elaborated on as the examiner's expertise grows.

The Eating Function Assessment form is designed as a checklist, but notations can be added as necessary. For guidance in administration of this assessment, see Chapters 12 and 15 to 17.

School readiness tests

School readiness is often assessed through performance on developmental, cognitive, and sensorimotor evaluations. However, therapists will frequently want additional data on hand use in activities. For this purpose the therapist is referred to the hand function measurements discussed in Chapter 10. In addition, an evaluation of upper extremity function developed by therapists at Colerain Elementary School provides a useful model. This test (Exhibit 11-4) assists with assessment of preferred hand use, school-related hand activities, prehension patterns, and functional range of motion patterns. Administration and scoring are self-explanatory on the form. Data collected can be used for descriptive purposes in assessment and treatment planning. There is overlap between this therapist-made test and the hand function and other motor tests discussed in Chapter 10. However, the emphasis here is on observed task performance rather than on underlying functions. Components of school readiness discussed in Chapter 14 are also recommended reading.

EXHIBIT 11-4

Evaluation of upper extremity function

Name _____ Date _____

Diagnosis _____

Code: 0 = Unable to perform
      1 = Difficult, accomplished, but only *with* assistance
      2 = Some difficulty, accomplished *without* assistance
      3 = Accomplished with ease

Preferred hand	Right		Left	
	0	1	2	3
1. Pencil/crayon				
a. Holding and marking randomly _____				
b. Dot to dot _____				
c. Color simple shape _____				
2. Blocks				
a. Tower _____ Number _____				
b. Bridge _____				
c. Train _____				
3. Pegboard				
a. Small (plastic) _____ Time _____				
b. Golf tees _____ Time _____				
c. One-inch diameter _____ Time _____				
4. Safety pin _____				

Comments:

Hand activities	Right		Left	
	0	1	2	3
1. Scissor cutting				
a. Holding and cutting randomly _____				
b. Straight lines _____				
c. Curved lines _____				
d. Star _____				
2. Pencil sharpening _____				
3. Opening book and turning pages _____				
4. Bead stringing				
1. Large _____ Number _____				
2. Small _____ Number _____				
5. Screwing and unscrewing jar lid _____				
6. Coin from coin purse _____				
7. Telephone _____				

Comments:

EXHIBIT 11-4, cont'd

Evaluation of upper extremity function—cont'd

Grasp, release, pinch

	Left				Right			
	0	1	2	3	0	1	2	3
1. Spherical grasp (2-inch diameter ball)								
Cylindrical grasp (1-inch diameter peg)								
2. Hook grasp (purse or bookbag handle)								
3. Active release								
Tip pinch (picking up ⅛-inch bead								

Lateral pinch (piece of paper) _____ pounds left

_____ pounds right

Palmer pinch (pencil) _____ pounds left

_____ pounds right

Comments:

Functional UE range of motion

	Left				Right			
	0	1	2	3	0	1	2	3
Reach or touch:								
Above head								
Top of head								
Back of head and neck								
Face								
Mouth								
Shoulders								
Waist (putting on belt)								
Back (fastening clothes)								
Knees								
Feet								
Floor								

Comments:

_____

Occupational therapist

THE MILLER ASSESSMENT FOR PRESCHOOLERS (MAP)

The Miller Assessment for Preschoolers[24] is a fairly new standardized instrument that shows promise. It was designed by an occupational therapist to determine school readiness and potential learning problems of children aged 2 years 9 months to 5 years 8 months. It may be administered in a short form that measures performance on 27 core items to assess sensory, motor, and cognitive abilities, and it examines behavior during the examination in terms of sensory reactivity, social interaction, and attention. A longer version assesses supplemental characteristics observed during performance of the core items and includes a developmental history as well. Specialized continuing education programs are available for therapists who wish to administer this test.[4,24]

Prevocational tests

A variety of tests are available through the literature and commercial resources to assess prevocational readiness. The tests that are included here have been found clinically useful in work with adolescents, and they appear to be particularly pertinent to the assessment questions asked by occupational therapists.

EXHIBIT 11-5

Adolescent Role Assessment

Test measures: The Adolescent Role Assessment uses information obtained from self-reports to determine adequacy of development in a variety of occupational roles. Information is gathered that relates to childhood play experiences; adolescent socialization in the family, at school, and with peers; and development of occupational choice and adult work motivation. The assessment is designed to serve as a tool for clinical treatment planning, although its content may also be used for diagnostic purposes by a knowledgeable clinician.

Population: It must be presumed that this evaluation may be used for the entire age range of adolescents. Black reported clinical application with individuals aged 13 to 17.

Test format: The Adolescent Role Assessment is administered as a semistructured interview. Six sets of open-ended questions are provided to open discussion in each of the areas mentioned above. Questions tend to produce information related to actions and feelings. The interviews can generally be completed within 1 hour. Scoring criteria are provided to interpret content elicited through the interview. According to criteria, information about performance in each area is rated with

+ = Indicates appropriate behavior
0 = Indicates marginal or borderline behavior
− = Indicates inappropriate behavior

A majority of "+" and "0" indicate no obvious role dysfunction. However, a majority of "0" and "−"

scores indicates a trend of inadequate development that requires intervention.

Advantages: This interview system can yield considerable data about the breadth of developmental performance in the adolescent. Although it was tested clinically by the developer with youths who had emotional and behavioral disorders, its scope lends itself to application with a broader population. The interview questions are carefully formatted in the vernacular to assist in establishing rapport with the teenage client.

Disadvantages: Black cautions that the validity of content obtained is dependent on the truthfulness and cooperation of the individual who is interviewed. In the experimental stage the test was administered as part of an evaluation battery. Black believed that, when combined with data from other evaluation tools, the Adolescent Role Assessment could be used to define clear patterns of behavior. However, it is not clear what the relative value of data from this instrument was in relation to information collected through other tools. The test was initially given to a small group of adolescents, and a case study that relates data from one such application was described by Black. However, there was no follow-up on the results of treatment planned through this evaluative process, nor was there any attempt made to establish validity or reliability.

Purchasing information: From Black, M.M.: Am. J. Occup. Ther. **30:**134, 1976.

BLACK'S ADOLESCENT ROLE ASSESSMENT

Black's Adolescent Role Assessment, a semi-structured interview, was designed to explore the individual adolescent's progress in the development of occupational role skills. The test was reported in 1976, including format and report forms.[6] A test analysis is shown in Exhibit 11-5. Unpublished field testing with normal adolescents suggests that the interview can be completed within 1 hour and that comprehensive descriptive information can be obtained if rapport is established early in the interview.

TESTS OF VOCATIONAL INTEREST

Two useful, commercially available tests that are easily administered by occupational therapists in clinical and educational settings are the California Life Goals Evaluation Schedules[18] and the Self-Directed Search.[19] Both tests use a self-assessment format in which the adolescent answers questions related to past and current interests, preferences, and dislikes. The subject can score his own test and by using obtained

scores can identify potentially appropriate vocational choices for further exploration. The therapist's assistance may be needed in the administration of the test with students who are unable to fill out the forms. With either procedure it is helpful to follow up on the testing with task analysis of the prospective job choices. Results can be reviewed with the student to determine the need for further study or training. A test analysis of the Self-Directed Search is found in Exhibit 11-6.

WORK PERFORMANCE SKILLS

Other prevocational tests that are of interest to occupational therapists include job samples and timed tests of manual dexterity. There are a number of elaborate commercial work sample evaluation systems that include work samples of varied nature and broad application. These are rarely administered by occupational therapists. Instead, therapists may use the information collected by vocational evaluation programs to assist in planning remedial programs.

However, therapists may wish to construct work

EXHIBIT 11-6

Self-Directed Search

Test measures: The Self-Directed Search is a test of vocational interests and aspirations. It is designed to clarify those interests according to a typology of six major work personalities that Holland developed to correlate with the U.S. Department of Labor *Dictionary of Occupational Titles* (DOT). The personality types are

1. *Realistic:* The individual who values mechanical skills and work with concrete objects. This individual tends to be conforming, persistent, and thrifty. Typical occupations include auto mechanic, farmer, and surveyor.
2. *Investigative:* The worker who enjoys tasks that require mathematical and scientific procedures, who tends to be analytical, independent, and introverted. Appropriate work may be found in chemistry, physics, or anthropology.
3. *Artistic:* A person who enjoys writing, musical, or artistic activities and tends to be emotional, imaginative, and nonconforming. Job examples include interior decorator, musician, or stage director.
4. *Social:* This individual has social skills and talents, but often lacks mechanical and scientific ability. Such persons are often cooperative, friendly, and responsible. Teachers, occupational therapists, and counselors would tend to be social personalities.
5. *Enterprising:* These individuals enjoy work that involves leadership and public speaking and may be described as adventurous, ambitious, and energetic. Typical jobs include sales persons, managers, and sports promoters.
6. *Conventional:* The conventional person engages in work that uses mathematical and clerical skills. This individual tends to be conscientious, conservative, and orderly and might be found in such occupations as stenographer, banker, or bookkeeper.

The Self-Directed Search was developed for use in vocational counseling programs, personnel offices, and research in vocational interests and personality typology. Administration of the test to an individual will yield a coded and ranked combination of type that may be used to explore vocational opportunities.

Population: The test has been developed with, and normative data are available for, a wide range of normal adolescent and work-aged men and women. Extensive normative tables are included in the test manual.

Test format: This is a pencil-and-paper test that is self-administered and scored in booklet form. It may be used with individuals and groups. The 228 test items are divided into categories that seek information about a person's activities, competencies, occupations, and self-estimates. In most questions the subject must make a choice between two preferences. Each choice is coded according to one of the types. Raw scores from the combined choices yield three predominating types and three low-preference types in codes. Permutations of the three preferred types, contrasted against an occupational classifications booklet, allow the subject to identify a number of vocational choices for further exploration with a counselor. The test may be administered in its complete form or in an adapted version for the individual with limited reading skills. Total test administration and self-scoring time may be 1 to 2 hours, with additional time spent with an occupational therapist or vocational specialist.

Advantages: The obvious advantage of self-administration and scoring is backed by extensive test development research. It is most useful because it provides immediate feedback to the subject. In addition to the 500 occupations included in the accompanying booklet, Holland also included a cross-reference to DOT codes in the test manual. The total package makes the test clinically useful without additional specialized study.

Disadvantages: Aside from the time requirements, it has been noted that information about job preparation requirements in the occupations booklet is not always accurate. Therefore individual counseling related to coded choices will be necessary.

Purchasing information: From Holland, J.C.: The Self-Directed Search, Palo Alto, Calif., 1979, Consulting Psychologists Press, Inc.

---

samples that will assess client skills in relation to employment prospects in a limited way. For example, if a high school student who is wheelchair bound expresses an interest in teaching, the therapist may wish to assess the student's ability to write on a blackboard, explain a math problem, and move around a school building freely. In this example the work samples are related to the physical demands of a specific job interest, rather than to comprehensive exploration of the student's skills in relation to the broad range of employment possibilities. The example demonstrates a method that is more typical of occupational therapy practice.

Assessment of work skills by occupational therapists usually involves activity analysis of the requirements of a specific job and sampling of the client's abilities to meet those job requirements. Often information from occupational therapy evaluation and treatment is synthesized to relate to job preparedness. Using the example just given, the therapist may note that the student has had difficulty keeping up with academic demands of his own high school program because of slow writing. If the student has been using a typewriter and tape recorder to aid in his completion of high school work, the therapist must consider how this equipment may be used to meet the demands of college preparation for a teaching career, as well as classroom duties. If it appears that the teaching career is beyond the capability of the student, the therapist might then work with vocational specialists to develop alternatives for the student.

CROMWELL'S PRIMARY PREVOCATIONAL EVALUATION

In 1960 Cromwell[11] published a manual that described the prevocational evaluation program used by occupational therapists at the United Cerebral Palsy Center in Los Angeles County. This assessment system was developed through a 4-year research project and includes three parts: the activities of daily living inventory, manual dexterity test battery, and the prevocational job sample test battery. Norms for performance of both handicapped (persons with cerebral palsy) and nonhandicapped individuals are included for all parts of the assessment system. Cromwell stated that the system was used clinically with individuals aged 14 years and older.

One of the useful features of Cromwell's manual is its survey of a variety of manual dexterity tests. The entire group of tests, which includes both commercial and therapist-designed tests, or the short version can be administered according to the needs and abilities of the individual client. Complete information is included about the construction of manual dexterity and job sample tests so that the therapist can safely apply norms. In addition to the evaluation's usefulness, Cromwell's job sample descriptions provide a model for the development of other task samples. This includes a description of the job sample, materials to be included in the sample kit, instructions for the examiner, instructions for the client, and rating-scoring information with norms. The manual is available from Cromwell.*

INTEGRATION OF EVALUATION FINDINGS

Through the course of formal and informal evaluation, occupational therapists compile extensive information about their young clients. The final, professional component of assessment is to organize, synthesize, and use these data to guide intervention. The American Occupational Therapy Association[3] defines assessment as

> . . . the process of determining the need for, nature of, and estimated time of treatment, determining the needed coordination with other persons involved, and documenting these activities.

Organization of data

From the beginning it is helpful to have some concrete tools to assist with the organization of data. Two resources have been found useful for these purposes. The Uniform Occupational Therapy Evaluation Checklist was adopted by the American Occupational Therapy Association's Representative Assembly in 1981.[3] It was developed with the use of the *Uniform Terminology for Reporting Occupational Therapy Services* and serves as a guide for baseline data collection (Exhibit 11-7). It is designed to be all inclusive, but each occupational therapy assessment in which this format is used is not expected to reflect all details. Instead, all evaluations should address the major categories. The checklist has proved to be especially useful in medical settings. Definitions of terminology are available.[3]

The Worksheets for Organizing Data Collection (Exhibit 11-8) were developed to organize results of assorted evaluative procedures by use of the defined parameters of occupational therapy practice identified by the American Occupational Therapy Association.[3] The terminology used in these worksheets is more in keeping with the model of practice described in Chapter 7, and it is perhaps more suited to educational settings. Information may be transferred from assorted measurements and evaluation resources with " + " and " − " notations regarding perceived strengths and weaknesses in the different areas. These worksheets can be adapted and tailored to the needs of the individual clinician, but the basic components of comprehensive occupational therapy should remain to serve as ticklers for overlooked areas. These worksheets are intended for internal use only; they do not constitute a formal evaluation report.

Assessment reports

Formal reports of occupational therapy assessment are usually filed in narrative form or on multipart and multipaged preprinted forms. Two sample reports that demonstrate the use of two formats to present information about the same child are shown in Exhibits 11-9 and 11-10. The preprinted form was originally adapted from an occupational-physical therapy screening tool designed by Taylor and Christopher,[17] but it has been subjected to considerable revision since. This format has been used in school system practice, so it would need further modification for a medically oriented setting.

---

*F.S. Cromwell, 1179 Yocum St., Pasadena, Calif. 91103.

Text continued on p. 214.

EXHIBIT 11-7

Uniform occupational therapy evaluation checklist

Procedure

I. *Demographic information*
   A. Personal information
      1. Name
      2. Address
      3. Telephone
      4. Date of birth
      5. Age
      6. Sex
   B. Referral related information
      1. Date of referral
      2. Reason for referral
      3. Referral source
      4. Date client first seen by OT
      5. Diagnosis
      6. Presenting problems/symptoms
      7. Date of onset
      8. Medications
      9. Precautions/complications
      10. Date of evaluation
      11. Evaluator
   C. Personal history
      1. Developmental history
      2. Educational history
      3. Vocational history
      4. Socio-economic history
      5. Medical history

II. *Skills and performance areas*
(See the AOTA *Uniform Terminology System for Reporting Occupational Therapy Services*, January, 1979, for definition of categories.)
   A. Independent living/daily living skills and performance
      1. Physical daily living skills
         a. Grooming and hygiene
         b. Feeding/eating
         c. Dressing
         d. Functional mobility
         e. Functional communication
         f. Object manipulation
      2. Psychological/emotional daily living skills
         a. Self-concept/self-identity
         b. Situational coping
         c. Community involvement

      3. Work
         a. Homemaking
         b. Child care/parenting
         c. Employment preparation
      4. Play/leisure
   B. Sensorimotor skills and performance components
      1. Neuromuscular
         a. Reflex integration
         b. Range of motion
         c. Gross and fine coordination
         d. Strength and endurance
      2. Sensory integration
         a. Sensory awareness
         b. Visual-spatial awareness
         c. Body integration
   C. Cognitive skill and performance components
      1. Orientation
      2. Conceptualization/comprehension
         a. Concentration
         b. Attention span
         c. Memory
      3. Cognitive integration
         a. Generalization
         b. Problem solving
   D. Psycho-social skills and performance components
      1. Self management
         a. Self expression
         b. Self control
      2. Dyadic interaction
      3. Group interaction
   E. Therapeutic adaptation
      1. Orthotics
      2. Prosthetics
      3. Assistive/adaptive equipment
   F. Prevention
      1. Energy conservation
      2. Joint protection/body mechanics
      3. Positioning
      4. Coordination of daily living skills

This outline was taken and adapted from the AOTA Uniform Terminology System for Reporting Occupational Therapy Services, prepared by AOTA Commission on Uniform Reporting System Task Force, Rockville, AOTA, January 7, 1979.

From The American Occupational Therapy Association, Inc., November 1981, Occupational Therapy Newspaper.

EXHIBIT 11-8

Worksheets for organizing data collection

Performance element	*Assessment process*	*Results (+ = Strength; − = Weakness)*

Component functions
Motor function
    Range of motion
    Gross muscle strength
    Muscle tone
    Endurance
    Functional patterns
    Postural stability
    Mobility
    Gross motor skills
    Prehension-manipulation
    Fine motor skills
    Expressive communication
 	
Sensory integrative function
    Body scheme
    Postural-bilateral integration
    Visual-spatial relationships
    Sensory-motor integration
    Reflex integration
    Visual and auditory functions
    Somatosensory awareness
    Somatosensory perception
 	
Cognitive function
    Comprehension
    Written communication
    Verbal communication
    Concentration
    Problem-solving
    Time management
    Conceptualization
    Ability to follow directions
    Integration of learning
 	
Social function
    Dyadic interaction
    Group interaction
    Cooperation
    Competition
    Task performance with others
 	
Emotional functions
    Ability to sublimate drives
    Sources of need gratification
    Tolerance for frustration and anxiety
    Impulse control
    Object relations		

EXHIBIT 11-8, cont'd

Worksheets for organizing data collection—cont'd

Performance skills	Assessment process	Results (+ = Strength; − = Weakness)
Age-specific developmental tasks (describe)		
Role performance		
Self-care		
Home living		
School living		
Community living		
Play		
Schoolwork		
Prevocational development		
Life space data collection		
Life roles		
Significant others		
Environmental requirements		
Cultural requirements		
Role requirements		
Resources		
Barriers to performance		
Alternatives		
Concurrent intervention goals and programs		

EXHIBIT 11-9

Case example: narrative report

Date of report: (month, year)

**Occupational therapy evaluation
(Any County Schools)**

Student: K.X.   Date of birth: XX/XX/76
Parents: Mr. and Mrs. X
School: Any City Elementary School
Class: Kindergarten, Mrs. Teacher

K. is a 6 year 9 month–old girl who is currently attending the half-day regular kindergarten program at Any City Elementary School. She was referred for occupational therapy evaluation by the psychologist and school personnel because of her delay in fine motor and social skills in classroom activities.

K. has been seen for evaluation one to two times weekly for ½-hour sessions since March 22, 198X. Because of immature social-emotional behavior, she has been difficult to test. Typically, when asked by her teacher or this therapist to leave the classroom with the therapist, K. sits on the floor or continues with her previous activity, avoiding the request. On several occasions she has agreed to come with the therapist when promised a reward. On other occasions it has been necessary to carry her to the classroom used by the therapist. By report of Mrs.

Teacher and other school personnel, this behavior pattern is occurring with increasing frequency when K. is directly asked to do something.

In the testing situation K. tends to cooperate fairly well but within a range of manipulative behavior. She refuses most activities initially, but eventually will try most things when a reward is promised. In general, she seems to like the test activities and often becomes engrossed in the activity once she accepts it. It should be noted that it would have been helpful to administer several additional performance tests to K., but her behavior patterns precluded this.

Tests administered: Any County Schools (A.C.S.) Occupational Therapy (O.T.) Developmental Skills Evaluation; Motor Free Test of Visual Perception; Ayres' Clinical Observations; Observation in classroom activities.

General performance skills: K. has been observed in class during preacademic sessions with Mrs. Teacher in singing and dress-up play groups and

Continued.

EXHIBIT 11-9, cont'd

Case example: narrative report—cont'd

when working at prewriting and visual perception activities. In singing and in the small group with Mrs. Teacher, she attended but did not participate. In an activity that looked for words that sounded the same, she pointed to the correct answer in her book but resisted answering the teacher. She finally gave the wrong answer even though her finger was still on the correct answer. When working on prewriting and visual perception worksheets, she focused on the task and did not interact with other children at the same learning station. When asked to share learning materials with other children after she had finished with a task, she refused.

K. seemed to enjoy the dress-up sessions and interacted more with other children during that time. She spoke with the other children in three-word sentences and tended to alternate between parallel and cooperative play. She tried to put on as many clothes as possible to make herself a fat man, after another child had done the same.

Because this is a half-day program, K. does not eat at school. Parents report that K. is independent in self-feeding with a spoon but requires considerable assistance with cutting, even soft foods. She can put on most clothing with supervision but needs physical assistance with fasteners and shoes. She washes her hands and toilets independently at school. She is unreliable in school hallways without supervision. At home she is generally supervised by other siblings or parents.

Based on expectations of child development and the observations noted above, her behavior was similar to that seen in a 4- to 5-year-old child during the first few weeks of a new preschool or kindergarten program. It is not typical of a child at the end of kindergarten.

Fine motor skills: K. is able to draw horizontal and vertical lines, a cross, circle, and square. She attempts a triangle and diamond, but the results look like her squares. She was able to draw a house with doors, windows, and roof but did not draw a recognizable human figure. She can cut a piece of paper in two, and she attempted to stay on a ¼ inch line with only one deviation. During the cutting activity, she shifted hands several times. Her left hand appears to be more accurate, and she tended to use this hand more in other activities as well. Cutting and prewriting skills appear to be just below the 5-year-old level.

K. is able to button and unbutton large and small buttons. However, her performance is quite slow. She can remove lacing easily but has considerable

difficulty inserting the lacing into holes. She could not tie a bow or her shoelaces—skills that are normally expected of a 6-year-old child. Lateral prehension patterns are adequate for manipulation of objects greater than ½ inch but fine tip prehension is not well developed.

Clinical observations: Throughout the testing K. showed a negative reaction to, and actively avoided being touched by, the therapist. It was necessary to eliminate several checks on gross motor function and muscular development that required direct physical manipulation.

Hand and arm functions: Muscle tone is slightly hypotonic, with some loss of cocontraction of arm, shoulder, and neck musculature. Again, she was defensive during this checkout, so results should be viewed accordingly. She was unable to rotate forearms smoothly and rapidly.

Reflex integration: K. was unable to hold the flexor postural and prone extension patterns for the minimum of 10 seconds. During administration of the arm extension test, she showed a slight loss of balance when her eyes were closed. In all patterns tested, she positioned each body part separately, that is, she could not initiate movements with both arms and legs at the same time.

Ocular pursuits: It was noted that K.'s preferred eye is her right, which contrasts with her left preferred hand. She was unable to cooperate with testing of oculomotor function-visual pursuits.

Gross motor functions: Gross motor function and coordination are typical of patterns seen in ambulatory children with Down's syndrome. K. has a broad-based, flat-footed gait with minimal reciprocal movement of the arms. Running is slow and lurching.

Sensory motor functions:

Visual perception: On the Motor Free Test of Visual Perception, K. passed 23 out of 36 items. Her best performance was on items that involved simple matching, form constancy, visual memory, and difference discrimination. She had difficulty on items that tested visual figure-ground discrimination and form-in-space visualization. It should be noted that K. often required more than the usual time limit to pass items. She tended to use a lot of finger tracing and verbalization to determine the correct answers.

Visual-motor function: K. easily replicates familiar designs but has difficulty reproducing drawings and constructions of unfamiliar forms. She pushes away such activities, saying that they are "too easy."

Tactile-kinesthetic processing: Formal testing of

EXHIBIT 11-9, cont'd

Case example: narrative report—cont'd

somatosensory awareness and discrimination was not possible. However, avoidance of touch has been noted on several occasions, and Mrs. Teacher reports similar observations.

Summary and recommendations: K. presently demonstrates the adaptive skill levels associated with a 4- to 5-year-old child. Her language development seems to be delayed. She requires one-to-one teaching-training situations with considerable repetition to learn new skills. Her social-emotional behavior is inconsistent and immature with peers and manipulative with adults. Although she is likable in a one-to-one situation, her immaturity and manipulative behavior tend to be disruptive in small group and classroom situations.

It would be to K.'s benefit to be placed in a very structured class with a low teacher-student ratio. Although Mrs. Teacher has worked very well with K. this year, it is doubtful that K. could receive the one-to-one attention that she needs in a regular first-grade classroom. Again, it would be to K.'s benefit to have her primary educational placement with a specialized Educationally Mentally Handicapped (EMH) teacher. Program needs include training in fine and gross motor skills, social skills, and language development. To supplement her special education program, K. could be seen by the occupational therapist one to two times weekly to develop fine motor skills and sensory integration.

Pat Nuse Clark, M.O.T., OTR/L
Occupational Therapist
Any County Schools

198X Occupational therapy goals and objectives

Goals: 1. Improve skills in school-readiness activities
2. Improve sensory processing

Objectives:

1. K. will cut out a simple geometric form along a ⅛-inch line using her dominant hand with no more than three deviations of more than ⅛ inch 80% of the time.
2. K. will draw a six-part human figure using her dominant hand 80% of the time.
3. K. will fasten three ½-inch button closures on a training board within 2 minutes 80% of the time.
4. K. will rotate both forearms simultaneously at least six times in 10 seconds 80% of the time.
5. K. will hold the prone extension pattern for a minimum of 10 seconds 80% of the time.
6. K. will permit the therapist to touch her arms three times in a row with vision occluded 80% of the time.
7. K. will identify the location of tactile stimuli given on her arms within 5 cm accuracy 80% of the time.

EXHIBIT 11-10

Case example: printed report form

Occupational therapy evaluation
Any County Schools

Student: K.X.   Date of birth: XX/XX/76   Chronological age: 6.9 years

Parents: Mr. and Mrs. X

School: Any City Elementary School

Class: Kindergarten, Mrs. Teacher

Meds-precautions: None stated

Referred by: Dr. Psychologist

Reason for referral: Delay in fine motor skills and social skills in classroom activities.

Pertinent history: K. was diagnosed as having Down's syndrome at birth. She has been seen in early intervention programs since infancy. Her parents are anxious for her to attend a local school.

Tests administered: A.C.S. O.T. Developmental Skills Evaluation; Motor Free Test of Visual Perception; Ayres' Clinical Observations; observation in classroom activities.

Evaluation summary-current levels and recommendations: As stated in narrative report.

Recommended therapy: One to two times a week, 30-minute sessions

Direct: initially   Monitor-skill support: check at midyear

Consult: Therapy not indicated:

Annual goals: As stated in narrative report.

Objectives: As stated in narrative report.

Pat Nuse Clark, M.O.T., OTR/L
Any County Schools

School-related performance skills:

0 = Normal

1 = Slightly impaired-delayed; independent with adaptations

2 = Moderately impaired-delayed; partial dependence

3 = Severely impaired-delayed; complete dependence

1. Self-feeding: uses spoon, needs maximal assistance with cutting	0 1 2 3
2. Dressing: difficulty with fasteners because of fine motor delay	0 1 2 3
3. Grooming and hygiene: needs reminder to leave bathroom	0 1 2 3
4. Toileting:	0 1 2 3
5. Transfers:	0 1 2 3
6. Movement around school: needs supervision.	0 1 2 3
7. Functional communication: uses words, phrases, three-part sentences	0 1 2 3
8. Age-level schoolwork: needs one-to-one training for new concepts	0 1 2 3
9. Age-level play and recreation: tendency toward parallel and imitative play	0 1 2 3

Fine motor skills:

0 = Normal

1 = Slightly impaired or delayed

2 = Limited performance

3 = Unable to perform

Preferred hand: *L* R (dominance not established)

1. Development of prehension-reach: **X**; grasp: **X**; release: **X**; ulnar grasp: ; radial grasp: **X**; tripod: **X**; lateral pinch: **X**; tip pinch: +/−	0 1 2 3
2. Accuracy of preferred hand use:	0 1 2 3
3. Use of nondominant hand: tendency to switch hands in middle of activity—midline?	0 1 2 3
4. Use of hands in bilateral activities:	0 1 2 3
5. Copying geometric figures: horizontal, vertical lines; cross; square; identifies triangle	0 1 2 3
6. Prints-writes: name: **X** letters: numbers: words: sentences: Check if problems noted in letter formation: **X**; spacing: **X**; directionality: **X**	0 1 2 3
7. Cutting skills: ¼ inch: **X** ⅛ inch: ¹⁄₁₆ inch:	0 1 2 3
straight lines: **X**; angles: ; curves:	0 1 2 3

Clinical observations:

0 = Normal
1 = Slightly impaired; needs improvement
2 = Moderately impaired; interferes with skills
3 = Severely impaired; prevents performance

1. Hand and arm functions: slightly hypotonic, some loss of cocontraction, unable to rotate forearms
   smoothly   0 1 <u>2</u> 3
2. Reflex integration: Unable to hold flexor and extension postures for 10 seconds; could not
   move body parts simultaneously   0 1 <u>2</u> 3
3. Ocular pursuits: unable to test; right eye preferred   0 1 2 3

Gross motor functions:

4. Oral-motor: lip closure: **X** slightly hypotonic; swallow: **X**; chew: **X**   0 <u>1</u> 2 3
5. Muscle tone: 0 <u>1</u> 2 3
6. Muscle strength: 0 <u>1</u> 2 3
7. Postural stability: 0 <u>1</u> 2 3
8. Balance-equilibrium: 0 <u>1</u> 2 3
9. Developmental skills (check highest pattern used below): Head control: ; rolling: ; creeping: ;
   sitting: ; kneeling: ; half-kneeling: ; standing: ; climbing: ; running: **X**; other: 0 <u>1</u> 2 3
10. Respiratory control: <u>0</u> 1 2 3
11. Hopping and skipping: 0 <u>1</u> 2 3

Sensory motor functions: vision: adequate; hearing: adequate

1. Visual perception: Scored 23/36 on MFTVF, required additonal time, finger tracing   0 <u>1</u> 2 3
2. Visual-motor function: see comments concerning fine motor   0 <u>1</u> 2 3
3. Tactile-kinesthetic processing: unable to test; however, noted defensive responses throughout
   evaluation; teacher agrees   0 1 <u>2</u> 3
4. Bilateral body integration: 0 1 <u>2</u> 3
5. Motor planning: requires considerable repetition to learn new skills   0 1 <u>2</u> 3
6. Vestibular functioning: unable to test; reportedly likes swinging and other vestibular stimulation activties   0 1 2 3

Prevocational skills:

1. Attention span: will stay on task once engaged   <u>0</u> 1 2 3
2. Ability to follow directions: 0 <u>1</u> 2 3
3. Ability to work with others: manipulative with adults, interacts minimally with peers—parallel
   play preferred   0 1 <u>2</u> 3

NOTE: Problems in performance appear to be primarily resulting from: motor impairment (#4); cognitive
impairment (#2); sensory-integrative impairment (#3); behavioral impairment (#1)

Adaptations and equipment needs:

Current status: one-to-one assistance from teacher or aide
    Environmental: recommend at least partial EMH placement
    Splinting: not indicated
    Wheelchair-mobility equipment: not indicated
    Small adaptive equipment: not indicated

SUMMARY

This chapter has reviewed a number of clinically useful instruments that allow an occupational therapist to assess age-related task performance. The tests presented include standardized and criterion-referenced developmental evaluations and assessments of self-maintenance, play, school readiness, and prevocational skills performance. Selections were based on use in the general range of occupational therapy treatment centers rather than on use in highly specialized locales. Although a number of commercial instruments are available for developmental assessment, occupational therapy concerns with activity performance usually require more detailed information about self-maintenance, school readiness, and prevocational skills. The majority of measurement tools used in practice for assessment of these areas are therapist made. Chapter samples of such clinical tools are considered representative and can be adapted to meet the needs of individual therapists and their clients. Credit to the designer of the original format should be retained on any adaptations.

The therapist is reminded that the focus of occupational therapy is on performance of observable everyday activities in the areas discussed. Therefore it is anticipated that the final assessment of a child before his discharge would include one of the tools presented in this chapter to determine progress and achievement of occupational therapy objectives.

REFERENCES

1. American Association on Mental Deficiency: AAMD Adaptive Behavior Scales, Monterey, Calif., 1981, McGraw-Hill Book Co.
2. American Association on Mental Deficiency: AAMD Adaptive Behavior Scales—public school version, Monterey, Calif., 1981, McGraw-Hill Book Co.
3. American Occupational Therapy Association, Inc.: Uniform terminology for reporting occupational therapy services and uniform occupational therapy evaluation checklist, Occup. Ther. Newspaper **35**(11):9, 1981.
4. Banus, B.J.: The Miller Assessment for Preschoolers (MAP): an introduction and review, Am. J. Occup. Ther. 1983, **37:**333, 1983.
5. Bayley, N.: Bayley Scales of Infant Development, New York, 1969, The Psychological Corp.
6. Black, M.M.: Adolescent role assessment, Am. J. Occup. Ther. **30:**134, 1976.
7. Brazelton, T.B.: Neonatal Behavioral Assessment Scales, Philadelphia, 1973, J.B. Lippincott Co.
8. Brigance, A.H.: Brigance Diagnostic Inventory of Basic Skills, Woburn, Mass., 1977, Curriculum Associates, Inc.
9. Brigance, A.H.: Brigance Diagnostic Inventory of Early Development, Woburn, Mass., 1978, Curriculum Associates, Inc.
10. Coley, I.L.: Pediatric assessment of self-care activities, St. Louis, 1978, The C.V. Mosby Co.
11. Cromwell, F.S.: Occupational therapist's manual for basic skills assessment or primary prevocational evaluation, Altadena, Calif., 1960, Fair Oaks Printing Co.
12. Currie, C.: Evaluating function of mentally retarded children through the use of toys and play activities, Am. J. Occup. Ther. **23:**35, 1969.
13. deRenne-Stephan, C.: Imitation: a mechanism of play behavior, Am. J. Occup. Ther. **34:**95, 1980.
14. Doll, E.A.: Vineland Social Maturity Scale: condensed manual of directions, Circle Pines, Minn., 1965, American Guidance Service, Inc.
15. Florey, L.L.: An approach to play and play development, Am. J. Occup. Ther. **25:**275, 1971.
16. Florey, L.L.: Studies of play: implications for growth, development, and for clinical practice, Am. J. Occup. Ther. **35:**519, 1981.
17. Gilfoyle, E.A., editor: Training: occupational therapy educational management in schools: a competency based educational program, module 3, vol. II, Rockville, Md., 1980, American Occupational Therapy Association, Inc.
18. Hahn, M.E.: The California Life Goals Evaluation Schedules, Los Angeles, 1969, Western Psychological Services.

19. Holland, J.L.: The self-directed search, Palo Alto, Calif., 1979, Consulting Psychologists Press, Inc.

20. Hurff, J.M.: A play skills inventory. In Reilly, M., editor: Play as exploratory learning: studies of curiosity behavior, Beverly Hills, Calif., 1974, Sage Publications. Inc.

21. Hurff, J.M.: A play skills inventory: a competency monitoring tool for the 10 year old, Am. J. Occup. Ther. **34:**651, 1980.

22. Knoblock, H., and Passaminick, B.: Gesell's manual of developmental diagnosis, revised, New York, 1980, Harper & Row, Publishers.

23. Michelman, S.: Play and the deficit child. In Reilly, M., editor: Play as exploratory learning: studies of curiosity behavior, Beverly Hills, Calif., 1974, Sage Publications, Inc.

24. Miller, L.J.: Miller Assessment for Preschoolers: manual, Littleton, Colo., 1982, The Foundation for Knowledge in Development.

25. Rogers, S.J., and D'Eugenio, D.B.: Assessment and application. In Schafer, D.S., and Moersch, M.S., editors: Developmental programming for infants and young children, vol. 1, Ann Arbor, 1977, The University of Michigan Press.

26. Snyder, C., Eyres, F.J., and Barnard, E.: New findings about mothers' antenatal expectations and their relationship to infant development, Am. J. Mater. Child Nurs. **4:**354, 1979.

27. Sprinthall, R.C., and Sprinthall, N.A.: Educational psychology: a developmental approach, ed. 3, Reading, Mass., 1981, Addison-Wesley Publishing Co., Inc.

28. Takata, N.: The play milieu: a preliminary appraisal, Am. J. Occup. Ther. **25:**281, 1971.

29. Tronik, E., and Brazelton, T.B.: Clinical uses of the Brazelton Behavioral Assessment. In Friedlander, B., Sterrit, G., and Kirk, B., editors: Exceptional infants. Vol. III: assessment and intervention, New York, 1975, Brunner/Mazel, Inc.

30. Vulpe, S.: Vulpe Assessment Battery: Developmental assessment performance analysis individualized programming for the atypical child, Downsview, Ontario, Canada, 1979, National Institute on Mental Retardation.

31. Walker, L.O.: The Brazelton Neonatal Behavioral Assessment Scales. In Humanick, S.B., editor: Analysis of current assessment strategies in the health care of young children and child-bearing families, Norwalk, Conn., 1982, Appleton-Century-Crofts.

32. Waters, E., Vaughan, B.E., and Egeland, B.R.: Individual differences in infant-mother attachment relationship at age one; antecedents in neonatal behavior in an urban, economically disadvantaged sample, Child Dev. **51:**208, 1980.

33. Widmeyer, S.M., and Field, T.M.: Effects of Brazelton demonstrations on early interactions of preterm infants and their teenage mothers, Infant Behav. Dev. **3:**79, 1980.

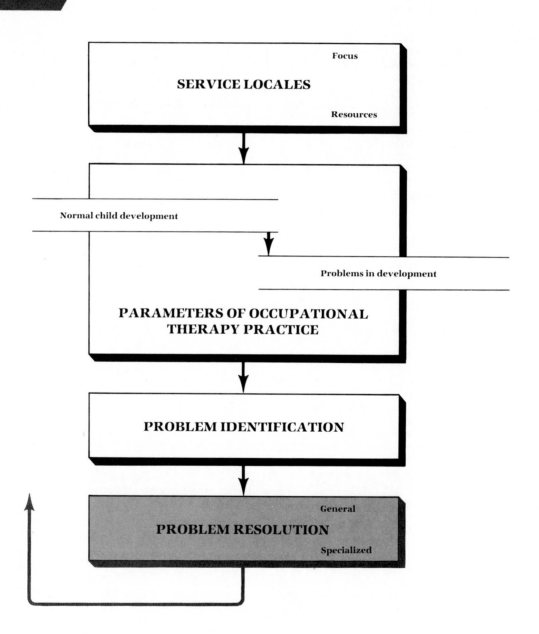

SERVICE LOCALES

Focus

Resources

Normal child development

Problems in development

PARAMETERS OF OCCUPATIONAL THERAPY PRACTICE

PROBLEM IDENTIFICATION

PROBLEM RESOLUTION

General

Specialized

Occupational therapy treatment: major areas of childhood performance

IDA LOU COLEY
SUSAN A. PROCTER

Self-maintenance activities

An early joy of parenthood is to observe the emerging independence of one's child, from the first gestures of holding a rattle to the fine hand manipulations seen in buttoning a shirt. Children are endowed with an innate drive toward mastery of their bodies and their environment.

For most parents their child's evolving competence is an assumed natural order of events, the result of maturation and the influence of surroundings. Occasional regression and unpredictable behaviors presented by children are to be expected as a part of their uniqueness. Overall, independence is an expectation within the family and society at large. When a baby is born with a physical or intellectual disability or acquires one after birth, the disruption in the lives of all family members can be intense.

FAMILY CONSIDERATIONS

Restructuring and adaptation necessarily may stretch over a period of months or years. Today, parents are increasingly expressive about the impact of restructuring lives and about their real needs for knowing the extent of their child's potential. They also express a need to understand the disability, to know specifically what they can do to help their child, and to know where they can receive assistance. They yearn to hear about their child's strengths as they come to grips with the handicap and cope with problems of medical expenses, energy output, time management, and underlying sadness.

Occupational therapists and other professionals are in a strategic position to help parents learn, to help create a partnership in problem solving, to demonstrate techniques that will facilitate care, to provide reading material, and to listen. Timing is an important factor in the adaptation process. Not all families respond to helping gestures offered by professionals. Their responses can be confusing to others and to themselves and may be tempered by a sense of inadequacy, guilt, embarrassment, or anger. They may need counseling and intervention by social service or, to a lesser degree, require reassurance and permission to ask questions again and again: as one parent expressed, "Until I can hear what is being said." Most individuals need time to master information, particularly when under stress.

There are a number of actions a therapist can take to assist a family in gaining a sense of direction:

1. Sharing knowledge of the child's self-maintenance function: what he can do and why he can do some things and not others. Copies of reports written in clear, understandable language help to reinforce verbal information.
2. Clarifying expectations and what responsibilities parents can realistically set for their child in self-care since this is often a source of parental indecision and inconsistency.
3. Outlining realistic programs that family members can carry out according to their capabilities, home environment, and life-style.
4. Presenting equipment options in such a way that parents' consumer rights are recognized and they are supported in making important decisions.

It is only when a therapist can view professional responsibilities as extending beyond the child—in a sense addressing the needs of the family as a whole—that it is possible to maximize the effects of efforts put forth in the child's treatment program. Above all, the desired goal should be to assist the child and family with the business of getting on with living full lives.

BASIC FACTORS
The activity setup

Thoughtful preparation is a first step toward a successful therapeutic session. The therapist must think through and organize the many details involved in assessment and treatment. A good way to begin is to consider immediate goals and then select activities that provide the child with specific experiences. One would want to question, In what order should the therapist introduce tasks? What supplies and equipment are needed? Is the equipment in good working order?

The degree to which the treatment environment influences the child's performance can range from minimal to striking significance. For some children a therapist will want to minimize stimuli and eliminate both visual and auditory distractions. Other children require environmental stimulation from color, music, and objects. The therapist is an influential part of the environment and must consider how to give reinforcement for the child's positive responses.

It is essential to be perceptive to parents and other persons who may be present and to address their needs and concerns, listen, give reassurance, involve them in making observations, and engage them in problem solving. A part of thoughtful preparation is to organize the information they need and have it in written form.

The functional position

An important concept to recognize is that there is no "one" position for function. An individual requires a variety of positions for various activities. Changing positions at intervals provides relief to skin areas and bony prominences and affords important changes in muscle length.

A therapist considers positions that will maximize independent task performance. The child with motor involvement may need to be positioned to break up mass patterns of flexion, extension, and asymmetry. Key points for stability that enable the child to use voluntary movement must be identified. When muscle weakness occurs, the therapist determines where support is needed or, for the child with muscle tightness, whether a preferred and comfortable position is contraindicated.

Looking carefully at the entire body of the child, one asks the following:

Where are the hips, shoulders, and head in relation to the trunk? Will more hip flexion in sitting break up extension patterns (Figure 12-1)?

What things increase trunk stability? Inserting lateral supports? A surface for supporting the feet? Widening the sitting base by abducting the legs?

If more head stability is needed, should the child be placed prone with a roll under his shoulders? Is the roll really under the shoulders or the chest? Are the elbows under the child's shoulders? Check the head position again (Figure 12-2, *A*).

Does sidelying break up strong extension in the prone position, and flexion in the supine position? Will a support pillow to the back prevent the child from rolling to the supine position? Will an anterior support pillow prevent rolling to the prone position? Is a roll between the legs needed to prevent adduction of the hips? Will a small wedge pillow position the head so that the child can see more efficiently with her eyes as her arm reaches out to contact a toy (Figure 12-2, *B*)?

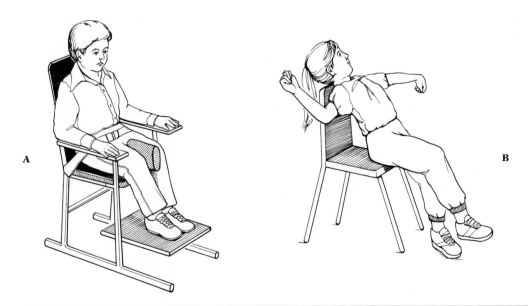

FIGURE 12-1

Sitting postures. **A,** Correct sitting posture. Weight equally distributed on the sitting base; feet and elbows supported. **B,** Incorrect sitting resulting from a massive extension pattern and an asymmetrical tonic reflex posture.

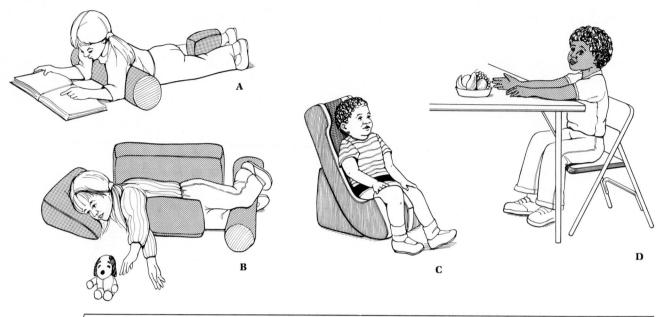

FIGURE 12-2

Adapted positioning for improved function. **A,** In prone position. **B,** In sidelying position. **C,** Grading sitting balance in a partial recliner. **D,** Increasing postural stability by elevation of working surface.

Will inclining the head and trunk prevent the head from falling forward (Figure 12-2, *C*)? Does the position facilitate eye contact between the child and persons in the environment?

The child with weak musculature should be viewed from the standpoint of the forces of gravity and what can be done to provide external support that will allow the use of the available muscle power. Postural security will allow the child to use energy more fully in arm and hand activity.

For the child whose problems are related to muscle tightness, one would need to consider giving required support to prevent fatigue, but a therapist should also question whether a continuous position will foster further contracture. Legs may need to be supported in maximal extension, rather than in a position of flexion.

The working surface

Having positioned the child, attention is next directed to the working surface that serves to give support at the elbows and provides an area for the objects the child will touch, manipulate, and use for self-maintenance. Here one looks more closely at the eye, arm, and hand at work and determines the surface height and angle that allow these body parts to work together more efficiently (Figure 12-2, *D*).

EATING
A bond with nurture

An infant's first experiences with eating usually occur in an atmosphere of tenderness. Nutritional nurture becomes a means for bonding between infant and mother and for building a sense of trust: the first stage of psychosocial development. During feeding, eye contact, touching, and talking reinforce the quality of social communication. It is a process of life that should be a part of awareness as attention is given to the more mechanical aspects of eating function.

Throughout this chapter, looking at the entire body and the whole child is emphasized. An experienced therapist put it another way, "When you evaluate an eating problem, be sure you don't just look at the mouth!" Like a camera lens, the trained eye of the clinician moves to view the child, focusing on details of posture, affect, movement, environmental stimuli, then it shifts to a close-up view of specific behaviors such as the subtle retraction of the upper lip as the child looks up at his feeder.

Eating is a complex function resulting in essential nutrition of the body. It requires a high degree of coordination of orofacial musculature and the vital functions of breathing and swallowing. Alternately and within boundaries, food and air share a common space. During eating the child opens his mouth, adjusts his lips, and gathers up the food, masticates it, moves it about in his mouth, forms a bolus, closes his mouth, and moves the bolus to the back of his throat for swallowing. Having an understanding of how eating occurs will clarify the kind of intervention that is needed when there is dysfunction.

Oral motor development

HOW GROWTH AND STRUCTURAL CHANGE AFFECT FUNCTION

The principle that development proceeds from proximal points to distal points applies to eating sequences. Initially consider the neck region as being proximal and the jaw as being distal. While the neonate is acquiring head control and stabilization in the shoulder region, nature provides reflexive mechanisms to assist him with acquiring food and protective mechanisms for his reclining posture.

SUCKING AND SWALLOWING

As the infant's lips grasp and close around the nipple and hold it close to the junction of the hard and soft palates, mucosal folds on the gums assist in sealing off the oral cavity. When the infant's lips develop more muscular control around 3 or 4 months of age, the folds disappear. The infant rhythmically suckles, and his cupped tongue moves in and out to bring the milk to the back of his throat. The tongue and jaw move together simultaneously and are lowered while the mouth is closed, thus creating a negative pressure. In addition, retrusion of the mandible facilitates the efficiency of the stroking action of the tongue.

When the tongue moves back during sucking and comes in contact with the tensed soft palate, the contact causes the milk to be directed into the lateral food channels.[29] The position of the epiglottis also directs the flow laterally. At this time the epiglottis and soft palate are in close approximation, and the larynx is high in close proximity. In this structural relationship the epiglottis provides a breakwater effect, and this protects the air passages. In addition, the tonsils and lymphoid tissue serve to keep the airway open and prevent food from reaching the posterior pharyngeal wall as the infant feeds in a reclining position.[29]

Because the oral cavity is small, the infant's tongue fills it, leaving little space for air to move in and out. But the infant now can breathe through his nose and can suckle, swallow, and breathe at the same time. The centers for these functions are located near one another in the brain stem. They coordinate their functions to allow liquid and air to cross the alimentary and respiratory passages in the pharynx. Respirations of the infant tend to be rapid and are accomplished by an abdominal breathing pattern. The chest at this time is barrel shaped, and there is minimal movement of the rib cage during breathing.

Cheeks are equipped with fatty tissue called *sucking pads*, which give the infant's face a rounded contour. It is thought that the sucking pads lend stability to the buccinator muscle of the cheek and contribute to the rigidity needed to maintain pressure for sucking.[28] The sucking pads also help to steady an unstable temporomandibular joint.

One of the most puzzling areas of dysfunction occurs within the swallowing mechanism. Therapists can observe the movements within the mouth, can check for the gag reflex, can palpate movement of the larynx, but according to some experts, conclusions must be considered an educated guess. What therapists observe is primarily the voluntary oral phase of swallowing. Cineradiography or videofluoroscopy is required for one to know what is happening in the pharyngeal phase.

In the older infant, child, and adult, the process of swallowing begins as a voluntary act and ends with a series of involuntary, automatic events. The time involved in the complicated process, from the oral phase through the pharyngeal phase, is a brief 2 seconds. Morris[23] states

> The majority of neurologically impaired children and adults who aspirate do not have an absent swallowing reflex. The reflex may be delayed, but the problem most likely lies with the coordination of the tongue, the lips, the cheeks, and the larynx. They may be unable to take food into the mouth, to maneuver it sufficiently to the back, and to trigger an efficient swallow reflex with appropriate timing of pharyngeal and laryngeal movements (p. 29).

In the *voluntary oral stage* (Figure 12-3, *A*) the tongue moves upward, pushes, strips along the soft palate, and propels the bolus to the back of the tongue. When the bolus reaches the area of the anterior and posterior pillars of fauces at the base of the tongue, the swallow reflex is triggered. Phrenic and intercostal nerves inhibit diaphragm and intercostal muscles, and respiration is inhibited.

In the *involuntary oral stage*, or automatic pharyngeal stage (Figure 12-3, *B*), the back of the tongue elevates and presses against the posterior wall. Meanwhile, the soft palate moves backward and upward, closing off the nasopharynx to prevent food from entering the nose. Simultaneously, the bolus stimulates nerve endings in the mucosal lining of the pharynx, and pharyngeal constrictors squeeze the bolus downward. Bronchial passages are protected by the epiglottis and the valving of the true vocal folds and the false vocal folds. The food passes downward into the esophagus as the cricopharyngeal muscle, or bottom pharyngeal constrictor, relaxes.

In the final *involuntary esophageal stage* the bolus stimulates nerve endings in the walls of the esophagus. Peristaltic movements then squeeze the bolus toward the cardiac sphincter. Relaxation of the cardiac sphincter allows the bolus to pass into the stomach.

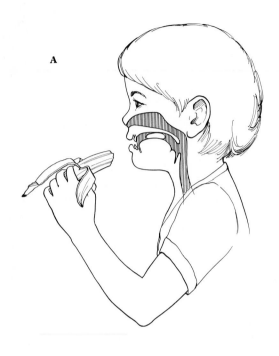

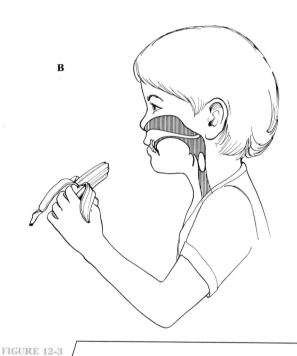

FIGURE 12-3

Swallowing. **A,** Voluntary oral stage. **B,** Involuntary oral stage.

FUNCTIONAL CHANGES

As head control and postural stability increase in the neck and shoulder region, structural changes within the oral cavity contribute to functional changes. The mandible enlarges and grows downward, enlarging the space within the mouth. Teeth erupt and will further enlarge the oral space vertically (p. 224). This allows the tongue to move more freely in an up and down sucking pattern. The tongue grows at the tip differentially, a good example of form following function.[29] It elongates and protrudes naturally to receive and carry semisolids between the gum pads.

With the more mature sucking pattern that now develops, a change in sucking, breathing, and swallowing functions is seen. They no longer occur simultaneously but alternately, and this is related to structural changes. Now the larynx is lower, exposing the airway to a greater degree. This necessitates a more mobile role for the epiglottis, which must move back and down to protect the airway. It is aided in its shielding function by the vocal folds. The soft palate rises to close the nasopharyngeal sphincter, and this interrupts nasal breathing. Now the infant accumulates fluid in his mouth and pauses in sucking and breathing while swallowing.

At 6 months, when the infant begins to spend more time sitting, gravity pushes downward on his body, elongating the thoracic cavity. The ribs, which have been at a right angle with the spine, begin to rotate so that the size of the thorax increases with inhalation. Now breathing is slower but deeper, and this allows babbling and longer, more controlled vocal sounds.

SEMISOLIDS AND THE SPOON

Initially when semisolids are introduced by spoon, there is a choking response as the child learns to handle a new texture and establish coordination between his tongue and pharynx. The food is drawn from the spoon by a suckling in and out movement. By 6 months the child is sucking more often, and the upper lip becomes active, closing down on the spoon. In time the lip will become mobile enough and isolated in movement to remove the food. Spoon-feeding becomes easier as the child learns to draw in his lower lip as the spoon is removed. Later the child's head comes forward to receive the spoon being presented by the feeder.

DRINKING FROM A CUP

The child starts to take liquid from a cup at about 6 months of age. In the first attempts, suckling movements may be evident along with up and down movements of both tongue and jaw. Choking responses are common as the child again learns to coordinate swallowing and breathing. The tip of the tongue may rest under the rim of the cup, and it now begins to elevate with swallowing. At first liquid leaks from the corners of the infant's mouth until he learns to purse his lips. The center of his top lip rises slightly to take in liquid. To maintain liquid in the mouth, the tongue forms a groove, while the cheeks press inward. Now the sucking pads are disappearing, and the cheeks become more mobile and autonomous in movement. To provide more external jaw stability, the child may bite down on the rim of the cup. Drinking will become a smoother function when the muscles around the jaw that control opening and closing can cocontract and the child can control opening.

BITING, CHEWING, AND SOLID FOOD

An infant begins to munch when crackers or cookies are introduced. Munching is the earliest form of chewing, and movements are up and down with mastication aided by a flattening and spreading of the tongue.[23] Because the infant cannot yet stabilize his jaw in a closed position, the feeder must break off the cracker as the infant maintains a bite position. When the infant eats, there is a suckling pattern, often in combination with sucking to move the food to the back of the tongue. A simple protrusion of the tongue may be present as well.

The infant also uses munching when ground food of lumpy texture is introduced. There may be choking again with accommodation to the new stimuli. The added stimulation of lumpy food contributes to the loss of hypersensitivity to touch within the mouth as the child experiences the additional sensory stimulation.

Next there is more movement of the tongue as it rolls the food to the sides. When the bolus is in the center of the tongue, the child may revert to a suckling pattern. The child begins to experiment with mouth play and uses the tongue to wipe food from the upper lip. When the tongue shifts to move food from the sides of the mouth to the middle, the jaw follows in a lateral and diagonal direction. By 12 months, the child may be able to transfer food from the center of the mouth to the sides through coordinated movement, rather than experimental rolling.

Lips too become more mobile and autonomous in movement. The corners begin to draw inward to control the movement of food and to prevent the loss of food or saliva while chewing. By 1 year, drooling is under better control. The upper incisors become useful for cleaning the lower lip of food, as well as providing the child with added sensory equipment to explore food. There are new possibilities for the child to enjoy mealtime as his skill with movement grows. By 2 years, the child chews with his mouth closed as he shifts food from one side of his mouth to the other. Jaw movement for breaking up solids is better controlled and by 3 years, the child shows the mature rotary pattern of chewing that is seen in adults.

HOW REFLEXES AFFECT FUNCTION

The relationship between reflexes and function has been described by Bobath,[4] Illingworth,[19] Peiper,[28] and others. At birth the newborn feeds by a sucking reflex. In 2 or 3 weeks he suckles and is directed to the nipple by a rooting reflex. With tactile stimulation to the perioral skin, including the cheeks and lips, the infant turns toward the stimulus in a food-searching manner. When there is stimulus to the lips, they respond with closing and pouting movements in preparation for sucking. These reflexes can be elicited when the infant is hungry, but they are diminished when he is satiated. The rooting reflex fades by 6 months, and by this time the child is sitting and taking swallows from a cup. He no longer needs the assistance of a reflex in searching out sustenance.

Similarly, the newborn shows a phasic biting reflex. When the newborn's lower gum is stimulated, his jaws open and close with rhythmic up and down movements. This response continues to be present until 3 to 5 months of age and is a component of the early munching pattern. It is gradually replaced by the more controlled volitional bite.

Moro's reflex is present at birth and is demonstrated by a strong abductor-extensor reaction of various parts of the body with loss of support that results in shaking of the head. The reflex fades and is integrated by 6 months when the infant begins to sit erect in a high chair and uses propping reactions of his arms. The startle reaction remains but with diminution. Otherwise, the infant would be unable to maintain sitting stability in the presence of stimuli.

Thus nature provides mechanisms for essential life-sustaining functions. With maturation of the central nervous system, primitive movement is inhibited and brought under control by higher centers. In addition, reactions appear that will be present for a lifetime. The labyrinthine righting reflex, optical righting reflex, propping, and equilibrium reactions assist voluntary, controlled movement that is needed for self-maintenance function.

Dental development

The primary, or deciduous teeth, erupt in a fairly predictable fashion, beginning with upper and lower central incisors. Most infants have a total of two upper and two lower incisor teeth by 7 months of age and thus acquire biting surfaces. Within another 4 months the biting surfaces will widen with the appearance of the lateral incisors. Sometime between 12 and 15 months the anterior (first) molars erupt, coinciding with the occurrence of refined lateral movements for chewing. Posterior (second) molars erupt between 24 to 30 months.

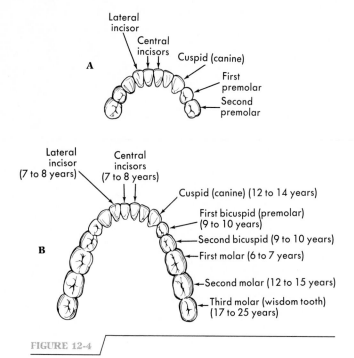

Dental development. **A,** Deciduous teeth. **B,** Permanent teeth.

Normally the shedding of primary teeth coincides with the eruption of corresponding secondary teeth, and this begins at the end of early childhood (between 6 and 7 years) with the appearance of the first permanent molars and the loss of the lower incisors. Permanent teeth are usually in place in early adulthood, from ages 17 to 22 (Figure 12-4).

Common problems of eating

Children with impaired neurological functions may show a combination of feeding difficulties that are not easily identifiable. Motor patterns may be a mixture of abnormal, primitive, and normal signs.

The child's body tone is indicative of the types of problems that may be seen. Newborns with neuromotor impairment are frequently hypotonic. They may show head lag and floppy extremities. Some rigidity may be seen, particularly at times of distress or with feeding. The infant may suck weakly or the sucking action may be arrhythmic and inefficient, resulting in excessive jaw movement and loss of liquid from his mouth. When the infant is in the supine position, gravity may contribute to his tongue retraction, and he may fix his tongue against his palate, making it difficult to accept a nipple. Lack of muscle tone may result in a flattened tongue without the capability of forming a central groove through which liquids can move easily.

As the infant grows and begins to deal with gravity, he must find ways to compensate for his low body tone,

and so he tends to lock in postures in his attempts to become functional. As he exerts more and more effort, muscle tone increases, and in time hypertonia may be seen.

Strong extensor tone of the neck, shoulders, and even hips can affect oral mechanisms and result in lip retraction and compensatory pursing, a jaw thrust, and tongue thrust. This is seen in children with spasticity who have difficulty developing isolated and independent oral movement patterns. Massive extension makes it difficult to close the mouth, chew, or use the tongue to move food in the mouth. A strong jaw thrust will inhibit the development of graded jaw movements for biting and chewing (Figure 12-5, *A*). Lip retraction will prevent use of the upper lip to draw food from the spoon (Figure 12-5, *B*). A tongue thrust will interfere with swallowing (Figure 12-5, *C*).

Children who have fluctuating tone have problems with stability in oral movement. Inefficient movement may result in poor timing, which delays the swallowing reflex, and results in coughing and choking responses. For example, the child may be unable to use his cheeks well in holding the bolus of food on his tongue.

When children have poor hand skills, have difficulty with grasp and cannot direct the hand, and have asymmetry such as is shown with the asymmetrical tonic neck reflex, they are also deprived of opportunities to explore properties with their mouths. It is characteristic of a child at about 5 months of age or earlier to grasp objects voluntarily and bring them to his mouth where he has abundant sensory receptors. This mouthing exploration is one means of reducing the hypersensitivity of the oral cavity. Without oral stimulation, hypersensitivity can contribute to a number of problems, including gagging, greater head extension, lip retraction, tongue thrusting, and jaw thrusting. Additionally, there may be sensitivity of the gums and teeth that trigger a bite reflex. Hypersensitivity may be so great that the child is unable to tolerate stimuli about the face, and he may find textured foods unpleasant.

Abnormal postural tone directly affects respiratory patterns.[18] When there is strong extensor spasticity with the head extended, the shoulders pulled back, even the abdominal muscles contracted, the rib cage becomes flared and flattened over a period of time and reduces the amount of air the child can inhale. The child's breathing is shallow, and his vital capacity is reduced. This, in turn, makes it difficult for him to sustain vocal production and to vary the sounds produced. Strong flexor spasticity also affects respiration. In this case, the head is lowered and the arms are forward and frequently are held tightly against the rib cage. This position also inhibits deep respiration and results in shallow breathing. When children have extremely low tone, they may develop asynchronous breathing. As they inhale, the sternum is indented and pulled inward. In addition

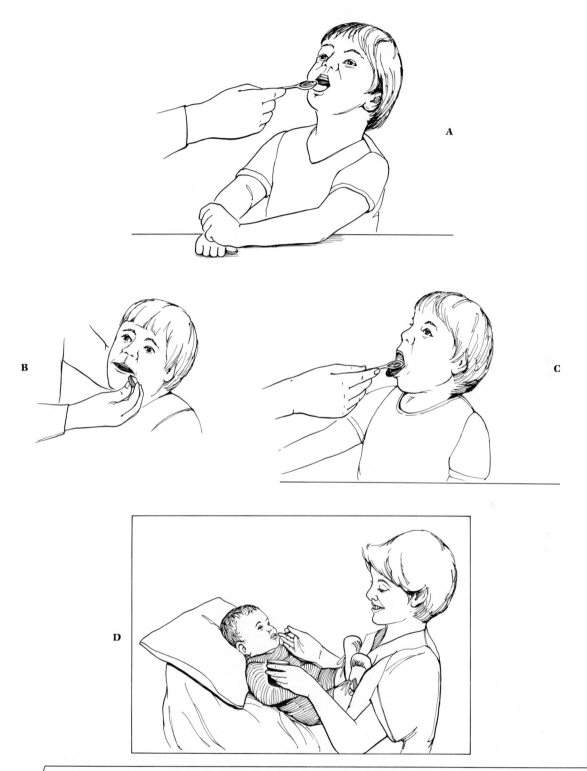

FIGURE 12-5

Feeding patterns. **A,** Jaw thrust: an abnormal downward movement of the lower jaw to an open position, making it difficult for the child to close his mouth and take in food. **B,** Lip retraction: an abnormal tightening of the lips horizontally, making it difficult for the lips to assist with sucking movements or to remove food from a spoon. **C,** Tongue thrust: an abnormal, forceful protrusion of the tongue from the mouth, causing utensils and food to be ejected. **D,** Symmetrical positioning for feeding with visual contact.

to influencing sustained vocal production, respiratory patterns influence quality, pitch, and loudness of the voice.

Finally, children with neurological impairment may be limited in their means to communicate and unable to indicate by word or gesture that they do not like a food, or that they would like more, or that they are satiated. If tone is low, they may not use facial expression and characteristically may show a sad, droopy face with little emotional affect. Communication is an integral part of the eating environment and should be addressed as a part of the program design (Chapter 18).

The following examples are presented to illustrate the questioning process as one seeks to identify the source of the eating problem. Questions and solutions may evolve together.

- Is the infant's difficulty in sucking related to poor tone? Can the nipple be removed from his mouth easily?
- Why can't the bottle be placed in the infant's mouth? Is his tongue retracted? Is it pressing against the hard palate? Does the infant sometimes tend to project his tongue? Is this a compensatory action to prevent obstruction of the airway? What happens if the infant is placed on his stomach?
- Why is the child not able to move food in his mouth? In his tongue flat and bunched? Can tongue control be improved by changing sensory stimuli during feeding or by presenting textured foods? Is the problem motor oriented, or sensory oriented, or both? Which exerts the greatest influence?
- If the child has an adverse reaction when a spoon is introduced to his mouth—such as lip retraction, tongue thrust, or jaw thrust—will allowing the spoon to remain there longer give the system more time to adjust?
- Does the child bite down on the cup for stabilization or because of a bite reflex?
- Is drooling related to poor tone, positioning, or increased motor output?

Answers may not be immediately available and may require investigation of the effects of changes in stimuli. The selection of remediation techniques will be based on the child's responses, rather than on a single

---

EXHIBIT 12-1

Summary of clinical observations for eating function

Position for eating:
In what position is the child usually fed? How well does the child maintain head and trunk control? Symmetry? Does the effort of eating affect postural tone? How often is adjustment in posture needed?

Response to sensory stimulation and environment:
How does the child respond to firm and light touches on legs, trunk, hands, arms, forehead, cheeks, lips? Does the child tolerate touch to gums, teeth, tongue, palate? To new tastes and textures? To temperatures? To sudden abrupt noises? Use smell to investigate food?

Sucking, swallowing, breast/bottle, spoon, cup:
What type of bottle nipple is used? How well does the infant grasp the nipple? What tongue pattern is used in sucking? Is sucking rhythmical? Is there excessive movement of the jaw with sucking? Does it take over 20 minutes to complete a bottle? Has the infant ever been tube fed?

What tongue pattern is used in sucking semisolids from a spoon? Does the child gag or choke? How well does the child coordinate sucking and swallowing? What is his head position when swallowing? Does the top lip come down on the spoon? Does the child use upper incisors to clean his lower lip?

Do the jaw and tongue move together in drinking?

Does the child choke? Bite down on the rim of the cup? Elevate his tongue tip in swallowing? Can the child purse his lips at the corners? What abnormal patterns interfere with sucking, swallowing, and drinking?

Biting, chewing solids:
Can the child stabilize with jaw closed while a cracker is broken off? Does the child use a munching pattern? Shift food from sides to center? Use his tongue to roll food to the sides of his mouth? Does the child cough and choke? Close his mouth when chewing? Show a rotary chewing pattern? What abnormal patterns interfere with chewing?

Drooling:
Is drooling under control? Is the chin wet or dry? Can the child keep his mouth closed? Does drooling increase with motor activity? With position change?

Respiratory patterns:
Does the child breathe through his nose or mouth? What is the postural tone of trunk, shoulders, and arms? What is the shape of the rib cage? Is the child's voice loud, soft, weak?

Communication:
Does the child communicate verbally? Or nonverbally through eyes, facial expressions, or hand gestures?

approach. To help therapists organize their questioning process, a summary of observations for eating function is shown in Exhibit 12-1.

Eating interventions

There are many remediation techniques described in the literature, and some are quite precise. Three approaches have been developed by Farber,[11] Morris,[23] and Mueller.[25] Farber uses neuromuscular facilitation for individuals with oral motor deficits. She suggests stretching the arches of the soft palate and uvula for the hypoactive gag response, using the walking back technique for the hyperactive gag response, vibrating the frenulum and stretching the tongue for tongue thrust, and using vibration and stretch techniques for sucking and swallowing. Morris uses a naturalistic approach and, among other things, looks to the total environment and normal development for therapy guidelines. Mueller advocates positioning and specific handling techniques, including jaw control and normalizing oral tactile sensitivity. All three authorities, plus others, offer valuable insights, and the reader is encouraged to become acquainted with varying points of view.

Clinicians in the field today are inclined to choose those techniques that they personally have found to be successful and with which they are most comfortable. The techniques included here are among the most commonly used approaches in eating intervention. Among the factors to be considered in a program are positioning; the eating utensils; the types of food in the diet; the normalization of orofacial hypersensitivity; and stabilization and control of the jaw, lips, and tongue for cup drinking, spoon feeding, and chewing.

POSITIONING

This chapter has thus far established the high priority of positioning in promoting more normal function and has emphasized looking at the total body in space. By way of review, specifically one looks for those positions that interrupt the motor pattern of asymmetry and massive hyperextension and hyperflexion. The key points of support are the neck and spine, shoulders, and pelvic area.

A variety of positions for eating are available and useful. It is important that those who feed the child share a common knowledge, understand the child's movement patterns, and recognize those postures that facilitate the child's function and those that interfere with it.

Sitting is the social posture for mealtime communication. Common guidelines include the following:

Keep the head and body aligned in midposition; the head forward in slight flexion; the shoulders slightly forward to bring the hands to midline; the hips flexed to 90 degrees or beyond with the legs slightly abducted and weight evenly distributed.

Avoid extension of the head that interferes with swallowing and elicits abnormal extension patterns in the mouth; asymmetry of the head that can affect the position of the jaw, the arms, the legs, and inhibit the child's visual fields; protraction of the shoulders that can contribute to flexion patterns and involuntary jaw clenching; retraction of the shoulders and extension of the hips that may trigger abnormal extension patterns in the mouth.

Good positioning should be based on what works for the individual child, what normalizes his tone, and what contributes to midline and proximal stabilization. This will permit the child to use the controlled movement available to him for distal refined movements of the jaw, tongue, lips, and the arms and hands.

Infants most frequently feed in their mother's arms, feeling the close contact with her body, gazing at her face. Insofar as possible, positioning that allows maximal contact with the mother or caretaker is to be encouraged. The mother's comfort in sitting is also a consideration, since feeding may be slow and time-consuming. A quiet uninterrupted time, as free from pressures as a household permits, helps to make the feedings as pleasurable as possible for mother and child.

Through simple adaptation the mother can use a large pillow or wedge to position her infant before her on her lap. She can then adjust the angle of the infant's body by propping her feet on a stool. She can check the infant's posture while he feeds, keeping his head slightly flexed in midline, his arms forward and at midline, and his legs slightly apart (Figure 12-5, *D*).

When the infant gains greater head and trunk control and is ready for a more upright posture, feeding can be carried out by sitting across his mother's lap. She can adjust the angle of the infant's hips and give stabilization and support where it is needed by bringing her arm around the infant's back.

When a child is ready to sit in a chair, the caretaker should provide postural security by inserting rolls in the seat if necessary. The child's spine should rest comfortably against the back of the chair, with the seat giving support along the thighs to a point just proximal to the knees, permitting full knee flexion to 90 degrees.

If strapping is necessary to maintain positioning, this should be applied across the pelvis. Added flexion of the hips to inhibit an extension pattern can be obtained by a rolled towel or a reversed wedged pillow under the child's thighs. The elbows should be supported; a tray suits this purpose well. The height of the tray may need to be raised if the child has trunk instability. If the child's legs tend to adduct, a small pillow between his legs will help to maintain abduction.

Weight should be distributed evenly on both hips, and symmetry maintained. Feet should be supported, if necessary by placing a box under the feet.

Prone lying is also an option to consider for the child with severe sucking and swallowing problems. This can be arranged in various ways, including use of a prone board or placement of a wedge pillow on the floor. Sidelying may be useful for a child who has a strong extension pattern in the supine position and a flexion pattern in the prone position.

The ultimate goal is to achieve as much independent movement for function as possible, and this requires practice and freedom to move. Static posture in most cases is not the end point.

FOOD PROPERTIES

Before discussing the selection of food for remediation techniques in eating, food terms according to texture and consistency need to be clarified. The following terms are commonly used:

Thin liquid Water, juice, or milk.
Thickened liquid Liquids thickened with cereal, pureed fruit, or other substances that make them less fluid.
Semisolids that are very smooth Solids that have been blended, strained, or pureed to obtain a smooth, thick consistency.
Semisolids that are lumpy Solids that have been passed through a food grinder or have been blenderized for a smooth and slightly lumpy texture; foods that have not been ground but are lumpy, including scrambled eggs, cottage cheese, and mashed cooked vegetables.
Solids Textures that are firm and tough, such as roast beef; crisp; or soft, such as cheese and skinless wieners that require minimal chewing.

Foods have specific properties that have significance for children with oral motor problems. Thin liquids are harder to manage than thickened ones. Because of their low specific gravity, thin liquids do not excite pressor receptors in the tongue and soft palate and tend to leak into the trachea, causing choking. Some therapists feel that acidic liquids, such as orange juice, increase saliva production; drooling is a common problem for children who lack tone or for some other reason have difficulty keeping their mouths closed. Dairy products, particularly milk rich in casein, produce mucus, which decrease sensation. This complicates the child's management of secretions still further. Above all, these children have difficulty handling mixtures of liquids and solids, as found in minestrone soup. The task of swallowing liquid while continuing to chew solids overburdens the poorly coordinated oral mechanisms.

Children may be able to demonstrate more normal oral patterns and show less coughing and choking when liquids are thickened. This can be done by adding yogurt or baby cereal. Thin purees can also be thickened, and nutritional substances such as bran and wheat germ can be added, depending on the child's tolerance. The thickened liquids slow down the swallowing process and give the child more time to organize the sensory information.

A cracker is usually one of the first solids an infant bites, and because it is soft, it mixes easily with saliva and can be easily swallowed.[2] Soft chicken or turkey pieces are also easily chewed and tend to stick together. Placing soft solids such as cubes of cheese in the sides of the child's mouth increases demands for chewing at a beginning level and also serves to inhibit the immature suckling and sucking patterns that occur when the food is resting on the center of the tongue. Morris[23] believes one should choose foods that put the system slightly under stress and challenge it through sensory input. Smaller, harder particles that do not mix with saliva, such as raisins, require greater manipulation by the tongue and increased chewing ability.

EATING UTENSILS

When determining the utensil that best serves the child's eating function, it is best to have an assortment of various shapes and sizes. This permits one to evaluate a number of them and determine which is more effective for the individual child. Parents appreciate seeing and knowing about products and learning about the availability, merits, and drawbacks of equipment on the market.

When an infant sucks weakly, mothers may attempt to help by enlarging the holes in the nipple. This is never recommended as a procedure, because it tends to elicit undesirable compensatory patterns. The preemie nipple, a soft one that compresses easily, is often selected in the hospital nursery. For an inefficient suck, the NUK nipple offers the advantage of keeping the infant's jaw further open than do regular nipples. This helps the lip maintain contact with the nipple. But the NUK nipple requires greater strength and coordination and may not be appropriate for the infant with a weak suck.[22] Some specialists feel that air swallowing may be prevented to some extent by use of a "banana" or "boat-shaped" feeding bottle that allows a slower, more even flow of milk. The nipple of choice is determined by the infant's response.

In general, spoons with a shallow bowl permit the child to have more success in pulling food from the spoon with the upper lip. Mothercare has a line of spoons that is functionally satisfactory and attractive. The sturdy plastic material is not vulnerable to shattering. Brittle plastic spoons should never be used with children who have oral motor problems, particularly when they have patterns of jaw clenching or exhibit the tonic bite reflex. For those children who are sensitive to warm and cold sensations, the sturdy plastic spoon offers the advantage of not conducting temperature as readily as a metal spoon. Some therapists and parents prefer the protective feature of the latex-coated spoon, while others feel that the added depth of the latex coating causes children to open their mouths wider. Additionally, they believe that the flexible plastic coating often stimulates a stronger bite reflex.[2]

When introducing cup drinking, many therapists choose to use a small, easily compressible plastic cup that can be held to form a spout. The cutout cup is usually satisfactory in preventing head extension as the cup is tipped for emptying, thus it allows the child to maintain slight flexion of the head. Therapists often choose cups that are translucent so that they, or the parents, can see the liquid levels in the cup, as well as the oral function of the child. Some children need the external stabilization provided by biting down on the rim of the cup. A thick-rimmed cup prevents this adaptation, but such a cup works very well for children not having problems with jaw stabilization.

NORMALIZING OROFACIAL HYPERSENSITIVITY

A guiding principle in reducing sensitivity to stimuli about the face, lips, and mouth cavity is to proceed slowly, kindly, and gently. It is a program that cannot be rushed, for the child's system must be given time to accommodate. The child is likely to be less defensive and apprehensive if tactile stimuli are presented through play, by use of firm, sustained pressure. Stuffed animals of various textures or furry puppets can reduce stress when they are used to converse with the child while taking imaginary journeys along the child's body, proceeding from the extremities toward the child's face, when tolerance for touch increases. Firm rubbing and stroking can be given with a washcloth during bathtime.

In approaching the face and mouth area, a good way to begin is by encouraging the child to explore his mouth with his own hands, providing he does not have a strong tonic bite or jaw clenching. The child may respond to soft squeeze toys that can even be used as utensils when it comes time to introduce food. Another natural activity includes wiping the mouth, but the method for this is to apply a slow, firm pressure in a blotting manner. Using a soft, damp, lukewarm cloth makes the stimulation more tolerable. Toothbrushing is a vigorous way of normalizing sensitivity.

Digital stimulation is a technique that can be used when touch about the face—the forehead, cheeks, and lips—is tolerated. It is introduced at the beginning of feeding to aid the child in accepting the sensory stimulation of food and utensils within his mouth. As an intrusion, the stimulation can be upsetting to the child and must be done slowly in a gradual manner. Again, by using play the therapist or parent can reduce the stress associated with this sensitivity. A suggested way to proceed is to invent a mouth game and during the game rub the child's outer gums on either side (not the front areas). Inner gums are then rubbed in a similar manner, and, if possible, stimulation may be given to the buccal and palatal regions as well. As discussed earlier, increasing food textures is another useful technique for reducing sensitivity.

Some children are sensitive to the point that the sight of an approaching spoon can result in a tongue thrust, jaw thrust, lip retraction, and extension of the head. Generally, tongue thrust should always be inhibited before presenting food in a spoon. This is commonly done by "walking the spoon back on the tongue," using an unfilled spoon. Starting at the anterior half of the tongue, the feeder gives downward pressure with the spoon and holds for a few seconds. This is repeated two or three times while continually moving back toward the middle of the tongue each time. An additional consideration for the child who is hypersensitive to spoon-feeding is to explore the use of a cup. When a child is spoon-fed, the spoon is repetitively inserted for brief periods, bombarding the system. On the other hand, in taking food from a cup, the contact is sustained over a longer period of time.

When a hyperactive gag response is present, stroking the tongue firmly, front to back by using an unfilled spoon is a step toward densensitizing the child's response. It is also helpful to press down on the center of the tongue with the spoon when food is presented to the mouth and to close the mouth to inhibit the gag response.

A number of interesting techniques have been proposed by therapists working with infants who show sucking problems. When an infant shows an arrhythmic suck, instilling a tempo of one suck per second is attempted by stroking the infant's tongue downward and forward at this tempo. Rocking the infant at a rock per second has also been suggested. When the infant's problem is a weak suck, measures include cuddling in flexion, since sucking is a flexion pattern. A pacifier can be used to facilitate the initiation of the suck, then at intervals semi-solid food by spoon can be introduced for suckling.

JAW CONTROL

Jaw control is a technique in which the therapist or other feeder gives external stabilization to the child's jaw and controls its opening and closing; it is frequently used when there are abnormal extension patterns and poor coordination of oral structures. Initially, a child may only be able to tolerate the control for a short period. It is advisable that the technique be introduced in a therapy session by a therapist, preferably during snacktime. In time the child should be able to accept the control during mealtimes as well. The person providing the jaw control must be aware of the degree of the child's function so that the amount of assistance can

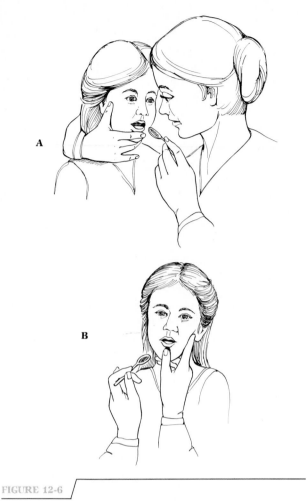

FIGURE 12-6

Jaw control. **A,** From the side. **B,** From the front.

be diminished as the child learns to function better.

Essentially, jaw control is given in two ways: sitting beside the child or sitting in front of the child. When sitting beside the child (Figure 12-6, *A*), put one arm around the back of the child's head. Place your index finger on the front of the child's chin; it assists with controlling the lip and jaw. Place your middle finger under the child's chin; it helps in controlling the jaw and closing the mouth. Use your thumb on the side of the child's cheek to stabilize his jaw. Try to position yourself so that you have eye contact with the child.

When sitting in front of the child (Figure 12-6, *B*), place your thumb on the front of the child's chin. Place your middle finger under the child's chin; it helps to control the movement of the jaw. Place your index finger along the side of the child's cheek to stabilize his jaw.

A therapist should always keep in mind that this technique will not work satisfactorily if abnormal oral motor patterns are being triggered by tonic reflex activity in other parts of the body. Careful monitoring of total body position should be maintained while jaw

control is given. The technique is used during spoon-eating, drinking, chewing, and swallowing. In addition to observing the steps outlined in the jaw control procedure, the following guidelines also facilitate better function.

With *spoon-feeding*, use a spoon with a shallow bowl. Present the spoon at midline. Introduce the spoon slowly, and encourage the child to use his upper lip to clean the spoon.

With *drinking from a cup*, position the child so that his head is slightly forward. Use a cut-out cup if there is head extension. Place enough liquid in the cup so that the child does not need to tip his head back. Close the child's mouth for swallowing.

Closing the lips helps to control drooling, to prevent loss of food from the mouth, to promote better chewing patterns, and to coordinate swallowing. Other techniques for closure include brushing the lips with your fingers, pinching the cheeks lightly, stretching the corners of the mouth, and having the child imitate the sound, "mmmmmm."

A technique sometimes used to teach *swallowing* is to fill a plastic straw halfway with a liquid the child likes. By placing a finger over one end of the straw, the feeder can keep the liquid in the straw. The other end of the straw is then placed in the child's mouth, and the liquid is released on the back of the tongue. To help the child close his mouth and swallow, the feeder gently strokes with a finger the child's throat. Upright posture and slight flexion of the head aid in swallowing. Some therapists have found that sour liquids facilitate swallowing as well.

A child normally acquires tonicity and lip control at about 2 years of age, but to be skillful at *straw drinking*, it may take an additional year or so. A play activity such as blowing bubbles or paper windmills helps the child to learn how to position his lips. Popsicles are useful to facilitate puckering of the lips and drawing in the liquid.

Other ways of managing feeding

In the acute medical setting one encounters a number of conditions that necessitate an alternative way of feeding. Although it is the nurse who is most closely involved in maintaining nutrition, an occupational therapist should be aware of the implications of the measures. Some of the methods of feeding are the following.

MEDICINE DROPPER

The medicine dropper is used with small premature infants who have a good swallowing reflex but who cannot suck with sufficient strength to draw the milk through the nipple or cannot swallow rhythmically as they suck. The tip of the medicine dropper is protected by a piece of rubber tubing. The infant is given a few drops of liquid at a time and allowed to swallow before the bulb is again compressed.

BOTTLE FEEDING

Bottle feeding is used with more mature premature infants or those with an unusually strong suckling swallow reflex.

NONORAL FEEDING

The infant who is unable to suck or swallow, or who becomes fatigued with the effort of nursing, or who is apt to become cyanotic after feeding on the bottle or medicine dropper is fed by *gavage,* a method generally performed by the nursing staff. A catheter is inserted through the child's nostril down into his stomach. The nurse holds a syringe above the infant and slowly pours nutrient into the syringe barrel. After feeding, the tube is cleansed with sterile water. The catheter is changed at least every 4 days. Problems presented by gavage feeding are a reduced gag reflex and irritation to the infant's nose and throat.

The tube poses a real problem to the caregiver who attempts to introduce oral feeding. Since the mouth became the place where the child was poked and investigated by strange objects, it would be understandable that he would reject food or intrusion from oral stimulation. Moreover, when the swallow reflex is triggered, the back of the tongue elevates and bumps into the tube—a negative reinforcer for oral feeding.

A *gastrostomy* makes it possible to avoid the potential hazards of prolonged nasogastric intubation. It is useful to prevent esophageal reflux and acts as a safety and outlet valve when vomiting occurs.

An incision is made into the abdominal cavity, and a tube is inserted directly into the stomach, halfway down the greater curvature. The tube is sutured firmly to the skin. A syringe is attached to the tube and is elevated for feeding.

Morris[23] points to a number of advantages this system presents. First, the child's clothing covers the area and eliminates the visual evidence of nonoral feeding, reducing the adverse reactions of others in the environment. Most importantly, it leaves the mouth free for oral stimulation while food enters the stomach. The feeder can reinforce the concept that the mouth is an enjoyable place through touching, mouthing, and sound play. Such measures help to prevent the hypersensitivity resulting from understimulation of a body part.

Morris further suggests a gradual progression from tube feeding to oral feeding as the child becomes nutritionally stable. She suggests allowing 20 to 30 minutes for oral feeding with the rest of the meal given by gastrostomy. She stresses the importance of holding, stroking, and engaging the child in other types of communication while the stomach is being filled. She also points to the advantage this system offers in conserving the child's energy, which was formerly required to maintain a borderline existence through oral feeding.

Problems presented by a gastrostomy include infection and skin breakdown.

Hyperalimentation is a medical procedure that introduces highly nutritional solutions directly into the bloodstream. It provides protein and calorie intake sufficient to sustain life and to promote growth in the absence of adequate gastrointestinal tract function. It is used for children with congenital bowel anomalies, extensive burns, intractable diarrhea, and cancer.

To be effective the fluid must contain protein, calories (dextrose), water, vitamins, minerals, and electrolytes. Since the high concentration of the solution makes it irritating to the blood vessel walls, a Silastic catheter through which the fluid is given must be placed into a vein large enough where blood flow is rapid to prevent sclerosis and thrombosis and to dilute the solution before it enters the peripheral circulation.

A surgical procedure is required and consists of inserting a catheter through the jugular vein and threading it down through the superior vena cava. The brachial artery also may be used. The catheter is secured by sutures.

An intravenous pump must be used at all times, since fluid will not drip by gravity. It is a continuously closed system. One of the complications that can occur is yeast and bacterial infection, since the hyperalimentation fluid is an excellent environment for the growth of organisms.

Self-feeding problems resulting from deficits in postural control

Before children are allowed to feed themselves alone, they should be able to swallow liquids and then solids without choking. They will also need a degree of sitting balance and some ability to control head movements.

There comes a time when a child is psychologically ready for self-feeding and desires to try. The dilemma for the therapist is that, although the child may have sufficient control to bring a spoon to his mouth or drink from a cup, his movement may trigger associated reactions leading to abnormal oral mechanisms. It is not unusual to see increased tension in the mouth as a result of the physical effort required in self-feeding.

Mueller[25] believes that when children have already been feeding themselves or are at an age when they feel a strong urge to do so, they should be allowed to pursue self-help efforts. Her approach is to assist them with a minimum of body control through key points, such as the shoulder or wrist, and with jaw control and lip closure for swallowing. She might assist the child with the first few bites by placing her hand over the child's hand as he holds the spoon, then gradually withdraw her help. Using this approach, a therapist gives support at the wrist and elbow, then just at the elbow, and finally the therapist withdraws support, allowing the child to eat unassisted.

Morris[22] gives examples of how associated reactions occurring with self-feeding can be minimized through repositioning and support at key points. Along with the action of a child's bringing a spoon to his mouth, there is overflow into the opposite arm that causes internal rotation and abduction of the shoulder and flexion of the elbow—the result of associated reactions in the arm. This has the effect of reducing the child's oral ability during feeding. When a therapist gives assistance through stabilizing and straightening and outwardly rotating that arm, there is relief of total body tension, and this allows more normal mouth patterns.

Another illustration is when the child attempts to drink from a glass. He brings his head forward and his trunk follows—the result of poor postural control. To compensate, the child stabilizes his elbows on the table and hyperextends his head, instinctively adapting to the effect of gravity as well. The therapist stops or inhibits this tendency to pull into a flexed pattern by providing a type of positional stability through elevating the elbows and thus supporting the shoulders in abduction. Less effort is then exerted by the child in holding the cup, and drinking improves.

Morris[23] also emphasizes that the success of techniques and adaptive equipment depends on the environment of the home and school. One must separate what will work in therapy, from what is possible at home, from what affects the child in a busy, stimulating atmosphere of a classroom or cafeteria. The therapist can convey his or her concerns and work with parents and school personnel in reaching the best possible solutions.

ADAPTIVE EQUIPMENT

To facilitate ease of feeding, one may first consider stabilizing the plate and cup. If the child is unable to grasp, a variety of handles can be evaluated. Some are built up or contoured to fit the hand or have straps to secure the spoon in the hand. To scoop food onto the spoon, the child may need a dish with a raised edge. These "scoop dishes" are available in many commercial designs. They make self-feeding easier by preventing the food from sliding off the plate. To bring the spoon to the mouth, further help may be needed in the form of a curved, extended handle. A cup with a handle on either side may be required initially so that the hands may be used bilaterally for greater stabilization. Further suggestions for equipment are included in Exhibit 12-2.

One piece of equipment sometimes considered is the cerebral palsy feeder. This device was designed for the child who has some gross arm function and limited grasp. The device assists the child in lifting the spoon to his mouth, and it can be lowered again by the child's simple arm movement. Manipulation of large wooden knobs raises and lowers the spoon and rotates the plate.

Self-feeding problems resulting from limitations in mobility and strength

Feeding difficulties may arise as the result of contracture, weakness, structural deformity, or lack of body parts. Such problems require a very different approach to feeding than those resulting from incoordination and poor postural tone. Here self-feeding is not so much a matter of remediation as it is of adaptation. To better understand why a child may have difficulties, let us look at the requirements for feeding from the standpoint of range and strength.

PROBLEMS IN RANGE AND ADAPTATION

Beginning with the neck, slight flexion is needed to look down at the table surface and monitor the hand as it manipulates utensils or finger foods. One has only to observe a child with severe involvement of the cervical spine in juvenile arthritis to appreciate how the lack of neck flexion can inhibit the visual field.

We are inclined to take for granted our ability to open and close our mouths and chew food, but this function is dependent on the range of the temporomandibular joint. With joint involvement, feeding can be painful and movement restricted.

The alignment of the vertebral column with its multiple joints can affect the position of the head relative to the body. For example, in severe scoliosis a child may need to support his trunk with at least one arm to maintain balance. This can slow and interfere with his ability to feed.

The elbow joint is the primary junction for bringing the hand to and from the mouth. A 60-degree arc of motion, between 60 degrees of flexion and 120 degrees of extension, is considered functional range. Contractures greater than this arc in either direction can compromise reaching the eating surface and reaching the mouth.

Lack of mobility and fixed contracture in the forearm, wrist, and fingers limit one's ability to grasp a utensil and to hold it at the required angle for food scooping and presentation to the mouth. An example of a feeding problem was presented by an adolescent whose wrist was subluxed and fused in flexion and ulnar deviation. She also had little supination available. This caused the spoon to approach her opposite cheek area rather than her lips. Limitations in supination can also result in spilling as the spoon is elevated.

EXHIBIT 12-2

Supporting function through adaptive aids

Function	Adaptive aid
Arm placement	*Suspension sling:* A device to support the upper extremity. Cuffs fit under the elbow and wrist and are spring-suspended from overhead bars. Assisted motions are shoulder horizontal abduction and adduction, shoulder external and internal rotation, shoulder abduction, and elbow flexion and extension.
	Mobile arm support (MAS): A frictionless arm support using the concept of the inclined plane. A trough supports the forearm and connects to a series of movable bars with adjustable stops. The unit fastens to a wheelchair with brackets. The MAS provides movement in space and helps weak shoulder and elbow muscles to position the hand.
Wrist support	*Cock-up splint:* A simple splint that extends from the distal palmar crease, supports the wrist, and ends two thirds up the distance of the forearm. It stabilizes and positions the wrist to provide mechanical advantage needed by fingers in prehension and grasp.
Grasp	*Universal cuff (utensil holder):* A cuff that fits around the palm, has a pocket for the insertion of handles of utensils, and can be used when grasp is not possible.
	Built-up handle: An enlarged handle that facilitates grasp.
	Modified handle for cup or glass: A projection on the utensil that will accommodate the child's grasping pattern. NOTE: Maintain low center of gravity when weakness is present.
Reach	*Curved handle:* A handle adjusted to angle so that the child can reach his body parts.
	Extended handle: An elongated handle that provides reach. It becomes less stable with length and weight.
	Sandwich holder: A plastic holder with rubber band that grips the sandwich; inserted in universal cuff.
Supination	*Swivel spoon:* Spoon with swivel mechanism that levels the bowl when wrist or finger motion is gone.
Stabilization of equipment or food	*Nonslip mat:* A nonslip plastic material that holds plates and glasses steady.
	Plate guard: A rim that clips onto a plate, provides a "wall" against which food is scooped by the fork or spoon.
	Scoop dish: A plate molded low in front and high in back to facilitate scooping food.
One-handed feeding	*Rocker knife:* A knife with curved blade; cuts with rocking motion provided by one hand. Other aids that can be used are the plate guard and nonslip mat.
Self-feeding	*Electric or battery feeder:* An expensive device that enables self-feeding without using the arms; requires only slight head motion to control switches; must be set up by caregiver.

PROBLEMS IN STRENGTH AND ADAPTATION

A child with weakness will often compensate and seek to stabilize body parts through external support, as in propping elbows on the table to keep the trunk from leaning forward. Then the neck is extended to bring it in line and out of the pull of gravity. Thus the child may tend to exaggerate postures to enlist or eliminate gravity. A child with a high spinal cord injury will sometimes use all available motion in his neck to reach toward a spoon of food with his mouth. By instinct, a child with weakness may first flex the elbow before raising the arm, thereby shortening the lever arm and changing mechanical forces. By raising feeding height, children lacking strength in the shoulder and elbows are able to bring the hand to the mouth by eliminating gravity. A higher surface on which arms are propped also serves to support an unsteady trunk.

Adaptive aids and techniques are among the most useful measures in helping children with these problems achieve greater independence. They offer the therapist the opportunity to work closely with parents and child, to enlist their help in evaluating equipment, and to choose the items that they determine to be the most useful in solving self-maintenance problems in the home setting.

EQUIPMENT CRITERIA

The choice of an adaptive aid is a cooperative decision to be made by the child, parents, and therapists as they evaluate its effectiveness together. Adolescents who are striving to identify with their peer group tend to reject aids that call attention to their disabilities. Younger children are easily frustrated if the aid's use exceeds their coordination abilities, their attention spans, or gadget tolerances. Some criteria to consider in selecting aids include the following.

1. The aid must be developmentally appropriate. It should not exceed the child's ability to manipulate it. Results from its use should be consistent, predictable, and fairly easily obtainable.
2. The aid should have a pleasing color, texture, and odor, with as close to normal appearance as possible and simple, flowing design lines.
3. The aid must be sturdy.
4. The aid should show good mechanical advantage and be well balanced with a low center of gravity.
5. The aid should be easily cleaned and stored.
6. The aid must be economical, replaceable, and easily obtainable.

Behavioral problems in eating and self-feeding

Children with developmental delays or motor difficulties are potential candidates for behavioral problems having to do with food, just as are children with primary emotional behavioral disorders. Parents, anxious about their child's nutritional intake, can easily fall into a pattern of urging, nagging, or bribing their child to eat. When parents are confused about appropriate expectations for their child, they may show even greater inconsistency in approaches and responses and feel even more stress in dealing with their child's behavior. Because no one can make a child eat, the child often assumes control of the feeding environment. Howard[17] stated, "Food becomes the vehicle through which the child expresses his feelings and attempts to gain control over an environment in which he may have little or no control" (p. 580). Moreover, if the child has an early history of being gavage or force fed, he may not have learned to establish a trusting relationship with the individual feeding him. Food may have been a symbol of frustration or conflict rather than love, and it initiates a host of feeding and behavioral problems.

FEEDING BEHAVIORS CAUSING CONCERN

A variety of behaviors can appear. Among those most commonly seen are refusal of the child to eat specific foods; bizarre feeding patterns; gagging; vomiting or rumination; unwillingness to finger feed or self-feed; limited attention span at mealtime; and disruptive behavior. Physical conditions that may result from feeding behaviors include slowed growth; in some cases, an excessive weight gain; anemia; lack of appetite or increased appetite; and constipation. These conditions are of concern to parents and professionals alike.

APPROACHES TO CHANGING BEHAVIOR

Professionals use a number of approaches to change eating patterns. One approach is the *mealtime assessment,* where mealtime behaviors of parent and child are observed. O'Neil[26] outlined the method by which interactions are analyzed in terms of the antecedent events, the behavior, and the consequences revolving around eating. Factors that contribute to behaviors include the parents' expression of attitudes, values, interests, beliefs, and their caretaking behaviors. On the child's side, behavior is influenced by intrinsic factors: the child's individual growth patterns, his learning potential, and his ability to incorporate increasingly complex experiences into his current state of thinking and functioning.

A basic concept in behavioral assessment is that behaviors are increased, maintained, or decreased by the consequences that immediately follow them. Through the observational assessment, parent-child mealtime interaction is analyzed according to most frequent eating and noneating behaviors. The team members help parents identify those child behaviors that they wish to change, as well as the appropriate eating behaviors that they wish to foster in their children. From the analysis, team members determine appropriate consequences that affect behavior; this can vary from child to child. Reinforcement and consistency are keystones for success in changing patterns.

Another approach is *teaching feeding behaviors.* This method is appropriate for the child who needs to have the feeding process broken down into sequential steps according to his developmental level. Reinforcement is given when the first step is learned, and other steps are added in succession as skill grows. This technique is sometimes referred to as *shaping. Fading* is a procedure in which one first gives maximal assistance and then withdraws help as the child's skill develops.

THE VALUE OF THE TEAM APPROACH

When behavior interferes with eating function, perhaps one of the most important things to remember is to seek help and collaboration with other professionals: the nutritionist, the social worker, the nurse, and significant others. Feeding is very complex, particularly when viewed within the framework of social interaction. Professionals need to be clear about their roles as they analyze behavior, design programs, and implement steps for change.

Other factors for a therapist to consider

COLLABORATION WITH THE SPEECH PATHOLOGIST

Speech pathologists specialize in identifying specific language deficits and help the occupational therapist in a number of ways. They are able to clarify the interrelationship between breathing patterns and phonation and can detect the fine, discrete coordination required of muscles for articulation. They are highly skillful in diagnosing language difficulties as a result of injury to speech centers and are able to obtain information about children's learning styles.

The *close tie between acquisition of feeding skills and later development of speech* is widely accepted among therapists. Indeed the tie is considered so close that in some settings it is the speech pathologist who evaluates eating problems and carries out the treatment program and consults with the occupational therapist on eye-hand motor function. Two of the leading authorities on eating problems, Morris and Mueller, are specialists in prespeech. Morris[23] believes the relationship between feeding and speech skills remains relatively unexplored and calls for more study. She describes how the function of feeding can be used to facilitate the movement required for speech. First, the child adds movement components before these are built into speech itself. The movements are facilitated at the automatic level, rather than the cognitive level. The therapist provides feedback and sensory awareness and facilitates a more volitional repetition of movement. Both food and the automatic feeding movements can be used to promote easier voicing and wider variety of articulatory movement.

Morris[23] provides examples of how this can be done. As the child approximates his lips to remove food from the spoon, the therapist may focus on the word *more*. The child is then able to immediately experience the proprioceptive feedback from the motor pattern to produce the word *more*.

If the child demonstrates good tongue tip elevation during the swallowing of pureed foods from the spoon, a spoonful of food can be used to reinforce correct tongue tip placement for words beginning with *t, d,* or *n*. Thus feeding movement facilitates speech movement.

Morris[23] emphasizes the *need for communication systems between feeder and child*. For the child who is developmentally above 18 months but unable to speak, Morris suggests such practical measures as a mealtime placemat containing pictures or symbols for concepts such as "more," "no more," "something else," "yummy," and "yuk." An older, nonverbal child with many persons who feed him benefits from a feeding procedure book with photographs that make the feeding process clear to others in terms of the child's comfort and function.

A speech pathologist and occupational therapist have much knowledge to share in mutually promoting functions of eating and speech.

COLLABORATION WITH THE NUTRITIONIST

Nutrients from food provide the raw material that allows the body to function and grow. Thousands of chemical compounds are broken down by the body to provide energy. Nutritionists are able to estimate the amount of nutrients needed for the individual child based on his size and motor dysfunction. Nutritionists understand the nutrient requirements at various stages of growth and identify the critical times for the introduction of foods with a variety of flavors and textures. They provide essential information for a feeding program that encompasses not only the function of the oral motor mechanisms but also the quality and amount of food required for health.

There are many insights to be gained from reviewing *nutritional research*. Some investigators believe the degree to which the mouth area is involved directly affects nutrition and that mouth involvement and general growth closely parallel one another.[28] A high calorie density diet has been recommended for those having poor oral skills. On the other hand, Hammond and others[16] found that the degree of mental retardation impeding self-help skills was a more significant factor in influencing dietary intake than the motor deficits imposed in neurological disorders. While studies may be debatable, they point to the overall effects of nutritional intake.

Two factors that affect children's eating performance are *medication* and *constipation*. Nutritionists can clarify the effects of medication on food intake. Medications can interfere with feeding in a global way: they can alter taste sensation, diminish appetite, promote insatiable appetite, and cause drowsiness. Anticonvulsant drugs prescribed to control seizures increase a child's need for vitamin D, alter folic acid metabolism, and interfere with riboflavin status.

One of the most frequently encountered problems in a disabled child is constipation. Fiber and fluid are important ingredients in ameliorating this common condition. Coarse fibrous foods such as raw fruits and vegetables are helpful, but when a child cannot chew, other preventive measures include the use of well-soaked bran, whole grain cereals, and foods with natural laxative effects.

In summary, there are many questions to present to the nutritionist who can help therapists make the eating program a nutritional model for parents to follow.

COLLABORATION WITH PARENTS

Successful feeding in early infancy is generally regarded as one of the measures of a parent's child-rearing competencies. It is no wonder that a mother can feel threatened by the professional who questions how she feeds the child and observes quietly as she struggles to place a spoon of food within her child's mouth. A sensitive therapist will recognize the potential for feelings of inadequacy on the part of the parents and will strive to *reinforce those good parenting behaviors observed.* The therapist will exercise caution in intruding on the mothering role but at the same time present a model for parents to follow. The goal is to improve the child's eating function and also to help parents acquire skill in management and to increase their feelings of competency.

There are *communication measures* to consider that can contribute to the parents' ease and receptiveness. First of all, determine what they perceive as the problem, what they want to change. Explore how this child's development differs from that of siblings. As one begins to investigate positioning, consult with the mother and father regarding the position for feeding that is comfortable for them. During the feeding, observe how well they perceive cues from their child and help them to be aware of communication gestures. Finally, provide the *environmental support* that enables the child and parents to relax, whether this be a quiet, dimly lighted room or one with privacy and free from distraction.

Data collection is an important part of the interview. Information is gathered on how long it takes to feed the child, the person or persons responsible for feeding, past successful or unsuccessful methods, utensils used, and whether there are behavioral problems and how they are handled. Investigation includes the kind of responses the child makes to new foods, their texture, smell, and temperature; how the child handles different kinds of food (liquids, semisolids, and solids); what preferences and dislikes exist; and how often the child feeds during the day.

It is unwise to spend the entire time presenting questions to the parents. For that reason, some therapists prefer the use of a questionnaire that parents can complete at their convenience. This allows time to carefully consider their child's eating patterns. Excellent examples of questionnaires are presented in works by Finnie[12] and Morris.[23]

During the evaluation session the therapist can also observe the *feeding environment:* the general atmosphere of parent-child interaction, the techniques used, the parental attitudes toward feeding, and the kinds of positive and negative reinforcing behaviors displayed. Above all, the therapist seeks to involve parents in the problem-solving process (Chapter 8).

TOILETING
Prerequisites for toilet training

In the literature there is a great deal of information and advice for parents on when and how to embark on a toilet training program with their child. Emphasis is rightly placed on the readiness of the parties involved. Certainly, parental attitudes are a strong factor in the ease with which progress is made.

Independent toileting is an important self-maintenance milestone with wide variation among individual children. It carries considerable sociological significance. Self-sufficiency can be a determinant when a school is considering whether to accept a child into a regular classroom program. Like other self-care skills, toileting is a complex task requiring a series of learning subskills. But before embarking on learning, a child must be physically, physiologically, and psychologically ready. Toileting consists of training sphincter reflexes and the volitional holding of urine and feces.

Physiological factors

At birth a newborn voids reflexively and involuntarily. Changes in position, handling by others, and other stimuli can trigger micturition. Voluntary control and restraint of the reflex, which is the method employed when control is established, is not available to the youngster until the spinal tract is myelinated to a level for bowel and bladder control at the lumbar and sacral areas. This is after the child is standing and walking alone. Bowel control precedes control over the bladder, and studies indicate girls are trained an average of 2.46 months earlier than boys.[10] Daytime bowel and bladder training is usually attained by 30 months, but bladder nighttime control may not be accomplished before 5 and 6 years of age.

The child's awareness

Another indication of readiness for toilet training is the child's awareness of discomfort after emptying bowel and bladder, as well as the ability to identify elimination as the cause of discomfort. There must be an awareness that characteristic sensations precede excretion. As early as 10 months the infant may begin to pay attention to the act of voiding. This can be detected by general facial expression and quieting behavior. By 14 months the need to eliminate may be indicated by gesture or action.

Other requirements for toilet training

The methods by which training is introduced vary, but most authorities agree on these fundamentals. First, there should be one or two significant people who are willing to devote time and effort to establishing patterns of toileting, and there must be a communication system between them and the child. Behaviorally, reinforcement is given for success, and harsh punishment for failure is avoided.

A gentle approach to toilet training

Brazelton[5] presents gradual steps for toilet training. He suggests that after 18 months of age, a child can be placed on a potty chair with all his clothing on, avoiding the cold surface of the seat. Introduction can begin pleasantly by talking or reading aloud as the child sits there. Within a week or so one can try having the child sit on the chair without diapers. This is followed by dropping the dirty diaper into the potty chair to build an association between the chair and elimination. Finally, efforts are made to catch the stool or urine while the child sits on the chair, and this is done several times a day. As the child's interest grows, independence can be made easier and more pleasurable if he is dressed in comfortable clothes, including training pants, that allow him to manage clothing adjustment alone.

Brazelton[5] also speaks of the fears that toddlers may experience with toileting and the anxiety they may have associated with giving up the bowel movement as a part of themselves. He points to the value of repetitive play to help children overcome such feelings. Brazelton notes that boys hold back their bowel movements much more frequently than do girls, even as they achieve urine training. He urges patience and reassurance from the parents to help the children relax and to master the task at their own pace.

Because of interest and motivation toward bowel and bladder control, toddlers demonstrate curiosity toward their own and other's genital organs. They observe and feel their own urinary stream and may touch and feel the feces, and touch and manipulate their own genitals. Parents can help a toddler satisfy tactile and perceptual curiosity by providing a simple explanation or by presenting play activities with clay and water and containment and release themes.

Tasks to be mastered

To be truly independent in toileting, the child will need to manage fastenings, get the pants up and down, and in the case of a girl wearing a dress, hold the dress away from the buttocks—subskills usually achieved at about 4 years. Children will need to climb on the toilet and seat themselves. This occurs at about 3 years. By 5 they are successful in cleansing after toileting, and they can wash and dry their hands efficiently without supervision. Progress is accomplished in sequence, according to each child's unique pace of development.

Considerations when posture is unstable

The child with postural control deficits must first acquire sitting balance or do so through the support of equipment. One can readily see that the child with increased tone would have difficulty. This is shown early when the mother attempts to diaper the infant. She may first need to place a pillow under the infant's hips, then flex them and spread the legs apart to break up the strong extensor and adduction patterns in his legs. With unstable sitting posture, the child will have difficulty relaxing and maintaining a position for pressing down and emptying the bowels. It has been said that unless the toilet seat is low enough so that the feet rest firmly on the floor and some flexion of the thighs is possible, the accessory muscles that normally aid in defecation have little opportunity to fulfill their function. Every effort should be made to help the child feel posturally secure. The feet should always be supported, and if the child needs to rely on his hands for balance, toilet bars should be considered.

Finnie[12] offers suggestions for adapting potty chairs and toilet seats for children with poor postural control. For example, she suggests placing the toilet in a corrugated cardboard or wooden box when the child's balance improves. Across the top of the box, attach a bar for the child to hold onto for added security. Commodes that feature such modifications as adjustable legs; safety bars; angled legs for stability; and padded, upholstered, and adjustable backrests and headrests are available on the market. Commodes are also available with seat reducer rings, seat belts, and adjustable footrests.

How range and strength affect function

Children with weakness and limited range of motion face a number of difficulties with toileting. They may not be able to manage fastenings because of hand involvement, or they may have problems in sitting down or getting up from the toilet seat because of hip and knee contracture or quadriceps weakness. In such cases a raised toilet seat is a consideration. Most distressful of all their problems is when they are unable to supinate the hand, flex the wrist, or internally rotate and extend the arm to cleanse after a bowel movement. An anterior approach may be tried. It is important to caution girls against contamination from feces, which can cause vaginitis. If at all possible, girls should wipe the anus from the rear. Solutions to cleansing problems are difficult and often discouraging.

Again, adaptive devices are among the most helpful measures available. A combined bidet and toilet offers a means for total independence. Several models are available that attach to any standard toilet bowl. A self-

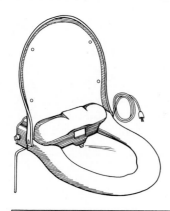

FIGURE 12-7

An electrically powered toilet bidet makes it possible to clean the perineal area independently without hands or paper.

contained mechanism spray-washes the perineal area with thermostatically controlled warm water, and dries it with a flow of warm air. Controls can be operated with the hand or foot (Figure 12-7). The unit is expensive but is worth considering, particularly for the sensitive adolescent. Other simple, inexpensive aids include various tong devices.

Loss of normal excretory function

Children with spinal cord injury or other conditions that produce a full or partial paralysis present a challenge for skin care when there is lack of sensation, and they require special management for bowel and bladder activities. Loss of control over these bodily functions can be infantilizing, producing embarrassment and decreased feelings of esteem. School-age children are characteristically modest about their bodies, and adolescents are struggling with identity issues and need to be like their peers.

BLADDER CONTROL

There are two types of bladder problems. When there is a lesion in the lumbar region or below, the bladder is flaccid. The reflex arc is not intact, and the bladder has lost all tone. The following terms are used for this condition: the lower motor neuron bladder and the atonic, or areflexic, bladder. When an injury occurs higher, above the level of bladder innervation, the reflex arc remains intact. Thus when the bladder is full, or its contents reach a critical level, it empties by reflex. In this situation the bladder is said to be a reflex bladder, an automatic bladder, or an upper motor neuron bladder. Training programs are undertaken to develop automatic responses in a spastic bladder. Children with a flaccid bladder cannot be trained because the bladder has no tone to empty. To determine if a child is a candidate for training, a number of tests may be carried out to measure the ability of the bladder to expel urine and to hold a particular amount of urine, depending on the size and age of the child.

There are a number of ways to manage urine collection. In boys one of the most common systems is by *condom drainage.* Boys are able to learn to apply and use this system independently, given sitting balance, hand dexterity, and alertness in following the procedure. With this external device system the condom is placed over the penis and is attached to a tube running down the leg to a collection bag that must be emptied at intervals. A common problem is skin breakdown where the condom is attached.

Managing the bladder can be more difficult for girls because of their anatomy. It is sometimes accomplished by an *indwelling catheter.* Boys may use this system as well. A Foley catheter consists of a small rubber tube and a balloon attachment. After the tube is inserted through the urethra to the bladder, the balloon is filled with sterile water, and this serves to keep the catheter in place. The tube drains the urine from the bladder to a collection bag. In some cases the catheter is clamped and unclamped at regular intervals to "train" the bladder to empty by reflex when the contents reach a critical amount. Bladder irrigation is a regular procedure when a catheter is used and is carried out periodically. This is done by injecting a benzalkonium (Zephiran) solution into the catheter to stir up sediment and prevent stopping up the catheter.

The catheter itself increases the likelihood of urinary infection and bladder stones, since it introduces a foreign body into the bladder. For this reason a high fluid intake is considered an important precautionary measure.

Credé's method is sometimes used to expel urine. With this method the hand is placed on the lower abdomen, on or above the bladder, and a gentle pressure downward is given. Balanced bladder function is attained if the amount of urine left in the bladder is 20% of bladder capacity or less. The Credé's method must be carefully executed to prevent reflux. When reflux occurs, urine goes up the ureters and then returns to the bladder, forming a pool for infection.

When urinary tract infection becomes chronic, a *suprapubic catheter* may become the system of choice. Here a catheter is placed directly into the bladder through the abdominal wall. Urine then drains through the catheter tube directly into a urinal bag.

Because of problems from infection and renal stones, an alternative method, *intermittent catheterization,* is increasingly used for management. The catheter is inserted into the bladder every 4 hours, then every 6 hours, to empty its contents and to promote an automatic bladder. It also offers the individual the advantage of being able to carry the catheter inconspicuously in a small bag. Self-catheterization has been successfully taught to children by nurses. A precaution to observe is to restrict fluid intake to prevent bladder distention. When there is partial control of bladder function, girls may wear disposable diapers or incontinence pants that are available in various styles and sizes.

When there are serious difficulties with the muscles or nerves controlling the bladder, congenital malformations of the urinary tract, obstructions, chronic infections, and scarring, physicians may recommend a surgical procedure, the *ileal conduit*. This is a detailed procedure, and children and parents need preparation and explanation. During the surgery a small section of the ileum (a few inches long) is resected, and the remaining ends of the small intestine are rejoined, leaving the digestive system intact. This separated section is then used to form a stoma in the abdominal wall. Ureters are severed near the bladder and are reattached so that the urine drains through the stoma into a collection pouch. The pouch must be emptied at intervals and periodically cleaned and replaced.

The procedure can have a deep psychological effect on children, especially the adolescent, since it represents a change in body image. Parents too express hostility and depression and question whether a daughter may bear children or whether it will impair a boy's masculinity. The surgery itself has no effect on sexual organs or childbearing.

BOWEL CONTROL

A basic principle for success in bowel reeducation is to have a regular, consistent evacuation of the bowel. The time for this is a matter of choice, but there should be a schedule that remains constant. In some cases, suppositories and a warm drink are given before evacuation. This stimulates contractions and relaxation of muscle fibers within the walls of the intestine that move the contents onward. Other techniques include digital stimulation, massage around the anal sphincter, or manual pressure by Credé's method on the abdomen.

Removal of the stool by hand may become necessary. Factors that contribute to ease in elimination include an adequate fluid intake and a regular diet. Stool softeners are sometimes used to maintain a stool of normal form and consistency.

Closely associated with bowel and bladder care is *care of the skin* in the perineal area. Skin should be cleansed thoroughly to protect the tissue against contact with waste matter and to eliminate odor. All children with decreased sensation are susceptible to decubiti, which are pressure sores that occur fairly rapidly when blood vessels are compressed, as around a bony prominence such as the ischial tuberosity. This can result in ischemia, or lack of tissue nourishment. Skin self-care for these children includes daily inspection of the skin by mirror and avoiding sitting in one position for long periods of time. There are also a variety of special cushions on the market designed to prevent tissue trauma.

A number of *surgical procedures* are carried out to construct alternative means for stool collection. One of these is a colostomy. An incision is made in the colon and a fistula, or tubelike passage, is made between the bowel and the abdominal wall. Special bags cover the opening and are emptied as needed. An ileostomy is a similar procedure in which the surgical opening occurs in the lower part of the small intestine.

SOCIAL ENVIRONMENT

To be socially acceptable, a child lacking bowel and bladder control needs to be helped with measures to eliminate odors. Odors can be produced by the collection devices, the collected urine, or stool. Appliances should be changed and cleaned regularly. They can be washed in a commercial cleanser or in a vinegar and water solution. Maintaining a good fluid intake will prevent a strong concentrated urine. If urine is alkaline, it is more likely to have a strong odor. Therefore keeping the urine acidic by drinking cranberry juice will not only cut down on odor, but it also prevents bacteria growth as well.

Of all self-care tasks, toileting may require the most sensitive approach on the part of those who work with the child on a self-maintenance program. Children may deny that they are unable to toilet themselves independently, or they may purposely restrict their fluid intake at school in an effort to avoid the need for elimination. Toileting can be a distressing, unverbalized problem that should be explored with great care after the child feels comfortable with the therapist.

Menstruation

Therapists should also be aware of a young girl's status regarding menstruation, which normally begins between 10 and 17 years of age. In particular, mentally retarded individuals may be viewed by others as never growing up, and their bodies, therefore, are viewed as remaining undeveloped too. Thus adults around mentally retarded adolescents neglect to prepare them for changes in their bodies and the onset of menarche. Consequently, its arrival can be traumatic and frightening. This undeniable indicator of puberty can be distressing to some parents, and their troubled feelings can be conveyed in a confusing way to their child. Families may require support and counseling in ways of giving their child reassuring, understandable explanations.

For the girl with a physical disability, it is also important that first experiences with menstruation be positive ones. Duffy[9] is an informative resource on the subject. She points to the possibility that the menses experience offers the young disabled female an affirmation of equality with her peers. Her body, though different in some ways, is operating normally in an area of particular significance, confirming her identity as a sexual being.

Duffy describes personal experiences of "differently abled" women, their feelings, problems, and solutions. For example, one subject who was cited found that using disposable diapers in the toddler size worked best during her menstrual period, because they were flat rectangles and the sticky tapes on the sides could be used to fasten them to the insides of underpants. Others report on the brands of tampons they find easiest to insert, as well as the best positions for insertion.

Another useful reference is the work of Friedman[13] who provides collective information on techniques and adaptive aids for bilateral high-level upper limb amputees. In general, there is still too little material available in the literature. This indirectly validates the expression of some young disabled persons that in this area of self-care there continues to be a lack of supportive assistance from medical and rehabilitation personnel.

DRESSING

An infant makes a first gesture to cooperate with dressing at about 1 year of age by holding out an arm or a leg while being dressed. By 18 months the child is beginning to remove his socks. At 3 years he is independent with pull-down garments but has some difficulty with turning the heel of a sock and does not know the front of garments from the back. Usually by 4 years of age he can turn clothing right side out and needs little assistance. By 5 years, he dresses with care except for some fastenings and tying bows. Normally it takes 4 years of practice—a combination of experimentation, repetition, and assistance—to master dressing.

It is easily understood that children must have the eye-hand coordination for manipulating fastenings, but in addition they must also have knowledge of their physical selves and how body parts are related.[6] They must know where their bodies are in space. As they attend to dressing tasks, they look at body movements. Kinesthetically they feel the position of their body parts and may even verbalize motor actions aloud. They consciously direct some body movements, whereas other movements are automatic and compensatory, enabling them to maintain equilibrium in the various positions they assume. They are aware of the two sides of their bodies and, because of neurological integration, are able to use their limbs cooperatively and reciprocally.

Children also look at the clothing they will wear and in doing so distinguish boundaries of the clothing article. They visually scan for details, and as the attention and focus of their eyes shift selectively, they separate foreground and background. Discriminatively, they recognize the form and totality of an article of clothing and categorize it as a sweater, shirt, sock, or other item.

This is an extension of the sensory process that involves concept formation. Having identified a clothing article, they maintain a visual form constancy of it, even if it is turned upside down. Through experience they accumulate space ideas.

The motor components of dressing—balance, range, strength, and control of movement—can be observed and, consequently, are more readily comprehended. What is less clearly understood are the internal mechanisms at work: the way the child receives and processes sensory information leading to a response in attending to the task at hand.

Common problems

PERCEPTUAL DYSFUNCTION

From the description of the dressing process one can begin to predict some of the problems that may occur with dressing. Among those children having perceptual deficits, difficulties may exist in distinguishing right and left sides of the body, in putting a shoe on the correct foot, or in turning the heel of a sock. A child may be unable to tell the front of his clothing from the back, or identify which leg goes with which pant leg or which sleeve goes with which arm. If one observes closely, there may be evidence that the child avoids crossing the midline by performing dressing tasks on the right side of the body with the right hand and those on the left with the left hand. At the other end of the spectrum, a child will most likely have great difficulty with fastenings and in tying shoelaces, tasks that require the two hands to work together.

INTELLECTUAL LIMITATIONS

Children with mental retardation tend to be chaotic in their organization of perceptual stimuli and, in addition to problems with left-right discrimination, may be unable to make connections with words such as "above," "behind," or "in front of" insofar as their own bodies are concerned.[7] Normally children become aware of these important dualisms between 2 and 3 years of age and are able to attach verbal labels to them between 4 and 5 years. Spatial relations are first mastered in the immediate areas of mouth, vision, and touch, and then they gradually extend out and away from the individual.

The child who has intellectual limitations cannot remember instructions and has a short attention span. Behaviorally there may be a low tolerance for frustration because the child cannot perform and dress himself as quickly as his siblings can. Language skills may be inefficient, which restricts the child's verbal capacity to express his frustration. This may increase when the child is faced with tasks that require fine manipulations. Coordination too may be impaired, as shown in attempts to button, snap, zip, or buckle.

To acquire independence, the child may require a special approach. After making a baseline assessment the therapist carefully analyzes each dressing task into its fine component parts so that the child can progress slowly in steps, in a chaining process, with reinforcement. Excellent examples of task analysis and teaching approaches are given by Copeland and others.[7] Their work is a valuable resource for those working with children who require great patience and consistency over a considerable period of time.

OTHER PROBLEMS

Children with various conditions may find dressing difficult because of the *coordination* and the range and strength required for pulling clothes on and off and connecting fasteners. Youngsters with arthritis who have painful fingers frequently require assistance during a flare-up of their disease. They may be unable to move their arms freely and to reach to areas of their body. Children with the use of only one hand will find it hard to zip trousers, tie shoelaces, and button shirts or blouses. Dressing is tedious and tiring. In most cases they learn adaptive techniques, often through their own experimentation. Tasks can be made easier by using simple measures such as dressing the involved extremity first or by using adaptive aids such as button hooks, rings on zippers, one-handed shoe fasteners, or Velcro closures (Figure 12-8).

Dressing infants and dysfunctional children

Although the common approach to dressing an infant is to do so while he is lying supine, the supine position frequently increases extensor tone in those infants with neurological impairment. For that reason, some therapists advocate placing the infant prone across one's knees with the infant's hips flexed and abducted, thus breaking up the extensor-adduction tone. As soon as the infant gains head and trunk control, there are advantages to the sitting position, with the infant's back resting against and supported by the caregiver's trunk. In this arrangement the infant has an opportunity to observe his body. Knowledge of the physical self is to be encouraged whenever possible. As early as 14 months some infants begin to point to a named body part.

During dressing, the caregiver carefully bends the infants hips and knees before putting on his shoes and socks (Figure 12-9), and brings the infant's shoulders forward before putting his arm through a sleeve. Attention is continually directed to positioning and to keeping the body in symmetrical alignment. When a child achieves sitting balance, a good way to proceed with dressing is to place the child on the floor and later on a low stool, continuing to provide support where needed from the back. Orientation to the body and its various parts should remain a focus in the social interaction. The caregiver can help the child understand how his body relates to his clothes and to the various positions—the arm goes through a sleeve and the head goes through the neck of a garment. There are many perceptual concepts to be explored and learned as a part of the dressing procedure.

When the child is older and heavier, there may be no alternative but to dress him while he is lying supine. Placing a hard pillow under the child's head, thus raising his shoulders a little, will make it easier to bring his arms forward and to bend his hips and knees. If it is

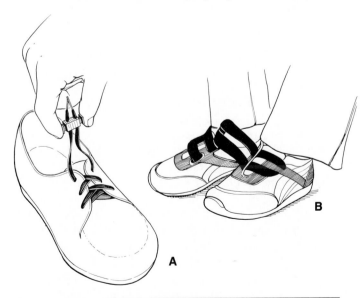

These shoelace fasteners can be managed with one hand. **A,** Spring tension blocks. **B,** Velcro.

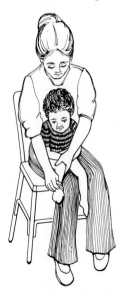

When dressing the child who is hypertonic, carefully flex the hip and knee before putting on socks and shoes.

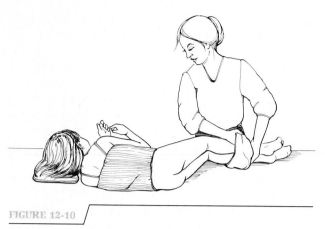

FIGURE 12-10

Sidelying may decrease tone and make dressing easier.

possible to maintain the child in a sidelying position, this posture may make it easier to bring his shoulders and head forward, to bring his arm forward, and to straighten his elbow (Figure 12-10).

Self-dressing techniques

A DEVELOPMENTAL APPROACH

Gesell[14] described with amusing accuracy the child learning backward rather than forward. Characteristically, one undresses before he dresses. This is an important guideline in setting expectations. Self-dressing can be introduced in a natural way, at bedtime, by allowing the child to complete the final step in pulling off a garment. Similarly, when the child becomes more goal directed and motivated to be independent, he is ready to try the more difficult tasks of learning to put on clothing. Again, the caregiver can begin by putting the garment on the child and then allowing the child to complete the action. Gradually the child learns to do a little more, eventually accomplishing mastery.

POSITIONING AND SUPPORT

The child who has hand skills but poor balance may be able to take advantage of the function he possesses when he is in a sidelying position with the effect of gravity lessened. For the child who can sit but is unstable, a corner of two adjoining walls or a corner seat on the floor may provide enough postural support for independent dressing. Finnie[12] suggests using chairs as supporting devices while the child either kneels on the floor or stands holding on, particularly when balancing on one leg, as when pulling on pants.

Associated reactions may occur as the child starts to use both hands. Thus one hand may be needed for holding on, while the other hand performs the task. Many dressing tasks require bilateral use of the hands. It is learned too that balance is more fragile as one reaches out with the arms, and this occurs frequently when donning overhead garments and reaching to the periphery of the body.

TASK ANALYSIS

When planning a dressing program, a therapist can assist the child and parents by refining procedures. Additionally, a part of good therapy is to increase the options for function by opening up a variety of ways to solve problems from which child and parents may choose. Perhaps the parents will elect to change the selection of clothing, finding this a better solution. Such a flexible approach has been suggested by Orelove and Gibbons.[27]

The following outline offers choices in problem solving, either through clothing selection and changes or by use of a technique that is feasible for the child.

Pull-up garments. Clothing aids that facilitate independence include loops sewn inside the waistbands of pants and skirts to assist with pulling; elasticized waistbands, provided the bands do not restrict pulling movements; and pressure tape as a substitute for conventional fastenings. If zippers are used, consider enlarging the grasping surface by adding a metal ring or fabric loop.

As previously noted, Finnie[12] advises that the task of donning garments will be difficult for the child who is unstable in standing or when required to balance on one foot. Sitting or lying on the floor is to be encouraged so that once the feet are through the pant legs or skirt band, the child can roll to either side while pulling up the waistband. If trunk balance allows, the child may kneel to pull up the garment once the waistband is above the knees. Having a chair close by is useful for support.

Pullover garments. The most important feature for ease in donning pullover shirts and sweaters is an easy opening for the head. It should be a neckline that expands, such as one made of rib-knit fabric. Again, consider flexible, elasticized waistbands and large sleeve openings. Stretchy knit fabrics allow children to experiment with movements as they gradually become more efficient in dressing.

For perceptual orientation it is helpful to have the child lay the garment on lap, floor, or table, front side down. Then, reaching out and opening the bottom of the garment, one arm can be pushed into the corresponding, or ipsilateral, sleeve, followed by the arm on the other side. After the arms are in the sleeves, the bottom of the garment can then be grasped with one hand and pulled over the head.

If the fabric has sufficient give and the child has adequate trunk balance, an alternate technique is simply to pull the garment over the head and then hold a sleeve open with one hand while pushing the other arm through. Repeat for the other side. An important point for making dressing easier is *always put clothing on the affected limb first.*

Front-opening garments. Selecting sleeves as loose as possible also applies to front-opening shirts, jackets, and sweaters. Fullness in the back of the garment through pleats, gathers, or gussets will allow more freedom in movement.

One of the most common techniques used by children with coordination or weakness problems is flipping the garment over the head. This is done by laying the garment on the lap, floor, or table, front side up, with the neck of the garment closest to the body. The child then puts an arm in each sleeve, working each down until the hand is visible. The next step is to duck the head forward while extending the arms over the head. Shrugging the shoulders and pulling down with the arms will help the garment fall down into place.

Buttons. If a child is learning to dress, avoid buttons in the early stage of training by selecting pullover styles or by sewing buttons on the right side of the garment and using pressure tape for fastening. When buttoning is introduced, provide flat buttons large enough to grasp and ones that are not sewn tightly. Buttons with shanks may be easier to grasp. The location of buttons will affect the child's success in fastening. They should be easy to see, possibly of a contrasting color, and easy to reach. Have the child begin buttoning with the bottom button so that is is possible to see the hands working. Having once secured the bottom button, it becomes easier to line up the other ones.

Zippers. A useful reminder is to test a zipper at the time a garment is purchased to be sure it glides easily. In general, nylon coil zippers are pliable and less likely to snag than metal ones.

When the child attempts to zip, give instructions on how to make the zipper taut by holding the garment below the zipper with one hand while pulling up the zipper tab with the other. To pull up a side zipper with one hand, hold the bottom of the zipper by leaning against a steady table or a wall.

Socks. Children are frequently frustrated when attempting to don socks because the socks may be too tight and unyielding or the tops may be edged with tight elastic. Soft, stretchy fabric and a larger size alleviate strain in pulling. Tube socks eliminate problems with heel placement. Sewing loops on both sides of the socks may make them easier to pull into place.

A technique that makes sock donning more successful for the child is folding or rolling down the upper part of the sock over the foot portion so that the toes can be placed directly into the foot of the sock.

Shoes. Styles that provide a broad, long opening will help children who have limited ankle motion. Tabs at the heel help the child to pull. Pressure-sensitive tape closures eliminate lacing and tying.

As previously suggested, shoes can be put on more easily if the leg is flexed and toes are pointing down. As the foot slides forward, encourage the child to push down at the heel. Keep the laces very loose when donning the shoe during the training period. Long-handled shoehorns are helpful, as are the tabs on the heels of some sport shoes.

Special considerations in clothing

FOR EASE IN TOILETING

For children who wear diapers, a full-length crotch opening with a zipper or Velcro closure will make changes easier. Girls may enjoy wearing wraparound skirts, and these are easy to put on and adjust for toileting. When children wear leg bags, they can reach and drain them with greater ease when their pants have zippers or Velcro along the seams.

FOR USE OF CRUTCHES

Children who use full-length crutches may tend to pull and tear their sleeves. Features to consider are double-stitched underarm seams or sleeves with gussets, knit inserts, or action pleats.

FOR CHILDREN SITTING

Most clothing is made for individuals in a standing position. For those who spend long hours in a wheelchair, the sitting position can cause pulling and strain on some areas of the garment and a surplus of fabric in others. Alterations can be made to provide more comfort in sitting, and directions to do so are presented by Kennedy[20] and Kernaleguen.[21] In general, moderate fullness in both skirts and trousers is recommended for children in wheelchairs.

FOR CHILDREN WEARING BRACES

The child who wears a brace may need to have clothing reinforced to protect against rubbing. Ideas include sewing fabric patches inside the garment where friction will occur and reinforcing all seams that will receive stress.

Other adaptive aids

Other tools to facilitate dressing include a dressing stick (particularly when range of motion is limited) and stocking aid. This latter device often proves to be frustrating to children and requires considerable ankle movement.

Increased attention to the needs of the disabled individual has been shown over the last decade, with some adaptive clothing becoming available through catalogue supply companies. Because of marketing volume, there is a limited range of choice and a higher cost per item factor, but a beginning has been made to provide attractive, functional clothing.

Even more promising is the literature with practical suggestions for those with sewing skills. Kernaleguen[21] presents sewing instructions for a variety of garments and aids. She is a strong advocate of providing attractive, fashionable clothing for the disabled, and she stresses that clothing should meet functional requirements, yet conform in appearance to peer group standards and fashion trends. Modifications should be inconspicuous, and, in general, the appearance of the clothing should not single out the wearer in any way. When possible, clothing should conceal the handicap or at least not attract attention to it. The clothing should contribute to the wearer's sense of well-being. Functionally the design of the clothing should enable the wearer to take care of personal needs as much as possible, help maintain proper body temperature, and provide freedom of movement.

GROOMING AND HYGIENE

Good grooming habits are important for all children but take on added significance for the disabled. At an early age the child with a disability needs to be encouraged and helped to achieve cleanliness.

Bathing

Bathing should be a pleasurable activity, but for the parent of a child who lacks balance it can be a tedious task that requires constant attention and alertness. The work involved multiplies as the child grows and becomes larger and heavier.

Finnie[12] outlines a number of measures to make bathing easier. As has been stressed repeatedly, positioning and handling are prime considerations. The child with a strong startle reaction should receive special mention, since triggering the reaction can result in sudden loss of balance. Keeping the child's head and arms forward before lifting and maintaining them there while lowering the child into the tub are advisable. Finnie suggests handling the child slowly and gently, and when the child is old enough, telling him what is going to happen next, including turning the water faucets on and off and draining water from the tub. It is a good idea to drain the tub and wrap the child in a towel before lifting him from the tub.

Making the child feel safe and secure can also be aided by special equipment that gives the support needed. There are bath hammocks that fully hold the body and enable the parent to wash the child thoroughly (Figure 12-11, *A*).

Various kinds of bath seats are available to support the young child. The Safa Bath Seat (Figure 12-11, *B*) is obtained through the Spastics Society of Great Britain.[15] There is also an inflatable chair made from strong waterproof canvas that gives support in the water when weighted down by the child. A simple, inexpensive way for giving security is to use a plastic laundry basket lined with foam at its bottom (Figure 12-11, *C*). Commercially, a light, inconspicuous bath support (Figure 12-11, *D*) offers good design features. The front half of the padded support ring swings open for easy entry and then locks securely, holding the child at the chest to give trunk stability. For the seriously involved youngster lying supine in the tub in shallow water, a horseshoe-shaped inflatable bath collar (Figure 12-11, *E*) serves to support the neck and keep the child's head above water level.

Some parents and children find a hand-held shower head useful in removing soap suds. A long-handled bath brush or sponge helps in reaching body parts. Children with limited grasp may be able to wash themselves with a bathmitt. If a child is unable to extend his fingers for washing, the parent may try to facilitate relaxation by stroking downward on the top of the child's hand with a washcloth and then trying to flex the wrist. As a last measure the parent could straighten each finger, beginning with the little finger.[8]

Nonslip bath mats are essential for safety, both beside the tub and in the tub. Grab bars and their placement require careful thought and planning in each individual case.

The parents' safety also should be addressed. They should be cautioned to protect their backs and be taught good body mechanics. To lessen strain, it is best for the adult to sit on a stool beside the tub or kneel on a cushion. Lifting is done with knees bent and the back straight, using the legs for power.

Oral hygiene

Toothbrushing can be especially difficult for the child with sensitivity. For that and other reasons, when assistance is given, the teeth should be brushed slowly and gently. This will help to prevent fear of the toothbrush. A small, soft brush is easier to move around in the mouth, especially if the child has a tongue thrust or gag reflex. When gums are tender, a soft sponge tip called a toothette can be substituted for a brush. This is a disposable product.

If a child has problems with a weak grasp, the handle can be enlarged with sponge rubber, or, if necessary, a Velcro strap can be added. When the difficulty is a matter of wrist coordination and arm movement, an electric toothbrush can be evaluated for use. This proves to be a good solution in some cases, but the unit may be too heavy for every child to manage. Some electric brushes have dual controls, moving from side to side and up and down, which allows for good cleaning of teeth and gums. To help with managing toothpaste, a

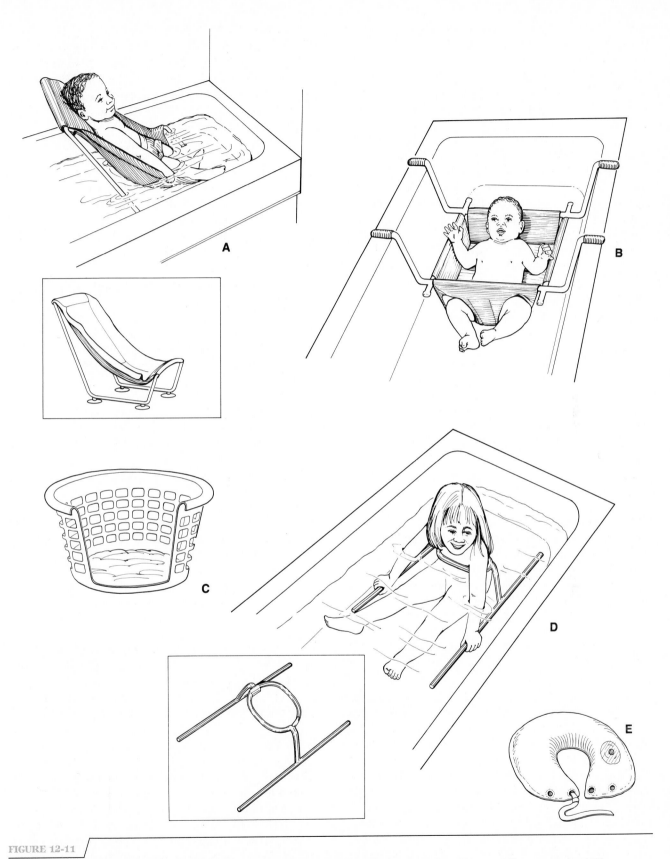

FIGURE 12-11

Adapted seating equipment. **A,** The hammock chair is adjustable and equipped with oversized suction feet. It fully supports the child who has no sitting balance and poor head control. **B,** The Safa Bath Seat is useful for bathing toddlers. **C,** The front of a plastic laundry basket is cut out to allow room for the child's legs. The basket gives security during first baths in a large tub. **D,** The trunk support is lightweight and compact and fits all bathtubs. **E,** The inflatable bath collar can be used when the child is either supine or prone.

long handle attached to the bottom of the tube helps in squeezing paste onto the brush.

Hair care

A simple style and good haircut are among the easiest ways to facilitate hair care, but children will want to identify with their peers and observe current fads. It is sometimes less tiring and gives greater stability when the child supports both arms on a table while combing or brushing his hair. A large comb or a brush with a thick handle may be easier for the child to use. A mirror at the proper height should be placed so that progress with personal grooming can be checked. When the child is unable to reach his head, extended handles can be tried. A hose attached to the faucet helps when washing hair over a basin or tub. If flexibility of the neck is a problem, a plastic shampoo tray can be fitted around the neck to direct water and suds away from the face.

Fingernail care

Caring for fingernails is often a trial for any child but is especially difficult when there are coordination problems or when the child has use of only one hand. Two styles of nailbrushes are useful. One is suction based and is used by rubbing the nails across the brush. The other has a curved handle that fits over one hand and then can be used to brush the nails of the other. A child may be able to file his fingernails if an emery board is taped to the edge of a table.

Confidence in one's appearance is essential to an individual's sense of worth. Good grooming and attractive clothing are strong allies in inviting positive responses from others. When children present an acceptable image to their cultural group, they in turn potentially receive stable, consistent, clear messages that help to shape a healthy self-concept.

MOBILITY
SUSAN A. PROCTER

The mobility of a child has a tremendous impact on his life experiences and overall development. The ability to move from one point in space to another enables the child to get to know his world and the people and objects in it. Mobility enhances physical development, perception, social interaction, autonomy, and knowledge of the environment. When a child's mobility is impaired, other areas of development can become delayed secondary to limited access to people, objects, and events. For instance, the child who is unable to roll or crawl over to his toys will forgo opportunities to manipulate and explore them unless they are brought to him. The child who takes 20 minutes to propel a wheelchair

to class and is fatigued on arrival misses parts of class and has expended energy that might otherwise go toward learning. The child who cannot effectively move toward his playmates, siblings, and parents is prevented from enjoying self-directed social experiences.

The therapist plays an important role by helping children develop independent and device-assisted mobility appropriate to developmental age level and physical, functional, and social needs. The therapist evaluates the performance capabilities of the children; their home, school, and community environments; and the desires of the parents. This information enables the therapist to select the system of mobility practical for the individual children, the families, and those people who interact with them on a daily basis.

Normal developmental sequence of mobility

Knowledge of the normal developmental sequence of mobility forms the basis for therapeutic intervention. In the course of normal development, children acquire postural and movement patterns that are the basis for functional mobility. Mobility develops first in a horizontal relationship to the floor. In an orderly sequential pattern children assume new postures and movement patterns leading to upright positions and vertical relationships in their movement in space.

Rolling is the first form of mobility that allows the child to change position in the horizontal plane. The ability to pivot on the abdomen to change position develops and is soon followed by the forward prone progression of crawling. As postural stability, righting, and equilibrium reactions mature, the child develops the ability to move onto all fours to creep. The rotational movement pattern from quadruped to sitting allows the child to attain the first independent vertical posture. When sitting can be maintained independently, the hands are free for object manipulation and tool use. From sitting, the child returns to his hands and knees to move through space. From all fours, progress is made to tall kneeling by holding onto furniture or the wall for stability. Moving further upward, the child develops the ability to pull to the standing position by using his arms and hands to attain and hold the vertical position. Mobility in the upright plane progresses from sideways cruising to walking by holding onto objects in the environment. The child then develops the ability to free his hands from external support and achieves independent standing and walking.

Mobility impairment resulting from disease or disability may limit the child's capabilities at any stage during the developmental progression of movement from rolling to walking. The degree of impairment is primarily determined by biological factors such as nervous system functioning, strength, coordination, physical structure, and cognitive functioning. Factors that can either facilitate or limit the ability or desire to move include the availability of experiences, activities, time, space, and assistive devices to augment mobility. Thus a combination of biological and environmental factors influence the functional level of mobility the child will attain.

Children need to develop effective methods of mobility in various physical settings to derive maximal benefit from childhood experiences. They learn by moving around and getting into situations where they can manipulate and explore, thereby experiencing the consequences of their actions. Participating as a member of a group, taking responsibility in school and at home, enjoying play with peers, and becoming independent are natural sequences to exploration.[1] Many children with disabilities learn adaptive ways to move by rolling or crawling. However, when the child's own abilities are insufficient to meet functional and environmental needs, assistive devices are used to help the child in a particular developmental stage to parallel or simulate the normal mobility milestones.[3,24,31]

Mobility for the nonambulatory child

Depending on the extent and severity of the disability, children who are nonambulatory move on the floor by using various patterns of rolling, crawling, creeping, or scooting in the seated position. Assistive devices, such as strollers and wheelchairs, expand the mobility capability of the child to traverse longer distances at home, at school, and in the community where floor-oriented mobility is not functional. Describing adaptive mobility and device-assisted mobility within the developmental sequence helps to point out the functional significance to the child.

ROLLING

The child who can roll is able to change position from prone to supine and to move on the floor. Rolling as a mobility mode is useful for making positional changes in bed regardless of age or disability. As a primary method of mobility, it is most suitable for short distance movement in indoor settings. The youngster who is eager to be amused and stimulated but who has severe limitations in moving toward and manipulating what he wants can have a more enriched environment when toys are placed on the floor with him and play activities are brought to him.

PRONE PROGRESS, CRAWLING

The child who crawls can go farther than one who rolls. Crawling is most functional on environmental surfaces where friction and abrasion forces are minimal, since the child has contact with the floor at his abdomen, arms, and legs. For example, the vinyl kitchen floor or the carpeted family room floor is more suitable for crawling than the asphalt driveway or playground. Mobility devices for children who are at the functional stage of crawling include scooterboards and crawligators that support the trunk close to the floor while allowing arm and leg use. Such devices can be homemade or purchased from therapy equipment catalogues for children. These devices are best used on hard surfaces that allow the small caster wheels to roll without excessive resistance. Some larger, ball casters are safer and roll with greater ease on carpets. The child's hands should be kept well in front of the wheels so that the device cannot roll over them. Supervised use of the device is important when the child cannot get on and off independently.[30]

CREEPING ON HANDS AND KNEES

Once off the abdomen, the child can venture further. Although rolling and crawling allow short distance mobility, for instance, within a room, the child who creeps independently may have wider access to the house and yard. Assistive devices for creeping are available. These support the trunk far enough off the ground to allow use of the arms in an extended position for weight bearing and use of the legs for weight bearing on the knees. They are best used in a training mode versus a functional mode. The child who creeps is often capable of attaining a sitting position by rotating onto the buttocks or by sitting back on the lower legs. These functional positions could be restricted by a creeping assistive device.

MOBILITY IN SITTING

Scooting on the buttocks while sitting on the floor is a mobility pattern used by some children who have adequate sitting balance, upper extremity strength, and control to move the body. The child may take weight on extended arms, unweighting the buttocks, sliding either forward or backward along the floor. Many children with physical disabilities such as meningomyelocele or traumatic paraplegia mobilize themselves using this pattern. Children who have some volitional leg function will assist their movement with their hips and feet. The upright position is more conducive to functional activities. Caster carts and wheelmobiles are available to facilitate floor-based mobility in the seated position. With these devices the child is seated in a long sitting position just off the floor. They are propelled by pushing wheels that are attached to the base in line with the child's shoulders (Figure 12-12).

Children whose mobility capabilities are floorbound will use these patterns and mobility devices for floor-oriented play in most settings where other children are frequently playing on the floor. Normal developmental progression and activity interests take the nondisabled child from floor-based activities to higher areas involv-

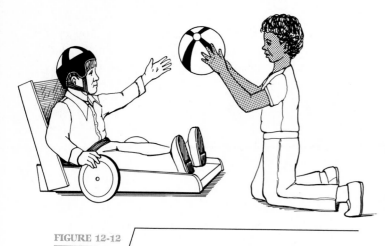

FIGURE 12-12

A caster cart provides seating and mobility for floor-oriented play.

ing sitting on furniture, participating in table-level activities, standing during play, and walking. The disabled child also has these needs and desires to be higher in space to pursue age-appropriate activities at a height and speed similar to those of peers. Children who are unable to achieve this through standing and walking will need mobility aids that provide support and mobility in the seated position. The growing child becomes larger and heavier and more difficult to lift off the floor. This too influences the transition from floor-oriented mobility devices to devices that place the child at a higher level.

WHEELCHAIR MOBILITY

Identification of the appropriate wheelchair is based on evaluation of a broad spectrum of factors, including the ability of the child, concurrent developmental tasks, environmental settings, and desires of significant others who interact with the child. The occupational therapist, the child, the parents, the physical therapist, the teacher, and other team members have valuable information to offer regarding the child's abilities and needs that will contribute to the selection of the device that will provide maximal function. The medical equipment dealer is an excellent source of information regarding new or improved items and features that may help solve unique problems relevant to the child's needs.

A wide variety of wheelchairs from different manufacturers are available for children. They may generally be categorized as the following:

1. Transport chairs, such as strollers and travel chairs, designed to be pushed by others
2. Manual wheelchairs propelled by the child or pushed by others
3. Electric wheelchairs for those children who have insufficient strength, coordination, or endurance

to propel a wheelchair manually, but who have the control and judgment to use power mobility safely

Young children (under age 3) are often transported in *strollers* designed for the normal population of infants and toddlers. Strollers are frequently used for transportation outdoors or in the community where carrying the child is impractical for the parents and the child's own method of mobility is inadequate for the distance or terrain. The umbrella stroller is popular because of the convenience, portability, and "normal" appearance. However, children with postural control problems are generally not supported adequately by the sling seats used in these strollers. The semireclined seat angle places the child in a passive position rather than upright, and this may hinder spontaneous postural responses, the feeling of comfort and security, and the ability to view the surroundings. Large strollers for children who have outgrown regular strollers are available from medical equipment vendors and are easily portable. The occupational therapist often helps the family adapt the stroller with solid seats and backs that provide improved postural support and seat angle for the child.

Travel chairs are highly specialized stroller systems with rear wheel retractor units that provide several adjustments of seat angle. For car travel the rear wheels fully retract to allow placement of the chair on a car seat while the child is still sitting in the device. These chairs are designed for the severely involved child who has positioning needs. The chairs come with a wide variety of accessory options to provide postural support and control, including solid seat and back units; knee abduction units; lateral supports for the trunk, hips, and thighs; head rests; trunk harnesses; and lap trays. Travel chairs provide postural stabilization and alignment during hand use activities, feeding, and transportation. Their capability of doubling as both car seat and wheelchair offers versatility. These systems are pushed and operated by others, making them appropriate only for children who are not capable of wheeling themselves. The chair should be tried in the family's car before purchase because some chairs do not fit on the seats of some vehicles. In most cars they will only fit on the front passenger seat.

Children who have sufficient upper extremity strength and control for self-propulsion are candidates for *manual wheelchairs*. Children around the age of 3 reach the size necessary to fit into Tiny Tot models offered by the major wheelchair manufacturing companies. Recently smaller chairs have become available for younger children who are ready to propel themselves. Most wheelchair companies have a series of models to meet the average size and functional needs of the growing individual from preschool to adolescent to adult.

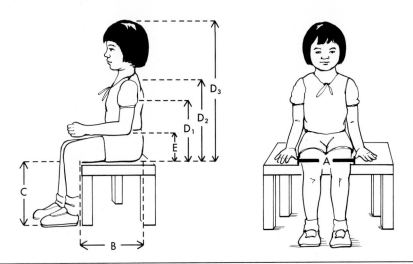

FIGURE 12-13

Measurements for the wheelchair. *A*, Hip width; *B*, leg length; *C*, Foreleg length; D_1, seat base to axilla; D_2, seat base to top of shoulders; D_3, seat base to top of head; *E*, arm height.

Modifications to meet individual requirements can be made by selecting different styles of armrests, footrests, wheel hand-rim options, and positioning accessories. The wheelchair size may be custom modified by upholstery, frame construction, or the addition of seat inserts. Selection of the appropriate size chair is based on body measurements and consideration of functional needs. The following measurements, taken while the child is in the seated position, determine the relationship between the size of the child and the chair (Figure 12-13).

1. Hip width: The measurement at the widest point across the hips or thighs plus 2 inches determines the width of the chair seat.
2. Leg length: The measurement from behind the knee to behind the buttocks determines the seat depth. For children there should be a clearance of 1 inch from behind the knee to the front edge of the seat.
3. Foreleg length: The measurement from the heel to under the thigh determines the height of the footrest system for foot support and weight bearing under the thighs.
4. Back height: Depending on the upper torso support needs of the child, the following measurements determine the seat's back height.
   a. Seat base to axilla: For children who require standard support.
   b. Seat base to top of shoulders: For children with additional trunk support needs.
   c. Seat base to top of head: For children who require head support.
5. Arm height: The measurement from the seat base to the elbow with the arm flexed determines the height of the armrests.

6. Seat height: The distance from the floor to the top of the seat base determines the seat height.

Functional activities that will be performed in the wheelchair have implications for the style of wheelchair and selection of components. For example, a lightweight model can be considered to increase the wheeling efficiency of the child or to help the parent who frequently lifts the chair in and out of the car. Removable armrests are needed for sliding transfers. Desk-type arms are an important feature for children who need to get close to tables for schoolwork, feeding, and play activities. The height of the seat base from the floor is critical for those doing standing transfers, and it affects access to tables and desks.

Electric wheelchairs should be considered for the child who is physically unable to propel a manual chair. Those who need to limit energy expenditure and joint stress, or whose wheeling capabilities prevent them from going fast enough or far enough to meet their needs for functional activities and exploration, are also candidates for electric wheelchairs.[32] The child's physical control, endurance, cognitive abilities, and judgment are essential considerations for safe use of power mobility. Assessment of the home, school, and community environments where the chair will be used, how it will be transported, and who will be responsible for its maintenance help to determine the feasibility of power mobility and will influence the type of system selected for a given individual.[3]

Most power wheelchairs are configured like manual chairs with the addition of electronic component systems, control unit, and batteries. They can be purchased as a complete power system from a variety of manufacturers. Separate power add-on systems designed to convert standard manual wheelchairs to electric wheelchairs are also available. Most models are equipped with a joystick for right- or left-hand use. Special controllers, electronic systems, or adaptations can be made for those who have insufficient upper extremity coordination or strength to manipulate the standard joystick. Joystick adaptation includes special knobs to promote grasp, templates to guide directional control, and special mounting and modifications to allow operation by the chin, head, or foot. Other control systems drive the power wheelchairs through puff-sip input, which includes an array of single switches that designates directional mobility, or through activation of a single switch on a directional scanning interface system. Voice and sonar control systems are being developed but are not ready for commercial application.

Frequently additional equipment, such as a van with a lift and tie-down system or ramps for the home, must be acquired to maximize the child's wheelchair use and independence. Such environmental modifications need careful consideration during the assessment process so that the family may plan to acquire additional systems that support the independent mobility of their child. Portable electric wheelchairs that can be dismantled and folded for transportation may be selected when a van and lift are not available. Those using power wheelchairs often have a manual wheelchair for use when the power system is being serviced or when the situation will not accommodate the electric wheelchair. There are also power units that can be used to adapt standard wheelchairs.

Mobility for the ambulatory child

WALKING BY HOLDING ON

The child who has adequate postural control and stability to stand and take steps while holding on to some support will use this method of mobility in the home or classroom where walls and furniture are available for the external stability needed to stay upright. The child's mobility is limited by the environment unless ambulation aids are provided. Orthotic devices, such as a shoe insert to stabilize the foot; an ankle foot orthosis (AFO); knee ankle foot orthosis (KAFO); or additional appliances that provide control at the hips, pelvis, and trunk, may be used to stabilize and align the lower extremities for ambulation according to the needs of the child. Walkers, crutches, and canes may be used to aid balance during ambulation. Children who can functionally use such ambulation aids are able to venture into open areas to determine their own route through space in contrast to being limited to the route determined by fixtures in the environment.

WALKING INDEPENDENTLY

The achievement of independent ambulation enables the child to move about with his hands free from body support functions. The disabled child often uses an abnormal gait pattern. Orthotic devices may be needed to align or support the lower extremity joints to improve the pattern. Those with congenital limb deficiency or amputation use prosthetic devices to achieve independent ambulation. The functional use of independent or device-assisted ambulation depends on the effort and energy it consumes, the time it takes to get from one place to another, and the distance that can be covered. Short-distance ambulatory children may walk within the home, school, and neighborhood, but use a wheelchair for long-distance community mobility.

• • •

Parents and professionals strive for a delicate balance with any adaptive aid, whether for mobility or for tasks such as eating or dressing. In general, aids should help children use their own skills as much as possible. Aids should not become substitutes for the children's efforts to learn to do things on their own.

Parents and professionals together need to observe children in their environments to clarify the goals to be accomplished with the particular aid. Once the goals have been established, efforts can be directed toward finding equipment that can be adapted to meet the goals. Regardless of what equipment is purchased, an ongoing review of the individual child's use of the equipment is essential to assess its value and to review whether modifications or changes need to be made.

SUMMARY

This chapter discussed the ways in which occupational therapists can help a child to become more independent. The processes of eating, toileting, dressing, and grooming were described, both from the aspect of evaluation and from that of training. Normal development of mobility and methods for building a child's ability to get around independently were also discussed. The child's treatment program must include the needs of the family as a whole. Adaptive equipment must be acceptable to the child's self-image and to the family's finances and life-style.

REFERENCES

1. Bergen, A.C.: Positioning the client with central nervous system deficits, New York, 1982, Valhalla Rehabilitation Publishers, Ltd.
2. Bigge, J.: Teaching individuals with physical and multiple disabilities, ed. 2, Columbus, Ohio, 1982, Charles E. Merrill Publishing Co.
3. Bleck, E.E., and Nagel, D.A.: Physical handicapped children; a medical atlas for teachers, New York, 1982, Grune & Stratton, Inc.
4. Bobath, K.: The motor deficit in patients with cerebral palsy, London, 1966, William Heinemann, Ltd.

5. Brazelton, T.B.: Toddlers and parents, New York, 1974, Dell Publishing Co., Inc.

6. Coley, I.: Pediatric assessment of self-care activities, St. Louis, 1978, The C.V. Mosby Co.

7. Copeland, M., and others: Occupational therapy for mentally retarded children, Baltimore, 1976, University Park Press.

8. Doyle, P., and others: Helping the severely handicapped child, New York, 1979, Thomas Y. Crowell Co., Inc.

9. Duffy, Y.: All things possible, Ann Arbor, Mich., 1981, A.J. Garvin & Associates.

10. Erickson, M.L.: Assessment and management of developmental changes in children, St. Louis, 1976, The C.V. Mosby Co.

11. Farber, S.: Sensorimotor evaluation and treatment procedures for allied health personnel, Indianapolis, 1974, The Indiana University Foundation.

12. Finnie, N.: Handling the young cerebral palsied child at home, ed. 2, New York, 1975, Dutton-Sunrise, Inc.

13. Friedman, L.: Toileting self-care methods for bilateral high level upper limb amputees, Prosthet. Orthot. Int. **4:**29, 1980.

14. Gesell, A.: The first five years of life—a guide to the study of the pre-school child, New York, 1940, Harper & Row, Publishers.

15. Hale, G.: The source book for the disabled, New York, 1979, Paddington Press, Ltd.

16. Hammond, M.I., Lewis, M.N., and Johnson, E.W.: A nutritional study of cerebral palsied children, J. Am. Diet. Assoc. **49:**196, 1966.

17. Howard, B.: Nutritional support of the developmentally disabled child. In Suskind, R., editor: Textbook of pediatric nutrition, New York, 1981, Raven Press.

18. Howison, M., Perella, J., and Gordon, D.: Cerebral palsy. In Hopkins, H., and Smith, H., editors: Willard and Spackman's occupational therapy, ed. 5, Philadelphia, 1978, J.B. Lippincott Co.

19. Illingworth, R.S.: The development of the infant and young child—normal and abnormal, ed. 3, Baltimore, 1966, The Williams & Wilkins Co.

20. Kennedy, E.: Dressing with pride, vol. 1, Groton, Conn., 1981, P.R.I.D.E. Foundation, Inc.

21. Kernaleguen, A.: Clothing designs for the handicapped, Edmonton, 1978, The University of Alberta Press.

22. Measuring the patient, Los Angeles, 1979, Everest & Jennings.

23. Morris, S.E.: The normal acquisition of oral feeding skills: implications for assessment and treatment, New York, 1982, Therapeutic Media, Inc.

24. Motlock, W.M.: Mobility for spinal cord impaired spina bifida patients, Paper presented at Conference on Mobility Aids, Toronto, 1974.

25. Mueller, H.: Facilitating feeding and prespeech. In Pearson, P., and Williams, C.A., editors: Physical therapy services in the developmental disabilities, Springfield, Ill., 1972, Charles C Thomas, Publisher.

26. O'Neil, S.: Behavior management of feeding. In Pipes, P.: Nutrition in infancy and childhood, St. Louis, 1977, The C.V. Mosby Co.

27. Orelove, F., and Gibbons, S.: A guide to independent dressing, Except. Parent 1981.

28. Peiper, A.: Cerebral function in infancy and childhood, New York, 1963, Consultants Bureau Enterprises, Inc.

29. Pipes, P.: Nutrition in infancy and childhood, St. Louis, 1977, The C.V. Mosby Co.

30. Robinault, I.P.: Functional aids for the multiply handicapped, New York, 1973, Harper & Row, Publishers.

31. Swinyard, C.: The child with spina bifida, Chicago, 1980, Spina Bifida Association of America.

32. Treffler, E., and Cook, H.: Powered mobility for children, Knoxville, 1979, University of Tennessee Center for the Health Sciences, Rehabilitation Engineering Center.

13

PAT NUSE CLARK

Play and recreational activities

This chapter addresses play as a generic modality and one outcome of occupational therapy intervention. A conservative estimate, based on clinical observations, is that at least half of occupational therapy services for children are delivered through the medium of play. Play is the preeminent occupational behavior of childhood and, as such, constitutes a major concern of occupational therapy. Services may be expected to promote the development of play behavior, as well as use play as the primary modality to facilitate change in the motor, sensory integrative, cognitive, emotional, and social functions of children. In observations of pediatric practice, play can readily be identified as the tie that binds occupational therapy assessment and treatment together.

Despite the manifestations of play in clinical practice, a cursory review of the literature from 1970 to 1983 by titles of articles suggests that play was of little concern to occupational therapists except as a theoretical concept. However, examination of the content of practice, as described in most articles about pediatric occupational therapy during that period, indicates that the treatment activities used most often may properly be described as play. Takata[27] noted that the focus of pediatric occupational therapy treatment from the 1950s until the 1980s was guided by the medical science orientation of the sensory integrative and neurodevelomental approaches. Because of the recent increasing shift of services from medical to educational environments, Takata proposed that the occupational behavior approach offered a more comprehensive framework because of its focus on human activity in environment rather than on dysfunction. It is questionable whether the two approaches are mutually exclusive. Again, clinical observation and written descriptions of treatment indicate that the activities used in sensory integrative and neurodevelopmental approaches most often serve as playful experiences for the children. The critical difference perhaps lies in the orientation of the therapist. In the neurodevelopmental and sensory integrative approaches, play is a modality that is used to develop improved performance in self-maintenance and schoolwork.[2,3] In the occupational behavior approach, play is an outcome as well as a modality.[26] The orientation of this text is in the direction of the occupational behavior approach: play is viewed as a generic modality and outcome of occupational therapy (Chapter 7).

SCOPE OF PLAY IN OCCUPATIONAL THERAPY

A thorough review of literature on play is impossible within the constraints of this chapter, but the references and suggested readings should prove helpful. For organizational purposes, however, a discussion of the scope of play in occupational therapy is warranted.

The theoretical foundation that is generally adopted for discussion of play is Reilly's explanation of play as an appreciative learning system[21] (Chapter 3). However, practice in occupational therapy demands more than a theoretical explanation of play. What is needed is a way to classify the myriad of usable activities that can assist the therapist with selection of appropriate play experiences according to the interests, capacities, needs, and ages of children seen in treatment. For this purpose, the works of Florey,[7] Michelman,[17,18] and Takata[26] provide a useful background.

Florey: a classification of play

Florey[7] defined play as the action on human and nonhuman objects that is engaged in for its own sake. Her concept that play is intrinsically motivated and rewarding was gleaned from, and continues to be supported by, a comprehensive review of play theories.[4,25] Florey[7] further described play as a learning process. This concept has been differentiated somewhat by other theorists. Piaget, as cited by Flavell,[5] defined play as those actions of the child that are dominated by assimilation, that is, when the child is able to direct actions with established mental schemes. In contrast, Piaget believed that playful actions that were dominated by accommodation are more properly described as imitation. Hutt[11] proposed a taxonomy of play that nicely integrates Piagetian theory with the more global view of Florey. Hutt stipulated that there are two major categories of play. *Epistemic play* behaviors are concerned with the acquisition of new information and knowledge. *Ludic play* includes those behaviors that are dominated by use of past experiences. This differentiation can be useful to the occupational therapist for selection and adaptation of activities.

Florey[7] developed a classification system that organizes the developmental sequence of play behaviors according to variations in actions with human and nonhuman objects. Actions with human objects include play with parents, peers, significant others, and the child's own body. Nonhuman objects are divided into three groups according to the inherent properties of the object for change as a result of the child's actions. Type I objects include creative and unstructured media that can be directly changed by the playful actions of the child. Objects that can be changed when combined with other objects are classified as Type II. Objects that maintain their original form in relatively stable condition regardless of play actions, such as bicycles and dolls, are referred to as Type III. Florey indicated through her classification that differential and preferential engagement in play with human and nonhuman objects will vary over the course of time. For example, during the preschool years, play with human objects is often directed toward the self and family. As the child matures, more action is directed toward peers and away from the self and parents. Similarly, involvement with an increasingly broad range of nonhuman objects occurs as the child ages.

Takata: a taxonomy of play

In work that enriches concepts of play presented earlier by Florey,[6,7] Takata[26] sought to identify critical patterns and representations of play and relate these to age and milieu. This was accomplished through the construction of a two-directional taxonomy that can be used to examine the content of play and to help prescribe areas for intervention. The taxonomy's elements will be reviewed here, and its content described through discussion in the practice section of this chapter.

Takata proposed that play evolves from a sequence of age-related *epochs*, and Takata characterized these in an integration of concepts developed by Piaget, Erikson, and Florey. Each epoch has representative elements, which Takata identified as materials, actions, people, and setting. The epochs are the following.

1. Sensorimotor epoch: During the period from birth to 24 months, the play of the child is characterized by exploration and manipulation of the self, parents, siblings, significant others, and common objects in the environment. The child engages in play for its sensory experience and comes to know the basic actions and sensory properties of people and things.

2. Symbolic and simple constructive epoch: Through the emergence and refinement of language, the child develops symbols for the actions and properties that he discovered during the sensory motor period. The ability to communicate through symbols, coupled with increasing gross and fine motor capacity, allows the child to construct relationships between objects. Relationships are established through the child's sensorimotor experiences but are extended through the developing imagination of the child.

3. Dramatic, complex constructive, and pregame epoch: The 4- to 7-year-old child learns to act out concepts and experiences through play and begins to put concepts together to form elementary rules of actions. Dramatic play replaces imaginative fantasy, since the child now knows better what is likely to happen. The putting together of objects through construction becomes increasingly important as the child's ability to represent reality increases. Peer interaction becomes pivotal as the child begins to test the validity of constructs and skills. This period is transitional from exploratory to competency play as defined by Reilly.[21]

4. Game epoch: The elementary school child is driven by the urge to control the actions of objects and events. Occupation in game playing predominates, because such activities offer the child increasingly complex variations of rules and thus increase the child's sense of control and mastery. Rules prescribe ways of doing things and show the child a way to increase competence. Competence is measured through competitive play with peers.

5. Recreation epoch: The play behavior of the adolescent assumes a more mature form through involvement in recreational activities. The balance

of occupation has shifted in the direction of work, and recreation allows the refinement of skills and interactions that will relate to or support the youth's performance in adult roles. The games and social activities of recreation demonstrate increasingly sophisticated rules, role functions, and patterns of cooperation with the team or group.

This play taxonomy was originally designed to be used in conjunction with Takata's play history (Chapter 9). The data on play and environment can be contrasted against the requisites defined by the taxonomy to identify the play status of the child. Areas of acceptable development and risk are highlighted.

Michelman: creative growth

The elements of symbolic and constructive play discussed by Takata and Florey were explored further in Michelman's study[17] of the development of children's creative interests. Michelman[17] wrote

> Art is a language of symbols and non-verbal communication. The child who freely explores with creative art media absorbs information through his senses which he assimilates and recasts into new symbolic forms (p. 88).

Drawing on the work of Lowenfield, Michelman identified six stages of creative growth and symbol formation that show differentiated development of human, color, and design schemata with stage-specific representation, motivation, media, and methods. Creative activities promote the self-expression of the child and are less rule-bound than other types of play behaviors. In a later work Michelman[18] proposed more specifically that creative interests are the route to intellectual growth.

A MODEL OF PLAY IN OCCUPATIONAL THERAPY

By using the studies of Florey, Takata, and Michelman in combination with Reilly's theoretical explanation of play and the other theoretical approaches discussed elsewhere in this text, a model of play in occupational therapy can be constructed. As an example, a developmental model of play activities is presented in Exhibits 13-1 to 13-5. This model provides an overview of play that is organized according to major types of play, and it analyzes some of the generic modalities of occupational therapy that are related to play. By using these tables, the therapist can determine what types of play experiences are most appropriate to the child's age and functional status.

Each major category of play activities is characteristic of an age group. However, it must be emphasized that engagement in play varies with the mood and motivation of the child. The competitive 8-year-old, for example, may well be found reading to stuffed animals as a respite from vigorous peer group play. The organization of the charts, therefore, is also designed to show a developmental progression of toys and activities in each category of play. There is recognizable overlap between many of the representative activities of each category, because analysis will indicate that each toy or play experience can serve several functions for the child. The examples of play activities are representative rather than all-inclusive. They should be interpreted and supplemented by knowledge gained from visiting toy stores and toy departments, observing children in play situations, and reviewing activity books for children in bookstores.

Use of the model for program planning

When considering assessment results, the therapist can determine which activities would help to meet intervention goals. For example, if a 4-year-old child has problems with fine motor function, the therapist would select symbolic and creative activities appropriate to the 4- to 7-year-old age range (Figure 13-1). If an 8-year-old child is developmentally delayed, the therapist might work toward engagement of the child in competitive games and activities at a slightly lower age level (Figure 13-2). The teenager who has become withdrawn might be directed toward some of the symbolic and creative activities appropriate to adolescence. This model is designed to appeal to the developmental interest level of the child or adolescent, as discussed by Frantzen,[8] and at the same time provide a wide range of therapeutically useful modalities.

PROGRAM DEVELOPMENT
Adaptation of play activities

Adaptation of play activities to promote the child's involvement, enjoyment, and success is another element of play in occupational therapy. Adaptations may be made to the position of the body and work surface; to the activity process itself; to the expectations for performance; and to the tools, materials, and equipment used in the activity process (Chapter 7). In addition, the therapist can use different interpersonal relationships to promote activity performance. Specific adaptive equipment and physical techniques are also used to enable the individual to participate in a larger range of activities. Ideas for activity adaptation may be found throughout this text in relation to specific problems; therefore, only selected activities will be discussed at this time. Suggestions will be presented through case examples and program reports from the literature.

Text continued on p. 260.

EXHIBIT 13-1

Exploratory play

1. *Description:* Play-recreational experiences through which the child develops a body scheme, sensory integrative and motor skills, and concepts of sensory characteristics and actions of human and nonhuman objects.

2. *Properties of activities:*
   a. Tools, materials, and equipment:
      Child's own body
      Significant others
      Environmental textures
      "Infant" toys with distinct sensory characteristics and actions
      Everyday household objects
   b. Human and object relationships:
      Strongest relationships occur through play between child and parents.
      Egocentric relationships occur with nonhuman objects as an extension of the child.
   c. Characteristic age level is newborn through 2 years.

3. *Representative toys and activities:*
   a. Newborn to two years:

Auditory toys: Rattles, play piano, and so on	Mobiles	Scarves, brightly colored
Balls: All sizes and textures	Pop-up toys	Scooters, scooter boards
Bells	Pots and pans	See N' Say
Blocks	Pull-and-push toys	Sensory play with parents
Busy boxes	Rolling, crawling, cruising activities	Spice bottles, empty
Containers and nesting toys	Sand and water toys and activities	Squeeze toys
Hammers and pegs		Teething toys
Inflatables		Textured surfaces

   b. Two to four years:

Amusement park rides	Magnets	Sand and water toys
Balance–rocker boards	Play tunnel	Seesaw
Blowing bubbles	Rocking horse	Slides
Finger paints	Rolling in the grass	Swings
Inflatables	Running	Tricycle riding

   c. Four to seven:

Amusement park rides	Obstacle courses	Simple woodwork
Balance beam	Playground equipment	Swimming
Bicycles and tricycle riding	Rocker boards	Swinging equipment
Dot-to-dot line drawings	Sand and water play	Tracing, templates
Inflatables	Scooter boards	Trampolines
Magnets	Simon Says	Visual perception worksheets
Mazes		

   d. Seven to twelve years:

Amusement park rides	Mazes	Simon Says
Dot-to-dot line drawings	"New" games	Stilts
Hopscotch	Parachute games	Swimming and water play
Hula hoops	Playground equipment	Throwing games
Jump rope	Obstacle courses	Visual perception worksheets
Kite-flying	Rough and tumble play	

   e. Adolescence:

Amusement park rides	Gymnastics	Swimming and water play
Calisthenics	Jogging, running	Wrestling
Dancing		

EXHIBIT 13-2

Symbolic play

1. *Description:* Play and recreational experiences through which the child formulates, tests, classifies, and refines ideas, feelings, and combined actions. Associated with the development of language.

2. *Properties of activities:*
   a. Tools, materials, and equipment:
      Gross motor play equipment
      Simple construction toys
      Simple art materials
      Toys for fantasy-imaginative play
   b. Human and object relationships:
      Play with peers begins with parallel imitation and develops into cooperative interaction.
      Parents validate products of play.
      Objects are given importance according to the child's ability to symbolize, control, change, and master.
   c. Characteristic age level is 2 to 4 years.

3. *Representative toys and activities:*
   a. Newborn to two years:

Dolls and stuffed animals	Mirrors	Scribbling with crayons
Imitative hand-body games	1- to 3-piece form puzzles	Shape boxes
Language play with parents		

   b. Two to four years:

Abacus	Dolls and stuffed animals	Put-together toys
Beads	Dollhouses	Puzzles
Blocks	Dramatic songs	Records
Cars, trucks, trains	"Dress up" materials	Sewing cards
Chalk and blackboard activities	Hand puppets	Simple storybooks
Clay, modeling dough	Household play items	Space stations
Colorforms	Miniature figures	Stacking toys
Construction kits	Musical instruments	Toy telephone
Crayons, paints, paper	Nesting toys	Tricycle riding

   c. Four to seven years:

Action figures	"Dress up" materials	Play house or store
Arts and crafts materials	Lemonade stands	Puppets
Building sets	Musical instruments	Records
Dolls and stuffed animals	Papier-mâché	Storybooks
Dramatic play		

   d. Seven to twelve years:

Action figures	Computer games	Mime
Arts and crafts materials	Mad libs	Reading materials
Charades		

   e. Adolescence:

Arts and crafts materials	Decorative arts	Mime
Charades	Diaries	Plays and skits
Computer programming	"Feelings" games	Role-playing

EXHIBIT 13-3

Creative play and interests

1. *Description:* Play and recreational experiences through which the child refines sensory, motor, cognitive, and social skills; explores combinations of actions on multiple objects; and develops interests and competencies that will promote performance of school-related and work-related activities.

2. *Properties of activities:*
   a. Tools, materials, and equipment:
   Arts and crafts
   Complex construction toys
   Dramatic play materials
   Household activities such as cooking, simple woodwork, pet care, and gardening
   b. Human and object relationships:
   Play begins in cooperative peer groups, with gradual emergence of competitive atmosphere; peer validation of play products becomes increasingly important.
   Parents assist and validate in the absence of peers.
   Nonhuman objects are valued according to outcome of play.
   c. Characteristic age level is 4 to 7 years.

3. *Representative toys and activities:*
   a. Newborn to two years:
   Blocks
   Crayon scribbling
   Pop beads
   b. Two to four years:
   Bead stringing
   Finger painting
   Mobile making
   c. Four to seven years:

Baking cookies	Gardening	Simple weaving—placemats, pot holders
Bicycle riding	Painting	Simple woodworking
Craft kits	Paperdolls	Stencils
Cutting and pasting		

   d. Seven to twelve years:

Cooking	Drawing	Painting
Crafts	Model kits	Science experiments
Decorative arts	Needle arts	Woodworking

   e. Adolescence:
   Crafts: jewelry making, woodworking, metalworking
   Creative writing
   Fine and decorative arts

EXHIBIT 13-4

Games

1. *Description:* Play and recreational experiences that have distinct rules and involve skill development and social interaction in a competitive atmosphere. Actions and results of actions are compared against those of peers.

2. *Properties of activities:*
   a. Tools, materials, and equipment:
      Sports equipment that requires refined control of gross and fine motor actions
      Table games
      Perceptual-motor games
      Cognitive-language games
   b. Human and object relationships:
      Peer relationship is most important.
      Attachment to nonhuman objects reflects importance in games in which the child can successfully compete.
   c. Characteristic age level is 7 to 12 years.

3. *Representative toys and activities:*
   a. Newborn to two years:
      Sensory-motor games with rules, for example, peekaboo
   b. Two to four years:

Checkers	Matching card games
Dominoes	Simple classification board games
Lotto	

   c. Four to seven years:

Same as above	Organized outdoor games at age level
Bicycle or tricycle races	Scooter board races

   d. Seven to twelve years:

Arcade games	Collections	Ping-Pong
Board games	Field days: races, tug-of-war	Roller-skating and ice-skating
Card games	Hangman	School plays, performances
Checkers	Jacks, marbles	Team sports
Clubs	Jump rope	Trading cards

   e. Adolescence:
      Individual or team competition
      School political activities
      Team sports

EXHIBIT 13-5

Recreation

1. *Description:* Play-leisure experiences that allow the youth to explore complex interests and roles to develop a sense of self-identity and achievement.

2. *Properties of activities:*
   a. Tools, materials, and equipment:
      Arts and crafts
      Collections
      Organized interest group activities
      Social activities
      Sports
   b. Human and object relationships:
      Peer group is still important for sharing of interests.
      Validation of outcome by self is increasingly important.
      Objects may have sentimental value but are viewed realistically.
   c. Characteristic age level is adolescence.

3. *Representative toys and activities:*
   a. Newborn to two years:
      Activities from other categories that represent individual interests and preferences
   b. Two to four years:
      Same as above
   c. Four to seven years:
      Same as above
   d. Seven to twelve years:
      Same as above
   e. Adolescence:

Collections	Musical instruments
Crafts	Performing arts
Dancing	Singing and choir
Decorative arts	Spectator sports
Fine arts	Social sports
Hiking and camping	Team sports
Individual sports	

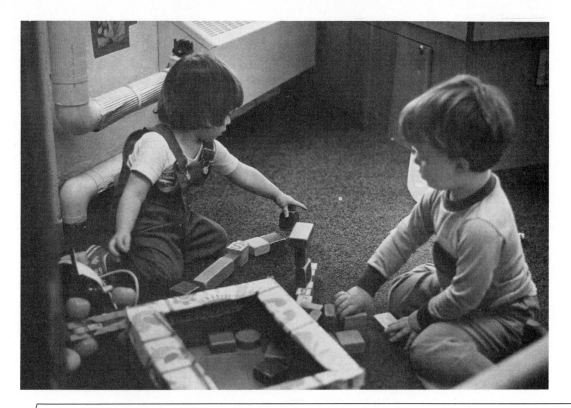

FIGURE 13-1

Preschool children develop fine motor, language, and role skills through play with toys that represent common objects.

From Weiser, M.G.: Group care and education of infants and toddlers, St. Louis, 1982, The C.V. Mosby Co.

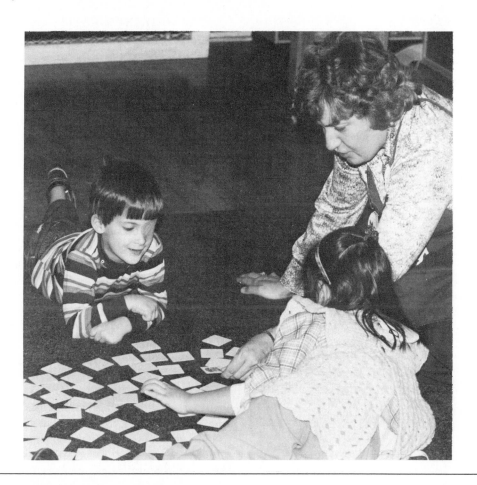

FIGURE 13-2

School-age children can strengthen visual processing skills through competitive game play.

From Hendrick, J.: The whole child: early education for the eighties, ed. 3, St. Louis, 1984, The C.V. Mosby Co.

MOTOR FUNCTION

Very often motor impairment may prevent the child's full participation in play. Through knowledgeable selection of activities, in cooperation with the child's interests and capacities, the occupational therapist can design a treatment program that will improve motor function and at the same time promote continuity in the child's development of play and related skills. The techniques that are used most with children who have motor problems include adaptation of position (of the body and work surface) and adaptation of the tools, materials, and equipment that are used for an activity.

CASE STUDY

Donna is an 8-year-old girl with moderate spastic hemiplegia who was referred to occupational therapy for improvement of gross and fine motor skills. Assessment indicated that her typical play behaviors were at the level of symbolic activities, although she was interested in participating in more creative play and games. She was able to use her uninvolved left hand in all fine prehension patterns, but precise manipulative ability was generally poor. She had difficulty drawing geometric figures, her printing was crude, and she needed assistance to hold paper when cutting. Results of her independent attempts in these activities were generally poor. Although her involved right hand was used fairly well as a gross assist and was relaxed at rest, she tended to become tight during concentrated efforts. In such instances, she became frustrated because she would lose control over her right hand as an assist.

Donna's sensory integrative function appeared slightly depressed, with fair localization of tactile and proprioceptive stimuli. Equilibrium responses were adequate against mild resistance, but she needed support to maintain positions against moderate resistance. Social skills were well developed. Although her articulation was not always clear, her speech and language development were generally age appropriate. She related well to others in her class and seemed to have a loving relationship with her divorced mother and siblings.

General goals of occupational therapy were to strengthen gross and fine motor skills to improve performance in schoolwork and age-appropriate play activities. Because of her age, she received her occupational therapy services two times weekly as a member of a group that included three age-mates who had similar problems. As a general rule, the group worked on creative activities once a week, with an emphasis on development of fine motor skills. The other weekly session was reserved for gross motor play through competitive activities.

One favorite activity was the puppet show, which was chosen to strengthen fine motor skills and symbolic representation. The therapist prepared two side outlines of simple animal shapes for felt hand puppets. The two sides were fastened together with a few paper clips over a slightly smaller cardboard template and set up in a table clamp. Donna sewed her puppet together by using a large needle and yarn in her left hand and by using the right hand to stabilize the edge near her stitches. Although she was unable to handle the felt with scissors, she traced and cut out paper patterns for the puppet's facial features. When the puppets were completed, the children worked together to develop a skit to present to the rest of their class.

Because each of the children had weak balance and underdeveloped gross motor control of their uninvolved arms, the therapist designed a beanbag toss game that would allow them to compete with each other and strengthen their gross motor skills. Together with the therapist, the children developed a set of rules that would govern the actions and scoring of the game. A rocker board was used for sitting, knee-standing, and standing. Each child was responsible for positioning the rocker board behind the starting line before each throw. Target distances ranged from 5 to 10 feet and were increased as individual improvement was noted. Initially, the target was a large square area on the floor that was bordered by masking tape. As the children became more proficient, the target was changed to a hula hoop, and later to a wastebasket. Donna began by using an underhand toss, and she progressed to an overhand throw. An overriding concern of the group was that each child should compete fairly with the others. Consequently, the children modified the rules according to the performance capacity of each group member. For example, because Donna was the best thrower in the group, her starting line was placed 1 foot behind the others. The children's positions on the rocker board varied according to their postural stability.

SENSORY INTEGRATIVE FUNCTION

Chapter 19 will present a thorough discussion of the activities that are used in sensory integrative therapy. As mentioned previously, much of this therapy is provided through the medium of play. Mack, Lindquist, and Parham[16] published a detailed study of the interactive relationship between play and sensory integrative treatment. They emphasized that sensory-motor play experiences normally mature through a hierarchical sequence of exploratory, symbolic, and creative activities. However, when the sensory integrative functions are inadequate, the child's ability to engage in more complex and mature forms of play is impaired.

Two critical areas for adaptation of play with such a child include the relationship between the child and the therapist, and the structure of tools, materials, and equipment in the play environment. Lindquist, Mack, and Parham[14] recommended that the therapist serve as a role model (Figure 13-3). When children lack the organization to direct their actions in new situations or with new play materials, they tend to withdraw from the activity. For example, the therapist can demonstrate how to get onto and ride a scooter board to a child whose interest in the play equipment results in awkward frustration. The therapist also serves as an extension of the child's body, helping the child to monitor movements. Once on the scooter board, or a piece of suspended equipment, the child may lack the capacity to make postural adjustments as his body shifts with the movement of the equipment. The resulting postural

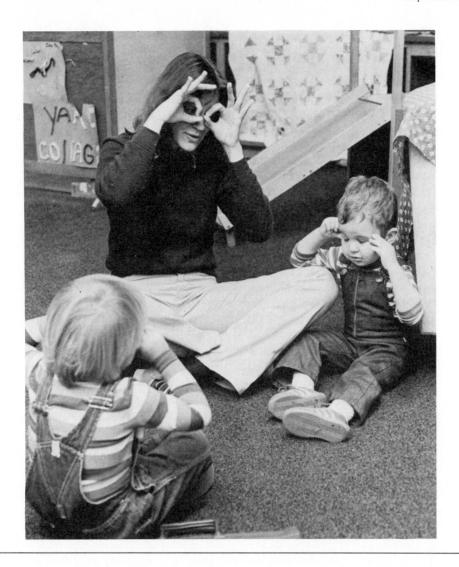

FIGURE 13-3

The therapist as role model.

From Weiser, M.G.: Group care and education of infants and toddlers, St. Louis, 1982, The C.V. Mosby Co.

insecurity changes the activity from a playful to a fearful experience. Verbal and physical cuing can be helpful in this instance. As the child's organization improves, the therapist may ask the child to explain what body parts must be moved to make postural adjustments.

Knickerbocker[13] also suggested that the therapist should serve as a role model, but in a more nondirective manner. Knickerbocker asked children to show what they could do when a piece of sensory motor play equipment was initially introduced to them. If a child demonstrated reluctance to approach the new play object, Knickerbocker advocated quiet play with the object by the therapist.

Structure of the play environment is always an important element of occupational therapy, because materials and equipment must always be organized to elicit maximal responses from children. However, the child with sensory integrative impairment has special needs for environmental structure because of diminished ability to handle competing stimuli. The treatment area or room can be attractive but sparse. Although a monotone barrenness can be depressing to a child, it is useful to set up the area with a minimum of colors. Cool but clear colors are usually manageable. Equipment should be neatly stored in closed cabinets whenever possible. It is helpful to have an open but raised shelf to hold the materials for a daily treatment session. Decorations on the walls should be neatly arranged, and too many decorations and distractible ones should be avoided. Treatment duration for each session should be determined by the child's ability to handle changing stimuli. Often two or three activities within a half hour are all that can be accomplished successfully by the child. Finally, sessions should be scheduled so that interruptions are held to a minimum.

As alluded to previously, it is important for occupational therapists to provide play activities that can be accomplished with a sense of success. This key ingredient can make the difference between a child who is intrinsically motivated to try out new play experiences[6,14] and a child who endures a program of meaningless, although potentially therapeutic, activities. Again, careful assessment of performance skills and interests before developing a program is necessary to achieve the preferred outcome. Reliance on measures of sensory integrative functions alone may yield impressive numbers but provides little guidance for actual treatment. The representative exploratory activities shown in Exhibit 13-1 provide a broad variety of suggestions for treatment. Each can be adapted to provide challenging and positive age-appropriate, play-learning experiences for the child or adolescent.

COGNITIVE FUNCTION

If the principles espoused by Piaget, Reilly, and Florey are accepted, then it is axiomatic that play experiences are critical to cognitive development and learning. The entire complement of play categories, activities, and toys presented in Exhibits 13-1 through 13-5 provides a range of self-directed experiences that will sharpen and expand the child's mind.

The mental development of children may be permanently impaired by neurological and metabolic problems. In such instances, special education services, including occupational therapy, will be needed to promote the child's achievement of optimal mental growth. However, therapists need to be aware that any problem that temporarily or permanently restricts the child's ability to engage in learning experiences can result in delay or depression of cognitive development. For this reason, therapists need to concentrate on the cognitive process and outcomes of treatment experiences for all children. Occupational therapists should select and grade treatment activities within the operative capabilities of the child.

Accordingly, the teaching skills of the therapist, in concert with knowledgeable activity analysis, will be of special importance to programs for children with cognitive impairment. The therapist's role-modeling as a player can assist the child's development of action schemes. Through imitation, the child can try out behaviors that have been demonstrated by the therapist.

One useful teaching technique is called *chaining*.[24] Through an activity analysis, the therapist identifies the sequence of steps required in an activity. Then the activity is taught to the child through his mastery of each successive step in the sequence. Although this basic method, called *forward chaining*, is often successful, its opposite, *reverse chaining*, tends to be more productive when cognitive impairment is present. In reverse chaining the therapist and the child work through the activity sequence together, with the child assisting as possible.

But the child is expected to perform the last step independently. When the last step is mastered, then the next-to-last step becomes the new target step for independent performance. From clinical practice, it appears that reverse chaining is more engaging to the child, because it allows the child more exposure to the complete process so that learning takes place through repetition. In addition, the child's experiences of success are tied into the outcome of the process. This appears to maintain higher levels of interest in the activity.

Sharp[23] developed a very useful series of Piagetian tasks that can be adapted for use in occupational therapy. Most of the activities are designed to support the development of classification, seriation, and conservation, and are typical of the symbolic play-learning experiences of the preschool and elementary school-aged child. Materials are prepared by the therapist from items readily available. For example, the children can play with glasses of water to develop volume conservation concepts or arrange shapes to form faces and objects. The activities are graded in a developmental sequence so that learning that is accrued from some of the earlier games will enable the child to master later activities more readily. Sharp[23] is an excellent resource for any occupational therapy program.

Rubin and others[22] reported a program for the remediation of cognitive-perceptual-motor dysfunction in primary grade children that emphasized skill development through exploratory, symbolic, and creative play and educational experiences. The activity program followed a developmental progression that allowed the children to proceed from mastered activities to more challenging ones. The investigators' approach to intervention also included the removal of the child from stress-evoking and stress-producing experiences in school on a part-time basis to obtain optimal results. The investigators found that children who participated in this program for one semester were able to return to home and to school with excellent adjustment and preparation for educational experiences.

Analysis of any toy or activity will suggest cognitive components. Color-matching games, for example, require the development of sensorimotor schema of color likes and differences. However, the child must also have a beginning ability to remember sequences of actions and to differentiate between a personal marker and markers of others and, for example, that a particular motion will cause an arrow to spin. These classification and causation operations may be expected and promoted in 4- to 5-year-children. Childen 3 years of age would have more ·difficulty playing such a game and would be likely to lose interest.

In Chapter 14, Stephens provides a clinical example of a jump rope activity that was unsuccessful because it was beyond the cognitive integration of the children for whom it was designed. She found it advisable to drop the activity entirely and concentrate on antecedent developmental skills. This type of situation will occur in practice daily; for every activity that is successful, there is likely to be another that is less so. Therapists need to remember that, although children's maturation follows a progressive course, there is a spiraling, cyclical nature to development that results in uneven functional states. This appears to be particularly true of cognitive development, because fluctuations of mood, restfulness, and other physical factors can influence the sharpness of the child's operative capabilities.

Construction toys offer a wide range of variations according to the cognitive development of the child. Young children engaged in exploratory play may examine the sensory and action characteristics of simple colored cubes and blocks. At this stage, blocks may be knocked, manipulated, dropped, banged together to produce noises, and placed side by side. Demonstration of the latter pattern on a repeated, purposive basis may be an indication of the child's transition to symbolic play. At this point, blocks take on additional characteristics through their relationships to each other and to the child's mental images. Through symbolic constructions, blocks become parts of a whole and are put together in increasingly complex patterns to represent real or imagined objects. As the child's fine manipulative skills increase, and schemata for interactions multiply, simple blocks are replaced by construction toys that have different shapes and properties. The variety of construction sets that are commercially available seems infinite, from shapes with simple projections that allow pieces to connect at random, to elaborate kits containing wheels, motors, connectors, and specialized parts. Even adolescents and adults may play for hours with the advanced technical kits.

EMOTIONAL FUNCTION

Clinical observations show children who are experiencing emotional difficulty to be characterized by diminished and regressed play behaviors. Children who are withdrawn usually withdraw from play as well. Children who demonstrate acting-out behaviors may use play objects in the course of such episodes, but the actions with such objects are not likely to be described as play. When children with emotional problems do play, their play tends to be perseverative, and the play objects are more appropriate to younger children. These observations indicate that engagement in play serves as a barometer of the emotional status of children.

Adaptation of play activities for the child with emotional problems is often accomplished through structure of the play environment and therapeutic relationship. Axline[1] reported on the use of a Rogerian form of play therapy with young children. She chose toys that, in general, lent themselves to symbolic play, such as action figures, dolls and dollhouses, and water play items.

Toys that did not elicit feelings and expression were not used in the program. As children explored, played with toys, and talked about their play, Axline used nondirective techniques to focus, clarify, and enhance the child's expressive capacity.

Vandenberg and Kielhofner[28] reported on the occupational therapy treatment of a 13-year-old boy with a diagnosis of adolescent adjustment reaction who demonstrated a tendency to withdraw from new situations. The boy resisted initial efforts to participate in a ceramics activity. Subsequently, the occupational therapist began to play with the clay, thus providing a role model for the boy. When the therapist dropped the clay, the situation was handled in a playful manner, subtly indicating to the boy that mistakes in new situations were permissible. Through this experience and subsequent treatment sessions with clay and other craft activities, the boy developed the capacity to approach and explore new situations with a sense of control and satisfaction. In this case, the therapist's structure of the interpersonal relationship was subtle. The choice of clay, a medium that lends itself to many different uses and forms, was complemented by the structuring of a playful atmosphere.

Llorens and Rubin[15] reported on a graded program of play activities that was used by occupational therapy for treatment of children with emotional disturbances. The core of the program was the children's involvement in activity groups. The "basic skills group" for children aged 6 to 12 emphasized free exploratory play with sensory-motor toys. When a child chose to play with an unfamiliar toy, the therapist instructed the child in one way to play with it. This technique was used, first, to provide the child with a successful play experience with the new toy and, second, through the success experience, to stimulate the child's motivation to explore the toy further and develop additional skills.

The "skill development group" was more structured, with specific training in performance of symbolic and creative activities. The children worked on projects in a large group. Although specific expectations for project completion were established, children were permitted to perform at their own individual rates. Interactive experiences with the other children in the group were fostered by the therapist.

The "advanced group" used craft activities and was highly structured. The therapist adopted the role of a teacher. Children were expected to work cooperatively and maintain a level of performance with the rest of the group. Activities ranged from structured kits to materials that demanded original designs. Increasingly complex techniques were taught through units, and children were graded on their productions.

Through this program, which used a variety of play activities that is similar to the model shown in Exhibits 13-1 through 13-5, the children progressed from free play to highly structured play. Expectations for performance were initially self-directed, with gradual increases in external controls. Play progressed from being parallel, to cooperative, to competitive. This program demonstrates well how occupational therapy can provide a microcosm of developmental play experiences for children.

SOCIAL FUNCTION

Many of children's social skills are developed through play experiences. The occupational therapist needs to be alert to this and to structure play situations to provide opportunities for social development.

Parten[20] was one of the early investigators of play. She identified six levels of social interaction in play that are generally regarded as definitive. As reported by Neumann,[19] the six levels are

1. Unoccupied: Playing with own body, random activity.
2. Onlooker: Watching others, but not entering into the situation.
3. Solitary: Plays with toys differently from children within speaking distance; interest centered on own play; independent activity.
4. Parallel: Plays independently but beside and not with others (Figure 13-4).
5. Associative: Group play with overt recognition by group members of common activity, interest, and personal association.
6. Cooperative: Most highly organized group activity; division of labor; group is organized to achieve some goal; control by one or more children (p. 97).

Through unoccupied play and the child's awareness of parental reactions to sensory exploration, the child begins to develop a sense of what actions are socially appealing. As the child watches the play and actions of others, she stores mental images for future consideration and imitation. Onlooker play is not limited to the very young child. It is apt to occur in novel situations, as when the child observes another playing with a new toy. In therapy the actions of the therapist with an unfamiliar toy may be repeated in the child's first experience with the object.

The child's play with a new object will often be solitary as the child obtains firsthand knowledge of characteristics and actions of the toy. The child may then imitate behaviors that were previously observed. Social behaviors in relation to sharing and cooperation are developed through parallel play experiences. Here also modeling and imitation are important, because the child will tend to do what he sees others do. The therapist can help by establishing simple rules for behavior and following up by clarifying to the individual child what behaviors are appropriate or not. Children will often want to play with a toy that another child is using. The therapist can develop skills of sharing and cooperation by structuring time limits and suggesting ways that two children can play together with the desired toy.

Associative and cooperative play experiences are easily promoted in the occupational therapy program. Craft projects and games are well suited to the development of interactive planning, decision making, and role-taking. In addition, children must take turns with

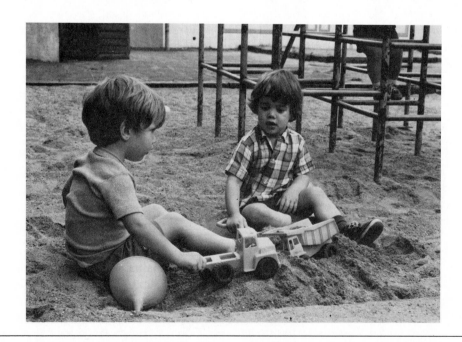

FIGURE 13-4

Exploratory play with sand and toy trucks in a parallel play situation.

From Weiser, M.G.: Group care and education of infants and toddlers, St. Louis, 1982, The C.V. Mosby Co.

tools and materials and develop and follow other cooperative rules. In the clinical example presented earlier, a group of children made felt hand puppets. Although adequate tools could have been made available, the therapist structured the situation to promote social skill development by providing a limited number of scissors, needles, and bottles of glue. The children had to pace their own work to share. The subsequent puppet show was written by the children, each taking turns to contribute lines for one's puppet character and offering ideas for each others' characters. Through this process the individual child's involvement was directed from his own puppet to the success of the group project.

The importance of play programs

In 1972 Gray[10] discussed the effects of hospitalization on work-play behavior. She proposed that, to a greater or lesser degree, the medical focus on the individual's disability and related intervention overrides concern for the life that has been disrupted. Through the course of intervention practices, the individual may experience loss of self-care, social, work, time, play, and decision-making skills. She speculated that these losses may be more of an impediment to the individual's recovery than the initial medical condition.

Although Gray's focus was on the hospitalized individual, her concepts may be readily applied to any individual who experiences a disabling condition. The well-meant reactions of significant others in a child's life tend to "do for" the child (Chapter 14). In addition, the child is often isolated from the mainstream of childhood play and interactions. Therefore it becomes increasingly important for occupational therapists to provide the types of play experiences that promote skill development in the areas cited by Gray.

Gralewicz[9] conducted a study that compared the play of small samples of nonhandicapped children and multihandicapped children who were 3 to 5 years old. Observations of play were recorded in the children's homes by their parents. Gralewicz found that the nonhandicapped children spent significantly more time playing, had more play companions, and engaged in a wider variety of play activities than the handicapped children. In addition, although data were not statistically significant, the multihandicapped children spent more time engaged in no observable activity at all.

A later study by Kielhofner and others[12] examined the differences in play of three nonhospitalized preschool children and three hospitalized children of similar ages who had spent more than 60% of their lives in hospitals. The children were videotaped at play in a hospital playroom and in a standardized play environment in which selected play objects were specifically set up before all videotape sessions. The investigators found significant differences in the level of play development

and the playfulness of the children. The nonhospitalized children were more advanced. The investigators noted that the hospitalized children used toys more simply, rather than trying out a variety of actions, and that they usually did not engage in symbolic and interconnected play activities.

These studies indicate that the children who are seen by occupational therapists in both educational and medical settings are likely to demonstrate deficiencies in both quality and quantity of play experiences. Therefore it is important that the therapist provide opportunities for children to engage in play for its own sake, exclusive of objectives for improvement of specific functional correlates. This may be done through the organization of hospital play programs, in-school and after-school play groups, and free play periods as part of occupational therapy treatment sessions. The role of the therapist as a player is critical. In the study described previously, Kielhofner and others[12] found that the attitude and engagement of adults in the play situation had specific effects on the playfulness of the children.

In addition, therapists can share their knowledge and appreciation of play and its developmental correlates with parents (Chapter 8). Again, the focus and range of play materials and experiences presented in Exhibits 13-1 through 13-5 may be useful for such purposes. Toys and materials can be demonstrated and made available for loan. Formal and informal parent education sessions, with opportunities for demonstration and practice, can be a productive addition to the occupational therapy service. Any program that results in the improvement of the play skills of the child may be considered a significant achievement.

SUMMARY

This chapter presented play as a generic modality in occupational therapy practice with children. Although play activities have long been used because of their therapeutic characteristics, occupational behavior theory has generated a renewed attention to the merits of play for its own sake. Based on the theoretical framework of play that was proposed by Reilly (Chapter 3), other occupational therapists like Florey, Takata, and Michelman have examined the development and content of play behaviors. Their ideas have been incorporated in this chapter in the development of a model of play development and activities for occupational therapy.

With this developmental model as a guide, occupational therapy programs may be planned and carried out that use play as both an adaptive modality and outcome of therapeutic intervention. Adaptation of play activities according to the functional needs of children was discussed in relation to the enhancement of motor, sensory-integrative, cognitive, emotional, and social skills. In addition, therapists were challenged to ensure the adequacy of play experiences for healthy development. Play is the preeminent occupational behavior of childhood and, as such, is a primary focus and modality for occupational therapists who work with this age group.

REFERENCES

1. Axline, V.M.: Play therapy, New York, 1969, Ballantine Books, Inc.
2. Ayres, A.J.: Sensory integration and learning disorders, Los Angeles, 1972, Western Psychological Services.
3. Bobath, K., and Bobath, B.: Cerebral palsy. In Pearson, P.H., and Williams, C.E.: Physical therapy services in the developmental disabilities, Springfield, Ill., 1972, Charles C. Thomas, Publisher.
4. Bruner, J.S., Jolly, A., and Sylva, K.: Play: its role in development and evolution, New York, 1976, Basic Books, Inc., Publishers.
5. Flavell, J.H.: Cognitive development, Englewood Cliffs, N.J., 1977, Prentice-Hall, Inc.
6. Florey, L.: Intrinsic motivation: the dynamics of occupational therapy theory, Am. J. Occup. Ther. **23:**319, 1969.
7. Florey, L.: An approach to play and play development, Am. J. Occup. Ther. **25:**275, 1971.
8. Frantzen, J.: Toys . . . the tools of children, Chicago, 1957, National Easter Seal Society for Crippled Children and Adults.
9. Gralewicz, A.: Play deprivation in multihandicapped children, Am. J. Occup. Ther. **27:**70, 1973.
10. Gray, M.: Effects of hospitalization on work-play behavior, Am. J. Occup. Ther. **26:**180, 1972.
11. Hutt, C.: Exploration and play (#2). In Sutton-Smith, B., editor: Play and learning, New York, 1979, Gardner Press, Inc.
12. Kielhofner, G., and others: Comparison of play behavior in non-hospitalized and hospitalized children, Am. J. Occup. Ther. **37:**305, 1983.
13. Knickerbocker, B.M.: A holistic approach to the treatment of learning disorders, Thorofare, N.J., 1980, Charles B. Slack, Inc.
14. Lindquist, J.E., Mack, W., and Parham, L.D.: A synthesis of occupational behavior and sensory integration concepts in theory and practice. Part 2: clinical applications, Am. J. Occup. Ther. **36:**433, 1982.
15. Llorens, L.A., and Rubin, E.Z.: Developing ego functions in disturbed children: occupational therapy in milieu, Detroit, 1967, Wayne State University Press.
16. Mack, W., Lindquist, J.E., and Parham. L.D.: A synthesis of occupational behavior and sensory integration concepts in theory and practice. Part 1: theoretical foundations, Am. J. Occup. Ther. **36:**365, 1982.
17. Michelman, S.M.: Research in symbol formation and creative growth. In West, W.L., editor: Occupational therapy functions in interdisciplinary programs for children, Rockville, Md., 1969, Maternal and Child Health Service, United States Department of Health, Education, and Welfare.
18. Michelman, S.M.: Play and the deficit child. In Reilly, M., editor: Play as exploratory learning: studies in curiosity behavior, Beverly Hills, Calif. 1974, Sage Publications, Inc.
19. Neumann, E.A.: The elements of play, New York, 1971, MSS Information Corp.
20. Parten, M.B.: Social play among school children, J. Abnorm. Psychol. **28:**136, 1933.
21. Reilly, M., editor: Play as exploratory learning: studies in curiosity behavior, Beverly Hills, Calif. 1974, Sage Publications, Inc.
22. Rubin, E.Z., and others: Cognitive-perceptual-motor dysfunction: from research to practice, Detroit, 1972, Wayne State University Press.
23. Sharp, E.: Thinking is child's play, New York, 1969, Avon Books.
24. Sieg, K.W.: Applying the behavioral model to the occupational therapy model, Am. J. Occup. Ther. **28:**421, 1974.
25. Sutton-Smith, B., editor: Play and learning, New York, 1979, Gardner Press, Inc.
26. Takata, N.: Play as prescription. In Reilly, M., editor: Play as exploratory learning: studies in curiosity behavior, Beverly Hills, Calif., 1974, Sage Publications, Inc.
27. Takata, N.: Introduction to a series: occupational behavior research for pediatric practice, Am. J. Occup. Ther. **34:**11, 1980.
28. Vandenberg, B., and Kielhofner, G.: Play in evolution, culture, and individual adaptation: implications for therapy, Am. J. Occup. Ther. **36:**20, 1982.

SUGGESTED READINGS

Play theory

Chance, P.: Learning through play, New York, 1979, Gardner Press, Inc.

Ellis, M.J., and Scholtz, G.J.L.: Activity and play of children, Englewood Cliffs, N.J., 1978, Prentice-Hall, Inc.

Kielhofner, G.: A model of human occupation. Part 2: ontogenesis from the perspective of temporal adaptation, Am. J. Occup. Ther. **34:**657, 1980.

Kielhofner, G., Burke, J.P., and Igi, C.H.: A model of human occupation. Part 4: assessment and intervention, Am. J. Occup. Ther. **34:**777, 1980.

Levy, J.: Play behavior, New York, 1978, John Wiley & Sons, Inc.

Parent, L.H.: Effects of a low-stimulus environment on behavior, Am. J. Occup. Ther. **32:**19, 1978.

Robinson, A.L.: Play: the arena for acquisition of rules for competent behavior, Am. J. Occup. Ther. **31:**248, 1977.

Takata, N.: The play milieu: a preliminary appraisal, Am. J. Occup. Ther. **25:**281, 1971.

Wehman, P., and Abramson, M.: Three theoretical approaches to play: applications for exceptional children, Am. J. Occup. Ther. **30:**551, 1976.

Play programs

Azarnoff, P., and Flegal, S.: A pediatric play program: developing a therapeutic play program for children in medical settings, Springfield, Ill., 1975, Charles C Thomas, Publisher.

Frost, J.L., and Klein, B.L.: Children's play and playgrounds, Boston, 1979, Allyn & Bacon, Inc.

Moersch, M.S.: Training the deaf-blind child, Am. J. Occup. Ther. **31:**425, 1977.

Morris, A.G.: Nationally speaking: parent education in well-baby care: a new role for the occupational therapist, Am. J. Occup. Ther. **32:**75, 1978.

Wehman, P., and Marchant, J.: Improving free play skills of severely retarded children, Am. J. Occup. Ther. **32:**100, 1978.

Play as a modality

Burnell, D.P.: Egocentric speech: an adaptive function applied to developmental disabilities in occupational therapy, Am. J. Occup. Ther. **33:**169, 1979.

Day, S.: Mother-infant activities as providers of sensory stimulation, Am. J. Occup. Ther. **36:**579, 1982.

DeGangi, G., Hurley, L., and Linscheid, T.R.: Toward a methodology of the short-term effects of neurodevelopmental treatment, Am. J. Occup. Ther. **37:**479, 1983.

Fahl, M.A.: Emotionally disturbed children: effects of cooperative and competitive activity on peer interaction, Am. J. Occup. Ther. **24:**31, 1970.

Farmer, R.: A musical activities program with young psychotic girls, Am. J. Occup. Ther. **17:**116, 1963.

Hindmarsh, W.: Play diagnosis and play therapy, Am. J. Occup. Ther. **33:**770, 1979.

Kohler, E.S.: The effect of activity/environment on emotionally disturbed children, Am. J. Occup. Ther. **34:**446, 1980.

Llorens, L.A.: Fingerpainting with an obsessive-compulsive organically-damaged child, Am. J. Occup. Ther. **17:**120, 1963.

McKibbin, E.H.: An interdisciplinary program for retarded children and their families, Am. J. Occup. Ther. **26:**125, 1972.

Montogomery, P., and Richter, E.: Sensorimotor integration for developmentally disabled children: a handbook, Los Angeles, 1977, Western Psychological Services.

Orem, R.C.: Montessori and the special child, New York, 1969, Capricorn Books.

Price, A.: Juvenile rheumatoid arthritis and occupational therapy, Am. J. Occup. Ther. **19:**249, 1965.

Rugel, R.P., and others: The use of operant conditioning with a physically disabled child, Am. J. Occup. Ther. **25:**247, 1971.

Tyler, N.B., and Kahn, N.: A home treatment form for the cerebral-palsied child, Am. J. Occup. Ther. **30:**437, 1976.

Tyler, N.B., Kogan, K.L., and Turner, P.: Interpersonal components of therapy with young cerebral palsied, Am. J. Occup. Ther. **28:**395, 1974.

LINDA C. STEPHENS
PAT NUSE CLARK

Schoolwork tasks and prevocational development

DEVELOPING SCHOOL READINESS SKILLS
Readiness factors

The occupational therapist who works with young children often must help them to cope adequately with schoolwork tasks. To do this, the child needs to develop academic readiness skills. These are the skills that educators deem important as foundations for learning academic skills such as reading and writing. Readiness has been described as the achieving of subskills along with the developmental maturity to integrate these subskills into a desired new skill.[18] The following is a discussion of motor, emotional, social, auditory-language, visual perception, and cognitive skills.

MOTOR SKILLS

Adequate physical developmental and physical health are considered important aspects of school readiness.[21] In the United States children generally enter an academic setting at age 6 and are assumed to have achieved physical readiness because of their chronological age. According to the Gesell Institute,[2] the average 6-year-old can stand on each foot alternately, make a 32-inch broad jump, catch a beanbag with hands only, tie shoelaces, and copy a divided rectangle. The 6-year-old likes to draw, color, paint, cut and paste, and can print most numerals from 1 to 11. In a study of prekindergarten screening,[9] the information processing of body awareness and motor control was considered to be an important predictor of readiness for first grade. This study also identified children with high activity

levels to be less likely to be ready for first grade.

Table 14-1 presents a developmental sequence of sensory integrative skills. The items in the third column can be considered functional readiness skills that are necessary for adequate performance of the activities listed in column four. Of particular importance as academic readiness functions are eye-hand coordination and ocular motor control.

EMOTIONAL SKILLS

Important emotional readiness skills include emotional stability and self-reliance.[21] Some normal 6-year-olds may not have developed this emotional maturity. The 6-year-old has been described as tumultuous and violently emotional, "typically brash and aggressive, ready for new adventure, falsely sure of himself" (p. 39).[16] To be ready for academic learning, the child should have achieved some degree of mastery of environment and developed feelings of adequacy (Table 14-1). Aggressive behavior has been identified as a factor likely to interfere with school readiness.[9] The abilities to self-direct and actively participate in schoolwork tasks are also important in the learning process.[18]

SOCIAL SKILLS

A child needs to develop the ability to function as a member of a group and to relate appropriately to authority figures to function in a formal learning environment. This social maturity has been identified as a preentrance variable necessary for school success.[21] Attentive behavior is another predictor of readiness for first grade.[9]

TABLE 14-1	Sensory integration development

The inherent function of the nervous system and information from the senses of	Are used to develop	These sensorimotor abilities are utilized to learn more concrete concepts and to develop	Use of these abilities develops an automatic level of function in
Touch	Body scheme	Eye-hand coordination	Reading
Movement	Reflex maturation	Ocular motor control	Writing
Gravity	Center of gravity aware-	Postural adjustments	Spelling
Vision	ness	Auditory-language skills	Number work
Hearing	Motor planning ability	Visual-spatial perception	Problem solving
Smell	Postural balance	Emotional stability	Sequencing
Pain	Awareness of two sides of	Mastery of environment	Ability to conceptualize
Temperature	the body	Feelings of adequacy	Independent work
	Balance between the pro-	Behavioral control	Spontaneous play
	tective and discrimina-		Creativity
	tive sensory systems		Ability to form meaningful personal relationships

From The American Occupational Therapy Association, Inc., Copyright 1980, Totems, Vol. 3, p. 37, Gilfoyle, E.M., and Hays, M.A.

AUDITORY/LANGUAGE SKILLS

Another important area of development is auditory-language function. Information processing of language and verbal reasoning ability have been identified as prerequisites for first grade. Verbal reasoning is defined as the ability to understand and express language.[9]

VISUAL PERCEPTION SKILLS

Some maturity of visual perception is a necessary factor in school readiness. There is evidence that the child who enters school with delayed perceptual development never catches up with his peers in academic achievement, although perceptual processing ability is believed to be fully developed by age 9.[22] Information processing in the visual perceptual-motor domain has been identified as one of the major factors that can predict readiness for the first grade. Adequate perceptual discrimination and visual-spatial perception are considered necessary for the development of reading and writing skills.[21]

COGNITIVE SKILLS

Cognitive function is also considered to be a school readiness factor. A child needs to have acquired a body of knowledge through experience and to be able to attach meaning to that experience.[21] Information processing in the areas of auditory-language skills, perceptual-motor skills, and body awareness must have meaning for the child to benefit from formal educational experiences.

Learning is considered to be a natural function of human beings; it takes place throughout life in and out of the classroom. Children approach new tasks eagerly and enthusiastically, enjoying the challenge of novelty.

Jensen[18] stated that "children do not have to be cajoled, persuaded, coerced, manipulated, or tricked into learning. Given the appropriate conditions, including readiness, children simply learn" (p. 7). The child whose development is delayed, or whose ability to learn is impeded by a physical or cognitive handicap, is also eager to learn. The challenge for the occupational therapist is to provide the appropriate conditions and activities to enable the child to learn at his own level. In this way the child can be helped to develop the necessary readiness skills for academic work.

Functional components of schoolwork tasks: subskill development

ACADEMIC LEARNING

Academic learning is a complex process that generally depends on the development of the readiness skills discussed earlier. In addition, the performance of specific academic tasks depends on the development of specific functional capacities and developmentally antecedent skills, or subskills. For example, a child who is attempting to print letters must have developed the abilities to maintain a sitting position at the desk or table and to grip a pencil or crayon. The child must also have sufficient eye-hand coordination and motor planning ability to direct the movement of the pencil; sufficient motor control to keep pencil marks in the appropriate space; and adequate visual perception, including perceptual constancy, spatial perception, and directionality. In addition, the child must have achieved a level of cognitive maturity that allows him to put together the subskills and abstract concepts needed to print letters. This is called integrated learning.[18]

It is possible that a child might have all the necessary subskills for a task, yet be unable to integrate them for successful performance. For example, a therapist recently attempted to teach two girls how to jump rope. Both girls were 11; one was mildly retarded and the other was learning disabled. Both girls were eager to learn to jump rope. The task was analyzed and broken down into subskills: standing, standing balance on one foot, jumping, jumping over a rope, jumping over a moving rope, and turning the rope with the arms. Each subskill was practiced and mastered. However, neither girl was able to achieve the necessary integration required to put the subskills together and jump rope independently.

When working with children to develop subskills, the therapist often reaches points at which the children's functioning seems to be limited by developmental level or integrative ability. It is of little benefit, and indeed might cause harm, to have the child continue to repeat the subskills in an attempt to learn the higher level skill. In the example given earlier, after several unsuccessful sessions, the jumping rope activity was deleted from the occupational therapy program unless requested by the girls. Meanwhile, other activities were substituted to help the girls develop integrated motor functioning. Perhaps later these girls will be ready to try again, or having mastered the subskills, they may try it on their own when they are developmentally ready.

EMOTIONAL FACTORS

It is important to consider emotional factors when planning occupational therapy programs to prepare a child to cope with schoolwork tasks. *Motivation* is a critical factor. Given the appropriate tasks, most children are eager and motivated to learn without extrinsic rewards. Some children, however, are considered unmotivated when presented with tasks that are beyond their capacities. When instruction persists beyond the child's level of learning, there seems to be a lack of motivation, and psychological turnoff may result.

This turnoff inhibits behaviors that promote learning, even learning for which the child is ready.[18] A teacher complained that a child in his multihandicapped class was unmotivated. The child did not finish her work, appeared uninterested, and persisted in printing her letters backward. The teacher insisted on completion of assignments and set up a reward system for good performance, using gummed stars and stickers. When the occupational therapist evaluated the child, the child was found to have a severe visual perception deficit. The occupational therapy program was planned, using simple perceptual activities and progressing to more complex ones in a small group setting. The child not only worked hard and enjoyed the activities, but also asked for more as homework. Was this an unmo-

tivated child, or had she merely withdrawn from the usual presentation of tasks beyond her readiness level? Jensen[18] stated that "the most effective reinforcement for learning . . . is the child's own perception of his increasing mastery of the skill he is trying to acquire" (p. 7).

Another important emotional component is *self-direction*. Ayres,[3] in discussing the art of therapy, stated that "the most therapeutic situation is that in which the child's inner urge for action and growth drives him towards a response that furthers maturation and integration" (p. 256). The skillful and effective therapist takes cues from the child and his approach to various activities. The self-directed child works with the activity presented by the therapist, needing little encouragment to perform. This child often repeats the activity a number of times, adding variations to it that require even greater organization and integration.

The therapist can frequently learn a great deal about the child by observing free play. Often the child chooses activities that are therapeutically appropriate and that provide both a challenge for growth and learning and also the opportunity for mastery. Certain other activities may be avoided, however, either because the child is not developmentally ready, or because earlier experiences with those activities have resulted in turnoff. The most effective therapy is a program that provides some guidance and structure, yet gives the child freedom to exercise self-direction.

Closely related is the concept of *active involvement*. For change to take place, positive emotional involvement with the activity is needed. The child who is coerced or performs an activity under threat of punishment may meet the requirements of the adult but never become actively involved in the therapy session. When a child works only because of extrinsic factors (that is, a reward, therapist's praise, or mother's insistence), it is extremely difficult for the therapist to determine if the activities are appropriate or to plan a progressively challenging program.

The child who lacks emotional involvement therefore poses a challenge to the occupational therapist. Frequently such children are older and have experienced failure repeatedly. They find it more comfortable to refuse an activity and experience the therapist's disapproval than to risk further failure and reinforce their feelings of inadequacy.

It is essential to work closely with parents when trying to develop active involvement of the child. If the therapist can find out what is important to a child or, for example, what aspect of the disability is particularly bothersome, then this can be used as a starting point for therapy. Sometimes a structured reward program that uses rewards that are meaningful to the child is necessary to encourage the child's cooperation at the beginning of therapy. As the child experiences successes in developmentally appropriate activity performance, the extrinsic reward program can be diminished gradually.

SPLINTER SKILLS

Often, through repetitive training or imitation, children learn to perform certain skilled actions without adequate development of subskills. Such splinter skills are characterized by an inability to generalize and the tendency to lose a skill if it is not practiced. A common example may be found among preschoolers who learn to recite numbers by rote but who are unable to count objects and forget the labels or sequence during a summer vacation.

Although reliance on splinter skill training should be avoided, this method may be useful on occasion in therapy. Most children are highly motivated to learn skills that they see their peers performing and will persist in their own attempts to imitate the behaviors. One intelligent boy with severe athetosis learned to ride a bicycle after many bumps and bruises, although he continued to walk with great difficulty and had no other functional hand use. Other children seen in practice who have extremely poor eye-hand coordination manage to become very adept at electronic video games.

Training to develop splinter skills as part of the occupational therapy program can help make a child more independent, or it can boost self-esteem. Learning to tie shoelaces is a good example. Some children can learn this skill by repetition, even though they do not have an adequate foundation of subskills and could not tie a bow anywhere else. Learning the splinter skill gives the child a sense of accomplishment and avoids the embarrassment of having untied shoes or having to ask the teacher for help. Of course, it is important to continue a comprehensive treatment program that will develop underlying functional capacities and developmentally antecedent skills so that the child will continue to progress in an integrated manner.

ATTENTION SPAN

Attention span is generally defined as the length of time a person attends to a task. Often the evaluation of a child's performance capacities will include a subjective appraisal of his attention span. The therapist (or teacher) observes the child's ability to attend to a task and compares this with the duration and nature of attention seen among other children of the same chronological age on the same task. Thus a child is often said to have a short attention span if he quickly becomes bored or distracted from a task. Efforts can then be concentrated on increasing the attention span. Making a subjective judgment that a child has a short attention span may be superficial and inaccurate. The therapist must question whether the presenting problem impairs the child's ability to attend or whether the activities are inappropriate. Most children become bored with and quickly distracted from activities for which there are no adequate subskills. The following case studies will illustrate this point.

CASE STUDY 1

Allen is a 7-year-old boy in a psychoeducational center for children with emotional and behavioral problems. He was referred to occupational therapy for evaluation and was described as hyperactive and distractible with a short attention span. He was difficult to test, because he concentrated very little on assessment activities presented, and he constantly turned around to grab something else. Several times he darted out of the room and ran down the hall. However, during administration of a standard developmental evaluation, the therapist presented him with a small bottle with a screw top and pellets inside. Allen sat quietly at the table, unscrewing the top, dumping pellets out, and putting them back inside the bottle. He would have continued longer if time had permitted. (Putting pellets in a bottle and dumping them out demonstrates a developmental level of approximately 15 months; screwing a 1-inch top is a developmental level seen at approximately 3½ years.) Does this child have a short attention span, or is his development delayed below age expectancy?

CASE STUDY 2

Kent is an 8-year-old boy who spends half a day in a language disorders class, and the rest of his school day is spent in a class for behavioral disorders. He was referred for an occupational therapy evaluation and was also described as hyperactive and distractible with a short attention span. Kent attempted the assessment activities presented by the therapist but constantly looked around the room, stoppng his activity to point and ask, "What's that?" When attempting gross motor activities, he frequently halted and ran to an object in the room. He fingered things excessively and went quickly from one object to another. Kent had many splinter skills (that is, he could print his name but could not copy a cross) and showed uneven developmental levels.

It is interesting to compare these two children. Allen's attention span deficit appeared to be, in part, a result of being expected to perform activities for which he was not developmentally ready. The occupational therapy program for this child should emphasize developmentally appropriate activities and treatment of other deficits found in the assessment process. In contrast, Kent's evaluation revealed that he probably had a sensory integrative deficit that prevented him from screening out irrelevant stimuli to concentrate on a task. The occupational therapy program for Kent would use a sensory integrative approach to deal with functional deficits. For each of these boys the poor attention span was only one symptom of the child's dysfunction. Therefore treatment was geared toward remediation of the dysfunction, rather than merely working to increase the attention span. Remediation of the dysfunction would have the effect of increasing the attention span.

Developing readiness skills: program goals

The occupational therapist can help young children develop school readiness skills in a number of ways by using selected activities. Many young children with handicaps become accustomed to being the center of a family's attention and to having things done for them. They do not have the social maturity, independent work skills, willingness to share, or ability to take turns that is needed to function in both formal and informal groups. By using group activity programs, the occupational therapist can help the young handicapped child develop these subskills that are needed in school settings.

The therapist, in guiding the child to complete a project that might be either a block tower or a clay figure, helps the child develop other skills that are important for schoolwork. Manipulating materials to make a tangible object helps a child gain mastery over the environment and develop feelings of adequacy. The development of self-reliance not only aids in performance of activities of daily living, but also promotes the child's feelings of capability.

By using carefully planned activities, the therapist helps the child attach meaning to experiences. Physically handicapped children do not have the spontaneous opportunities to explore their environments that normally developing children have. Sensory stimuli and physical activity are needed to promote body awareness and motor control that are prerequisites for academic work.

The therapist can also provide the child with opportunities for problem solving. Often the dependent status of a child with handicaps precludes experiences in making choices, repetition of trial and error, and taking responsibility for one's decisions. The child needs to experiment with different ways of doing activities and to develop the capacity to predict the results of various actions.

RECOMMENDED PROGRAM ACTIVITIES

The pediatric occupational therapist has an infinite variety of activities to use for planning and directing programs to develop school readiness skills. Many traditional childhood games can be used or adapted to meet defined needs. The therapist can also get many ideas by observing normal preschool children at play and determining what developmental needs are met by the activities seen. Why do young children love to play

TABLE 14-2	Eye-hand coordination activities	
Activity	*Adaptations*	*Purposes*
Punch the ball Hold stick with both hands and punch small ball suspended by string (Figure 14-1).	Use cutoff broomstick or long cardboard tube. Try to hit spot marked on wall. Hit while prone or supine. Two children hit ball to each other.	Bilateral coordination Eye tracking Motor planning
Bleach bottle toss Make scoop from bleach bottle. Attach wiffle ball with string (Figure 14-2).	Toss in air and catch in scoop. Use unattached ball. Toss ball to another child to catch. Catch ball in scoop while sitting on T-stool or while walking across room.	Motor planning Eye tracking
Bead stringing	Use varying sizes of beads. Pick out all one shape or color. Copy sequence of beads on another string or on pattern card.	Bilateral coordination Fingertip pinch Grasp and release Figure-ground perception Form perception Sequencing
Rubber band board Make board with rows of nails sticking up 1 to 2 inches. Use colored rubber bands.	Stretch rubber band from one nail to another. Make rows of horizontal, vertical or diagonal bands. Copy pattern card. Superimpose rubber bands over shape made by another rubber band. Try to find hidden shape.	Bilateral coordination Fingertip pinch Form constancy Spatial relationships Figure-ground perception

in large boxes? Why does the toddler enjoy playing with Mom's pots and pans, and what variations does he introduce into the play? Activity analysis, guided by an understanding of child development, can help the therapist relate the use of these everyday activities to the needs of special children.

The following listed material describes a sample of games and activities that can be used with children in treatment programs. The emphasis here is on developing school readiness skills that every child needs, regardless of the presenting problem or disability. Activities for specialized treatment are not included here but may be found in Part VI. In recent years the number of commercially available products for therapists to use in pediatric programs has increased dramatically. Some of the companies offering these products, as well as some useful commercial program packages, are listed in educational catalogs. However, the therapy program can be adequately equipped at little expense. Basic materials and equipment might include the following:

Balls of several sizes	Rope (a 50-foot clothes-
Beanbags	line is good)
Cardboard cartons of	Large wooden, plastic,
various sizes	or cardboard blocks
Carpet samples	Velcro dart board

Beads to string (large	Crayons and large
and small)	marking pens, assorted
Pegboards and pegs	Children's scissors,
(large and small)	assorted
One-inch cubes in colors	Paper, assorted
Formboards with various	
shapes	

With the above materials and thoughtful activity analysis, the variety of program ideas is limited only to the therapist's imagination. Tables 14-2 and 14-3 and Exhibit 14-1 show some sample activities and suggested adaptations that can be used for various purposes in occupational therapy programs.

SCHOOLWORK PROBLEMS

The occupational therapist is frequently asked to evaluate and remedy certain functional problems that interfere with a child's ability to perform schoolwork activities. The most common reasons for referral are (1) uncertain hand dominance, (2) poor visual perception, (3) problems with handwriting, and (4) inadequate ability to use scissors.

Hand dominance

Although a preference for one hand may be evident early in life, hand dominance is often not evident until a child reaches school-age, and it is not stabilized until

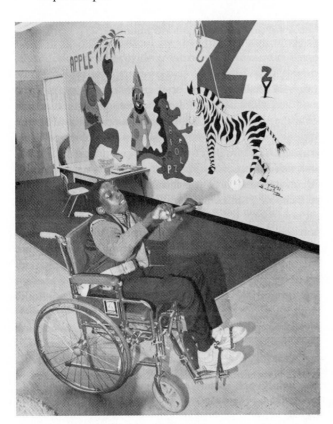

FIGURE 14-1

This eye-hand coordination activity is positioned to encourage trunk and arm extension.

Courtesy Atlanta Public Schools, Atlanta, Ga.

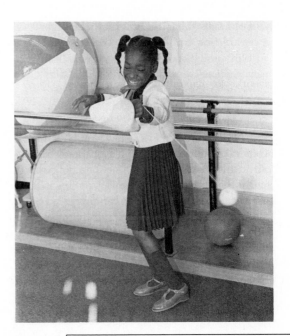

FIGURE 14-2

This girl demonstrates use of the bleach bottle scoop.

Courtesy Atlanta Public Schools, Atlanta, Ga.

TABLE 14-3 / **Gross motor activities**

Activity	Adaptations	Purposes
Pass the beanbag	Imitate manner that beanbag is passed (for example, under one leg, behind back). Sit on floor or on T-stools. Use only right or left hand. Play "hot potato." Person holding beanbag when music stops is loser.	Grasp and release Cross midline of body Motor planning Sitting balance Body scheme Right-left discrimination
Animal walks (Exhibit 14-1)	Use for relay races or "Mother may I." Include in obstacle course. Walk along rope or line on floor. Do it blindfolded.	Motor planning Bilateral integration Body scheme
Cross the river Child must step on "stepping stones" to "cross river" (walk across room) without "getting feet wet" (missing stepping stone and putting foot on floor) (Figure 14-3).	Use carpet squares, cardboard pieces, tape marks, and so on, for stepping stones. Jump or hop on squares. Color code for right and left. Vary placement of squares. Step on rope laid across floor. Walk across by stepping in shoe boxes.	Motor planning Cross midline of body Balance Bilateral integration Right-left discrimination
Obstacle course Arrange course to go over, under, around, through, between, and so on (Figure 14-4).	Examples: under chair or table; step in boxes; roll on carpet or mat; step between rows of blocks; jump over boxes; crawl around desk; and so on.	Motor planning Body scheme Bilateral integration Tactile input Sequencing
Hopscotch	Use jumps instead of hops. Reduce size or number of squares. Use beanbag as marker.	Motor planning Equilibrium Sequencing Bilateral integration
Hit the target Throw beanbag or ball in box or trash can, or use Velcro dartboard (Figure 14-5).	Throw from different positions: all fours, prone, and so on. Sit on T-stools. Throw with both hands simultaneously. Cross midline when throwing. Throw while swinging. Throw with right or left on command.	Motor planning Eye-hand coordination Crossing midline Sitting balance Right-left discrimination

EXHIBIT 14-1

Animal walks

Frog jump	Squat on floor, placing hands on floor in front of you. Move both hands forward, then bring feet up to hands in jumping motion (remain in squatting position).
Bear walk	With hands and feet on floor, move right arm and leg forward simultaneously, then move left arm and leg. If this is too difficult, try it on hands and knees (homolateral creeping).
Inchworm	Squat on floor with hands in front. Keeping feet stable, walk hands forward as far as you can so that you are stretched out. Then keep hands stable and walk feet up to hands back to squatting position.
Elephant walk	Bend over with arms dangling toward floor. Clasp hands together to form trunk. Maintain position while walking, swinging trunk from side to side.
Kangaroo jump	Squat on floor, hands at sides. Raise up and jump forward, sinking back into squatting position as you land.
Crab walk	Lean back and put hands on floor (supine with buttocks off floor). Walk backwards, using hands and feet alternately.
Duck walk	Squat on floor with hands at sides. Remain in position while walking (waddling) forward.

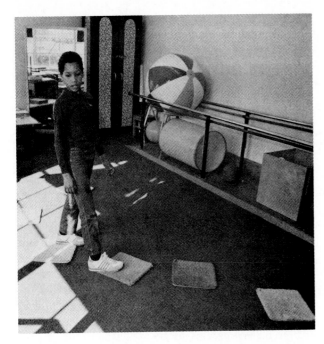

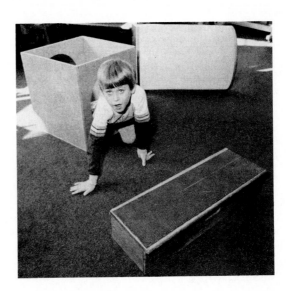

FIGURE 14-3

Stepping on rug squares can be a challenging motor planning activity.
Courtesy Atlanta Public Schools, Atlanta, Ga.

FIGURE 14-4

This obstacle course requires the child to go through the box and
jump down from the step.
Courtesy Atlanta Public Schools, Atlanta, Ga.

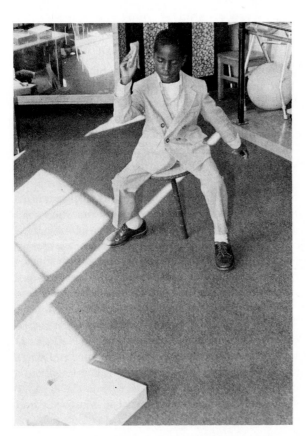

FIGURE 14-5

The addition of a T-stool adds an element of balance to a beanbag game.
Courtesy Atlanta Public Schools, Atlanta, Ga.

age 7.[3] Hand preference, and dominance, are indications of a well-established maturation and differentiation of the two cerebral hemispheres. In general, there is a hereditary predisposition toward hand preference. Of all children with two left-handed parents, 42% will be left-handed. Of children having one left-handed parent, 17% will be left-handed. When both parents are right-handed, only 2% of the children will be left-handed.[5]

The significance of cross dominance (right-handed and left-eyed, or vice versa) has probably been overemphasized as a contributing factor to learning problems. It is estimated that as many as 50% of normal children exhibit cross dominance.[5]

However, in an academic setting, the child must learn to write. If the child does not show a clear hand preference, then it becomes necessary to make a decision regarding hand use so that the child can keep up with the rest of the class. The occupational therapist may be asked to provide data on which a decision can be based and also to provide program activities to aid the child in establishing hand dominance.

One of the first things that the therapist must consider is that lack of established dominance may be a symptom of a more pervasive dysfunction. Children who lack a cerebral dominance may also display inadequate postural mechanisms, hesitancy to cross the midline of the body, a tendency to use each hand on its own side of space, and other indications of an underlying neurodevelopmental problem. Ayres[3] recommended investigating the underlying causes, ameliorating them, and allowing the brain to establish its own dominance.

ASSESSMENT

As a practical matter, however, it is sometimes necessary to make a decision regarding handedness for classroom activities while therapy is progressing. The therapist who has been trained to administer the Southern California Sensory Integration Test battery can obtain useful information through this instrument. The comparison of differences between right-hand and left-hand scores on the Motor Accuracy Tests and left-right differences on the somatosensory tests can be especially helpful when detecting dominance trends.[3]

Knickerbocker[19] offers several methods of assessing hand dominance in children. Timed hammering and coloring samples offer data regarding efficiency of hand use through observation of hand and shoulder control, facial stress, overflow, attempts to change hands, and finished sample products.

PROGRAM ACTIVITIES

Lack of hand dominance in school-aged children rarely occurs as an isolated phenomenon. Therapy for this problem must occur in conjunction with remedia-

tion of the underlying dysfunction. However, activities for exploring dominance, such as those suggested by Knickerbocker[19] (hammering, pounding clay, punching bags, and so on), are also helpful in establishing dominance.

Visual perception

Adequate development of visual perception is crucial, not only for academic learning, but also for coping with and adapting to the environment. Ayres[3] suggested that visual perception is one of four interactive sensory integrative and motor functions that are essential to survival:

1. Perception of gravity and motion through space
2. Extraocular muscle control
3. Locomotion and postural responses
4. Visual perception of space

This section will present a developmental sequence of visual perception and a description of types of visual perceptual dysfunctions to guide the therapist in planning intervention for children with these problems. It is beyond the scope of this chapter to present various theories of dysfunction, nor will the countless research studies related to visual perception be reviewed. Methods of assessing visual perception are found in Chapters 10 and 19, and intervention for visual perception problems associated with sensory integrative dysfunction is discussed in Chapter 19.

SEQUENCE OF VISUAL PERCEPTION DEVELOPMENT

At birth the infant has rudimentary visual fixation ability and brief reflexive tracking ability.[4] Even very young infants have some shape perception and are particularly aware of the human face. Infants as young as 1 week have been shown to have a differential response to patterns. Complex designs, such as the bull's eye, stripes, and checkerboard squares, receive more attention from the infant than simple circles and triangles.[7]

The infant of 2 months or younger has the ability to organize visual information in a meaningful manner. There is some evidence to indicate that visual form perception results from an interaction of innate ability, maturation, and learning, with a critical period for the development of a given visual behavior.[7] At the critical period, or age, the child is physically and mentally ready to develop the perceptual function with little or no training.

In the developmental process of organizing space the child first acquires a concept of vertical dimensions, followed by horizontal dimensions. Oblique and diagonal dimensions are more complex, and perception of these spatial coordinates matures later. The 3- to 4-year-old child can distinguish vertical lines from horizontal ones but is unable to discriminate vertical, horizontal, and oblique lines until about age 6.[5] The ability to discriminate between asymmetrical numbers and letters, such as *b* and *d* and *p* and *q*, does not mature until around age 7.[5,17]

The ability to recognize shapes and forms matures much earlier than the visual motor ability to draw those shapes, or the cognitive-language function of labeling the same. Around 15 months the child begins to make random marks and scribbles on writing surfaces. Most 3-year-olds are able to draw a circle.

The Gesell Institute[17] found that children could draw certain geometric forms at the following ages:

Circle: 3 years
Square: 4 to 5½ years
Cross: 4 years
Triangle: 5 years
Divided rectangle: 6 to 7 years
Diamond: 7 years

Preschoolers and primary grade children continue the developmental process of organizing and defining concepts of form and space by drawing pictures to represent the world around them. Circles with sticks (oblique lines) radiating from them are "suns," squares are houses with triangle roofs, and two vertical lines with circles are trees.

VISUAL PERCEPTION PROBLEMS

Perception may be defined as the ability to recognize, differentiate, and ascribe meaning to information received from the senses. Visual perception can be categorized into several areas: figure-ground perception, size and shape constancy, position in space perception, and spatial relationships.

Figure-ground perception is the ability to differentiate a stimulus from its background or the ability to attend to one stimulus without being distracted by irrelevant visual stimuli around it. Children with figure-ground problems may have difficulty attending to a word on a printed page because they cannot block out other words around it. Inattentive, distractible children may feel compelled to respond to visual stimuli around them (such as a colorful bulletin board or movement in the room) rather than attend to the task at hand.

Size and shape constancy are important aspects of perception that allow a person to develop stability and consistency in the visual world. *Size constancy* enables a person to make assumptions regarding the size of an object, even though visual stimuli may vary under different circumstances. A visual image of a car in the distance is much smaller than the image of the same car at close range, yet the person knows that the actual sizes of the cars are similar. In fact, as adults we learn to gauge speed and the distance between cars by the varying size of the distorted visual image of the cars.

Shape constancy enables the person to recognize objects even when there are differences in orientation or detail. Children with perceptual constancy problems may have difficulty recognizing geometric shapes presented in different sizes or orientations in space. This interferes with the child's ability to organize and classify perceptual experiences for meaningful cognitive operations (Piaget, Chapter 3). This may result in a problem recognizing letters or words in different styles of print or in making the transition from printed letters to cursive ones.

Position in space perception is the ability to perceive the relationship of an object to the self.[8] This perceptual ability is important in understanding directional language concepts such as *in, out, up, down, in front of, behind, left,* and *right*. Children with problems of position in space perception may have difficulty differentiating among objects that differ because of their direction in space. They will also have difficulty planning their actions in relation to the objects around them. These children may continue to show letter reversals past the age of 8, or they may be confused regarding the sequence of letters or numbers in a word or math problem. For example, they may read *was* instead of *saw*. Such children may also have difficulty with the left-to-right, top-to-bottom orientation needed for reading and writing.

The perception of positions of two or more objects in relation to each other and to oneself is called *spatial relationships*. Dysfunction in this area impairs the individual's ability to make judgments when moving through space, because the individual cannot tell if there is sufficient space to walk between two objects. The child might have difficulty catching a ball, because he cannot prepare his body in relation to the ball's movement through space. Adequate spatial relationships are necessary for writing and spacing words and letters on the paper.

OCCUPATIONAL THERAPY INTERVENTION

Visual perception problems are frequently encountered among the handicapped children with whom the occupational therapist works. Such children can benefit most from the activities discussed in this section. However, it is recommended that the treatment for learning disabled children who have visual perceptual difficulties follow the sensory integrative model presented in Chapter 19. Ayres[3] wrote that "irregularity in development of form and space perception is seldom seen independently of other sensory integrative problems" (p. 191) in the learning disabled population. Other children such as those with cerebral palsy, spina bifida, mental retardation, and behavioral disorders should be able to improve their capacity in schoolwork performance through the use of a simple visual perception training program.

Many gross motor activities and games that are

| TABLE 14-4 | Activities for visual perception | | | |

Materials	Figure-ground discrimination	Shape constancy	Position in space	Spatial relationships
Beads to string—assorted sizes, shapes, and colors	Pick out all one color (or shape) from box of assorted beads	String beads of one shape that vary in size or color	String beads in specified sequence (red, blue, yellow or square, circle, oval)	Copy pattern card showing different shapes and sizes
Blocks (1-inch color cubes)	Arrange blocks of one color in a pattern with several colors surrounding it; identify pattern		Copy set of four, six, or nine blocks with colors in correct positions	Copy pattern cards showing three-dimensional block designs
Puzzles	Puzzles with figures having competing background	Formboard puzzles; outline of one shape or picture	Puzzles of graded difficulty requiring rotation to fit in hole	Interlocking puzzles
Pegboards of different sizes	Pick out one color or size from box of assorted pegs	Make different shapes for child to copy on pegboard (square, rectangle, etc.)	Copy pegboard patterns emphasizing left and right, top and bottom	Copy abstract pegboard patterns from pattern cards

used to improve movement and body scheme will also aid in developing basic visual perception abilities. Examples are the following:

Simon Says: Imitating body postures to develop position in space perception and spatial relationships.

Hokeypokey: Concepts of right and left directionality.

Obstacle course: Position in space concepts of *in, on, through, around,* and so on.

Many activities for eye-hand coordination help develop visual perception (Table 14-2). Additional activities for visual perception are shown in Table 14-4 (Figure 14-6).

Handwriting

Occupational therapists concerned with developing independent living skills and functional hand use are often involved in program planning for children with significant handwriting problems. A discussion of the developmental stages in writing and some approaches to remediation are presented here.

Cratty[5] described a series of stages of written expression through which children progress:

1. Holding a writing instrument; making marks on paper and other surfaces
2. Crude scribbling and random marks
3. Reaction to stimuli on paper; the child may "balance out" a figure on one side of the paper with lines or scribbles on the other side
4. Drawing of simple geometric figures such as crude spirals and crosses
5. Drawing of more exact geometric figures; combining two or more figures
6. Drawing of objects familiar to the child, such as people, houses, trees
7. Printing and cursive writing
8. Drawing of three-dimensional figures and pictures

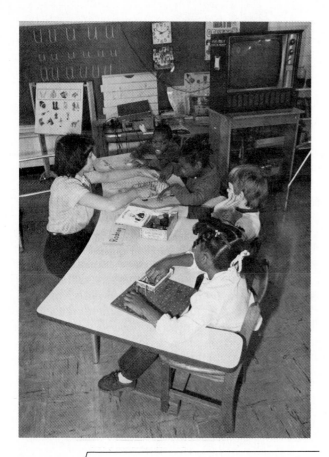

FIGURE 14-6

An occupational therapist guides orthopedically handicapped children in activities for visual perception.

Courtesy Atlanta Public Schools, Atlanta, Ga.

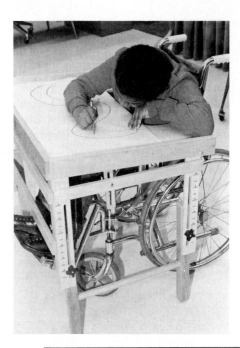

FIGURE 14-7

Proper positioning is essential for this prewriting activity.

Courtesy Atlanta Public Schools, Atlanta, Ga.

OCCUPATIONAL THERAPY INTERVENTION

In general, planning for remediation of handwriting problems follows the same general principles of treatment for other problems encountered by the occupational therapist. The child's handwriting is evaluated, during which specific problem areas are identified. By use of activity analysis, components of the needed skills are determined, and a program of graded activities is planned to develop subskills. The development of prewriting skills can enable the child to accomplish smooth and efficient handwriting (Figure 14-7). Several authors have developed specific programs for dealing with handwriting problems. The methods described by Olsen,[24] Knickerbocker,[19] and Frostig and Horne[8] are summarized here.

Olsen[24] described a method of teaching both printing and cursive writing that emphasizes letter formation. Olsen specified readiness skills needed before learning writing. She presented a logical method of teaching writing based on the kinds of strokes used in each letter. The use of specially prepared paper that has large spaces, directional orientation cues, and simple lines is recommended. This method has proved to be especially useful with older children who have already learned how to write but who are unable to write legibly because of poor eye-hand coordination and improper formation of letters.

Knickerbocker[19] described a program for developing writing skills that stressed the development of sensorimotor skills as prerequisites for learning to write. The progression from gross motor coordination and sensory functioning to fine movements of the dominant hand is described in the program plans which include a section on manuscript printing and cursive writing. This section spans "the development of pencil skills from the early scribbling stage and beginning finger prehension of preschoolers to the refinements of script writing" (p. 223).[19] In Knickerbocker's approach, large writing motions are initially used with scribble board activities, bimanual circles, templates, and large figure eight patterns. Such motion patterns help develop the basic motions for formation of letters in writing. Directional orientation of letters and numbers is emphasized with specific training in letter formation and sequential patterns of movement.

Frostig and Horne[8] described an approach for teaching writing in which premanuscript exercises and precursive writing activities are presented to help the child practice the basic components of letters and numbers. For example, "cat's tails" become the stroke for the printed *j* and *g*, while "giant's upper teeth" are the basic motions for the cursive *i* and *u*. The use of grids is recommended to aid the child in producing letters

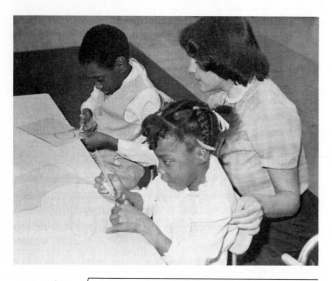

FIGURE 14-8

Cutting activities are often used as part of programs to improve eye-hand coordination or fine motor function.

Courtesy Atlanta Public Schools, Atlanta, Ga.

correctly without reversals. Frostig and Horne mentioned the need for adequate form perception and form constancy before developing the ability to form letters correctly.

Cutting with scissors

Children in kindergarten and primary grades are frequently involved in coloring, cutting, and pasting activities. These are necessary readiness skills that also promote visual-motor coordination and perception. The occupational therapist often includes cutting activities as part of programs to improve eye-hand coordination or fine motor function (Figure 14-8).

DEVELOPMENTAL SEQUENCE

When the motor and perceptual functions of a child have developed normally in the first 2 years, cutting skills will generally progress in the following manner[4]:

2 years: Holds scissors with fingers in correct holes.
2½ years: Holds paper with nondominant hand; makes snips or single cuts.
3 years: Makes continuous straight cut close to or on the line to cut paper in two.
4 years: Cuts along lines to cut out triangle.
5 years: Cuts curved lines; cuts out circle.
6 years: Cuts cardboard and cloth.
7 years: Cuts out complex designs and pictures.

OCCUPATIONAL THERAPY INTERVENTION

Careful assessment of the child's scissor-cutting skills is necessary before occupational therapy can be planned. Is the child correctly positioned and supported sufficiently for optimal hand use? Is the child developmentally ready for the activity? Does the child have sufficient supination to hold the scissors correctly? Is there sufficient isolation and differentiation of movement of the fingers to open and close the scissors?

The therapist can then make decisions regarding appropriate activities and adaptations for the child. Although some left-handed children can use regular right-handed scissors, left-handed scissors are preferable. Right-handed scissors cause pressure and pain in the metacarpophalangeal thumb joint area of left-handers, and under the best of conditions this can reduce motivation for cutting activities.

A number of types of special training scissors are available from educational supply companies. One type has a large, single loop to control the blades rather than smaller finger loops, and it is useful for children with immature fine motor control. Cutting is achieved by using gross grasp and a squeezing motion on the loop. Other training scissors have extra loops for the therapist to control the scissor movement. For some children it may be necessary to use some type of holding device to facilitate one-handed cutting.

Using scissors is not only important as a developmental and school readiness skill, but also as a life skill necessary for independent living. Graded cutting activities can be included as part of a prevocational program. For example, a retarded, blind teenager progressed from snipping rolls of therapy putty, to cutting small pieces off a strip of paper, to cutting yarn for a weaving project. The overall goal was to develop adequate prevocational skills for employment in a sheltered workshop setting.

PROGRAM EXAMPLE

An effective program to develop cutting skills that is interesting to children has been developed by Carol Leaman, Fulton County School System, Ga. Initial testing of cutting skills is done to identify

1. *The width of line that the child can stay within while cutting.* This may be ½ inch, ¼ inch, ⅛ inch or 1⁄16 inch. Normal performance is demonstrated when a child can cut along a 1⁄16-inch line with few deviations.
2. *The form of line that the child is able to control hand movements to cut.* These are sequenced from straight lines, to angles, to corners, to large and small curves. The ability to cut along all of these forms constitutes normal performance.
3. *The number of deviations from the line (into the white space of paper) made by the child during testing on the width and form of line that represents the upper limits of cutting skills.* This precise measurement of cutting skills assists both with the formulation of objectives and the plan of treatment activities. Variations in training

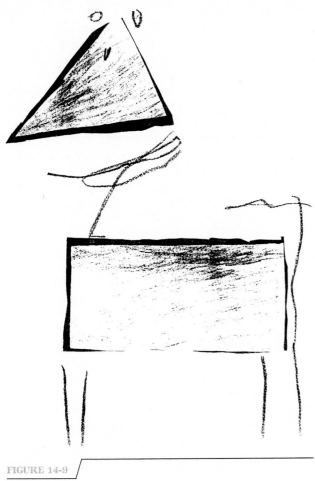

FIGURE 14-9

Sample of cartoon made by cutting and coloring.

PREVOCATIONAL DEVELOPMENT
Vocational development processes in early and middle childhood

It is generally agreed that the ability to work constitutes a primary indication of mature adult functioning in our society. Therefore a major goal of the growing child's socialization is to develop work attitudes, goals, and behavior. This is particularly true of the formalized socialization experiences that occur within educational institutions.

However, most vocationally oriented instruction begins at the junior high and high school levels. In most instances, satisfactory performance of related classwork is dependent on the prior development of adequate manipulative, cognitive, and interpersonal skills. For adolescents with chronic developmental, physical, or emotional disorders, such instructional programs can be particularly stressful, because the assumed foundation of skills is generally not well developed. The youth with an acute condition may have less difficulty with developmentally antecedent skills but still be limited in participation in vocationally oriented classwork by the constraints of a presenting problem.

Clinical observations

Observation from occupational therapy practice suggests that the difficulty encountered by children with chronic disabilities is caused by a paucity of appropriate play and prevocational-directed experiences during the preschool and elementary school years. People around a handicapped child tend to "do for" him or her, thus eliminating opportunities for decision making, problem solving, and development of perceptual, manipulative, and interpersonal skills to full capacity. Parents frequently place a larger burden of household chores on other siblings because of the more extensive care needs of the handicapped child. Too often they tend to overlook the possible assignment of feasible household responsibilities to the handicapped child. In fact, both teachers and parents often relieve the handicapped child of many of his achieved self-care tasks in the interest of time. Although children with emotional or behavioral problems may be expected to assume more self-care and household responsibilities than the child with motor impairment, expectations are still limited by time, tolerance, and temperament. The short-term result of these childrearing methods is that the child never acquires enough practice to become proficient in those tasks for which he has the capacity.

The described problems are coupled with fewer opportunities for free play experiences with other children. The child with behavioral or emotional problems tends to be rejected by his peers because of his poor play skills. The child who has an acute illness or injury

scissors and other adaptive techniques are made according to the cause of the child's cutting problems.

A series of geometric shapes that uses the described line forms are preprinted with different line widths. Each child is presented with a booklet of pictures that uses the same basic geometric shapes and coloring to produce animal cartoons. The child selects a cartoon to copy and then colors in the geometric shape with specified line width that is used for that cartoon. Shapes are then cut out and pasted to construction paper; coloring completes the cartoon details (Figure 14-9). This activity aids in the development of writing skills as well when necessary adaptations are made in the selection of drawing and coloring tools. Leftover paper from the geometric forms are taped together and deviations are checked in red pencil to maintain a record of skill development. Original cartoons can also be made with the shapes according to the skills of the child. Children like this activity, because they have a finished product to share with their parents that has been more enjoyable to perform than rote cutting exercises on strips of paper.

may have, through hospitalization or confinement at home, severely diminished play experiences. The child with motor impairment is dependent on others to transport him to playmates. Increased time spent on self-maintenance and transportation activities results in less time available for play. In addition, because the child cannot engage in many of the play activities of neighborhood peers, he may be excluded from other activities for which capability does exist. Often the simple fact that a child does not attend the local school or preschool is enough to preclude development of play relationships with other children in a neighborhood. The end result of these limiting factors is often a disabled adolescent who is poorly prepared to enter the competitive labor market.

The following section will identify some of the specific differences in the vocational development experiences of handicapped and nonhandicapped children in early and middle childhood. Examination of such differences will allow the therapist to design pediatric occupational therapy programs that can help to promote more adequate vocational development. A continuum of prevocational programming and recommended modalities are also proposed.

Development of work behaviors

Regrettably, there is only minimal information available that is specifically related to prevocational and vocational development of handicapped children during the preschool and elementary school years. Occupational therapy is the only discipline that has a history of identifying this early development as important, yet there is no clinical research to support our hypotheses. Pertinent information is available, however, about general vocational development and vocationally oriented programs for handicapped adolescents. There is also a large body of research related to attitudes toward handicapped children that has bearing on the problems described earlier.

VOCATIONAL DEVELOPMENT

There is general agreement among theorists of work behavior that vocational development is already in process during middle childhood. Ginzberg and others[10] identified middle childhood as a fantasy period for occupational choice, in which the child daydreams and role-plays with future possibilities. At about 10 years of age the child enters a tentative stage of occupational choice, and begins to consider vocational opportunities in terms of personal interests, skills, and values. By late adolescence the choice process becomes realistic. The older teenager is able to more accurately determine his capabilities and interests in terms of job options and settle on a specialized course of vocational skill development.

Super[30] proposed that the first stage of vocational exploration occurs in early adolescence, with the recognition of a number of possible vocational choices. Both Super[30] and Ginzberg and others[10] believed that more realistic matching of vocational interests and aptitudes occurs later in the teen years. However, Roe[27] proposed that the antecedents of occupational interests and aptitudes could be found in the activities and relationships of preschool children.

One of the most comprehensive and recent texts on work behavior is by Neff,[23] who was interested in vocational rehabilitation of psychiatric clients. Neff believed that work is a learned behavior, and that immediately on entry into school, children are socialized into being productive. They develop a need to achieve that is reinforced by families.

Hershenson[15] proposed that work adjustment involves three domains that develop in the following sequence:

1. Work personality, including self-concept and personal motivation for work
2. Work competencies, including habits, physical, cognitive, and interpersonal emotional and social skills
3. Work goals that are specific and appropriate

There are some differences in Hershenson's model when applied to handicapped individuals, which will be discussed later in this chapter.

In a cross-sectional study of children's knowledge, attitudes, and experiences of work, Goldstein and Oldham[12] surveyed 905 children in first, third, fifth, and seventh grades. They found that children were very aware of work behaviors, even in first grade, although their knowledge became increasingly specific and realistic by seventh grade. Of particular interest was their finding that most of the children already had direct, personal work experiences. Even first graders typically had at least two household chores for which they were held responsible. Many had been paid for chores that assisted neighbors, such as feeding pets or helping with gardening.

In the field of occupational therapy, play is viewed as the exploratory arena for the development of work skills, competencies, and roles[26] (Chapter 3). Shannon[29] stated that

> Play provides for the development of the child's physical and intellectual capabilities and is therefore a major force in shaping self-concept. Play teaches discipline, responsibility, and citizenship. Cooperation, competition, loyalty, and respect for others are learned in the play milieu. Play encourages risk-taking, trial and error, and commitment, essential to the development of problem-solving or decision-making skills. Play also provides for identification with the worker role through the simulated experiences of role-playing and day dreaming (p. 290).

In essence, play and childhood chores promote the development of a foundation of readiness skills commonly regarded as being prevocational. This includes such elements as motor, sensory-integrative, and cognitive skills for task performance, problem solving, ability to follow directions and work with others, and decision-making.

PREVOCATIONAL PROGRAMS FOR HANDICAPPED ADOLESCENTS

Although there is an abundance of literature related to vocational rehabilitation of handicapped adults, only recently has attention turned to programs for youth. Hershenson[15] stated that a handicapping condition affects work competencies and that this in turn reflects back on components of the work personality. Because an individual does not have adequate competencies for the work environment, self-concept and motivation to work are affected. The self-concept does not include identification with the worker role, and motivation to work is hindered by expectation of failure. Although Hershenson's remarks were related to the adult with an acquired disability, his concepts seem applicable to children with chronic disabilities.

Similarly, Neff[23] defined work as a learned complex of behaviors and stated that

> An early disability may have the effect of denying the person those experiences, interactions, and environmental pressures which gradually transform most of us from nonworking children to working adults. . . . They have either never learned to play the role of a worker or have been desocialized for so long a period that the work role has become alien (p. 264).

Most reports of work-oriented programs for handicapped youth are available to high school students only. In a comprehensive review of services for adolescents, Goldberg[11] declared the need for enriched prevocational experiences. He reported on a number of new programs in the metropolitan New York City area that included field trips to businesses and industries, part-time work experiences, and counseling. Perhaps the best developed of these programs was under the direction of Haraguchi[14] at the New York University Institute of Rehabilitation Medicine. Although the program was designed to serve adolescents only, similar types of experiences seem feasible for younger age groups. Haraguchi[14] noted that

> The family has no immediate experience with living life as a disabled person. . . . They are often more likely to try to protect a more vulnerable disabled teen from additional physical harm and the stresses of life than to urge the teenager to creatively make maximum use of his or her assets (p. 76).

This statement supports speculations made earlier regarding parental limitations of the handicapped child's activity competencies. This should not be misconstrued as a negative attitude toward parents; the behaviors noted are typically demonstrated by concerned and caring parents.

ATTITUDES

No reports have been found that investigated early prevocational development among preschool and elementary school-aged handicapped children. However, another body of relevant literature is concerned with attitudes of others toward disabled children as playmates and classmates. Westervelt and Turnbull[31] reported on a review of such attitudinal studies and concluded that as the physical or behavioral manifestations of a child's disability increase, so does the child's social isolation.

Popp and Fu[25] asked normal preschool children to indicate whether handicapped and nonhandicapped children could participate in a variety of play and self-care activities. The children were shown a series of line drawings accompanied by audiotaped verbal descriptions. The subjects were then asked to point to one of two pictures of children (nonhandicapped and wheelchair-confined or walking with a crutch) to indicate which child was capable of performing the activity. Popp and Fu found that, to a significant degree, even preschool children judged the handicapped child as being less capable. Even more pertinent was the fact that when the subjects had the opportunity to choose a representational child as playmate for the various activities, they most frequently chose the least disabled child.

It may be concluded that a child with a chronic or severe disability who manifests many observable signs of the disabling condition is likely to suffer from a deprivation of play and other socialization experiences that normally promote vocational development. Occupational therapy appears to be the only human service discipline that has historically demonstrated a concern with programming related to this phenomenon before the adolescent years of the handicapped youth. Regardless of the theorist, any developmental model of occupational therapy indicates that the problem must be addressed in the formative years of readiness skills. The same readiness skills for schoolwork that were discussed earlier permit the maturation of vocational readiness. It may be hypothesized that prevocational programming for handicapped chidren that begins at the high school level is too late to achieve even minimally adequate results.

Activities to promote prevocational skill development in early and middle childhood

Shannon[29] developed an inventory of occupational choice skills that rates an individual's experience with various play and household chore activities that are be-

EXHIBIT 14-2

Composite list of play-leisure and household activities that promote vocational development

1. Construction sets: erector sets, Tinkertoys, Lego sets
2. Toy cars and trucks
3. Doll play
4. Household odds and ends
5. Toy tools
6. Handcrafts
7. Collections
8. Dress up
9. Cops and robbers
10. Doctor-nurse-patient
11. Space fantasy games
12. Other dramatic play
13. Races
14. Contests
15. Model building
16. Photography
17. Playing cards
18. Sketching
19. Drawing and coloring books
20. Painting
21. Scrabble
22. Dramatics
23. Musical instruments
24. Creative writing
25. Inventions
26. Experiments
27. Videogames and computer play
28. Soccer
29. Basketball
30. Baseball and softball
31. Aerobic exercises and dancing
32. Care for pets
33. Care for younger siblings
34. Help with housework
35. Clean own room
36. Make own bed
37. Wash and dry dishes; help load dishwasher
38. Remove trash
39. Help with yardwork
40. Set dinner table
41. Prepare simple foods
42. Run errands for parents
43. Do chores for neighbors and teachers

Adapted from Goldstein, B., and Oldham, J.: Children and work: a study of socialization, New Brunswick, N.J., 1979, Transaction Books; and Shannon, P.: Occupational choice: decision-making play. In Reilly, M., editor: Play as exploratory learning: studies in curiosity behavior, Beverly Hills, Calif., 1974, Sage Publications, Inc.

lieved to promote self-discovery, decision-making skills, and work role experimentation. Activities included playing with erector sets, painting, dramatic play, caring for pets, and many others. Although the ratings that Shannon presented are inadequately normed, it is believed that the chosen activities do constitute an appropriate variety of prevocational development experiences for the elementary school-aged child. These activities can form the basis of a prevocational program for children when combined with some of the activities identified by Goldstein and Oldham[12] as routine chores of children. Exhibit 14-2 provides a composite list of activities from these two sources, with the addition of computer play. Certainly, not every child will perform all of these activities because of variable interests and capabilities. However, activity adaptation by the occupational therapist should enable each child to participate in a number of these choices.

HOUSEHOLD ACTIVITIES THAT PROMOTE VOCATIONAL DEVELOPMENT

One of the critical elements will be persuading parents and teachers to use the adapted activities in the daily routine of a child. For example, a child in a wheelchair might easily carry daily attendance sheets from the teacher to the principal's office. A child at home can sort through fresh fruits as easily from bed as at the kitchen table, if parents are alerted to the relationship of such activities to future vocational skill development. Similarly, the parents of a developmentally disabled child may need periodic encouragement to continue their efforts to involve the child in self-care activities, with the reminder that skill development comes through prolonged repetition.

CASE EXAMPLE: LEARNING DISABILITY GROUP

Handicrafts offer an excellent medium for occupational therapy programming to develop work skills. Children's motivation to do and make things is particularly evident with crafts such as leather kits, simple jewelry making, popsicle stick projects, embroidery, ceramics, and the ubiquitous plastic-lacing activities. Exhibit 14-3 details the task analysis objectives for a prevocational program that was designed for a group of 8- to 10-year-old children in a class for severe learning disability. For the 2 years before initiation of this program, the children participated in individual and small group occupational therapy programs that emphasized sensory integrative and academic skill development. The occupational therapists felt that these children could not wait until high school to begin programs that would relate to career development, so they chose to shift the focus of therapy services.

EXHIBIT 14-3

Prevocational program objectives for elementary school children with learning disabilities

Annual goal: The student will complete several prevocational skill development activities that will use elementary marketing, taking written orders, measuring, sequencing, money skills, counting, adding, construction, and fine motor dexterity. Activities will be completed with decreasing supervision and assistance and increasing accuracy.*

Media: Prevocational work task kits and projects, including alphabet bead bracelets and necklaces and rainbow link belts. Graded puzzles will also be used as enabling activities for practice of skills.

Objectives: The student will
1. Correctly count and record the number of all parts in a designated set of 1 to 20 parts, with 90% accuracy
2. Correctly identify and record the type and number of missing parts in a designated set of 1 to 15 parts, with 80% accuracy
3. Follow a three- to five-part verbal instruction sequence through completion of a designated task, using written cuing, with 80% accuracy
4. Complete two product samples with 100% accuracy, and 90% independence of assistance from the therapist
5. Approach at least five customers, following a prescribed verbal sequence with 90% accuracy
6. Measure size of product for individual customer orders, using a string and measuring instrument, with 100% accuracy and minimal assistance from the therapist
7. Plan out and place parts of product in correct sequence to prepare for construction of order, with 100% accuracy and minimal assistance
8. Complete five orders, with 100% accuracy and minimal assistance
9. Count the number of components used in the product, and by using price of 1¢ per component, determine cost of product and write out a "bill for service," with 100% accuracy and minimal assistance
10. Return to customer for payment by following a prescribed verbal sequence, with 90% accuracy and minimal assistance from the therapist.

*Percentages for accuracy and independence are varied according to the ability of each child in the group.
Courtesy Carol Leaman, OTR, Fulton County Schools, Atlanta, Ga.

The goal of the next yearlong program was to begin to develop prevocational skills, and the medium chosen was stringing alphabet bead bracelets. This activity was selected because of its appropriateness to the sensory-integrative and academic status of the children, and because it lent itself to practice of a wide range of vocationally useful skills. A review of the objectives (Exhibit 14-3) indicates that to complete the alphabet bead bracelet project the children were involved with elementary marketing as they approached school staff to show samples and take written orders. Their measuring skills helped determine the proper length for the finished bracelet, and their money concepts and money-changing skills were developed as well. The development of sorting, counting, sequencing, and math skills was also intrinsic to the activity. Finally, the actual production of the bracelets strengthened prehension and manipulative abilities of the hand and challenged visual and tactile perception. As the program progressed, the success of its objectives was increasingly apparent through improved interest levels, self-confidence, and organization of work.

Vocationally oriented occupational therapy with older children and adolescents

PREREQUISITES FOR VOCATIONAL TRAINING

In an unpublished paper Sarkes,[28] a vocational educator, prescribed a list of readiness skills expected of entering students before the initiation of specific job skill training. This list included awareness of and adherence to safety rules, work motivation, understanding of the importance and purpose of work, ability to follow rules, positive self-image, and specific perceptual and motor skills needed for job performance. Table 14-5 contrasts these criteria with areas of a standard occupational therapy assessment through which vocational readiness data can be obtained. Specialized prevocational evaluation instruments are discussed in Chapter 11, along with a number of tests that can be used to elicit relevant information. However, most useful information can be obtained within the format of an ordinary occupational therapy assessment, if the therapist looks at the data in terms of these criteria.

TABLE 14-5	Comparison of prerequisites for vocational training with data collected through a standard occupational therapy evaluation

Factor	*Occupational therapy evaluation items*
Awareness of and adherence to safety rules	Judgment
	Ability to follow directions
	Problem-solving ability
	Knowledge of safety rules
Work motivation	Psychological functions
	Performance motivation
	Social and cognitive functions
Understanding the importance and purpose of work	Same as above, plus—
	General pattern of activity involvement
	Independence in self-care, home, and community living skills
	Ability to describe purpose of work
Ability to follow rules	Cognitive functions
	Same as first section above
Positive self-image	Psychological functions
Perceptional motor skills needed in vocational arena	Sensory-integrative functions
	Motor functions
	Activity analysis

Adapted from Sarkes, A.: Unpublished paper presented to the Cobb County School System, Marietta, Ga., 1979.

OCCUPATIONAL THERAPY PROGRAM OBJECTIVES

It should be reiterated that occupational therapy services should be directed to developing readiness for vocational exploration and training. There are a number of well-trained disciplines that can provide specific training for job performance. Occupational therapy is not one of these. Instead, the focus of the occupational therapist is on total task performance within the developmental requirements of the individual's daily routine. For the adolescent this includes preparation for the worker role. In the middle (junior high) and high school levels, most curricula provide opportunities to explore different vocational opportunities and develop specific work skills. Related services may include guidance counseling, industrial arts, vocational education, career days, cooperative work experiences, home economics, and office or library aide programs. School systems typically require several related courses and offer other options as electives.

In a discussion of occupational therapy and vocational education, Creighton[6] noted that the therapist is best qualified to provide the following services: task analysis of specific job training activities for student placement purposes, pretraining assessment of student skills, and modification of equipment and facilities. These services may be used in the computer labs, home economics and typing rooms, as well as in sheltered workshops and day training centers. An American Occupational Therapy Association position paper[1] on the role of occupational therapists in vocational rehabilitation stressed that services should be used to ensure the potential worker's smooth transition from the evaluation phase to the work environment. Again, this rests on the therapist's use of the processes of activity analysis and activity adaptation.

CONTINUUM OF OCCUPATIONAL THERAPY SERVICES

The suggestions from Sarkes[28] and Creighton[6] may be used to support the development of a continuum of occupational therapy services in prevocational and vocational skill development. At the beginning of the continuum, which is directed toward promoting independence in self-maintenance skills, the occupational therapist is heavily involved in the planning and training aspects of the program. However, as the adolescent participates more in specific work-related training and performance, the therapist's role becomes more consultative.

1. *Increasing independence in self-maintenance skills.* As part of gaining independence in the world of work, the adolescent is first expected to assume increasing responsibility for self-reliance in personal care, home management, school responsibilities, community living, and communicating for himself. Occupational therapists can provide practice experiences in related activities for the child or adolescent with a disability in cooperation with other service providers in an educational or rehabilitative setting. The therapist can ensure

that the youth can make telephone calls, order food from a fast-food restaurant, establish a morning routine for personal care and household chores, and get from one place to another by using appropriate transportation resources.

2. Developing work skills through leisure activity groups. Assuming that not all adolescents will have had the benefit of a vocationally oriented rehabilitative program during elementary school years, the therapist may often need to intervene at the middle and high school levels. The focus of treatment is to develop those same skills identified by Sarkes[28] and discussed earlier. Again, the use of craft activities and graded individual and group chores can be adapted and used.

At a training center a group of young adults with severe cognitive impairment were referred to the occupational therapist. Their age range was 18 to 23 years, and all were independent in ambulation or wheelchair locomotion. Several had lived at home exclusively and participated through the years in training center programs directed toward developing partial independence in feeding, developmental, and perceptual-motor activities. Others had participated in similar programs at a state residential facility for the retarded before discharge in a deinstitutionalization phase. The training center had a well-established sheltered workshop program doing industrial subcontracts on a piecework basis. However, the referred group members were unable to adapt to this program because of their poorly developed work skills.

The therapist felt that a daily program was needed that would allow the clients to learn to produce tangible objects. A group program was chosen that had gradually increasing requirements for adherence to rules and independent task performance. The training center aides were instructed in the use of various structured, repetitive crafts, such as mosaic tile designs and leather link belts. Initial sessions were held for 30 minutes daily, including time for clean up of work space. As general abilities improved, the sessions were lengthened to one hour daily, and clients were expected to help prepare materials as well as clean up cooperatively. The program continued well over a year for a number of clients before they were able to transfer to the subcontract program. Rather than using a variety of activities, this program concentrated on developing increased skill in performance of a small number of tasks. This focus seemed more appropriate to the repetitive nature of piecework jobs that would be done in the sheltered workshop. The therapist monitored the program on a twice monthly basis and spent additional on-site time with staff training and client evaluation.

3. Improve function in specific work activities. As the adolescent reaches the point of specific vocational education-preparation, the therapist's role becomes generally consultative. The selection and the direction of training activities are likely to be done by a rehabilitation specialist, industrial arts teacher, or other personnel specialized in job skill training. The occupational therapist is called on when problems arise in the performance of training activities that appear generally appropriate to the client. The occupational therapist's use of activity analysis according to functional components of task performance may assist in the selection and grading of work assignments.

Often the occupational therapist is asked to assist with adapting the job so that it can be at least partially performed by the client without assistance. This may involve adapting the position of the body, work surface, or task materials; grading the tools, materials, or equipment that are used to do a job; altering the training methods or work process to meet the capabilities of the client; or establishing graded sublevels of expected task performance (Chapter 7). Very often the therapist merely needs to help design a "jig," that is, a small piece of equipment that will assist the work trainee in doing a specific task.

For example, a young man placed in the sheltered workshop program discussed earlier was hemiplegic. The primary subcontract of the workshop was packaging parts for silk flower kits in small plastic bags. Trainees who had use of both hands would hold the bags open with one hand while sorting and stuffing with the other. Because the hemiplegic hand of this trainee was immobile, he had tried to work one-handed much without success. Because he was highly motivated to produce, and had attained a high production rate on previous subcontracts, the trainee became highly frustrated and began a pattern of absences. The case was referred to the occupational therapist who designed a simple Orthoplast jig to hold the plastic bags upright and open. Within one day the young man learned how to use the jig efficiently enough to match piecework rates of other trainees.

Occasionally a client in job training or preparation requires specific remedial programming to improve his function before he can satisfactorily meet the demands of one or more tasks. In such instances it may require backing away from the specific vocational preparation program to concentrate on improving component functions. The occupational therapy treatment program will be time-limited: activities should be age-appropriate and clearly related to subsequent performance of the desired work.

CASE STUDY 3

A 19-year-old college student had grown up in a small town where her family was well-known. She participated throughout her school years in church-related activities. She reported that she had always had difficulty with academic work, but, with family and teacher assistance, she graduated from high school. She chose a career in religious education and attended a small junior college for her first 2 years because her fiancé was going there. Because of various external social pressures, she decided to earn her associate degree in arts and sciences before transferring to another school for her junior and senior years in religious education. She was referred to the occupational therapist by another therapist at the end of her freshman year.

Confronted by the demands for technical reading and writing, as well as time-limited tests in the sciences and math, the student experienced overwhelming failure in her freshman courses. After reviewing the student's self-reported history and observing her postural patterns, the occupational therapist decided to thoroughly assess her work interests, sensory-integrative function, and study skills. The therapist referred the student to speech therapy evaluation of cognitive language development and auditory perceptual functions. Evaluation results indicated that the student had impaired postural and bilateral integration, including poorly developed dominance, visual figure-ground discrimination deficits, and very poor auditory and visual memory. Her chosen occupation as a religious teacher was well in line with her interests and capabilities, and it appeared that the required coursework for her junior and senior years would be manageable. However, results of the vocational interest tests indicated that her associate degree curriculum courses were far removed from areas that interested her.

The combined occupational and speech therapy programs included a modified Montgomery-Richter[20] home program to improve postural and bilateral integration. Every 2 weeks the therapist would demonstrate a set of exercises to the student and send materials home with her with check-off instruction charts to document the exercises that she practiced 15 minutes daily. The activities began at the apedal level in prone and supine positions and progressed to the standing position in which balance activities on one foot were to be done. To provide a higher level of difficulty, selected activities from the first 8-week sequence were then to be done on a large inflatable. The student reported that she often did the activities with her roommate, and both girls tended to think of it as a physical fitness program rather than an occupational therapy program.

In addition to the home exercise program, treatment activities also included giving the student drills to improve her auditory and visual memory and giving her assistance with developing her study skills. The student was advised to meet with professors of courses to review reading and writing requirements before selecting courses for registration. By underlining sentences as she read, the student eliminated some of the difficulties she had with figure-ground discrimination and visual memory. A number of other compensatory methods were suggested and adopted, and the student's grades gradually improved. She was discharged at the end of her sophomore year after 6 months of therapy with the option to return if she had difficulty meeting academic requirements of the religious education curriculum.

PLANNING AHEAD FOR VOCATIONAL DEVELOPMENT

Developing work-related skills is a long-term process, even for normally functioning children. Parents have to make conscious decisions about when to require independence of their children, when to assign them a new responsibility, and when to intervene in their interactive play situation. The occupational therapist who intervenes in this process with children who have handicaps must create and simulate developmental experiences. This requires working and planning ahead with other service providers, agencies, work-related resources, and parents.

Most often services will be provided in coordination with educational facilities and staff. In an average high school, space and curriculum schedules are determined 1 or more years in advance. Practically speaking, this means that, although an occupational therapist may decide that a group of physically handicapped high school students need to learn to make sandwiches, the home economics room and teacher may not be available for such a program until the following year, if that soon. Industrial arts classes cannot be readily moved from an inaccessible basement, even if they are nominally open to students with any disability. A whole year may be necessary to survey vocational resources in a school and community before the therapist can begin to develop a program framework to present to administrators. Transportation, teacher, and room resources and schedules; alternatives to on-site programs; and capital improvement costs need to be considered. Useful alternatives include area vocational-technical schools, state vocational rehabilitation programs, and state independent living programs. These agencies are already developed to assist with the handicapped teenager, but each has individual constraints in service delivery. The therapist and colleagues are faced with sorting through resources and needs, and they must use careful planning to design a program continuum that will foster the development of work readiness.

SUMMARY

This chapter has presented an overview of school and prevocational skills that are considered basic outcomes of occupational therapy programs for all children. The therapist has a responsibility to ensure that children will be prepared to undertake the requirements of appropriate academic and vocational training opportunities. To ensure children's preparedness for schoolwork, the occupational therapy program will emphasize the development of visual perception skills, cutting skills, and writing skills, as well as the establishment of hand dominance. Occupational therapists are aware that these skills also support the development of vocational abilities, and they design programs that provide graded experiences to promote work skills and knowledge of occupational choices. This is accomplished through activity selection in general occupational therapy programs for preschool and school-aged children, as well as in specific, vocationally oriented programs for adolescents. Occupational therapy services in vocational programs include increasing independence in self-maintenance activities, developing work skills through leisure activity programs, and improving function in specific work activities. Collaboration with teachers and vocational specialists is basic to service delivery.

REFERENCES

1. American Occupational Therapy Association, Inc.: Official position paper: the role of occupational therapy in the vocational rehabilitation process, Am. J. Occup. Ther. **34:**881, 1980.
2. Ames, L.B., and others: The Gesell Institute's child from one to six, New York, 1979, Harper & Row, Publishers.
3. Ayres, A.J.: Sensory integration and learning disorders, Los Angeles, 1975, Western Psychological Services.
4. Brigance, A.: Brigance Diagnostic Inventory of Early Development, North Billerica, Mass., 1978, Curriculum Associates, Inc.
5. Cratty, B.J.: Perceptual and motor development in infants and children, New York, 1970, Macmillan, Inc.
6. Creighton, C.: The school therapist and vocational education, Am. J. Occup. Ther. **33:**373, 1979.
7. Fantz, R.L.: The origin of form perception, Sci. Am. **204:**66, 1961.
8. Frostig, M., and Horne, D.: Frostig Program for Development of Visual Perception, Chicago, 1963, Follett Publishing Co.
9. Gallerani, M.O., and Reinherz, H.: Prekindergarten screening: how well does it predict readiness for first grade? Psychol. Sch. **19:**175, 1982.
10. Ginzberg, E., and others: Occupational choice: an approach to a general theory, New York, 1956, Columbia University Press.
11. Goldberg, R.T.: Toward an understanding of the rehabilitation of the disabled adolescent, Rehabil. Lit. **42:**66, 1981.
12. Goldstein, B., and Oldham, J.: Children and work: a study of socialization, New Brunswick, N.J., 1979, Transaction Books.
13. Reference deleted in proofs.
14. Haraguchi, R.S.: Developing programs meeting the special needs of disabled adolescents, Rehabil. Lit. **42:**75, 1981.
15. Hershenson, D.B.: Work adjustments, disability, and the three R's of vocational rehabilitation: a conceptual model, Rehabil. Couns. Bull. **26:**91, 1981.
16. Ilg, F.L., and Ames, L.B.: The Gesell Institute's child behavior, New York, 1981, Harper & Row, Publishers.
17. Ilg, F.L., and Ames, L.B.: School readiness, New York, 1965, Harper & Row, Publishers.
18. Jensen, A.R.: Understanding readiness: an occasional paper, Urbana, Ill., 1969, ERIC Clearinghouse on Early Childhood Education.
19. Knickerbocker, B.: A holistic approach to the treatment of learning disorders, Thorofare, N.J., 1980, Charles B. Slack, Inc.
20. Montgomery, P., and Richter, E.: Sensorimotor integration for developmentally disabled children: a handbook, Los Angeles, 1978, Western Psychological Services.
21. Moore, R.S., and others: School can wait, Provo, Utah, 1979, Brigham Young University Press.
22. Morency, A., and Wepman, J.: Early perceptual ability and later school achievement, Elemen. Sch. J. **73:**323, 1973.
23. Neff, W.S.: Work and human behavior, ed. 2, Chicago, 1977, Aldine Publishing Co.
24. Olsen, J.Z.: Handwriting without tears, Brookfield, Ill., 1980, Fred Sammons, Inc.
25. Popp, R.A., and Fu, V.: Preschool children's understanding of children with orthopedic disabilities and their expectations, J. Psychol. **107:**77, 1981.
26. Reilly, M.: Play as exploratory learning: studies in curiosity behavior, Beverly Hills, Calif., 1974, Sage Publications, Inc.
27. Roe, A.: The psychology of occupations, New York, 1951, John Wiley & Sons, Inc.
28. Sarkes, A.: Unpublished paper presented to the Cobb County School Systems, Marietta, Ga., 1979.
29. Shannon, P.: Occupational choice: decision-making play. In Reilly, M., editor: Play as exploratory learning: studies in curiosity behavior, Beverly Hills, Calif., 1974, Sage Publications, Inc.
30. Super, D.E.: The psychology of careers: an introduction to vocational development, New York, 1957, Harper & Row, Publishers.
31. Westervelt, V.D., and Turnbull, A.P.: Children's attitudes towards physically handicapped peers and intervention approaches for attitude change, Phys. Ther. **60:**896, 1980.

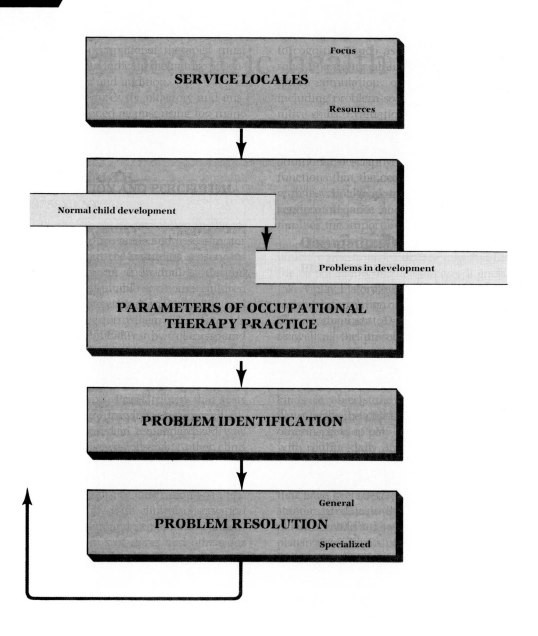

Occupational therapy treatment: specialized areas

JUDITH M. PELLETIER
ALISA PALMERI

High-risk infants

A dvances in medical technology have resulted in higher survival rates for gestationally younger, smaller, and sicker infants. Improvements in obstetrics now enable medical and nursing staffs to monitor infants through complicated gestations, to postpone premature births, and to make difficult or high-risk deliveries safer for both mother and infant. Concurrent improvements in pediatrics have increased the ability to prolong and maintain the lives of sick infants. One of the by-products of such medical advances has been the development of special care nurseries that are equipped to provide specialized treatments needed by these high-risk infants.

CONCEPT OF RISK
Identification of infants at risk

A number of biological and sociological factors that appear to indicate high-risk status have been identified in the literature[53] (Table 6-1). Concern with early identification of these factors has resulted in the development of several screening devices. These include Parmelee's Obstetric Complications Scale,[34] which is used to predict the effect of maternal factors on the unborn child. The Apgar Scoring System[32,52] (Chapter 9) is used to assess fetal and perinatal factors. A number of developmental and neurobehavioral assessments, such as the Brazelton Neonatal Behavioral Assessment Scale[9] (Chapter 11), the Dubowitz Neurological Assessment of the Preterm and Full-term Newborn Infant,[19] and Als' Assessment of Preterm Infant Behavior (APIB),[2] are used to monitor the progress of the infant beyond the delivery room.

High predictive value of neurological and neurobehavioral assessments of newborns has not been well established.[52] Instead, it appears that long-term outcome depends on a large number of variables. Examples include severity of an initial traumatic insult, plasticity of the central nervous system, potential for recovery, and hereditary and environmental (including socioeconomic) factors. Research in this area continues in an effort to provide comprehensive, accurate, and useful assessment of the newborn.

Who is at risk?

The term *at risk* has been discussed at length in Chapter 6. For purposes of this chapter, it shall refer to an infant who has suffered prenatal or perinatal complications that might contribute to later developmental delays or deficits.[21] Such infants have a certain probability of showing sensory-motor deficits or cognitive handicaps in childhood.[39]

Traditionally, birth weight and gestational age have been major determinants of the risk status of the newborn.[32] Concern with these factors has given rise to the terms *small for gestational age (SGA)*, *appropriate for gestational age (AGA)*, and *large for gestational age (LGA)*, as well as *preterm*, *term*, and *post-term*. In general, the shorter the gestation period, or the lower the birth weight, the greater the infant's risk status.[16]

Without the addition of other complications, shortened gestations per se are not necessarily risk-producing. However, a preterm delivery may be symptomatic of dysfunction in the maternal, fetal, or placental systems. It is these complications that can interfere with a smooth transition from fetal to extrauterine life.[23] The more common medical problems to which premature infants are susceptible vary according to the degree of prematurity (Table 15-1). Other medical problems of high-risk infants that are not necessarily related to prematurity are described in Table 15-2.

Because of the variety of individual differences, as well as the variations in postnatal complications, it is difficult to make generalizations regarding the developmental outcome of preterm infants. Variable definitional criteria of prematurity in different studies in the literature[8,12,48] have led to the investigation of heterogeneous populations, and therefore comparisons of these

studies are difficult to make. However, it is evident that young, sick preterm infants are a vulnerable group who may be at risk for neurodevelopmental deficits.

Although *at risk* and *vulnerable* are often used interchangeably in this and other writings, some authors do make a differentiation. In such instances, vulnerability refers to those intrinsic characteristics of the infant that increase susceptibility to complications, and at risk is related to extrinsic, environmental factors. These distinctions are supported by increasing evidence from follow-up analysis of groups of preterm infants at older

---

TABLE 15-1 Common medical problems of premature infants

	Description	Potential associated disorders of developmental significance
Respiratory		
Respiratory distress syndrome (RDS)	A respiratory disorder that affects immature lungs and is characterized by grunting, retractions, nasal flaring, tachypnea, and cyanosis.	May require prolonged mechanical ventilation that results in decreased movement, decreased stimulation or interaction, and decreased parent-infant interaction.
Atelectasis	Incomplete expansion of lungs at birth resulting from poor development of lung tissue and weak respiratory muscles.	There is an increased incidence of neurodevelopmental deficits in infants who have required prolonged ventilation resulting from respiratory complications. The infant may also develop secondary feeding problems.
Hyaline membrane disease (HMD)	A respiratory disorder in which there is inadequate amount of pulmonary surfactant lining the terminal respiratory units of the mature fetal lung, and subsequently inadequate fetal lung development.	
Bronchopulmonary dysplasia (BPD)	A chronic lung disease characterized by abnormal development of the lung and bronchi that occurs in many survivors of respiratory therapy for HMD.	
Meconium aspiration	Inspiration of meconium, a fetal fecal substance passed during delivery when hypoxia occurs; can result in obstruction of the airway, interference with gas exchange, and respiratory distress.	
Apnea	The transient cessation of breathing.	
Cardiovascular		
Patent ductus arteriosus (PDA)	Failure of the fetal heart openings to close. The most common cause of congestive heart failure in the newborn.	Inadequate nutrition resulting from fluid restriction. There is a risk of chronic pulmonary abnormalities and prolonged ventilation.
Hemorrhage	Bleeding resulting from deficiency of several clotting factors in the blood combined with the fragility of the capillary walls, especially in small vessels as in the brain, which leads to intraventricular or intracranial hemorrhage.	Neurological insults and subsequent neurodevelopmental deficits.

Adapted from Dorland's illustrated medical dictionary, ed. 25, Philadelphia, 1974, W.B. Saunders Co.; and Paxson, C.: Van Leeuwen's newborn medicine, ed. 2, Chicago, 1979, Year Book Medical Publishers, Inc.

Continued.

TABLE 15-1	**Common medical problems of premature infants—cont'd**	
	Description	*Potential associated disorders of developmental significance*
Metabolic		
Hyperbilirubinemia	An excess of bilirubin (a red bile pigment) in the blood causing infants to appear jaundiced.	Neurological deficits in severe cases.
Metabolic acidosis	A pathological condition resulting from accumulation of acid or loss of base in the body, characterized by decreased pH.	Jitteriness. Neurological deficits in severe cases.
Hypocalcemia	Reduction of the blood calcium below normal.	Jitteriness, convulsions.
Hypoglycemia	An abnormally diminished content of glucose in the blood.	Hyperirritability, jitteriness, apnea, cyanosis, irregular respiration, convulsions.
Nutritional and gastrointestinal		
Necrotizing enterocolitis (NEC)	An acute superficial necrosis of the mucosa of the small intestine and colon characterized by profound shock and dehydration.	Long-term feeding problems and behavioral complications.
Temperature regulation		
Subnormal body temperature	Results from poor heat production or increased heat loss. Cold exposure can cause an increased metabolic rate and oxygen consumption with subsequent acidosis, apnea, hypoglycemia, and pulmonary hemorrhage.	Possible neurological deficits in severe cases.
Immunity		
Pneumonia	Inflammation of the lungs.	Respiratory distress, temperature instability, acidosis, poor feeding, lethargy, seizures. Potential hearing loss secondary to ototoxic antibiotic medication.
Septicemia	Presence in the blood of bacterial toxins.	
Meningitis	Inflammation of meninges of the brain.	
Urinary tract infection (UTI)	Infection of the urinary tract.	
Ophthalmological		
Retrolental fibroplasia (RLF)	Characterized by the presence of opaque tissue behind the lens, leading to retinal detachment and arrest of eye growth; generally attributed to use of high concentrations of oxygen in the care of the premature infant.	Myopia, poor central acuity, retinal detachment, blindness.

ages. The literature suggests that as the child ages, perinatal factors assume considerably less importance, while environmental factors become more significant. There is reason to believe that the detrimental effects of prematurity are exacerbated in nonsupportive environments and ameliorated in supportive, caregiving environments.[16,17,50] Retrospective studies now indicate that the four factors that relate to subsequent deficits include social conditions, as well as anoxia, delivery complications, and prematurity.[50]

Despite a rich body of literature, a well-developed conceptual model of risk remains elusive.[30] A combination of prenatal, perinatal, postnatal, and genetic conditions offers the best definition of cause. Recent data show that the proportion of children who demonstrate serious sequelae as a result of preterm birth is markedly

TABLE 15-2	Other common medical problems of high-risk infants

	Description	*Potential associated disorders of developmental significance*
Neurological		
Asphyxia	Anoxia and increased carbon dioxide tension in blood and tissues.	Abnormal tone, poor interactive skills, irritability, feeding problems, decreased spontaneous movement.
Intraventricular hemorrhage (IVH)	Bleeding into the ventricles of the brain.	
Seizures		
Congenital anomalies		
Trisomies	Presence of an additional chromosome of one type in an otherwise diploid cell, as in Down's syndrome.	Abnormal muscle tone; mental retardation.
Limb deficiencies	Absence at birth of a portion of one or more of the extremities.	Temporary movement and functional disorders.
Cleft lip or palate	Longitudinal opening or fissure (occurring in the embryo) in the lip or palate.	Feeding problems, speech difficulties.
Tracheal-esophageal fistula	Abnormal passage or communication between trachea and esophagus.	Feeding problems.
Birth weight		
Small for gestational age (SGA)	Weight for age falls in the 0 to 10th percentile range.	Impaired attachment process. Jittery, irritable.
Large for gestational age (LGA)	Weight for age falls in the 90th to 100th percentile range.	Frequently poor tone.
Birth trauma		
Head injuries		Neurological sequelae, depending on nature of injury.
Nerve injuries		
Fractures		Temporarily impaired movement.

Adapted from Dorland's illustrated medical dictionary, ed. 25, Philadelphia, 1974, W.B. Saunders Co.; and Paxson, C.: Van Leunwen's newborn medicine, ed. 2, Chicago, 1979, Year Book Medical Publishers, Inc.

reduced from prior years. While studies indicate continuing problem areas, such as learning disabilities, we cannot clearly identify causal mechanisms, early precursors, or onset periods. What has become more apparent is that the hazards and stresses that were thought to have specific, definitive, and direct influences on development are in fact more complex in their interactions and effects.

Research on early intervention

The significance of early identification of risk status lies in the implication that early intervention may lead to improved function and outcome. Much has been written on the effects of early experiences on behavior, especially with regard to the nature-nurture controversy, the plasticity of the central nervous system, criti-cal periods, and effects of sensory stimulation and deprivation. General conclusions from a review of the literature are that

1. The vulnerability and responsiveness of the innate elements of the central nervous system are heightened during critical periods.
2. The significance of both stimulation and deprivation varies with the type, length, and time of the experience, as well as other factors.

One view that may be postulated is that the preterm infant who is placed in an Isolette is deprived of the opportunity to complete fetal maturation in the protected environment of the womb and is deprived of its normal intrauterine sensory experiences as well. Moreover, life in an Isolette deprives the infant of many human interactions and the opportunity to receive organized stimuli. Such deprivations may contribute to later problems. In contrast, it may be hypothesized that the infant in an Isolette is exposed to additional, different experiences, particularly of a visual and auditory nature, that can affect behavioral development in a detrimental way. Although no definitive body of knowledge clearly supports either proposal, it seems clear that deprivation or experience must be considered within the context of the infant's maturational level. This means that either deprivation or stimulation can be expected to have less impact on an immature infant than on a more mature infant. This concept can be applied both neurologically and behaviorally, and requires thorough knowledge of the embryological development of the central nervous system, as well as postnatal neurobehavioral development.[31,36,38,49]

It is also apparent that extrauterine experience does have some influence on development. Review of the literature seems to indicate positive effects of infant stimulation programs with preterm babies.[13,22,51,59] However, because of variations in research design, types of stimulation provided to study groups, and measurement techniques, it is difficult to draw specific conclusions. More research is necessary with clearly defined groups, special attention to individual differences, and measurement of responses at multiple age periods. The most critical issue at this time is the identification of more specific types of intervention that are appropriate for each particular infant.

THE NEONATAL INTENSIVE CARE UNIT

The neonatal intensive care unit is a busy, often crowded place where the atmosphere is frequently high-pressured. Emergency life-and-death decisions are interspersed throughout the daily care routines for infants. A visitor to the unit is immediately struck by the complicated equipment (Figures 15-1 to 15-4). Each infant lies in an open warmer, an Isolette, or a crib. The open warmer allows easy access to the infant during the initial period after admission to the unit when many medical interventions are necessary. It also contains a heat source to keep the infant warm. The Isolette provides a neutral thermal environment for temperature maintenance, and as a contained area it allows the provision of supplementary oxygen when necessary. Mechanical ventilatory assistance (via respirator use) can be provided to infants on open warmers or in Isolettes. Once the infant is able to maintain his own body temperature and to tolerate room air, he will be moved to an open crib. Parents and staff then have easier access to the infant, and the infant can be more easily moved to other locations within the unit or outside the unit, for example, to and from the parents' visiting room. Often attempts are made by parents and staff to personalize each infant's space through placement of toys and pictures.

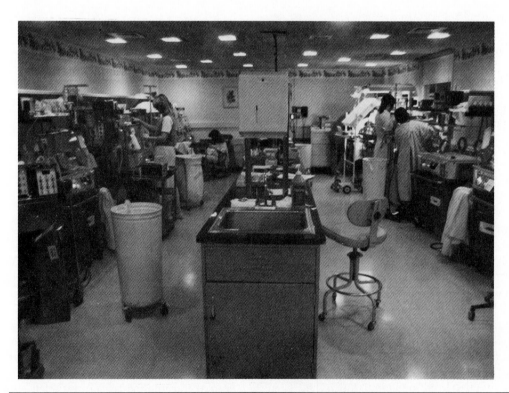

FIGURE 15-1

The neonatal intensive care unit.

Photo courtesy Newborn Intensive Care Unit, University of Connecticut Health Center's John N. Dempsey Hospital, Farmington, Conn.

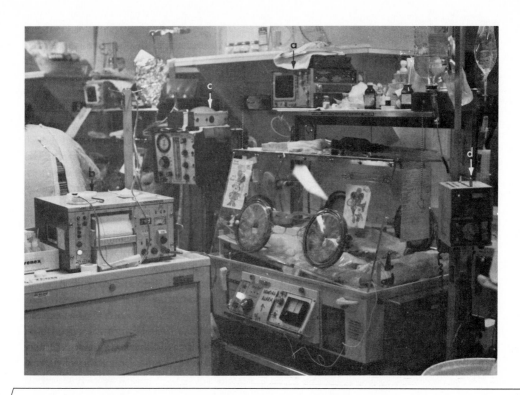

FIGURE 15-2

Isolette *(center)* with other neonatal equipment as indicated: *a,* heart monitor; *b,* oxymonitor; *c,* respirator; *d,* infusion pump on intravenous pole.

Photo courtesy Newborn Intensive Care Unit, University of Connecticut Health Center's John N. Dempsey Hospital, Farmington, Conn.

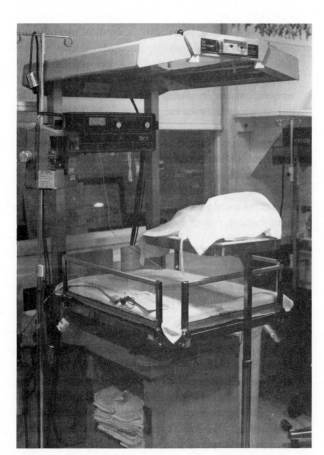

FIGURE 15-3

Open (radiant) warmer.

Photo courtesy Newborn Intensive Care Unit, University of Connecticut Health Center's John N. Dempsey Hospital, Farmington, Conn.

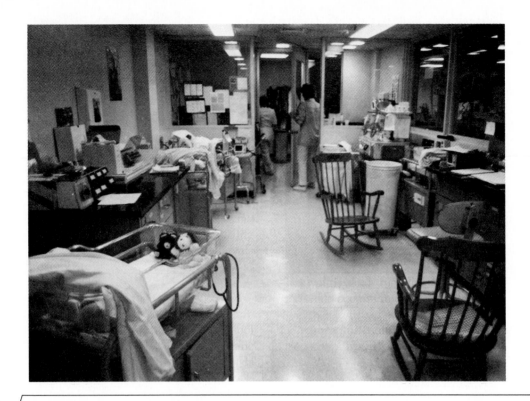

FIGURE 15-4

Newborn step-down nursery houses "graduates" of the neonatal intensive care unit. Of note are the more open environment, the quieter atmosphere, and open foreground.

Photo courtesy Newborn Nursery, University of Connecticut Health Center's John N. Dempsey Hospital, Farmington, Conn.

There is an abundance of additional equipment that is used in caring for these infants and that adds to the complexity of the unit. Ventilators provide respiratory assistance to infants who are unable to sustain adequate respiratory patterns on their own. Heart monitors, apnea monitors, and oxygen monitors assist the staff with constant monitoring of vital signs. Since many infants are unable to receive adequate nutrition orally because of illness or immaturity, volumetric infusion pumps may be used to provide nutritional requirements through continuous nasojejunal (tube) feedings or through central alimentation (intravenously).

While some of the additional equipment has a diagnostic purpose (for example, the transilluminator, portable x-ray machine, electroencephalography [EEG] and ultrasound equipment), other equipment (for example, bright lights that provide phototherapy in the treatment of hyperbilirubinemia) is used in the treatment of specific medical problems. The infant himself, being necessarily attached to some of this equipment, most likely has skin electrodes placed on him to monitor his heart rate; may have an intravenous tube; may be on a respirator; or may have an orogastric or nasogastric tube in place for feeding. Obviously the effect may be overwhelming for parents who are already faced with the stress of the unexpected birth of an ill or premature infant.

Although the environment of the nursery is lifesaving, it can also be potentially overstimulating to the infant. The intense medical care required by the sicker infants often necessitates bright lighting around the clock. The various sounds and alarm signals of monitors and ventilators combine with ringing telephones, voices of staff and visitors, and cries of infants to maintain a fairly high noise level. The infants are also subjected to a variety of procedures, such as multiple examinations, radiography, and other tests including blood work, some tube feedings, and surgery, that can be considered invasive.

The general activity level of the nursery is high because of the multitude of services required by the infants. The subsequent number of personnel involved may include physicians, nurses, respiratory therapists, occupational therapists, physical therapists, aides, and unit clerks. The number of people in the unit at any given time may be increased intermittently by the presence of parents taking advantage of the 24-hour visiting privileges.

Although the primary focus on the neonatal intensive care unit historically may have been on medical care for survival, growing concern has developed regarding more qualitative issues, many of which relate directly or indirectly to the ultimate question of developmental outcome. What are the long-term effects of the medical problems that caused the infant's hospitalization in an intensive care unit? What effect might such a difficult introduction to life have on growth and development? What is the role of early experience and, in this case, the early experiences provided by prolonged hospitalization? How does the infant respond to the many and varied sensory stimuli, such as bright lights and loud noises, provided in the special care nursery? And what kinds of interventions or environmental adaptations can we make to provide the infant with an optimal setting for growth and development?

OCCUPATIONAL THERAPY INTERVENTION
Practice settings

With the increasing recognition of the importance of early identification and treatment of developmental risk factors, the services of allied health professionals, especially occupational and physical therapists, have been more consistently employed at facilities providing health care for high-risk infants. Earliest contact with these infants is made in the neonatal intensive care unit. Most neonatal intensive care units are attached to larger medical centers that can provide a variety of specialized services and follow-up care. After the initial intensive care hospitalization, infants requiring long-term hospitalization, but not continued intensive care, may be transferred to another unit within the facility such as a pediatric inpatient floor where occupational therapy services may continue to be provided. Further follow-up care is provided after discharge through the neonatal follow-up clinic. Here the services of an occupational therapist may be employed to provide developmental assessment at regular intervals during the early years of life. Typically, follow-up visits to the occupational therapist might be scheduled at the ages of 4, 8, 12, 18, and 24 months and annually until school age.

Because of the high level of technology required, special care nurseries most often function on a regional basis. This means that admissions to a particular nursery may be from a widespread geographical region. Therefore, although a certain percentage of infants come from the immediate local area, a number of others are from outlying areas and have either been transported to the unit shortly after birth or have been delivered at the unit's medical center after maternal transport. Since parental visiting is often more difficult in these cases, the goal with such infants who need continued medical care is to transfer them back to local hospitals as soon as medically advisable. Therefore the length of stay at the neonatal intensive care unit or its related step-down nursery may be relatively short. Follow-up occupational therapy services may be necessary at the outlying hospital.

A certain number of infants seen in the neonatal intensive care unit have specific and identifiable deficits that may require continued intervention after discharge from the hospital. In some cases occupational therapy services can be provided on an outpatient basis at the medical center where often the same neonatal therapist can follow the child. In other cases occupational therapy services are most efficiently provided through local early intervention programs.

Role of the occupational therapist

In whatever setting, the multiple and varied needs of high-risk infants necessitate the involvement of a variety of professionals: physicians (including neonatologists, neurologists, ophthalmologists, and often other medical specialists), nurses, occupational therapists, sometimes physical therapists, and social workers. Continuous interaction among these professionals is essential to providing complete and efficient care.

Because the professionals involved must work so closely, there is at times an overlap of specific caregiving roles. A concrete example is feeding. Although feeding is routinely an integral part of the nurse's role in caring for the infant, it often becomes an area of primary concern to the occupational therapist when the infant is having some difficulty in this area. The occupational therapist, nurse, and parents must collaborate in dealing with the problem. However, the specific responsibilities of the occupational therapist can be identified and categorized into four major areas: assessment, consultation, referral, and intervention. This categorization is applicable to both inpatient work in the neonatal intensive care unit itself and to follow-up care of infants after their discharge from the hospital. The individual importance of each area may vary in different settings.

ASSESSMENT

A primary service provided by the occupational therapist in the neonatal intensive care unit is assessment. When the infant reaches a point of medical stability, initial evaluation from a developmental perspective can begin. A single evaluation visit is almost never satisfactory, and repeat visits invariably provide valuable additional information from which to determine a more accurate overall picture of the infant. For very small or young infants it is often impossible to complete a full developmental assessment in one visit because of the infant's intolerance of prolonged handling and stimulation. In this sense, *prolonged* may be a matter of only a few minutes.

Developmental assessment is also a primary role of the occupational therapist in the follow-up clinic. Specific assessment techniques are discussed later in this chapter.

CONSULTATION

As information is gathered through the assessment process, sharing this information with parents and other staff and, at the same time, making suggestions for encouraging or facilitating appropriate responses and inhibiting abnormal responses becomes perhaps the second most important role of the occupational therapist. In this way the occupational therapist fulfills the role of consultant. Since interventions that may be appropriate for infants often seem to resemble or fit best into routine caretaking procedures, and since such interventions are most effective when provided on a consistent basis in a relaxed or routine environment, providing the infant's consistent caretakers—parents and nurses—with the information and skill that will be of benefit to that infant is the most efficient use of the therapist's time and the most effective means of reaching the infant. Specific areas often addressed are positioning, feeding, and sensory stimulation.

While in most settings a social worker will be available to help parents work through their feelings of anger, rejection, and mourning, it is not unusual for the occupational therapist to be called on to fill such a role. Working with the parents may involve helping them deal with their feelings of helplessness by providing them with instructions for specific activities that can be therapeutic. Involvement with the infant through such activities may assist them in overcoming feelings of helplessness, hopelessness, as well as the fear that can be generated because of the apparent fragility of the infant. Such therapeutic activities may include simple acts such as gentle stroking, or slow rocking, or holding (cuddling). Experience shows that parents are in general very eager to actively contribute to their infant's care by providing developmentally relevant stimulation, and they are pleased to find that many of their own attempts to reach their infant through touching, holding, and cuddling are in fact appropriate and beneficial. In addition, the occupational therapist is often the most appropriate resource person to answer the many questions posed by parents regarding the current and future development of their infant. This can be done individually or in a group. Parents' groups afford the opportunity for parents to voice and share their questions and concerns among other parents whose infants are at various stages in their neonatal course. In this way the group can be a supportive and helpful resource to its participants. Developmental issues can be addressed by the occupational therapist at parent group meetings.

REFERRAL

Specific neurodevelopmental deficits that are interfering with normal function and development—for example, increased or decreased muscle tone, abnormal reflex activity, lack of alertness, and feeding problems—

are identified in some infants during the course of their hospitalization. When these deficits continue at the time of discharge, it is appropriate to refer the infant for treatment after discharge. Questions regarding parental ability to provide nurturing experiences for their infant are also appropriate reasons for referral. Most often such referrals are made to local early intervention programs and more specifically to the home-based infant program component. Infants being discharged to other hospitals may need referrals for occupational therapy follow-up through those hospitals.

INTERVENTION

There are some instances when direct intervention, other than assessment, is necessary. For example, an occupational therapist can be most effective in working directly with an infant who is medically and developmentally ready for feeding but experiencing difficulty because of poor sucking, swallowing, or some other neuromuscular, behavioral, or structural disorder. Other areas of direct treatment or intervention include organization of sensory stimuli for a specific sensorimotor deficit, positioning, facilitation and inhibition techniques, and range of motion for immobilized infants. In all cases, infants are assessed individually, and treatment programs are prescribed based on specific needs.

It is important to note that direct treatment never occurs in isolation. In any case in which direct treatment is necessary, it is always appropriate and also necessary to consult with staff and parents to assure carryover of the techniques prescribed and to facilitate continuity of care for the infant.

Characteristics of the therapist

Completion of an accredited professional curriculum is a basic requirement for eligibility for employment in a facility treating high-risk infants. Prior pediatric experience should be a prerequisite. Furthermore, given the nature and complexity of this field, it is recommended that therapists contemplating employment in such a setting become further acquainted with the field of fetal and infant development, as well as the psychology of parent-infant relationships.

The neonatal intensive care unit can be a demanding, stressful, and often unpredictable place. Although there is a certain amount of regularity in the routine care of the infant in the nursery, these routines are subject to unexpected change for a variety of reasons. Because of the nature and severity of the medical problems of many of these infants, the infants themselves are often unpredictable. As such, working with high-risk infants requires flexibility on the part of the therapist. It is necessary to schedule occupational therapy visits around medical procedures, feeding schedules, and parent visits. It is absolutely essential to maintain a working relationship with the many other professionals involved, as well as with parents.

A final suggestion is that therapists working in intensive care nurseries should continue to see normal infants periodically to maintain an appropriate perspective regarding the developmental process.

NEONATAL ASSESSMENT

During the last 20 years our understanding of the newborn has undergone a tremendous change. Instead of being considered helpless, passive, reflex-bound and capable of little more than eating, sleeping, and crying, newborns are now considered to possess a number of well-organized behaviors and to be capable of molding their own environments. What then are some of the inborn capacities that the newborn child brings into the world?

The traditional, standardized neurological examination, such as that of Prechtl and Beintema,[45] was the prevalent tool available for looking at newborns. It considered only the physical and neurological status of the infant. With the increasing recognition of innate behavioral capacities, interactive behaviors and organized responses of the newborn came to be recognized to be as significant as the neurological findings. Pioneering work in identifying, organizing, and quantifying these behavioral components has been done by Brazelton,[9] culminating with the Neonatal Behavioral Assessment Scale.[9]

As medical technology improved, the focus shifted to the increasing numbers of low birth weight, preterm infants and the surviving distressed infants who filled the intensive care nurseries. Although the primary concerns regarding these infants will always be survival with minimal medical complications and subsequently adequate growth, more attention is being given to the preterm infant's *adaptive* behaviors[3] and his ability to meet the challenge of the extrauterine environment. The Assessment of Preterm Infant Behavior (APIB)[2] is an assessment tool created for research purposes. It defines and organizes these behavioral findings into a meaningful and useful schema. These, as well as some other measures, will be described more fully later in this chapter.

General considerations

A number of considerations apply to the administration of assessments in general. Any examination, however noninvasive, should be recognized as having a potential impact on the infant. While the goal of the examination is to gather valuable clinical information, for the infant the experience can be either therapeutic or stressful. Therefore procedures may have to be modified and carefully administered, depending on the individual infant's particular medical problems.

In addition to the infant's clinical problems, there are additional elements that need to be considered before each examination and noted so as to aid in the interpretation of findings:

1. State of the infant at the time of examination by use of Brazelton's definition of six states of sleep and arousal.[9]
2. Timing of the examination in relation to feeding. Specific recommendations may vary with each measure. About two thirds of the way between one feeding and the next, irrespective of the frequency of feeding, is generally considered an advisable time for many infants. However, this may not be true of the very premature infant who may be more likely to become alert one-half hour just before feeding.
3. Medication. There are some drugs frequently used in the intensive care nursery; their effects may vary according to amount and time of administration in relation to examination.
4. Unusual physical or environmental conditions. This includes many elements such as intravenous tubing or other elements the examiner feels may have limiting effect on the examination.

There is general agreement in the literature that a single examination may, at best, offer a glimpse of an infant's clinical state. Repeated examinations, whether partial or complete, offer a much greater opportunity for accurate assessment and should be preferred whenever possible, for it is the cumulative data over time that serves diagnostic and monitoring tasks of the occupational therapist.

In summary, a complete assessment should include the following:

1. Pertinent medical information, including history, physical and neurological data, and a list of present problems
2. Reported observations, as related by staff and parents
3. Observations of the infant at rest and during routine procedures, such as feeding, and diapering
4. Results of the examination
5. Summary of findings with a resulting impression

Specific neonatal assessments

There are a number of infant assessments available that require varying degrees of expertise and training. The specific type of assessment performed by occupational therapists may vary, depending on the needs within each nursery. Some of the more well-known tools with which the therapist should become familiar are described here.

The Brazelton Neonatal Behavioral Assessment Scale[9] was designed for the purpose of measuring the interactive capacity of the full-term infant. It differs from many other measures in that it strives to bring out the best of the rich repertoire of interactive behaviors of the newborn. Thus the examiner is encouraged to make every effort in that direction, rather than be bound to format. The scale measures the newborn's capacity to habituate to stimuli, regulate changes in state of consciousness (sleep and arousal), and respond to both animate and inanimate objects. It also measures the neuromotor integrity and physiological stability of the newborn. The scoring system is complex with 27 behavioral items to be scored on a 9-point scale and 20 reflex items scored on a 3-point scale. Reliability training is recommended for formal use of this scale.

The Neurological Assessment of the Preterm and Full-term Newborn Infant developed by Dubowitz and Dubowitz[19] is a comprehensive scale designed to measure the functional state of the central nervous system of the preterm and full-term infant. It considers the various stages of neurological maturation of the premature infant, as well as interactive capacity of the newborn. This assessment was found to be more comprehensive than the classical neurological assessments like that of Prechtl and Beintema[45] because of the addition of the interactive behavior component. Directions and scoring are well-illustrated and simplified to make it more accessible for routine examinations by medical staff.

The Assessment of Preterm Infant Behavior (APIB)[2], which was based on Brazelton's work, is a rather complex instrument designed for research purposes. It requires extensive training for its administration and scoring. The underlying concepts, however, contribute very valuable information regarding the preterm infant's early stages of behavioral organization. It also provides a rich and comprehensive description of the vast array of observations in the physiological, motor, attentional-interactive, and regulatory systems, and general state of the infant by interpreting and organizing them meaningfully. The scale is divided into six packages, each one placing specific graded demands on the infant and measuring the effect of these on a number of subsystems.

Other neonatal assessments not described here include the Clinical Assessment of Gestational Age in the Newborn Infant,[18] the Neurological Examination of the Full-term Newborn Infant,[44] and the Graham Rosenblith Behavioral Examination for Newborns.[47]

Although there are no published or formal occupational therapy assessments of the newborn, the following was developed to meet the needs of the occupational therapists at the University of Connecticut Health Center intensive care nursery. The Occupational Therapy Neonatal Assessment (OTNA) represents one system of organizing a number of findings that are considered relevant and appropriate to the role of the occupational therapist in the intensive care nursery. Many of the items are derived from Brazelton's work.[9] A number of other authors[1,39,54,56] have contributed to our understanding of the significance of developmental assessment findings. The assessment form of the Occupational Therapy Neonatal Assessment (not provided here) is divided into four parts, each one outlined and clarified:

1. Part 1 includes any pertinent medical history and information about the infant.
   a. Name, sex, and date of birth
   b. Gestational age (GA) at birth
   c. Conceptional age: Refers to gestational age plus time in weeks since birth.
   d. Prenatal complications: Refers to any fetal or maternal factors, such as maternal history of drug abuse or intrauterine growth retardation of the fetus, which have occurred before the birth process and are likely to be related to the infant's present state.
   e. Birth information: Refers to the type of delivery and any complications at or around the time of birth.
   f. Apgar scores: Refers to the scoring system devised by Apgar.[5]
   g. Medical complications: Refers to any of the common medical problems listed in Table 15-1 and their supporting diagnostic data.
   h. Present medication
   i. Other factors affecting assessment
2. Part 2 consists of the list of observations made during the examination. It is separate from the rest, and it may be used for repeated or periodic examinations.
   a. Habituation: Refers to the "infant's capacity to decrease responses to repeated disturbing stimuli."[9] Lack of this function may be indicative of hyperexcitability of the central nervous system and should be considered worrysome.
   b. State transitions or patterns: State refers to the infant's state of consciousness. There are six states as defined by Brazelton[9] that cover the continuum between sleep and crying. Observations regarding rapidity of buildup and smoothness in transition between one state and another, as well as observations regarding regularity and predictability of sleep-wake cycles, are noted here. It is not uncommon for preterm infants to have irregular sleep patterns. Such information may be particularly helpful to parents.
   c. Alertness: Refers to state four according to Brazelton's scale,[9] a period when the infant is most available for interactive behavior. Periods of alertness may vary from fleeting moments, which is

characteristic of the very premature infant, to sustained periods exhibited by the more intact and mature infant.

d. Orienting behavior: Refers to the infant's capacity to turn toward the examiner (or other person) in response to a combination of sensory stimuli. An orienting response may be useful in facilitating the attachment process for infants with decreased visual and auditory responses.

e. Sensory responses: Auditory, visual, tactile, vestibular, pain, and olfactory. The infant's responses in each of the sensory systems are considered separately. For the visual and auditory responses, animate or inanimate stimuli may be presented. Observations regarding the tactile and vestibular senses are arrived at by noting the infant's responses to handling and changes in position during the examination. Observations regarding pain can be reported by nurses. A bottle of common extract such as orange or mint can be used to assess olfactory responses.

f. Muscle tone: Passive and active; trunk and shoulder; lower extremities; and upper extremities. Passive tone refers to the infant's position at rest as described by Dubowitz.[18] Active tone refers to the infant's general tone following handling. There is usually a significant change in tone in response to a number of sensory experiences. Proximal muscles (trunk, neck, and shoulders) are examined separately from the extremities. Consistent signs of asymmetries as well as hyper-hypotonia are described.

g. Motor responses: Spontaneous activity, quality of movements, and reflexes. Spontaneous activity refers to the amount or frequency of activity exhibited by the infant in between specific maneuvers. Jittery, flailing, smooth, clonic, and organized movements are terms used in describing the quality of movements. A number of neonatal reflexes as described by Barnes, Crutchfield, and Heriza[6] are tested. These include the asymmetrical tonic neck reflex (ATNR), Moro reflex, gag reflex, rooting reflex, sucking-swallowing, palmar grasp, plantar grasp, Galant reflex (trunk incurvation), positive supporting, stepping, and placing. Absent or significant decrease in motor response is often seen in very distressed infants.

h. Consolability: Refers to the infant's capacity to quiet following a period of crying. The degree of intervention necessary to help the infant to quiet is usually noted, and it may be indicative of the infant's ability to regulate state changes.

i. Feeding: Refers to the infant's ability to take adequate amounts of nutritive liquid by sucking (at times observations may be initiated before actual use of a nipple). All aspects of feeding are considered, including appropriate oral reflexes, muscle tone, and interactive behavior.

3. Part 3 includes pertinent family and social information.
   a. Family composition (includes ages)
   b. Significant information about the family
   c. Availability of family members for visits to the nursery

4. Part 4 provides space for a descriptive paragraph to cover summary findings and recommendations.
   a. Summary
   b. Impressions and recommendations

In addition to the general considerations discussed earlier, there are some specific guidelines for using Part 2 of the Occupational Therapy Neonatal Assessment regarding procedure and scoring. Although the items are listed in the sequence in which they are usually presented to the infant, the examiner need not feel bound to the order or the number of items to be presented at any given time. Descriptive scoring is used in this form, although a quantifiable scale could be added.

Indications for use of assessment measures

Although each individual test may have been designed for a specific purpose, the examination of the infant and the findings may be used to implement a number of different objectives.

DIAGNOSTIC CONSIDERATIONS

Diagnostic interpretation of findings is never an easy task, particularly with preterm or distressed infants whose changes in status are very unpredictable and occur more rapidly than in any other newborn population. As indicated before, findings derived from a single examination should be interpreted with more caution than those derived from repeated observations over time. It is not uncommon for the examiner to encounter variations of responses in the same infant, but the cumulative data will help to identify the typical as well as the optimal responses of any given infant. This approach will require scheduling flexibility and may be less efficient, but in the end it will provide more reliable and useful information for discharge planning.

Although most therapists agree that the continuum between what is considered normal and abnormal cannot be easily defined, some guidelines for recognizing this continuum in relation to infants is necessary.

1. Normal: This qualifier should be used to describe all those findings that are consistent with the expected level of function for the conceptional age (the gestational age of the infant at birth with the number of weeks since birth added to it) of the infant. For information regarding age-appropriate behaviors, reference

can be made to a variety of authors who have described the normal process of development[4,6,26,49] (Chapter 4).

2. Worrisome or suspect: This term should be used to describe most of the findings that are not considered appropriate for conceptional age. They may range from minimal to significant.

3. Abnormal: This term should be used only with observations obtained from repeated examinations over a prolonged period of time to describe the pathological extreme of any given response. This term should be used preferably when observations are supported by additional diagnostic data, for example, electroencephalography or computerized tomography (CT scan).

CONSIDERATIONS FOR REFERRAL

The plasticity of the central nervous system and its ability to recover from a number of insults is the basis for most of the therapeutic intervention theories. Recent advances regarding fetal development of the central nervous system suggest periods when certain neurological functions may be more vulnerable[26] and therefore more susceptible to trauma. With the information available to date, it has not been possible to predict accurately the severity or degree of the sequelae. However, some of the findings suggest the possibility of problems in certain functional areas such as with hypotonia, which is likely to affect motor development.

Yet, like many other professionals involved in the discharge planning of the vulnerable or at-risk infant, the occupational therapist is often asked to make decisions regarding intervention, implying a predictive value to the assessment information.

Both abnormal and worrisome findings should be considered valid reasons for recommending therapeutic or other intervention. Thus, depending on the degree and nature of the problems, as well as on parental preference, the therapist may recommend: (1) making a referral for early intervention, (2) instructing parents until a later reassessment, or (3) recommending an early follow-up appointment. The importance of considering the readiness of the parents when making discharge plans cannot be overemphasized. The parents' understanding of the nature and ramifications of the problem, as well as their psychological readiness, will play an important role in making the referral more meaningful and acceptable to the family. The eventual success or failure of intervention may depend on the family's attitude and understanding.

THERAPEUTIC CONSIDERATIONS FOR THE INFANT AND PARENTS

Intrinsic to each examination is its therapeutic potential. This is often not given due consideration by those whose primary objective is to gather accurate and sufficient observation. It is possible, however, to carry out examinations that provide the infant with a positive and organizing experience. Recognizing the many and varied signs of stress that may be very subtle in the preterm infant is the first step in that direction. Allowing for sufficient time between maneuvers to permit the infant to reorganize himself and to return to an "available" state[3] is one technique that will more likely result in a therapeutic experience.

Widmayer and Field[62] describe how enriching an experience it is for parents to observe the assessment of their infant with the use of the Brazelton scale. In fact, it has been described as the single most useful form of intervention with some parents who are considered to be at risk for disturbances in the attachment process. While this is generally true in the case of healthy term infants, there are also many instances when it can be beneficial in the neonatal intensive care unit. It is important that the therapist recognize that such an experience, while informative, may be distressing or delightful, depending on the parents' interpretation of responses and their general perception of their infant. It is advisable to omit certain items when examining preterm or distressed infants in front of their parents because of their obvious distressful effect. This may include response to painful stimuli and a number of reflexes including the gag and Moro reflexes.

Specific maneuvers from various test items can be used to teach parents ways of eliciting certain responses in their infants. For example, alertness can be increased with vestibular stimulation. With infants who are exhibiting some worrisome findings, such as obligatory asymmetrical tonic neck reflex, irritability, and inefficient sucking, the examination may provide an opportunity to give the parents suggestions for positioning and other facilitating or inhibiting techniques that may be appropriate to the situation.

Although research considerations will not be discussed here, the opportunities for research in the field of neonatology are vast and should be considered by the occupational therapist engaged in observing infant behavior.

CONSIDERATIONS FOR INTERVENTION WITH HIGH-RISK INFANTS
Precautions

Two major considerations must be taken into account in dealing with the high-risk infant: temperature regulation and stress tolerance. Cold exposure can cause increase in metabolic rate and oxygen consumption with resulting increase in oxygen requirement, acidosis, apnea, hypoglycemia, and possibly pulmonary hemorrhage. To keep the infant warm, it may be necessary to be sure he is adequately covered when out of the Isolette. Or, in some cases, it may be necessary to work with the infant inside the Isolette.

Many high-risk infants can tolerate only limited amounts of handling or stimulation. Therefore the therapist must be sensitive to each infant's level of tolerance and to watch for signs of stress. Some of these signs are color changes, including circumoral cyanosis and mottling of the skin; marked increase or decrease in respiratory rate; change in heart rate; sudden limpness; and sudden fussiness. At the point of occurrence of one or more of these signs, it may be necessary to terminate the assessment or treatment at least temporarily. Unnecessary stress or fatigue should not be permitted.

Guidelines for intervention

There is much controversy in the literature regarding the effectiveness of "infant stimulation." There is some evidence that supplemental stimulation has positive clinical and developmental effects. There is also evidence that eliminating some noxious stimuli and organizing caretaking activities may also have positive effects. However, there is not enough data as to the type, amount, and timing of such experiences that would be of most benefit for each infant. It is apparent that the answers to these questions will vary for each infant and his individual needs. In any case, it would seem desirable to provide treatment to encourage developmentally appropriate responses and to reduce inappropriate responses. This type of approach to intervention with developmentally vulnerable infants has been referred to as "developmental support."[57]

The goals of early developmental support as such are to "1) enhance parent/infant interaction thus providing a secure base for a future parent/child relationship; 2) facilitate the infant's own adjustments to his environment; and, 3) facilitate the infant's acquisition of developmental skills" (p. 3).[57] In a more specific sense, we might add to this list the facilitation of normal patterns of movement and muscle tone, as well as the enhancement of appropriate sensory and motor responses. Specific intervention techniques, outlined in the following sections, can be accomplished at different levels by therapists, parents, and nurses. These suggestions are by no means all-inclusive. It should be remembered that each infant must be considered individually, and only those techniques appropriate to each infant's gestational age, medical status, and central nervous system maturity should be used.

LEVEL OF ALERTNESS

Premature infants spend the greatest portion of each day in a sleep state. There are, however, brief periods of alertness that occur periodically. It is during these periods of alertness that the infant is available for interaction with caregivers and ready to receive some type of sensory stimulation, particularly visual stimulation. With maturation, the normal developmental process allows for increasingly frequent and more sustained periods of alertness. For many high-risk infants, this process is delayed, altered, or interrupted. Small for gestational age infants and infants who have suffered specific neurological insults frequently fall into this group of infants who demonstrate less than optimal levels of alertness.

At one end of the continuum may be infants with infrequent or lack of sustained periods of alertness. These infants may also be difficult to arouse. At the other extreme, an infant may be hyperexcitable, hyperresponsive, or hyperirritable. These infants commonly experience significant difficulties in the interactive area. Self-quieting behaviors, such as hand-to-mouth movements and positional changes, may also be diminished. In either case, the result of deficits in the ability to sustain alert periods can include interactive difficulties, feeding problems, and sensorimotor deficits.

Intervention guidelines for arousal and state transition (alertness)

1. To facilitate a quiet-alert state.
   a. Swaddle.
   b. Gently restrain flailing arms across chest.
   c. Work in dimly lit, quiet room.
   d. Gently rock into a more upright position.
2. To facilitate self-quieting and behavioral organization.
   a. Swaddle.
   b. Help infant suck on his hand, fingers, or on a pacifier.
   c. Reduce level of stimulation in the environment (lights, sounds).
3. To bring infant to an alert state.
   a. Unwrap.
   b. Bring to semi-upright position.
   c. Provide sensory stimulation through voice, touch, and movement.

MUSCLE TONE

Muscle tone develops in a caudocephalic (toe to head) direction and is a function of maturity of the neuromuscular system. The more immature infant is characterized by hypotonia or reduced muscle tone. Because of this hypotonia, the premature infant assumes a relatively extended posture that, with the added effects of gravity, leads to the development of a predominance of extensor tone. The full-term infant is born in a flexed posture with a predominance of flexor tone (Figure 15-5). The premature infant rarely develops this same degree of flexor tone but can still develop normally.

High-risk infants (term and premature) are often prone to abnormal tone patterns. These abnormalities may result from prolonged immobility resulting from medical complications, from specific neuromuscular disorders, or from other causes. Persistence of abnormal

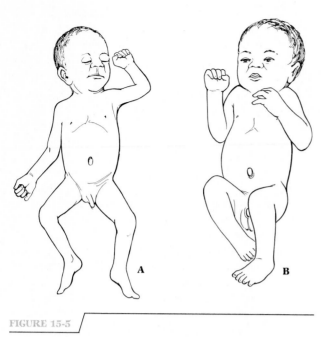

FIGURE 15-5

Resting posture: **A,** Premature infant; **B,** Full-term infant.

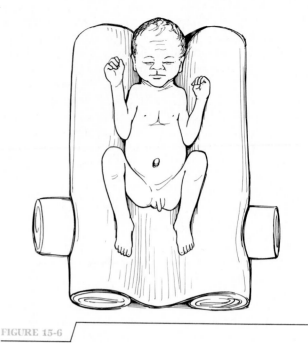

FIGURE 15-6

Supportive positioning in supine position. Infant positioned in blanket with sides rolled to form "blanket cradle."

postures can interfere with later development of normal head control, oculomotor skills, eye-hand coordination, mobility, interpersonal interaction, sitting, and standing. It is therefore essential to interrupt abnormal posture patterns through positioning and other techniques. Many of these techniques are appropriate also for the normally developing premature infant (the growing preemie) to facilitate the development of flexor tone and prevent the development of abnormal patterns that may potentially result from the imbalance of flexor and extensor tone. It should be noted that many of these positioning techniques also have an organizing effect on the behavior of the infant and subsequently allow better potential for self-quieting, developing body awareness, and developing organized movement patterns.

Intervention guidelines for muscle tone

1. To facilitate the development of flexor tone and prevent overstretching of joints resulting from generalized decreased tone.
   a. Position in sidelying. Use rolled blanket behind infant's head and trunk. For additional support, add smaller roll in front of infant's chest and abdomen over which top leg can be placed. A blanket over infant and tucked under mattress will keep infant in position.
   b. Place infant in semiflexed position in the supine position. Low tone infant will need considerable support. Place infant on a blanket, each end of which has been rolled. Place rolled diaper under bottom of blanket to support knees (Figure 15-6). Side rolls will support head near midline. Keep shoulders semiprotracted, and prevent external rotation of lower extremities (frog-leg position). Can use stuffed animals instead of rolls.
   c. In infant seat, rolled blankets should also be used at sides to keep head in midline and prevent excessive abduction and external rotation of upper and lower extremities, as well as retraction of shoulders.
   d. Swaddle.
   e. Place rolled diaper under chest and hip area to facilitate flexion in the prone position.

FEEDING

Although sucking and swallowing begin very early in fetal life, it is not until 32 to 34 weeks gestational age that a coordinated pattern of sucking and swallowing is strong enough and can be sustained for a long enough period to allow adequate nutritional intake. (This does not imply that preterm infants should be introduced to the nipple at this time.) Medical complications and certain treatment procedures may interfere with this process. Immature infants who require tube feedings or nonnutritive treatment procedures, such as suctioning, may develop hypersensitivity in the oral area, which may develop into later feeding problems (refusal of nipple). Normal sucking patterns may be interrupted by medical equipment used in treatment, for example, the endotracheal tube that is placed in the provision of mechanical ventilatory support. Sucking that does occur may disappear because of lack of use or lack of reward from use. An acutely ill infant may not be able to suck and swallow because of poor tone or rapid fatigue. Other infants may lack the muscle coordination required for sucking because of neurological or other impairments, or both. The potential causes for impaired oral feeding with an infant who is otherwise medically and gestationally ready are many and varied. Some fairly simple facilitation techniques can be easily incorporated into the infant's routine care to facilitate the normal development of sucking and at the same time perhaps enhance the digestive process in general.

Intervention guidelines for feeding

1. To facilitate sucking-swallowing in premature infant
   a. Encourage sucking during tube feedings (pacifier).
2. To facilitate use of the nipple for the infant who is developmentally ready for oral feeding.
   a. Position infant semireclined with head in neutral, arms and shoulders forward, and lower extremities semiflexed (swallowing will be difficult if not impossible if the head or neck is excessively flexed or extended).
   b. Select nipple of appropriate size for the infant's mouth and of the appropriate resiliency to allow moderate flow of liquid into the mouth.
3. To prevent fatigue.
   a. Allow rest periods in between sucking bursts. Do not push too hard. Rest periods are normal.
4. To facilitate sucking when infant appears unresponsive but not fatigued.
   a. Gently move nipple partially in and out of mouth.
   b. Rotate nipple in mouth.
   c. Stroke firmly under chin (back to front) during feeding.
   d. When indicated, provide supportive jaw control by placing your thumb and index finger on either side of the mandible with your middle finger flexed under the infant's chin.
5. To facilitate swallow.
   a. Stroke gums to increase saliva flow and facilitate swallow.
   b. Stroke *gently*, bilaterally on front of throat.
6. To facilitate lip closure.
   a. Intraoral and perioral stimulation before feeding (stroking, tapping, quick stretch to lips)
   b. Supportive jaw control as described above.
7. To reduce tongue thrust.
   a. Supply firm pressure by finger or nipple on tongue.
   b. Avoid stimulation of tip of tongue when approaching mouth with nipple.

SENSORY RESPONSES

One of the first questions asked by many parents is "When will my baby be able to see?" We know that full-term infants are able to visually fixate on and follow objects and that they prefer faces to objects. This behavior is very rewarding to parents and others who are interacting with the infant. This ability is not consistently seen in premature infants, and some high-risk infants actually tend to exhibit more gaze-averting behavior. As a result, parents' interactions with their high-risk infants often are not rewarding and can be frustrating. Their concern can be alleviated somewhat by the knowledge of the course of normal development in this area and perhaps by suggestions of activities to enhance the infant's alertness and visual responsiveness.

The high-risk infant can be hyperresponsive or hyporesponsive to other types of sensory stimulation. Some infants appear to be oversensitive to sound, touch, or movement. Others appear to respond very little, if at all, to these types of input. Olfaction is another sensory function that is often overlooked. Close observation is necessary in this area. In some cases, carefully graded presentation of such stimulation singly or in various combinations, perhaps coupled with environmental adaptations, may enhance appropriate sensory responses. In addition, various types of sensory stimuli can be used in treatment to enhance appropriate functional responses in many areas. For example, tactile stimuli can be used to enhance muscle tone; olfactory stimuli can be used in the treatment of feeding disorders.

Intervention guidelines for sensory responses

1. To decrease hypersensitivity to touch or movement.
   a. Avoid sudden movements.
   b. Approach infant in slow, gentle manner.
   c. Swaddle.
2. To decrease hypersensitivity to sound.
   a. Avoid loud noises that may startle infant, for example, slamming Isolette porthole doors.
   b. Gradually introduce different sounds—use musical toys.
3. To increase visual responses.
   a. Place toys in Isolette in infant's line of vision.
   b. Encourage parents, staff, and others to move their faces in infant's line of vision when interacting with infant.

Intervention guidelines for other responses

1. To facilitate parent-infant interaction.
   a. Encourage early, active involvement of parents by teaching them developmentally appropriate stimulation techniques, for example, stroking, rocking, oral facilitation.
   b. Encourage positioning during feeding that allows eye-to-eye contact.
   c. Demonstrate to parents the infant's interactional capacities as they develop.
   d. Allow for the parents' expression of negative feelings.
2. To prevent flattening of the head from prolonged positioning on one side.
   a. Support head closer to midline by using props at various points of contact (use rolled blankets, stuffed animals, and so on).

CASE STUDY

Susie was born at a local hospital at 30 weeks' gestational age after a pregnancy that was uncomplicated until the onset of premature labor. The delivery was vaginal with breech presentation. Apgar scores were 1 at 1 minute, and 5 at 5 minutes. Birth weight, length, and head circumference were appropriate for gestational age. Susie was transported to the neonatal intensive care unit because of prematurity and respiratory distress.

Susie required mechanical ventilatory support for 2½ months because of chronic lung disease. She remained on supplementary oxygen after extubation and after discharge from the hospital. She developed cardiac problems shortly after birth and went into respiratory arrest at 10 days of age. Initial diagnosis was patent ductus arteriosus, which was resolved without surgical treatment, but cardiomegaly persisted. Intermittent seizurelike activity was noted early on, and treatment consisted of anticonvulsant medication. Although initial electroencephalograms and CT scans were abnormal (showing evidence of an intraventricular hemorrhage), at the time of discharge both were within normal limits, and head circumference was growing appropriately. Grade II-III retrolental fibroplasia was diagnosed by the ophthalmologist, but it was improving by discharge time. Results of audiology evaluation were age appropriate. Susie also had hyperbilirubinemia, which was treated with phototherapy.

In summary, Susie's major perinatal problems included prematurity; breech presentation; respiratory distress; hyaline membrane disease with bronchopulmonary dysplasia (chronic lung disease); respiratory arrest; recurrent cardiac arrhythmia; cor pulmonale; patent ductus arteriosus; intraventricular hemorrhage; asphyxia; and retrolental fibroplasia. Among the procedures used in her treatment were endotracheal intubation, oxygen therapy, mechanical assisted ventilation, umbilical catheterization, echocardiogram, electrocardiogram, electroencephalogram, CT scan, phototherapy, lumbar puncture, multiple blood gas tests, and multiple medications.

Susie was referred to occupational therapy 6 weeks after birth (at 36 weeks conceptional age) because of concern about motor development and general level of responsiveness resulting from her complicated medical course and apparent neurological symptoms. Initial assessment was limited, because she was on a respirator at the time. Muscle tone was generally decreased with the exception of increased trunk and neck extensor tone noted during intermittent arching. Findings were discussed with the nursing staff, and various methods of positioning were suggested to decrease trunk arching and to maintain Susie in a more functional position by facilitating a semiflexed posture.

Susie was followed almost daily over the next several weeks so that organized patterns of sensory stimulation, maintenance of appropriate positioning, and continuing evaluation could be provided. The parents were involved early, and the results of the evaluation as well as treatment recommendations were discussed. The parents were eager to participate in Susie's care in anyway they could, and they were responsive to the suggestions made.

Susie had early problems with nutrition secondary to fluid restriction imposed during treatment of cardiac problems. She was maintained on intravenous hyperalimentation until 3 to 4 weeks after birth when nasojejunal feedings were begun. Approximately 2½ months after birth intermittent orogastric feedings were started, and oral feedings began soon after at 3 months. Susie initially had some difficulty accepting the nipple, as well as difficulty handling the fluid once in her mouth. She frequently gagged on the formula. During this time occupational therapy goals were expanded to include improvement of feeding skills. Susie's treatment program included oral facilitation techniques and positioning recommendations (semiupright, semiflexed with extremities toward midline), since she continued to assume a position of neck and trunk hyperextension, which is not a suitable feeding position. Changes were made in the consistency of the formula

(by thickening it with rice cereal) to facilitate the swallowing process. She made slow progress but finally began to accept all feedings orally. She continued, however, to be a slow feeder.

In summary, the major focus of occupational therapy with Susie centered on the following areas:

1. *Personal-social-emotional.* As a long-term patient, Susie was generally at high risk for developmental problems in this area. The active participation of her parents was very important in this regard. Additional concerns during her hospitalization included decreased level of alertness, decreased interactive ability, and decreased tolerance for interaction-stimulation. The gradual introduction of playful handling at times other than feeding times and the gentle introduction of various types of stimulation, such as slow rocking, were used by her parents, therapist, and nurses in an effort to improve her function in this area.

2. *Orientation.* Because of early inconsistent auditory and visual responsiveness and the subsequent diagnosis of retrolental fibroplasia, there was a period of serious concern in this area. It was suggested that Susie have toys in her Isolette and that auditory stimuli be combined with visual stimuli in approaching her, for example, using combined face and voice or musical toys. Concern was resolved by discharge time, and Susie was following face and objects 180 degrees and responding appropriately to sounds. Some strabismus did continue but was later corrected by surgery.

3. *Motor development.* Trunk arching; generally decreased tone with increased extensor tone during arching and later increased extensor tone in the lower extremities; decreased head control with poor trunk and neck stability; and some tongue thrusting were some of the specific findings leading to concern in this area. Parents and staff followed through with suggested activities, such as positioning, swaddling, and playing with her in the reclined position and later in the more upright position. These activities aimed to reduce the effects of the motor problems that continued at the time of discharge.

4. *Feeding.* Intermittent tongue thrusting, apparently increased oral sensitivity with refusal of the nipple, and gagging on formula led to concern in this area. Perioral and intraoral stimulation and other oral facilitation techniques were coupled with changes in formula consistency to improve feeding ability. Basic positioning during feeding was also addressed. By discharge time, Susie was feeding slowly but acceptably.

After a long and complicated medical course, Susie was discharged home 6 months after birth at which time she was 3½ months corrected age. Muscle tone continued to be slightly decreased with continued intermittent trunk arching. Head control was poor to fair. Reflex responses were generally within normal limits; however, bilateral sustained ankle clonus continued. Sensory responses (including visual, auditory, tactile, and vestiblar) were within normal limits. Although periods of lethargy continued, general level of alertness had improved, and Susie was able to maintain sustained periods of alertness at times. Activity level remained low to moderate. She had begun to coo and make sounds, but no laughing or squealing was noted. She had established consistent hand-to-mouth movement with insertion of her thumb in her mouth. There was no midline hand activity. She had begun to show interest in toys and reached for them with no grasp.

Follow-up plans included participation in a neonatal follow-up clinic with the first visit scheduled 1 month after discharge (earlier than the routine 4-month visit), referral to a home-based early intervention program, and cardiac and ophthalmological follow-ups.

At the time of this writing, Susie is chronologically 2½ years old. Since her hospital discharge she has had five rehospitalizations for respiratory problems and one for corrective eye surgery (for bilateral strabismus). Home visits by team members of the early intervention program to which she was referred were discontinued after about 1 year but were reinstituted about 1 year after that. She has made slow but consistent developmental progress, monitored through regularly scheduled visits to the neonatal follow-up clinic.

Susie is currently ambulating independently, feeding herself (prefers finger foods but can use a fork and spoon), saying a few words (some clearly understood), and is developing appropriate self-care and social skills. A generalized developmental delay of about 4 to 6 months is apparent at this point. Poor fine motor skills, poor eye-hand coordination, continued decreased muscle tone, and speech delay are signs of generalized delay. It is noted that it is the poor quality of many of these skills, rather than their existence or nonexistence, that contributes to her developmental findings.

Susie's parents are considering preschool nursery placement to provide for her programming needs and to help all three of them (Susie, Mom, and Dad) with the separation-individuation process. Follow-up through the neonatal clinic will continue until age 3, at which time special services will be continued through the local school system.

SUMMARY

In considering the role of the occupational therapist with the high-risk infant, the controversy that exists over the effectiveness of early intervention must be recognized, particularly as it relates to the growing involvement of allied health professionals in nurseries and neonatal intensive care units. The neonatal intensive care unit is a busy, at times hectic, stressful place where the greatest precautions must be taken to protect vulnerable infants already at considerable risk because of prematurity and medical problems.

Although attention to the infant's medical status and survival rightfully takes priority, it should not be to the exclusion of other needs more closely related to the quality of life. While there are genetic and maturational bases for individual differences in both rate and pattern of development, there is growing evidence that environmental conditions during the prenatal and perinatal periods and the early years of life have a determining impact on the intellectual, affective, and sensorimotor development of the human infant. This is particularly relevant for the increasing numbers of infants born at risk with central nervous system dysfunction associated with such conditions as malnutrition, drug effects, prematurity infection, respiratory distress, and hyperbilirubinemia. Initially the high-risk infant is exposed to a somewhat distorted somatosensory environment, and often the crucial mother-infant interaction is severely disrupted. Both somatosensory experience and maternal-infant attachment have been identified as playing crucial roles in infant development.

Although further research is needed in this area, the implication is that the environment must make available the right type of stimulation at the right time for the optimal development of the infant. The role of the health care provider, in particular the occupational therapist, is to provide organization in the amount, quality, and kinds of stimulation to maximize developmental potential. For intervention to be consistently effective, it must be individualized to the requirements of each situation.

Occupational therapists have extensive knowledge of developmental processes and the sensory systems influencing those processes. They can contribute to the neonatal intensive care unit primarily by providing (1) individual assessment from a neurodevelopmental perspective by identifying the infant's unique pattern of strengths and vulnerabilities in terms of both rate and adequacy of developmental trends; (2) consultation with other nursery staff to adapt the environment and manipulate the infant's early experiences with the understanding of his needs and response capabilities to provide for optimal development; (3) consultation with parents to give additional information at their level regarding the neurodevelopmental status of their infant, to provide support to facilitate parent-infant attachment, and to use parents as the primary intervenors; (4) information to the team to assist in the early identification of risk status and the potential need for early intervention both on the unit and in the community after discharge (making referrals to community agencies as appropriate); and (5) direct service in cases of "functional deficits" (for example, feeding disorders, specific neurological deficits, and orthopedic deformities), therapeutic programs, and instruction of parents and staff on appropriate therapeutic techniques. With these considerations in mind, the role of an occupational therapist on the neonatal intensive care unit is a positive step toward the delivery of more comprehensive health care.

REFERENCES AND SELECTED READINGS

1. Als, H., and Brazelton, B.: A new model of assessing behavioral organization in preterm and full term infants, J. Am. Acad. Child Psychiatry **20**:239, 1981.
2. Als, H., and others: Manual for the Assessment of Preterm Infant Behavior (API). In Fitzgerald, H., Lester, B., and Yogman, M.,

editors: Theory and research in behavioral pediatrics, vol. 1, New York, Plenum Publishing Corp. (In press.)

3. Als, H., and others: Toward a research instrument for the Assessment of Preterm Infants' Behavior (APIB). In Fitzgerald, H., Lester, B., and Yogman, M., editors: Theory and research in behavioral pediatrics, vol. 1, New York, Plenum Publishing Corp. (In press.)

4. Andre-Thomas, A.J., and others: The neurological examination of the infant, Little Club Clinics in Developmental Medicine, No. 1, 1960.

5. Apgar, V.: A proposal for a new method of evaluation of the new born infant, Curr. Res. Anesthes. Analges. **32:**260, 1953.

6. Barnes, M., Crutchfield, C., and Heriza, C.: The neurophysiologic basis of patient treatment. Vol II: Reflexes in motor development, Morgantown, W.Va., 1979, Stokesville Publishing Co.

7. Bowlby, J.: Grief and mourning in infancy and early childhood, Psychoanal. Study Child **15:**9, 1960.

8. Braine, M., and others: Factors associated with impairment of the early development of the prematures, Society for Research in Child Development, Monograph No. 31, vol. 4, 1966.

9. Brazelton, T.B.: Neonatal Behavioral Assessment Scale, Philadelphia, 1973, J.B. Lippincott Co.

10. Bronfenbrenner, U.: When is infant stimulation effective? In Glass, D., editor: Environmental influences, New York, 1968, Rockefeller Press.

11. Bronfenbrenner, U.: Is early intervention effective? In Ffiedlander, B., Sterritt, G., and Kirk, G., editors: Exceptional infant, vol. 3, New York, 1975, Brunner/Mazel, Inc.

12. Caputo, D., and Mandell, V.: Consequences of low birth weight, Dev. Psychol. **3:**373, 1970.

13. Cornell, E., and Gottfried, A.: Intervention with premature human infants. Child Dev. **46:**32, 176.

14. Dorland's illustrated medical dictionary, ed. 25, Philadelphia, 1974, W.B. Saunders Co.

15. Drillien, C.: The incidence of mental and physical handicaps in school age children of very low birth weight, Pediatrics **27:**452, 1961.

16. Drillein, C.: The growth and development of the prematurely born infant, Baltimore, 1964, The Williams & Wilkins Co.

17. Drillien, C.: Causes of handicap in the low weight infant. In Jonxis, J., Visser, H., and Troelstra, J., editors: Aspects of prematurity and dysmaturity, Leiden, Holland, 1976, Stenfert Droese.

18. Dubowitz, L., Dubowitz, V., and Goldberg C.: Clinical assessment of gestational age in the newborn infant, J. Pediatr. **1:**10, 1979.

19. Dubowitz, L., and Dubowitz, V.: The neurological assessment of the preterm and full-term newborn infant, Philadelphia, 1981, J.B. Lippincott Co.

20. Erikson, E.: Childhood and society, New York, 1963, W.W. Norton & Co., Inc.

21. Field, T.: Infants born at risk, New York, 1979, Medical and Scientific Books.

22. Field, T.: Supplemental stimulation of preterm neonates, Early Hum. Dev. **4:**301, 1980.

23. Field, T., Dempsey, J., and Shuman, H,: Developmental follow-up of pre- and post-term infants. In Friedman, S., and Sigman, M., editors: Preterm birth and psychological development, New York, 1981, Academic Press, Inc.

24. Francis-Williams, J., and Davies, P.: Very low birth weight and later intelligence, Dev. Med. Child Neurol. **16:**709, 1974.

25. Freud, A.: The concept of developmental lines, Psychoanal. Study Child **18:**245, 1963.

26. Gilfoyle, E., Grady, A., and Moore, J.: Children adapt, Thorofare, N.J., 1981, Charles B. Slack, Inc.

27. Haskins, R., Finkelstein, N., and Stedman, D.: Infant stimulation programs and their effects, Pediatr. Ann. **7:**2, 1978.

28. Hommers, M., and Kendall, A.: The prognosis of the very low-birth weight infant, Dev. Med. Child Neurol. **18:**745, 1976.

29. Knoblock, H., and Pasamanick, B.: Prospective studies in the epidemiology of reproductive casualty: methods, findings and some implications, Merrill-Palmer Q. **12:**27, 1966.

30. Kopp, C., and Parmalee, A.: Prenatal and perinatal influences on infant behavior. In Osofsky, J., editor: Handbook of infant development, New York, 1979, John Wiley & Sons, Inc.

31. Langworthy, O.: Development of behavior patterns and myelinization of the nervous system in the human fetus and infant. Contrib. Embryol. **24:**139, 1933.

32. Lipsitt, L., and Field, T.: Perinatal influences on the behavior of full-term newborns. In Lipsitt, L., and Field, T., editors: Infant behavior and development: perinatal risk and newborn behavior, Norwood, N.J., 1982, Oblex Publishing Corp.

33. Lipton, R., and Provence, S.: Infants in institutions, New York, 1962, International Universities Press.

34. Littman, B., and Parmelee, A.: Obstetric Complications Scale (a modification of the Prechtl Obstetrics Optimality Scale) and the Postnatal Complications Scale. Unpublished manuscript, 1964.

35. Lubchenco, L., and others: Sequelae of premature birth: evaluation of premature infants of low birth weight at ten years of age, Am. J. Dis. Child. **106:**101, 1963.

36. Moore, J.: Concepts from the neurobehavioral sciences in relation to rehabilitation of the mentally and/or physically handicapped, Dubuque, Iowa, 1973, Kendell/Hunt Publishing Co.

37. The nature and nurture of behavior, Readings from Scientific American, San Francisco, 1973, W.H. Freeman and Co., Publishers.

38. Parmelee, A.: Neurophysiological and behavioral organization of premature infants in the first months of life, Biol. Psychiatry **10:**501, 1975.

39. Parmelee, A.: Early intervention for preterm infants. In Brown, C., editor: Infants at risk: assessment and intervention for health care professionals and parents, Piscataway, N.J., 1981, Johnson & Johnson.

40. Parmelee, A., and Heber, A.: Who is the risk infant?, Clin. Obstet. Gynecol. **16:**376, 1973.

41. Parker, S., and Brazelton, B.: Newborn behavioral assessment: research prediction and clinical uses, Child. Today **10:**2, 1981.

42. Paxson, C.: Van Leeuwen's newborn medicine, ed. 2, Chicago, 1979, Year Book Medical Publishers, Inc.

43. Phillips, M.: Prediction of scholastic performance from perinatal and infant development indices, Dissert. Abstr. Int. **33:**1526, 1972.

44. Prechtl, H.: The neurological examination of the full-term newborn infant, ed. 3, Philadelphia, 1977, J.B. Lippincott Co.

45. Prechtl, H., and Beintema, D.: The neurological examination of the full-term newborn infant, Little Club Clin. Dev. Med. **12:**entire issue, 1964.

46. Rabinovitch, M., Bibace, R., and Caplan, H.: Sequelae of prematurity: psychological test findings, Can. Med. Assoc. J. **84:**822, 1961.

47. Rosenblith, J.: The Graham/Rosenblith behavioral examination for newborns: prognostic value and practical issues. In Osofsky, J., editor: The handbook of infant development, New York, 1979, John Wiley & Sons, Inc.

48. Rubin, R., Rosenblatt, C., and Balow, B.: Psychological and educational sequelae of prematurity, Pediatrics **52:**352, 1973.

49. Saint-Anne Dargassies, S.: Neurological maturation of the premature infant of 28 to 41 weeks gestational age. In Falkner, F., editor: Human development, Philadelphia, 1966, W.B. Saunders Co.

50. Sameroff, A., and Chandler, M.: Reproductive risks and the continuum of caretaking casualty. In Horowitz, F., and others, edi-

tors: review of child development research, vol. 4, Chicago, 1975, University of Chicago Press.

51. Schaefer, M., Hatcher, R., and Barglow, P.: Prematurity and infant stimulation: a review of research, Child Psychiatry Hum. Dev. **10:**199, 1980.

52. Self, P., and Horowitz, F.: The behavioral assessment of the neonate: an overview. In Osofsky, J., editor: The handbook of infant development, New York, 1979, John Wiley & Sons, Inc.

53. Sell, E.: Follow-up of the high risk newborn—a practical approach, Springfield, Ill., 1980, Charles C Thomas, Publisher.

54. Solnit, A., and Provence, S.: Vulnerability and risk in early childhood. In Osofsky, J., editor: The handbook of infant development, New York, 1979, John Wiley & Sons, Inc.

55. Taub, H., Caputo, D., and Goldstein, K.: Toward a modification of the indices of neonatal prematurity, Percept. Mot. Skills **40:**43, 1975.

56. Thoman, E.: Affective communications as the prelude and context for language learning. In Schiefelbisch, R., and Bricker, D., editors: Early language: acquisition and intervention, Baltimore, 1980, University Park Press.

57. Thurber, S., and Armstrong, L.: Nurses' guide—developmental support of low birth weight infants, Houston, 1982, St. Luke's Episcopal Hospital.

58. Tjossen, T.: Early intervention: issues and approaches, In Tjossen, T., editor: Intervention strategies for high risk infants and young children, Baltimore, 1976, University Park Press.

59. Touwen, B.: The preterm infant in the extrauterine environment: implications for neurology, Early Hum. Dev. **4:**287, 1980.

60. Usher, R.: The special problems of the premature infant. In Avery, G., editor: Neonatology—pathophysiology and management of the newborn, Philadelphia, 1981, J.B. Lippincott Co.

61. Usher, R., Allen, A., and McLean, F.: Risk of respiratory distress syndrome related to gestational age, route of delivery, and maternal diabetes, Am. J. Obstet. Gynecol. **111:**826, 1971.

62. Widmayer, S., and Field, T.: Effects of Brazelton demonstration on early interactions of preterm infants and their teenage mothers, Infant Behav. Dev. **3:** 1980.

63. Wiener, G.: Psychologic Correlates of premature birth: a review, J. Nerv. Ment. Dis. **134:**129, 1962.

16

NANCY J. POWELL

Children with cerebral palsy

Early in the development of the profession, occupational therapy assumed a major role in the assessment and treatment of children with cerebral palsy. In 1929 Paisley[78] recounted the early work of occupational therapy in the schools with spastic hemiplegics. Treatment emphasized (1) the use of activity in bimanual activities, (2) positioning the upper extremity for relaxation before activity, and (3) the use of activity, including craft and academic skills that required "correct position and the use of weak muscles" (p. 88).[78] Recreation (play), including dancing and motion songs, was included along with activities that were related to student work skills. In this early article it is interesting to note the blending of physical restoration, work in the form of school skills, and play.

In 1950 Abbott[1] noted and described the variety of neuromuscular restoration techniques developed by Fay, Kabat, and Phelps that had recently begun to be used in the treatment of cerebral palsy. Concurrent with these neuromuscular approaches, occupational therapy was aimed at *activity* to correct upper extremity movement patterns and to establish "the habits of arm use in play" (p. 65).[46] Specifically, treatment was given in the sitting position by use of (1) repetitive motion and conditioning for the spastic child, (2) eye coordination activities for the ataxic child, and (3) relaxation followed by motion for the athetoid child. Wheelchair positioning and training in self-care were also stressed.[46,68,71] Toys were adapted to encourage specific movements, increase hand coordination, and motivate the child to productive self-care and other hand functions.[108]

Since the 1950s occupational therapy intervention in the developmental, occupational, and self-care functions of children with cerebral palsy has expanded be-cause of developments in occupational therapy theory, in neurophysiological techniques, and in technological innovation in therapeutic equipment. Bax[13] pointed out that during the 1970s there were major advances in early diagnosis and assessment of cerebral palsy. However, in the 1980s findings about the effectiveness of different intervention methods still remain inconclusive.

To lay a foundation for developing more effective occupational therapy services in the treatment of cerebral palsy, students need guidance in synthesizing existing theories and practice. All major approaches to occupational therapy for the child with cerebral palsy should be examined. The purposes of this chapter are

1. To present the overall scope of cerebral palsy, including types and associated functional problems of concern to occupational therapy
2. To present a model that integrates theoretical approaches to guide occupational therapy intervention for children with cerebral palsy
3. To review the contributions of occupational therapy in the assessment and treatment of cerebral palsy within the context of that model

SCOPE OF THE PROBLEM
Definitions, tonal patterns, and related problems

In Chapter 6 cerebral palsy was defined as a nonprogressive disorder primarily characterized by aberrant motor control and posture resulting from brain insults or injuries occurring in the prenatal, perinatal, or infant period of development. Cerebral palsy is generally described according to (1) the predominating muscle tone pattern present in the individual and (2) the distribution of the motor dysfunction throughout the body. Bobath[18] described three distributions of motor dysfunction. He defined quadriplegia as total body involvement with the upper extremities usually affected more, or at least equally affected as the lower extremities. Diplegia is total body involvement with the lower extremities more affected. Hemiplegia is involvement of one side of the body, for example, the right arm, trunk, and leg.

Spasticity, or hypertonia, is a muscle tone disorder affecting movement where an increase in tone creates an imbalance between muscle groups. Spasticity is characterized by hyperactive deep reflexes, abnormal plantar reflexes, and clonus[31] (Chapter 6). Spasticity can occur in all three of the distribution patterns previously described. A severely spastic child is fixed in a few postures because of increased cocontraction at proximal joints.[18] Jones[56] described the typical posture of spastic quadriplegics: trunk flexion, shoulder adduction, elbow flexion, forearm pronation, thumb adduction, and finger flexion. The lower extremities show flexion, internal rotation, and adduction at the hips, flexion at the knees, plantar flexion at the ankles, and inversion of the feet. Bobath[18] described the functional abilities of the spastic child. The child with spastic quadriplegia has difficulty moving from one posture to another, such as from the supine position to the prone position, or from lying to sitting. The spastic child is unable to rotate about the body axis, so righting reactions cannot develop. Equilibrium reactions usually develop to some degree in sitting but are decreased in kneel standing or standing. Gross and fine movements are slow and laborious. The child will be delayed in self-care and play because of restricted range of movement and lack of manipulation skills. Drooling and feeding problems are common because of the lack of tongue control, the presence of primitive suck-swallow reflexes, and the lack of coordination between breathing and swallowing.[56] The child with spastic diplegia typically has more involvement in the lower extremities than in the upper extremities. Bobath[18] cited insecurity, withdrawal from the environment, resistance to change, and passivity as personality traits of the spastic child. Deformities that may result from improper positioning of the spastic child are scoliosis; flexion contractures of the hips, knees, and ankles; and subluxation of the hip.[18]

Hypotonia is characterized by decreased muscle tone and a failure of the muscles to respond to volitional stimulation.[31] Hypotonic, or floppy, infants often develop spasticity later.[31,60] Problems of the hypotonic child include the lack of the development of stability patterns for gross motor function.

Spastic hemiplegia is characterized by spasticity in either the right or left side of the body (for example, the right arm, trunk, and leg). Bobath[18] described the involvement of the spastic hemiplegic. The hemiplegic child will frequently ignore the involved side, preferring to use the noninvolved side for activity. Bilateral hand use in play and self-care is often absent or decreased. Sensory disturbances, including impaired proprioception and stereognosis, are often found on the affected side. Delays in motor development and lack of equilibrium reactions will be evident. Deformities involving the upper extremity associated with spastic hemiplegia include flexion contractures of the elbow, wrist, and fingers with pronation of the forearm, ulnar deviation of the wrist, and thumb adduction. Scoliosis and talipes equinovarus or talipes equinovalgus of the ankle are other deformities often noted. Aggressive behavior and frequent temper tantrums are often social-emotional components of this disorder.[55]

Disordered movement can also take the form of dyskinesia, that is, involuntary extraneous motor activity accentuated by emotional stress.[31] Athetosis, the most common type of dyskinesia, is characterized by fluctuating muscle tone; predominating extensor tone; and uncontrolled, jerky, twisting movement of the extremities.[31,56] Bobath[18] described movement and functional problems of the child with athetosis. The child with athetosis is unable to cocontract the proximal muscles to stabilize joints; therefore, the stability required for gross motor development is lacking. Such a child will have difficulty maintaining proximal fixation to allow hand use. The child with athetosis has less control in the midranges of movements. Activities that require head and eye control, such as feeding, are difficult. Drooling and speech problems often occur. Bobath[18] also pointed out the personality traits of children with athetosis. They demonstrate unstable and somewhat unpredictable responses to stimuli, and they show quick and extreme physical and emotional changes. Other characteristics of dyskinesia include choreiform movements, dystonic movements, tremor, rigidity, and ataxia.[31]

Often the movement disorders just described present themselves in combination.[49] For example, some degree of spasticity can be found in children with athetosis. When this occurs, the occupational therapist must be aware of the distribution and type of tone present in different body areas so that treatment is appropriate. For example, treatment procedures must be aimed at providing stability in areas having fluctuating tone, and mobility for areas where hypertonia is present, not vice versa.

Although motor disorder is often cited as the definitive symptom of cerebral palsy, Levine[65] believed there is no single finding that is definitive of cerebral palsy. He noted the lack of minimal criteria to make an early diagnosis. A retrospective study by Levine indicated that children of 1 year of age or older are likely to be diagnosed as having cerebral palsy if they have abnormalities in four or more of the following areas: (1) posture and movement patterns, (2) oral motor patterns, (3) strabismus, (4) muscle tone, (5) postural reactions or motor milestones, and (6) reflex development. Cruickshank[29] and Swartz and others[101] explained that cerebral palsy includes a wide collection of symptoms: psychological, neuromuscular, behavioral, sensory, and other symptoms.

Occupational therapists working in schools and clinics will rarely, if ever, see a child with cerebral palsy whose limitations are only motor in nature. The occupational therapist will most often note a unique grouping of handicaps in every child with cerebral palsy in the cognitive, affective, and motor areas. A definition of cerebral palsy that might clarify the occupational therapist's role in the treatment of the child with cerebral palsy is a disorder in motor function with subtle or pronounced associated sensory, affective, physical, or cognitive handicaps.

Cruickshank[29] noted that some associated problems, such as blindness, may have no etiological relationship to cerebral palsy. In other cases, such as deafness, a viral agent may cause both the deafness and the cerebral palsy.[76] Other disabilities commonly associated with cerebral palsy include visual impairments, auditory problems, seizures, mental retardation, sensory integrative disorders, perceptual-motor problems, and social-emotional disorders.[29,30,84]

Relationship to occupational therapy

The occupational therapist possesses expertise in the assessment and treatment of the motor, psychological, and social dysfunctions of the individual with cerebral palsy and in each of the possible associated disability areas as well. Occupational therapists therefore can combine their knowledge and clinical skills in each disability area to develop a comprehensive and tailored approach for each child with a unique pattern of problems. Even after a minimum of clinical experience in treating children with cerebral palsy, the occupational therapist will realize that no two individuals with cerebral palsy are alike in all the manifestations of the disorder. Theoretical approaches in physical function, as well as mental health areas of occupational therapy and their practical application, must be applied with creativity and ingenuity. The occupational therapist must synthesize knowledge to formulate a unique intervention plan for each child. In a sense, the whole of each occupational therapy plan is greater than the sum of contributed skills in specific disability areas. The difficulties that arise with multiple handicaps in the child with cerebral palsy demand a special pooling of resources both from the environment and the therapist. The goal of maximal adaptation for the patient depends on this collaboration.

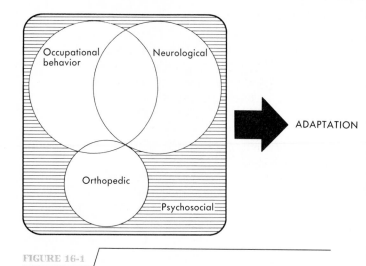

Theoretical model of occupational therapy for children with cerebral palsy.

THEORY

To aid in comprehensive evaluation and treatment of children with cerebral palsy, a holistic model synthesizing related occupational therapy theory and approaches is presented. The model contains neurological, sociocultural, psychosocial, and orthopedic elements. Occupational behavior is the sociocultural concept specific to occupational therapy and is so named in the model (Figure 16-1).

First, a description of these theoretical approaches will be presented. Next, major assessments, treatment objectives, and treatment methods related to each approach will be described. The explanation of treatment methods will also illustrate how the theoretical components can be combined. The goal of this integrated approach describing occupational therapy for cerebral palsy is to formulate fundamental and logical relationships between theory, assessment, practice, and research. This model should be viewed as a flexible framework that will require research to demonstrate its effectiveness in intervention for the child with cerebral palsy. It is hoped that the model will stimulate the reader to develop assessment and treatment procedures and critically analyze current ones.

Description of the model components

THE NEUROLOGICAL APPROACH

The neurological approach is based on neurophysiological principles and was described by Kielhofner and Burke.[59] This approach has emphasized the use of sensory input to produce adaptive behavior. Proponents of different systems of neurophysiological treatment have emphasized particular neurophysiological principles. They have used different kinds of sensory stimuli to improve motor and other functions in patients with central nervous system damage.

Price[83] also described major neurological approaches, or neurotherapies, used in occupational therapy: (1) sensorimotor approaches, (2) perceptual motor approaches, and (3) the sensory integration approach. The sensorimotor approaches are the neuromuscular facilitation approaches of theorists such as Bobath and Bobath,[19] Brunnstrom,[22] and Rood[91] and are distinguished by their emphasis on motor behavior and posture resulting from sensory stimuli (usually tactile and proprioceptive) and the feedback mechanisms of movement. Perceptual motor approaches teach specific skills in deficient areas.[7] For example, balance is taught by having a child learn to walk heel-toe on a 2- by 4- inch board; or specific visual-motor skills are taught such as sorting triangular forms from square forms. It is hoped that such balance and visual-motor skills will be applied to academic and other necessary life tasks. The sensory integration approach emphasizes the organization of sensory information for perception, learning, and adaptive responses.[5,7] There is an emphasis on vestibular stimulation during treatment, because the vestibular system is viewed as contributing a large part to the sensory organizational mechanisms of the central nervous system.[5,83] (See Chapter 19 for more detail on sensory integration as distinguished from other neurological approaches.) Other examples of neurological systems of therapy include the multisensory approach (neurorehabilitation) described by Farber[35] and the spatiotemporal adaptation model described by Gilfoyle, Grady, and Moore[43] (Chapter 3).

Traditionally, the sensorimotor approaches have been used most widely in the management of cerebral palsy, since motor behavior is recognized as the major problem in cerebral palsy. The most prevalent sensorimotor system of therapy for cerebral palsy is Neurodevelopmental Treatment (NDT) developed by Bobath and Bobath.[20,21] Bobath[17] and Bobath and Bobath[21] emphasized early assessment of the infant with cerebral palsy so that treatment could be initiated by at least 6 months of age. At this early age normal movement can be facilitated and hypertonia prevented. The infant is assessed for the presence of abnormal tone by observation for tonic patterns that are provoked by spontaneous movement and special handling. For example, tests in the supine position detect extensor hypertonia; the infant is lifted from the supine position by placing the hand behind the infant's head or shoulder. The examiner notes extensor tone in the trunk and neck and notes shoulder retraction. Other tests in the supine position, as well as tests in the prone and upright positions, allow evaluation of tonic patterns (reflexes) and maturing righting and equilibrium reactions.

The treatment techniques developed by Bobath[17] and Bobath and Bobath[20,21] for the child with cerebral palsy are called handling. The aims of treatment were outlined[17] in 1967:

1. To develop normal postural reactions and postural tone against gravity for support and control of movements.
2. To counteract the development of abnormal postural reactions and of abnormal postural tone.
3. To give the child, by means of handling and play, the functional patterns he will use later on for feeding, dressing, washing, etc. for self-help.
4. To prevent the development of contractures and deformities (p. 374).*

For a child with increased tone, the use of reflex-inhibiting patterns counteracts abnormal tonic reflex activity in a particular body position (for example, supine) and modifies abnormal postural tone.[21] More normal movement can then occur. Active movement in normal patterns is facilitated at key points: usually the head, neck, shoulder, and hips. Inhibition of abnormal postural and movement patterns and facilitation of normal movement patterns are effected by handling the child at the key points and avoiding stimulation of distal body parts. These normal movement patterns include righting and equilibrium reactions. As normal reflex activity develops, the child is advanced in motor development abilities.[21] For example, the occupational therapist might begin to work on proximal stability, progress to gross arm movement, and then concentrate on hand function.

Neurodevelopmental treatment also incorporates proprioceptive and tactile stimulation techniques to normalize muscle tone and to balance agonists, antagonists, and synergists. In selected children with hypotonia and impaired reciprocal movement, such as those with athetosis, Bobath and Bobath[21] recommended

1. Weight-bearing, pressure, and resistance
2. Placing and holding
3. Tapping

Weight-bearing involves weight transfer to obtain automatic adjustments of the trunk and limbs. Placing is passive movement of a limb with minimal support into a position that the patient holds. Holding is maintaining control of body and limbs after being placed in various positions. When combined with placing, tapping helps to increase muscle tone, to activate antagonists to spastic muscles, and to activate synergists by using a sweeping stroke in the direction of movement. Caution in using these techniques must be employed to prevent triggering spasticity by stimulating abnormal

*Reprinted with permission from Bobath, B.: Dev. Med. Child Neurol. **9:**374, 1967, Spastics International Medical Publications, London.

reflex activity. Bobath and Bobath[21] recommended using these techniques with reflex-inhibiting patterns, applying the stimulation carefully and only when tone is low, as well as applying these techniques to obtain localized responses.

Courses in the theory and application of Neurodevelopmental Treatment are given throughout the United States and the British Commonwealth countries on a regular basis. Certification in the use of Neurodevelopmental Treatment can be gained through some of these courses. The above description is a brief overview of the original therapy system presented by Bobath and Bobath.[21] Many therapists[38,43] have expanded the application of the approach.

Perceptual motor approaches are often used by occupational therapists in school systems and clinics to support the educational process. The use of the sensory integration approach with cerebral palsy patients is controversial. Occupational therapists, such as Price,[84] are currently investigating the use of sensory integration evaluation and treatment methods for children with cerebral palsy.

The research base for using the neurological approach for the treatment of cerebral palsy is limited in size and contains contradictory evidence. Tyler and Kogan[111] devised a study to examine the effectiveness of occupational therapy for the treatment of cerebral palsy. They attempted to assess the effects of occupational therapy, including Bobath techniques and others, on the use of the upper extremities in manipulative and self-help skills. Seventy-seven children with various types of cerebral palsy ranging in age from 10 months to 6 years were included in the study. Most children were tested at 9- to 15-month intervals. Gain scores on the manipulative and self-help skills test were analyzed in relation to age, IQ, diagnosis, past therapy history, initial scores, and amount of therapy. IQ was found not to be related to gain scores. Other tentative findings from the study were that children less affected, younger children, and children receiving 1 year less of treatment made greater gains. Amount of therapy was related to higher gain scores in self-help skills. Interpretation of these results is difficult, because there was no control group used. Also, the type of therapy was not designated, so questions remain as to the impact of sensorimotor therapy per se.

Carlsen[23] did a pilot study to compare the effectiveness of two occupational therapy approaches: one emphasizing sensorimotor facilitation, the other a functional skills program. Twelve young children with cerebral palsy were matched for developmental age and type of motor involvement and randomly assigned to treatment groups. They were pretested on the Denver Developmental Screening Test (DDST) and the Bayley Motor Scales. The facilitation treatment consisted of activity to promote sensory organization, postural stability, and controlled movement. The functional treatment consisted of positioning, adaptive hand skills, and self-care skills. After 6 weeks of treatment in the clinic and daily home programs, the children in the facilitation group made significant improvement on the Bayley Motor Scales and the gross motor subsection of the Denver Developmental Screening Test. The facilitation group also had greater gains on the Denver Developmental Screening Test in the personal-social, fine-motor adaptive, and language subsections, although these were not significant. The results of the study indicated "that for the age group studied, a program that is primarily based on facilitation of gross sensorimotor integration, but does not exclude training in fine motor activities, may be the most effective" (p. 272).[23] The lack of a control group and blind evaluation limit the generalizability of the study.

In a study evaluating a combination of sensory integrative and neurodevelopmental treatment, Norton[77] found that three children diagnosed as profoundly retarded with multiple handicaps achieved higher developmental levels in posture, emotion, perception, and cognition. Treatment consisting of handling and positioning, arousal stimulation, respiration, prefeeding facilitation, and vestibular and tactile stimulation was administered by the mothers of the children for 9 months. Small sample size and the lack of a control group are the major limitations to interpreting the results.

Scherzer, Mike, and Ilson[93] gathered data on 22 infants under 18 months of age who had a definite or presumed diagnosis of cerebral palsy. In a double-blind study an experimental group received neurophysiological physical therapy consisting of positioning, movement to inhibit abnormal reflexes and to facilitate normal motor development, and a home program. A control group received only passive range of motion exercise. Medical and physical therapy evaluations of motor status, social maturation, and home management revealed a definite correlation between change and experimental group status. They found a trend of positive change in more intelligent children who received the neurophysiological treatment.

Studies aimed at assessing the vestibular function of children with cerebral palsy and measuring the effectiveness of vestibular stimulation on the motor deficit in cerebral palsy have shown similar nonconclusive findings. Torok and Perlstein[107] found in a study investigating vestibular function in 518 children with cerebral palsy that 34% had vestibular abnormalities. Hyposensitivity was most common in children with athetosis. Hypersensitivity to vestibular stimulation was most common in spastic hemiplegics. These findings may have prompted researchers to ask the question: Does treatment involving the vestibular system affect motor behavior of children with cerebral palsy?

Twenty-three preambulatory children with cerebral

palsy, ages 2 to 6, were pretested by Chee, Kreutzberg, and Clark[24] on a gross motor skills test and a reflex test. Twelve children were assigned to a treatment group that received vertical and horizontal semicircular canal stimulation for 4 weeks. Two control groups were established. One group received no treatment, and the remaining children were handled but received no vestibular input. The treatment group showed greater gains in gross motor skills and reflex development. Subjective evaluations by therapists and mothers also indicated improvement in equilibrium, gross motor control, alertness, curiosity, and social-emotional status.

A similar study by Sellick and Over[95] involving 20 children with cerebral palsy aged 8 months to 56 months did not support the findings of the study of Chee, Kreutzberg, and Clark.[24] The treatment group in the Sellick and Over study that received controlled vestibular stimulation over a 4-week period showed no significant improvement on the Bayley Infant Developmental Scales when compared to a control group. The children were posttested in the week following treatment and 3 months later.

Ayres[6] conducted a study of children with learning disability and choreoathetosis, a motor disorder characterized by mild involuntary motions interfering with fine motor coordination. She found no significant improvement in eye-hand coordination in a group who received sensory integrative therapy when compared to a control group who did not receive therapy.

In summary, the research studies investigating the effectiveness of neurological approaches for the treatment of cerebral palsy present contradictory evidence. Although some of the studies mentioned earlier are flawed in methodology, they do indicate trends toward improvement by use of sensorimotor techniques.

THE OCCUPATIONAL BEHAVIOR APPROACH

The occupational behavior approach is derived from the frame of reference called occupational behavior and was originally proposed by Reilly.[85] The approach focuses on individuals in life roles and is studied through work and play phenomena.[70] Adult work and social recreation roles are viewed as evolving from play (Chapters 3 and 13). Development of occupational behavior involves "the translation of skills to habits for a sequence of life roles beginning with preschooler, progressing to student and worker, and culminating in the retiree role" (p. 101).[89]

Matsutsuyu[70] explained three concepts in occupational behavior. The first is occupational choice, a developmental process of choosing an occupation. The second is occupational role, the specific tasks and social position of an individual, such as housewife or preschooler. The third is socialization, a process that allows the learning of occupational behaviors. A motor disorder such as cerebral palsy may interfere with the

development of skills and habits related to achieving occupational choice, occupational role, and socialization. Matsutsuyu[70] emphasized the aim of occupational therapy as "one of identifying the nature of adaptations or the renewal of acquisition of new skills needed to maintain, support, or raise the daily living performance of patients in their current life roles" (p. 292).

The occupational behavior approach has been expanded to include self-care skills as important habits to acquire in relationship to life roles. Shannon included[97,98] self-maintenance as a part of work. This included self-care, as well as sleep and rest. He recommended a balance of work and play in an individual's life. Pezzuti[79] cited mastery of self-help skills in childhood as a factor in the development of occupational choice. Play produces the motor, cognitive, and social skills that contribute to the development of self-care. Abnormal motor development of children with cerebral palsy produces interference in play experiences and thus may affect self-care and work.

Reilly[86] proposed the three hierarchical stages of play: exploratory behavior, competency behavior, and achievement behavior (Florey, Chapter 3). Cerebral palsy may restrict exploratory motor behavior, such as object manipulation and locomotion. Knox[64] pointed out that a disability can inhibit exploration. Thus the process of exploration, which discovers the meanings of objects, motions, and people in the environment, and the assessment of one's assets and limitations may be delayed or hindered by cerebral palsy. Competency or adaptation will not develop because of the lack of feedback from both the environment and the child's own actions. Children with cerebral palsy often do not persist in mastering difficult motor tasks. Hence, feelings of self-reliance and self-confidence are affected. Difficulties in exploratory and competency behavior will have an accumulative effect on achievement behavior. Gunn[48] noted the relationship between the inability of the handicapped to play and their decreased ability to cope with novel, complex, and dissonant situations. These kinds of situations often arise in the lives of handicapped individuals; therefore, the inability to play may affect coping mechanisms related to the handicap.

Takata[102] described aspects of "play deprivation" of multihandicapped children. These include (1) sedentary and passive experience, (2) limited, or the lack of, available raw materials, (3) an emphasis on either large or small motor actions, and (4) parental expectations that are either too high or too low. These factors upset the balance of four important elements that nurture play. According to Takata, these are (1) human elements, (2) nonhuman elements, (3) qualitative aspects of who and what is played with and how the child plays, and (4) the quantitative aspects (time spent at play). In a study comparing multihandicapped (including cerebral palsy and other types of handicaps) and nonhandicapped preschool children, Gralewicz[45] found that the multihandicapped child played less with related adults and had less total playtime than nonhandicapped children.

In summary, because of deprivation of play experiences and the inability to play, the child with cerebral palsy is likely to have difficulty in achieving competancy in life roles. The severity of the motor disorder, the number of associated disorders, the support of the family, and the medical community will all affect the child's play development and the subsequent acquisition of self-care and work skills. The occupational therapist needs the knowledge of play and its development; the knowledge of the motor, affective, and cognitive problems related to cerebral palsy; and the understanding of the effect of cerebral palsy on play to assess and develop an intervention plan to normalize the development of occupational behavior.

THE ORTHOPEDIC APPROACH

In a facility that uses the orthopedic approach, the occupational therapist works directly with an orthopedic surgeon in the management of the child with cerebral palsy in the preoperative and postoperative phases of care. Although orthopedic specialists may also endorse nonsurgical methods of care, such as neurological approaches, most believe that surgery has a definite place in management of the child with cerebral palsy. Goldner[44] and Zancolli and Zancolli[120] stated that for carefully selected patients upper extremity surgery can be helpful. Goldner[44] stated that most children with cerebral palsy are not surgery candidates because they can adapt to their motor deficit and have limited potential for improvement. Pollack[82] reviewed the results of surgery in cerebral palsy and reported that in one group of patients who had upper extremity surgery, 36.8% had results that were considered failures. Although the occupational therapist may be involved in the orthopedic management of the lower extremities, the present discussion of assessment and treatment will be limited to the upper extremity.

The orthopedic component in the present model for occupational therapy for the child with cerebral palsy is defined as all the assessment and treatment used in conjunction with orthopedic surgery. This approach is related to the biomechanical approach used by occupational therapists in physical dysfunction as described by Trombly[109] and Trombly and Scott.[110] This approach uses kinematic and kinetic assessment and treatment for orthopedic problems. These problems involve loss of range of motion, strength, and endurance that are necessary components of movement to enable the child to perform functional life tasks. This approach is applicable to patients who have voluntary muscle control.

Orthopedic surgeons state that children with purely spastic paralysis are the best candidates for surgery but that it is important to have at least some voluntary control of the spastic muscles to be treated by surgery to assure functional results.[44,49,120] The objectives for performing hand surgery in children with cerebral palsy include the following:

1. To increase hand function to optimum[92]
2. To increase hygiene[15]
3. To increase cosmetic appearance[15,44]
4. To assist in the psychological adjustment of the child and the parents[120]

Green[47] noted that surgery is aimed at changing "the relative agonist-antagonist action and to establish better balance of muscle power" (p. 3).

THE PSYCHOSOCIAL APPROACH

The psychosocial component of the model includes two areas specified in the American Occupational Therapy Association's Uniform Terminology for Reporting Occupational Therapy Services:[114] (1) psychological-emotional daily living skills and (2) psychosocial skills related to self-management and dyadic (relating to another person) and group interaction. Psychological-emotional daily living skills include developing self-concept, coping with life situations, and the ability to interact with the community, including organizations and social systems. Psychosocial skills related to self-management include adequate self-expression and self-control.[114]

Versluys[115] described psychosocial adjustment to physical disability. She described the effects of chronic illness, some of which pertain to the cerebral palsy patient. These are reduced self-esteem, security, independence, and social contacts. The child with cerebral palsy lacks the ability to manipulate and cope with the environment and the behavior of others.[62] Therefore social adjustment is threatened, and the ability to establish effective relationships with peers and adults is impaired.

Abnormal motor behavior may interfere with developing an adequate self-concept, and therefore perception of one's needs, feelings, physical performance abilities, and sexuality may be disrupted. Coping with stress and solving life problems will be difficult for the child with cerebral palsy. Because of decreased self-expression skills, such as speaking, writing, and perceptual abilities, the developing individual is likely to be hindered in learning how to deal with social organizations, social systems, and individuals with different social norms. Adjusting behavior to situational demands is a problem area for children with cerebral palsy.

Research by Imperio, Cullinan, and Riklan[53] suggested that physically disabled young adults may be at higher risk for developing a maladaptive personality. A representative group with mild physical dysfunction showed a trend toward greater pathology. Imperio, Cullinan, and Riklan suggested the use of counseling and psychotherapy that includes paying particular attention to the areas of sexual behavior and sex-role adaptation.

In a report on public and professional attitudes toward the sexual and emotional needs of the handicapped, Shearer[99] described the lack of sex education for physically handicapped children in schools and at home. She stated that handicapped children are denied knowledge about their own sexuality and the means of expressing sexual and emotional needs. Society prefers to keep handicapped people in a childhoodlike state, thereby ignoring sexual needs.

Teplin, Howard, and O'Conner[105] studied self-concept of young children with cerebral palsy. Two measures of self-concept were adapted and administered to a group of 15 mainstreamed children with cerebral palsy, ages 4 to 8, and to a control group. Findings indicated a tendency for the handicapped group to have lower self-concepts. Teachers also rated the handicapped group as having lower self-concepts. The authors concluded that self-concept and its subsequent effect on self-esteem is an important factor in the primary grades, particularly for boys.

Tyler, Kogan, and Turner[113] studied interpersonal components displayed during therapy by young children with cerebral palsy and their mothers. In therapy they found that mothers displayed a controlling and negative affect that was not manifested during play. The child also demonstrated greater amounts of negative behavior during therapy. The authors speculated that children with cerebral palsy are delayed in their interactive abilities. This delay interferes with the establishment of a normal mother-child relationship. They concluded that professionals need to assess the mother-child relationship before determining a mother's role in therapy.

A later study by Tyler and Kogan[112] investigated the effect of behavioral instruction given to mothers of children with cerebral palsy on stressful and conflicted interactions. By analyzing behavior via videotape, they found that 8 weeks of behavioral instruction was sufficient to reduce stressful and conflicted behavior. Most of the change was shown by the mothers, and the change was maintained as long as 1 year later. There was no gradual decrease in expressions of positive feelings. The authors concluded that "physically handicapped children have a more difficult time participating in reciprocal interaction" (p. 155)[112] and that the mothers experience a nonrewarding interaction that does not proceed at as rapid a rate as it would with a nonhandicapped child. Mothers may cope by using various forms of disengaging behavior with their handicapped child.

ADAPTATION

Ayres,[5] King,[60] and others[43,63] have explained adaptation as the goal of therapeutic intervention. King[60] stated that individual adaptation involves active participation, responsiveness to environmental demands, an outcome orientation, and self-reinforcement. The goals of individual adaptation are described as the enhancement of personal survival and actualization of potential. Kleiman and Bulkey[63] have expanded the adaptation concept to a continuum. On one end of the continuum are basic homeostatic reactions. These include basic survival mechanisms such as reflexes and breathing. Next are the adaptive responses that are active, self-reinforcing, goal-directed, and integrated actions, such as grasping. Adaptive skills are next on the continuum and include combinations and repetition of adaptive responses. Playing baseball is an example of adaptive skills. Finally, at the end of the continuum (opposite homeostatic responses) are large, complex behavioral units called adaptive patterns such as balanced leisure time activity.

Depending on the severity of the motor handicap, the child with cerebral palsy will need variable amounts of intervention to achieve the goals of individual adaptation. This child is often dependent on others for personal survival, and he needs assistance in achieving his potential. The child with cerebral palsy may have difficulty at all points along the adaptation continuum. The reactions linked with basic survival may be impaired, such as breathing and feeding reactions. Adaptive patterns might not include smooth coordinated movement and can be too laborious to be functional. The child with cerebral palsy may gain very few adaptive skills that can be executed in a normal manner. Playing games in the usual manner will be impossible for many children. Without proper intervention, a well-balanced adaptive pattern, such as recreational activity, may only be achieved with limited success and independence by most children with cerebral palsy. The elements presented in the model—neurological, occupational behavior, orthopedic, and psychosocial—are the main therapeutic ingredients included in the occupational therapist's theoretical and practical repertoire to facilitate maximal adaptation for the child with cerebral palsy.

Discussion of the model

The model illustrated in Figure 16-1 is a graphic representation of (1) the major theoretical approaches in occupational therapy related to intervention in cerebral palsy and (2) the interaction of these theoretical components in terms of their contribution to the goal of occupational therapy, which is adaptation.

In the model a significant amount of interaction is shown between the neurological and occupational behavior components. Play is an integral part of neurological treatment. Lindquist, Mack, and Parham[67] described the synthesis between sensory integration (a subcategory of the neurological approach) and occupational behavior. They suggested that play is a process in achieving competence. Competence, a component of adaptation, is the ultimate goal of both approaches.

Other similarities between the two approaches that the authors describe are (1) concepts of hierarchical development, (2) the influence of the environment on development, and (3) self-directed, active participation on the part of the child in therapy. The authors described how sensory integration can influence play and how play is the therapeutic process for sensory integrative development. This idea can be expanded: play brings out certain characteristics, including movement, self-direction, purpose, and intrinsic motivation, that activate sensorimotor, sensory integrative, and perceptual-motor mechanisms.

Florey[41] noted that the role of play provides feedback necessary for change. Therefore the occupational therapist needs to incorporate appropriate play activities into treatment (1) to promote behavior that a specific neurological approach, such as Neurodevelopmental Treatment, is trying to elicit and (2) to develop play skills that will contribute to the development of skills and habits necessary for occupational roles. DiJoseph[32] emphasized the use of activity in occupational therapy to elicit desired movement patterns. Self-care skills and school skills are also developed through play and can be used as treatment activities to produce specific movement.

As sensorimotor processes are normalized in the child with cerebral palsy, play, self-care, and school skills will be improved. Ayres[9] stated that sensory integration helps to organize occupational behavior. She cited motor planning ability as necessary for performing those self-care tasks that are enacted in the programmed sequence of events involved in getting ready for school.

Orthopedic treatment also overlaps with the occupational behavior approach. The child with cerebral palsy who undergoes orthopedic surgery will require intervention by the occupational therapist to prevent disruption of the development of occupational behavior. Work, play, and self-care skills should improve as a result of orthopedic surgical management. Representative tasks can be used as activities to increase motor function in occupational therapy after orthopedic surgery.

Assessment and treatment in the neurological and orthopedic approaches show minimal overlap. The assessment of sensation and treatment for inadequate sensory awareness in the hand can be included in both approaches. Sensory function in an extremity is related to regaining movement, whether the means to that end is obtained through orthopedic surgery or obtained through a neurological treatment method. Combining surgery and sensorimotor approaches in the treatment of cerebral palsy is controversial. As previously discussed, the orthopedic approach is believed to be applicable in only a few carefully selected cases; therefore, the component is represented as being smaller in Figure 16-1.

The psychosocial approach is a component that is related to all the other approaches in the management of cerebral palsy and must be used in combination with other approaches. The other three approaches may contain some of the same processes within them. An example is socialization that is related to the occupational behavior, as well as the psychosocial, approach. The outcomes of the neurological, occupational behavior, and orthopedic approaches contribute to the achievement of psychosocial objectives. For example, Ayres[7] hypothesized that self-esteem is an end product of sensory integration therapy. Other principles and methods in the psychosocial approach in occupational therapy can be used in conjunction with the other approaches to maximize their effect on the child with cerebral palsy. The ultimate goal of all the assessment and treatment components is adaptation. The challenge for the occupational therapist is to select and combine appropriate assessments and treatment methods from each of the appropriate theoretical approaches to provide a holistic intervention plan tailored to the changing needs of each developing child with cerebral palsy.

ASSESSMENT

Occupational therapists assess children with cerebral palsy by using a combination of instruments and techniques related to the theoretical approaches described previously. Howison, Perella, and Gordon[51] pointed out that there is no single evaluation that will thoroughly assess a particular child. It is usually necessary to use a combination of measures. Some of the factors that can influence what instruments are used include (1) the age of the child, (2) the degree and type of motor disorder, (3) the associated disorders, such as mental retardation, and (4) the philosophy of the treatment team. Early assessment followed by treatment is viewed by most in the field to be essential to later function. Neurological assessment and treatment is usually recommended for the infant and very young child with cerebral palsy. Bleck[15] recommended that children about 5 years of age or older may be candidates for orthopedic surgery. It is speculated that neurophysiological (neurological) approaches are less effective for the child over 5 years of age. However, the time to stop neurological approaches and to begin orthopedic care, if appropriate, is controversial. In all cases, therapists must assess psychosocial function and occupational behavior.

Major assessment techniques related to each of the theoretical approaches are described here. There is some overlap between methods, or techniques, used in the four approaches, such as the use of sensory evaluation in the neurological and orthopedic approaches. It is important to reemphasize that the assessment used by the occupational therapist will reflect all of the approaches discussed.

Neurological assessment

MUSCLE TONE

Bobath and Bobath[21] suggested that a child's muscle tone be tested with the child placed in certain postural patterns, including supine, prone, sitting, kneeling, and standing positions. Abnormal muscle tone is assessed by moving the child's limbs, head, and trunk in patterns in these positions and by noting the amount of resistance to movement. An example of a position and pattern is placing the child in the supine position, abducting the legs with outward rotation in flexion and in extension. Also, the adjustment of muscle tone while assuming a new position from the previous position is noted. For example, children often show resistance to sideturning from the supine position. In the authors' assessment, tonic reflex patterns are noted, such as the asymmetrical tonic neck reflex pattern.[21]

Bobath and Bobath[21] assessed muscle tone in postural patterns as being severely, moderately, or slightly resistive or having irregular, transient, or a complete lack of resistance. If spasticity is present, an abnormal amount of resistance to postural patterns will be felt during testing. Characteristic of the child with athetosis is intermittent abnormal resistance alternating with complete lack of resistance. Hypotonic or flaccid tone is noted by an abnormal lack of resistance to a postural pattern.

Passive movement of joints through total ranges of motion is another method of testing tone. Joint mobility and deformity, contractures, and muscle shortness can be noted in this method. Bobath and Bobath[21] cautioned that this method does not take into account that muscle tone varies over time, from part to part, with changes in excitability and with changes in the position of the head in space and of the head in relationship to the trunk. Observation of movement can also contribute to assessing muscle tone.

REFLEX ASSESSMENT

In cerebral palsy stereotyped, primitive reflex movements may persist. The influence of residual primitive reflexes delays the development of righting and equilibrium reactions. The occupational therapist must test for the presence of persistent primitive reflexes to determine their interference with normal development of movement. One of the first reflex testing systems was developed by Fiorentino.[39] This is a comprehensive test of reflexes and righting and equilibrium reactions. Another assessment by Milani-Comparetti and Gidoni[73] assesses reflexes and motor patterns on a single form, thus showing the relationship between reflexes and motor milestones.

SENSORIMOTOR DEVELOPMENT

The child with cerebral palsy must be tested to determine the level of achieved motor development, as well as any abnormal movement patterns that interfere with normal motor development. Semans and others[96] have devised a Cerebral Palsy Assessment Chart that tests muscle tone and basic motor control in 20 test postures and movements related to functional activity arranged in a developmental sequence that includes the supine position, the prone sitting, kneeling, standing, and walking.

There are several developmental tests that are used to assess motor development (Chapters 9 and 11). These include the Bayley Scales of Infant Development, the Denver Developmental Screening Test, and the Gesell Developmental Schedules. Lewko[66] reported on dissatisfaction with the use of published tests to evaluate motor performance. Important problems noted were (1) too much subjectivity in the interpretation and scoring, (2) insufficient number of items per age level and category, (3) lack of measurement of quality of performance, (4) lack of useful information to guide treatment planning, and (5) the inappropriate design of the test for children with neuromuscular impairment. Erhardt[34] developed a prehension assessment that can be used with children with cerebral palsy who are severely, mildly, or moderately involved.

Responding to the lack of appropriate motor tests for children with cerebral palsy, many therapists have constructed tests they feel give a better picture of current sensorimotor and cognitive ability. Lewko[66] questioned whether these self-made tests were appropriate, since they borrow items and change the format of standardized tests. These unpublished tests may include (1) a combination of functional categories, such as gross motor, fine motor, self-care, oral-motor, play skills; social-emotional skills; and perceptual skills and (2) scoring that gives additional qualitative information, such as "accomplishes activity, with some assistance" or "accomplishes activity, but in more than average time, or in an awkward manner."[75]

ORAL-MOTOR ASSESSMENT

Oral-motor function influences feeding and communication in work and play. Related assessment includes evaluation of oral-motor reflexes, muscle tone, oral movement synergies and motor control, head and shoulder control, respiration, sensation, and upper extremity control (Chapters 9 and 12).

SENSORY EVALUATION

With cerebral palsy children who have developed a high enough level of communication skills, the occupational therapist can perform a sensory evaluation to determine the kind and amount of sensory input that is getting through to the central nervous system. Trombly and Scott[110] outlined a gross sensory evaluation procedure that can be adapted for the child with cerebral palsy. The kinds of stimuli to be evaluated in this assessment include touch, deep pressure, temperature, sharp-dull (pain), proprioception, kinesthesia, stereognosis, and two-point discrimination. Tizard, Paine, and Crother[106] found the discriminative senses including stereognosis, two-point discrimination, and position sense, to be the ones most often affected in patients with cerebral palsy. Children with athetosis have been found to have fewer discriminative sensory disturbances than those with spastic cerebral palsy.[57] With young children and infants, the occupational therapist must rely on clinical observation to indicate the nature of sensory abilities, such as vision and audition.

Farber[35] outlined procedures for olfactory and gustatory evaluation. She cautioned against using too many different sensory stimuli at one time during evaluation and consequently overstimulating the child's nervous system.

SENSORY INTEGRATION AND PERCEPTUAL-MOTOR ASSESSMENT

Occupational therapists assess perception in the visual, tactile, and proprioceptive areas and assess motor abilities to hypothesize about the nature of sensory integration occurring within an individual.[5,8] Certain standardized tests may be suitable for some children with cerebral palsy who have enough motor ability and communication ability to perform them. These include the Motor-Free Visual Perception Test by Colarusso and Hammill,[27] the Test of Visual-Perceptual Skills by Gardner,[42] and parts of the Southern California Sensory Integration Tests[8] such as those on space visualization and figure-ground perception. Price[84] noted that tests which require manipulation, drawing, or sustained sitting at a table cannot be used in a standardized way with many children. She suggests observing other clinical signs, such as how the child plans movement, to assess praxis.

A history of the child's sensory integration is an important assessment tool along with clinical observation to evaluate sensory integration and perception. Hyland[52] adapted sensory history forms of Ayres and others for the collection of subjective data from parents that indicated the child's reactions to sensory inputs (for example, "Did your child enjoy being rocked as an infant?") and perceptual performance ("Does your child make reversals when copying?"). Some of the items on these tests, such as the last example given, may not be appropriate for very involved children with cerebral palsy because of their lack of fine motor control. A form could be adapted for children with severe involvement.

COGNITIVE ASSESSMENT

Cognitive assessment is included under the neurological approach, because cognition is theorized to result from sensory integration, a neurological approach. Ayres[7] cited the capacities for abstract thought, reasoning, and academic learning as examples of higher mental functions emerging from the integration of sensation. The contribution of the occupational behavior approach, the psychosocial approach, and, to a much lesser degree, the orthopedic approach to cognition should not be overlooked. Indiana University Hospitals use a Mental Scale[71] that is a checklist of skills related to cognition, such as visual regard of objects and persons, fine motor abilities, vocalizations, response to auditory stimulation, object permanence, and cognition including problem-solving ability and various basic cognitive skills. Evaluation of cognition by the occupational therapist should supplement evaluation by a psychologist. Clinical observation during activities can provide additional descriptive, qualitative data about cognitive functions that the occupational therapist can use, along with psychological testing information, to plan intervention.

Occupational behavior assessment

PLAY HISTORY

A play history, as described by Takata,[103] is used to obtain information to use in planning occupational therapy treatment. Data from previous play experiences, as well as the present play of the child with cerebral palsy, are analyzed and compared to play experiences of normal children. Finnie[38] used a questionnaire to gather similar data. Both assessments ask about what kinds of objects the child plays with, who the child plays with, the child's body positions during play, and other aspects of play (Chapter 9).

PLAY ASSESSMENT

Florey[41] outlined the pilot instruments, or guides, that have been developed to assess play. These are nonstandardized tests that assess the changing nature of play in a child's development and that guide the therapist in providing a play milieu and proper play experience. Florey[40] suggested two play observation screening devices: the Guide to Play Observation[88] and the Guide to Observation of Play Development.[40] Various play scales[16,64] and other measures may be appropriate to assess mildly involved children with cerebral palsy (Chapter 11). These scales were developed for children without motor handicaps; therefore, some of the items are inappropriate for severely involved children. The play milieu of the child can also be assessed to indicate necessary changes in the environment.

SCHOOL AND WORK SKILLS

The occupational therapist who works with school-aged children in a school system needs to evaluate functional tasks related to learning. (See Chapter 24 for the evaluation of school skills.) Some school therapists might evaluate and treat a child by using sensorimotor approaches, but functional assessment of the ability to perform learning tasks is usually unique to the school occupational therapist. Developmental, cognitive, and adaptive behavior scales usually contain items related to school tasks, such as writing. An interview with the child's teacher and classroom observation would add to the data in this area. In later childhood skills related to occupational roles subsequent to the student role may be assessed by use of prevocational tests. Descriptive information about the older child's engagement in activity can also be used to assess work skills. In the less involved older child performance on physical capacities evaluations and standardized prevocational tests might be employed.[58]

SELF-MAINTENANCE

Most comprehensive evaluations of children with cerebral palsy include parental questionnaires to gather data in regard to the child's eating, toileting, and sleeping habits, among others. Age appropriate self-care skills such as feeding, dressing, and grooming are generally included in items on developmental scales. One example is the Bronson Methodist Hospital's Motor Development Test.[75] Such activities of daily living scales usually require direct observation to gather criterion-referenced data on self-maintenance, which is considered to be a more reliable method than interviewing parents.

ACTIVITY CONFIGURATION

By completing an activity configuration assessment for the child with cerebral palsy, the occupational therapist can assess the child's amount and quality of play, his self-maintenance, and his work (school) activities. As described by Mosey,[74] this tool assesses the child's and parents' ideas, "feelings, need satisfaction, and values relative to his typical weekly activities" (p. 101).

Orthopedic assessment

Orthopedists have stressed the importance of the occupational therapist in preoperative and postoperative assessment.[15,120] Preoperatively, to select candidates for whom good functional recovery may be expected, orthopedists emphasize assessment in three main areas: (1) sensation, (2) psychosocial functions, such as cognition and motivation, and (3) movement-related factors, such as range of motion, strength, and functional abilities (dexterity). These factors are most often cited

as being related to functional outcomes. Occupational therapy assessment of the child for upper extremity surgery will include the following:

1. Sensory evaluation. Gross sensory testing before surgery involving the upper extremity is critical. Stereognosis, graphesthesia, proprioception, and two-point discrimination are important to assess. Without adequate sensibility, the functional results of surgery are likely to be poor.
2. Passive range of motion testing to evaluate muscle tone and to note joint deformities, contractions, and muscle shortness.
3. Active range of motion testing.
4. Manual muscle testing, if the child is able to cooperate.
5. Hand function assessment, including voluntary control of gross and fine motor coordination; speed and dexterity in activity; and use as assistive hand in bimanual play, self-care, and school skills.
6. Endurance and dexterity.
7. Cognition. Orthopedic physicians recommend assessing cognition in candidates for upper extremity surgery. Hoffer[49] stated that children with an IQ below 50 are not good candidates. The occupational therapist can contribute to the psychologist's assessment of cognitive ability through observation of the child in activity and by the use of assessment tools, such as the Mental Scale.[71] Also, through observation and interview of the child and his family, the occupational therapist can assess attitude, motivation, and emotional status.
8. Self-maintenance. The child's use of his arm and hand before and after surgery in self-care and communication should be evaluated as well as their assistive use in mobility.

Psychosocial assessment

Psychosocial assessment is done through a questionnaire, an interview, and observation. The data gathered by the occupational therapist will supplement the psychological evaluation.

During the initial evaluation by the occupational therapist, the parents of the child with cerebral palsy may be given a questionnaire covering family information, behavioral and attitudinal data, and other information related to self-care, play, and sensory motor function. An example is Finnie's questionnaire referred to earlier. Through observation the occupational therapist can identify delays in psychosocial behavior and language skills through the use of the Denver Developmental Screening Test. The Cerebral Palsy Clinic in Indianapolis has developed an Annual Psycho-social

Evaluation[3] that is aimed at school-aged children and assesses school experience, peer relationships, adjustment to authority, mood state, outside interests, attitudes, and other factors.

The occupational therapist may need to interview the entire family of the child with cerebral palsy to assess values, attitudes, accuracy of information and perceptions about cerebral palsy, and feelings of family members that will influence the carryover of treatment to the home. An interview conducted in the home where the occupational therapist can also observe interactions among family members can provide valuable information about sibling interactions, cultural influences, socioeconomic status, and family roles that could influence treatment.

TREATMENT GOALS

From a comprehensive evaluation, the occupational therapist derives specific treatment goals to meet the needs of the child with cerebral palsy. The goals of treatment are outlined in the following paragraphs in each of the areas presented in the model: neurological, occupational behavior, orthopedic, and psychosocial. The reader is reminded that approaches, and therefore goals, derived from assessment data are combined to produce a holistic treatment approach.

Neurological goals

Several neurological approaches to the treatment of cerebral palsy were outlined earlier. Occupational therapists who use specific treatment methods, such as Neurodevelopment Therapy, need specialized study in those approaches, including the specific evaluation and treatment methods involved. There are, however, general goals of neurological approaches that can be formulated and presented here.

1. To provide controlled sensory stimuli through positioning and activity to adjust tone and promote normal movement patterns
2. To provide postural stabilization as necessary in work, play, and self-care
3. To facilitate the development of righting and equilibrium reactions through selected activities
4. To promote, through activity, the development of sensorimotor milestones leading to fine motor skills
5. To provide planned, controlled sensory input to promote sensory integration, perception, and cognition leading to adaptive work, play, self-care, and affective responses

Occupational behavior goals

The following are treatment objectives for occupational behavior approaches.

1. To develop play skills and, through play, develop the skills and habits necessary for occupational roles
2. To develop self-maintenance functions to their fullest potential
3. To maintain an age-appropriate balance of work (school-related activities and self-maintenance) and play by assisting parents and other caregivers with selection and direction of play and work activities
4. To assist the child to maintain or improve performance in his current life roles

Orthopedic goals

General treatment goals for the child who requires orthopedic surgery of the upper extremities are listed here. However, the occupational therapist must tailor these goals to follow the prescription of the orthopedic physician for the child who has had surgery.

1. To provide orthoses postoperatively
2. To prevent edema through positioning
3. To increase active range of motion of all joints of the upper extremities through graded exercise and activity
4. To increase muscle strength and endurance
5. To integrate actions of transferred muscles into movement patterns through gross to fine motor activity
6. To increase function of the affected extremity in self-care, work, and play
7. To teach the use of adaptive equipment and adapted techniques during the acute postoperative phase and as necessary thereafter
8. To reassess all pertinent areas on a regular basis to provide information to the orthopedic physician that will document the results of surgery

Psychosocial goals

Psychosocial goals in occupational therapy for the child with cerebral palsy are achieved to a large extent through the neurological, occupational behavior, and orthopedic goals. If sensorimotor functions are improved, appropriate play and work skills developed, and hand function and appearance improved, these results will contribute to the attainment of psychosocial goals. In addition, drawing from the psychosocial area of occupational therapy, several goals can be specified. These are related to specific intervention methods in occupational therapy for psychosocial problems. Intervention by these methods will support the contribution of the other approaches.

1. To improve the child's self-concept, self-control, and coping skills
2. To promote satisfying peer relationships
3. To provide support to family members through education about the problems of the child with cerebral palsy and intervention related to occupational therapy
4. To assist the child's adjustment to authority

Specific objectives related to each of these goals should be written in behavioral terms for each particular child. Chapter 7 describes the construction of behavioral objectives.

TREATMENT METHODS

To plan an integrated occupational therapy program for the child with cerebral palsy, the therapist must be sure to coordinate programming with other disciplines. Reevaluation should be conducted at regular intervals to assess the effectiveness of treatment, as well as the changes in the child's status resulting from maturation and the development of secondary problems. The occupational therapist also will need to consider evaluation in response to institutional and governmental documentation requirements. The occupational therapist will provide an individualized treatment program for each child by combining goals and objectives in the specific methods used.

Combined neurological and occupational behavior treatment

The occupational therapist treating the child with cerebral palsy needs to combine treatment methods derived from the theoretical approaches described in the model. Activities provided for the child at a developmentally appropriate level to elicit adaptive motor, psychosocial, and cognitive behavior can combine many objectives from the theoretical approaches. The theoretical interaction between the neurological approach and the occupational behavior approach was discussed previously (see also Chapter 19). The changes that neurological approaches can elicit in the motor, affective, and cognitive functions of the child with cerebral palsy will also enhance the child's ability to perform life roles and habits. In turn, work, play, and self-care activities can be used to elicit movement, a necessary component in neurological approaches.

An occupational therapist can use play activity in two ways. The first method is to provide the initial sensory stimulus. For example, the child can maintain a reflex inhibiting pattern as part of a game. Second, the activity can be used after initial sensory stimulation to elicit feedback through more normalized movement patterns. For example, a hypertonic child might be en-

couraged to roll over, feel, and explore a stuffed animal after excessive tone has been inhibited. In a similar manner self-care and sometimes school activities can be used as part of neurological treatment procedures.

A description of how neurological techniques and occupational behavior can be combined in the occupational therapy process is presented in the following paragraphs. The purpose of the description is to illustrate some neurological treatment methods in combination with play and self-care. The example should not be considered a formula for treatment, but rather a guide for application of theoretical concepts to a variety of cases.

METHODS TO ADJUST MUSCLE TONE, PROMOTE NORMAL MOVEMENT PATTERNS, AND PROVIDE STABILIZATION

The methods described in this section combine neurological goals 1 and 2 and occupational behavior goals 1, 2, and 3 discussed previously.

For the hypertonic child, Farber[35] described a variety of inhibition techniques that begin with maintained touch and progress to slow stroking, neutral warmth, slow rolling, and slow rocking. Precautions should be taken with slow rocking to avoid excessive inhibition of the vestibular system. Watch for unconsciousness and cyanosis.[5] Positioning of the child is used to inhibit tone. The use of commercial or homemade devices for sidelying (Figure 16-2) and the use of wedges or rolls for the prone position are examples of techniques to inhibit tone. A number of play activities can be done in these adapted positions.

Michelman[72] described three hierarchical play

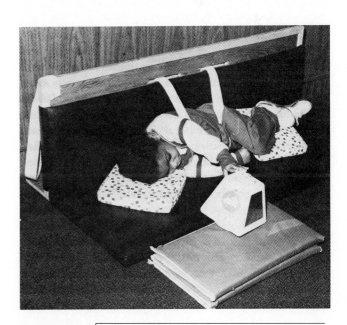

FIGURE 16-2

Child in a sidelyer.

stages: (1) the sensory-motor stage of play practice, (2) the symbolic, imaginative play stage, and (3) the stage of play where children learn to play games with rules. The sensory-motor stage is characterized by play that attracts the eyes, ears, senses, and muscles as they challenge growth. An inhibitory activity that uses slow rocking at this level is rocking in a rocking chair or on a rocking horse. The symbolic, imaginative play stage involves play "for strengthening large muscles, for stretching the mind and activating problem-solving, for make-believe, pretending and practicing grown-up role behavior, for creating and expressing feelings and ideas, and practicing symbol formations" (p. 196).[72] A child at this stage of play could pretend to be a boat captain and slowly rock on the "sea" in a "boat." Children in the stage of play where they are learning to play games with rules need activities that require risk-taking and decision-making social interaction and skill building. An inhibitory activity for a child in this stage might be slow rocking with another child while singing a counting or number concept song. There is considerable overlap between stages, and much play content from a previous stage is retained as the next stage emerges.[72]

Children with cerebral palsy who exhibit other types of muscle tone problems also require sensory stimulation to adjust their tone in conjunction with play activity. For the hypotonic child, for example, to provide sensory stimuli that will increase tone, activities that involve bouncing may be graded to the appropriate level.[2] In the sensory-motor and symbolic, imaginative stages the child can "ride" an inner tube to act out a fantasy story about cowboys rounding up cattle.

The athetoid child with fluctuating muscle tone needs activities that reinforce proximal stability, decrease involuntary movement, and increase controlled movement in the midranges of joint excursion. "Freeze like a statue" games can be used for a child in the symbolic, imaginative play stage to encourage proximal stability and control of movement. Many creative and expressive activities requiring symbol formation for children at this play stage can be structured to require controlled motion in the midranges. For example, after enough control of movement is established, finger painting can be structured to require midrange movement. The child may need support from wedges and other equipment to help with stability.

Many children with cerebral palsy show a mixed tonal pattern. For example, the child may exhibit spastic tone in the lower extremities and low tone in the trunk, neck, and upper extremities. Also, tone can change rapidly in an opposite direction. For example, a hypertonic child can lose too much tone through inhibitory activity. The occupational therapist must be alert to muscle tone changes and adjust the play activity as necessary.

METHODS TO FACILITATE RIGHTING AND EQUILIBRIUM, NORMAL MOVEMENT PATTERNS, AND PROGRESSION OF SENSORIMOTOR MILESTONES

The methods described in this section correlate with neurological goal numbers 1 to 3 and occupational behavior goal numbers 1 to 3 discussed previously.

Abell and others[2] described the desired movement patterns for the hypertonic child to be extension and rotation of the trunk and abduction and external rotation at the hips. After tone has been reduced, Abell and others recommended the use of activities that require trunk extension or reaching activities with trunk rotation and extension, leg extension, abduction, and external rotation. Such activities can be done by placing the child on a prone board with an abduction block between the legs. The occupational therapist provides various toys for the child to reach, touch, and explore during the sensory-motor stage of play. In the symbolic, imaginative play stage, a child might play a song using chimes, if the therapist positions the instrument so that the child must reach up and rotate the trunk to contact the chimes. Exploration activities done on a scooter board or games including mazes and follow-the-leader activities can be used with the child at the symbolic, imaginative stage and at the stage of learning play rules.

Activities that require rolling to normalize trunk rotation patterns and righting reactions can be added once tone has been reduced in a hypertonic child. The child in the sensory-motor stage can make a game of rolling from side to side to put objects into containers. The child at the symbolic, imaginative stages can help to cut "cookies" from Play-Doh while lying on one side and then rolling over to the other side to put them in the "oven."

Abell and others[2] recommended the use of games that require the manipulation of large objects from side to side while the child is seated astride a bolster to obtain body rotation and stimulate equilibrium reactions. A child in the rule-learning stage might make a model spaceship by placing and glueing large objects such as blocks or paper milk cartons from one side of the bolster to a spaceship frame on the other side. Children with cerebral palsy who have other types of tone and movement problems will require positioning, support, facilitation, or inhibition appropriate for their motor problems.

Activities that help a child to progress from quadruped to kneel-standing would involve placement of an appropriate play activity on an adjustable table set at the desired height. Making shapes with clay at a table positioned at the proper height for kneel-standing might be appropriate for the child in the symbolic, imaginative stage.

As part of oral-motor treatment, a play activity can be used to promote lip closure, to increase respiratory capacity, and to control respiration. A musical instrument that requires blowing, such as a simple flutaphone or kazoo, might be appropriate for a child who is learning to play games requiring rules, risk taking, and decision making.[36] In the sensory-motor state, oral exploration of objects, such as a textured ball, can be encouraged.[36]

Playing dress-up is a form of symbolic play. This activity fosters practice of sensorimotor and prevocational skills, as well as movement patterns.

After sensory stimuli have been used to normalize tone and movement patterns, the occupational therapist can incorporate activities of daily living tasks into the treatment program. Fine motor ability and bilateral hand use are required to open a milk carton. Therefore this might be an appropriate treatment activity for a child with spastic hemiparesis, if these are neurological goals of treatment. In her discussion of activities and the neurophysiological approaches, DiJoseph[32] described positioning of materials and equipment so that the desired motion can occur. Positioning of the child is also important.

In summary, the above methods illustrated show how neurological techniques that are used to improve motor ability can be combined with play and self-care to achieve competency and adaptation. The main idea is to incorporate an occupational activity that represents the appropriate play level to elicit a desired movement pattern or posture.

Recently there has been an increase in the development and use of adapted equipment in both the neurological and occupational behavior approaches. Adapted equipment enables body positioning that is in concert with neurophysiological principles. Such equipment also can permit the child to carry out life roles and habits.

Bergen and Colangelo[14] noted the importance and dynamic nature of equipment to affected motor behavior. Adapted equipment allows proper body positioning to "normalize tone, decrease the influence of pathological reflexes, increase range of motion, decrease the tendency toward deformities, increase stability, and facilitate components of normal movement in a developmental sequence" (p. 3).[14] They also emphasized that the functional goals of body positioning are performance of self-maintenance activities and schoolwork activity. They point out that proper positioning and assistance from equipment can free the child with cerebral palsy from problems associated with instability and difficult movement resulting from poor body position. Once positioned properly and once stabilized, the child can engage in cognitive-directed activity. Also, they suggest that proper positioning will increase self-esteem by enabling increased function and more independence. Drawbacks that should be pointed out include decreased sensory feedback from static positioning, as well as the stigma that may be attached to the appearance of equipment for a handicapped individual. Mainstreaming of handicapped children in public schools may be contributing to a change in the attitudes of the nonhandicapped about adapted equipment.

Seating and wheelchair adaptations are important for nonambulatory children with cerebral palsy. Several occupational therapists and physical therapists have developed adaptive chairs to position the child for better motor control of the upper extremities and to prevent deformity.[33,87,90] Bergen and Colangelo[14] stressed the following requirements for wheelchairs to be used for children with tone problems: a firm seat and chairback, a 90-degree angle between the back of the chair and the seat, proper angulation of the seat belt or harnessing, proper tilt of the seat back, proper trunk alignment, proper head support, and positioning the arms forward in a position to allow functional upper extremity movement. Also, foot supports and abductor pommels or wedges to keep the thighs in a position of abduction are important.

Armrests and lapboards are of special interest to the occupational therapist. Lapboards provide a work surface for fine motor activity, self-feeding, and school-related work. Armrests should allow access to a regular table, if such access does not interfere with support and motor control of arms.

There are many specialized wheelchairs available. The one pictured in Figure 16-3 has molded plastic inserts* on a Pogon Buggy frame.† This system consists of plastic seats, backs, foot supports, head and neck supports, and straps of different sizes that can be put together in a unique "system" for every child. A simulator unit is available that allows for quick, easy interchange of parts for assessment. The chair is considered dynamic because it has features to normalize tone, such as an anterior roll in the seat, and to increase symmetry, such as the side projections on the back. These can complement the motor development program. This chair, as many others, has a more natural, furniture-type appearance that lessens the stigma that has been attached to conventional wheelchairs. The new plastic materials are also easier to maintain than some of the older woven fabric types. The Molded Plastic Insert System can also be used on conventional wheelchair frames.

Children who need more custom-fitted chairs be-

---

*Molded Plastic Insert System (MPI), Medical Equipment Distributors, Corporate Office, 1701 S. First Ave., Maywood, Il 60153.

†Pogon Buggy, Genac, Inc., 1700 S. 120th St., Lafayette, CO. 80026.

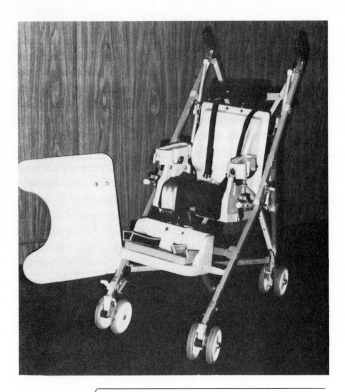

FIGURE 16-3

Molded Plastic Insert System (MPI).

cause of their fixed spinal curvature deformities, for example, may need seating made from one of the moldable support materials such as Foam-in-Place,* a foam substance that can be molded around a child. The Desemo† seating system consists of a bag of polystyrene beads and an expoxy resin that are individually molded to support the patient in needed areas. The Desemo moldable seating material can also be used to make custom toilet seats and sidelying supports.

Other major positioning equipment includes sidelying positioners (sidelyers), abduction scooter boards, specialized chairs and benches, and therapy rolls. Sidelyers (Figure 16-2) are used to position the hypertonic or hypotonic child for play and other activities. These devices prevent head and trunk extension, keep the body symmetrical, and place the shoulders forward and the hands together in the midline.

Bergen and Colangelo[14] and others have noted that placement in the prone position allows for development of head control (specifically neck extension); weight bearing on the upper extremities for shoulder and upper trunk stability; bringing the hands to the midline for play; eye-hand coordination; and visual involvement in

---

*Foam-in-Place, Rehabilitation Engineering Center, University of Tennessee, Center for Health Science, 682 Court Ave., Memphis, TN 38163.

†Desemo Customized Support Kit, Desemo, Inc., P.O. Box 22, 309, Savannah, GA 31403.

the environment. Chest wedges and adjustable prone standers are typically used to support the prone position.

Benches and specialized chairs can be custommade to place children in positions that inhibit abnormal positional and movement patterns. For children who show an extensor abduction pattern of spasticity in the lower extremities that interferes with sitting, therapists[28,38] have recommended a straddling type of sitting apparatus. Use of this seat promotes hip flexion, abduction, external rotation with 90 degrees of flexion at the hips, knees, and ankles. This wide, stable sitting apparatus enables the child to sit comfortably and to engage in bilateral hand skills.

The role of sensory feedback in sensorimotor functioning has been emphasized by many.[5,21,43] The use of biofeedback techniques to increase the motor ability of individuals with cerebral palsy is now being researched. External feedback in the form of a buzzing auditory signal was found to have a positive effect on eye-hand coordination of spastic children ages 7 to 21.[104] In a study involving two children with cerebral palsy and mental retardation, Ball, McCrady, and Hart[10] demonstrated that head posture was strongly controlled by using music as feedback. Basmajian[12] also reported positive results with biofeedback techniques that were used with patients with cerebral palsy. The influence of feedback from external sources on performance of specific play, work, and self-care tasks is an area open to investigation by occupational therapists. More research is needed to indicate whether this technique can be used to increase the function of children with cerebral palsy.

METHODS TO PROMOTE SENSORY INTEGRATION AND PERCEPTION

The methods discussed in this section relate to goal number 5 of the neurological approach and goal numbers 1, 2, and 3 of the occupational behavior approach.

Price[84] noted that sensory integrative disorders may exist in children with cerebral palsy, possibly from the same source as the primary motor deficit. If the motor deficit is severe, deprivation of sensory experience may add to the problem. The existence of sensory integrative disorders as secondary disorders in children with cerebral palsy is not yet documented by research. Analysis of preliminary data from Price[84] supported the effectiveness of treatment of associated sensory integrative disorders in children with cerebral palsy. Possible changes reported were an increase in academic abilities, a decrease in tactile defensiveness, and an increase in motivation and attention. Until more research regarding the nature of sensory integrative disorders in children with cerebral palsy and the effectiveness of treatment is completed, the use of sensory integrative therapy will remain controversial. However, since sensory integrative therapy is being used both experimentally and in practice as treatment for children with cerebral palsy, a brief discussion of its application will be included.

The occupational therapist using sensory integrative therapy with cerebral palsy patients must combine this treatment with the sensorimotor treatment that the child may be receiving. For example, vestibular input, a major component of sensory integrative therapy, should correlate with the type of input being used in a sensorimotor approach. In the hypertonic (spastic) child, vestibular stimuli to inhibit tone is the recommended treatment, whereas facilitative vestibular stimuli, such as fast spinning, is to be avoided, since it may increase tone.[35] Price[84] recommended caution with the use of vestibular treatment with children who have a history of seizures. The child's physician should always be consulted. She also cautioned about the use of light touch stimuli, as well as treatment in the inverted (head down) position and the use of persevering treatment for adaptive responses.

The typical methods of administering sensory integrative treatment (Chapter 19) must be adapted for children with cerebral palsy and special precautions must be used. Price[84] suggested using a pillow in a hanging net for more support and security. Extra support and special positioning may be needed on scooter boards, such as positioning the legs in abduction (Figure 16-4).

The therapist must be aware of muscle tone changes that might lead to faulty positioning and adjust the stimulation activities and position as necessary. Price[84] also suggested giving the child more time to respond and letting the child do as much as possible within the confines of support. In addition to support given by the therapist, environmental arrangements such as floor mats and an environment that is free of unnecessary equipment can prevent injury from falling.

Play as an integral part of sensory integration has been explained by Ayres[5] and Lindquist, Mack, and Parham.[67] The environment should be structured as a play milieu that incorporates equipment to give sensory input. Although sensory integrative therapy is self-directed, materials that relate to the play stages are also most appropriate for eliciting desired adaptive responses. Much of the sensory integrative equipment can be used for play activities of all levels or stages.

Occupational therapists, especially those practicing in school systems, may provide perceptual-motor experiences for the child with cerebral palsy. Ayres[7] defined perceptual-motor training as teaching specific perceptual skills, such as walking a balance beam or sorting shapes. The aim of perceptual-motor therapy is the generalization of these abilities to academic skills like reading. Perceptual-motor activities can be used in combination with the other neurological treatments described earlier. Perceptual-motor activities are incorporated as play activities in the play agenda. For example, after

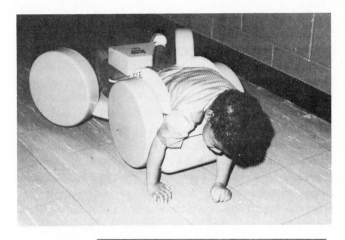

FIGURE 16-4

Scooter board that provides special positioning.

sensorimotor treatment to reduce tone and normalize movement patterns, the child with hypertonia may perform a perceptual-motor activity, such as doing a puzzle or stringing beads in a shape sequence. Activities such as these are appropriate if the child has reached the symbolic, imaginative stage. A body image training doll was designed by Waters[117] to assist the development of a realistic body image. The doll's body parts are attached together with Velcro. The child for whom fine motor coordination activities are appropriate can play with this perceptual-motor toy. Other activities may be selected on the basis of teacher feedback about classroom performance. Craft activities that incorporate perceptual-motor tasks, such as eye-hand coordination activities and left-to-right orientation sequences, would be used by the occupational therapist in preference to pencil-and-paper perceptual-motor work. For older children, games involving decision making, rule learning, and problem solving might be appropriate.

Occupational behavior treatment

METHODS TO DEVELOP SELF-MAINTENANCE AND MAINTAIN OR IMPROVE PERFORMANCE IN OCCUPATIONAL ROLES

The methods described in this section are related to goal numbers 3 and 5 of the occupational behavior approach.

Equipment to assist feeding the cerebral palsy child starts with appropriate seating supports. The child must be positioned and supported adequately to allow oral mechanisms to function optimally. Feeder seats (Figure 16-5) give support and position the severely involved child during eating and play activity. Equipment for self-feeding is pictured in Figures 16-6 and 16-7. Common equipment pictured in Figure 16-6 promotes

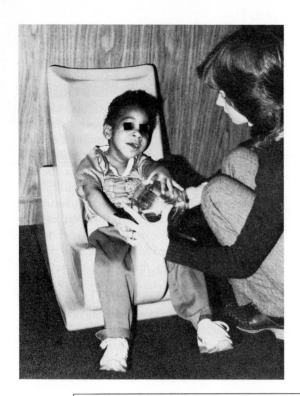

FIGURE 16-5

Feeder seat.

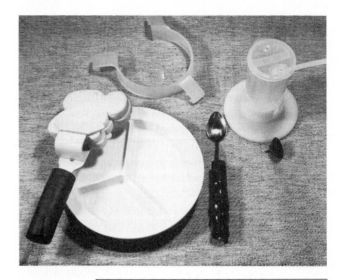

FIGURE 16-6

Self-feeding equipment.

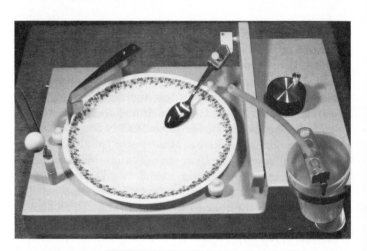

FIGURE 16-7

Winsford Feeder.

stabilization of the extremities during self-feeding by the child with athetosis. The heavy, weighted dish on a nonskid surface, the divided plate to separate and stabilize food, and the cup with a weighted base and a clip-on flexible straw help to secure the environment. The suction cup screw can be driven into the plastic cup holder. When suctioned to a table surface, it provides further stabilization. A plastic plate guard can fit many size plates and helps keep food on the plate when a child scoops. A weighted spoon with a large handle can assist with stabilization for the child with lack of manual control. A sandwich holder can also help the child with increased tone and control problems to prevent his crushing a sandwich. Weiss and Weiss[118] constructed a napkin holder–type sandwich holding device with suction cups to stabilize it on any surface.

When motion is very restricted because of impaired tone, or when movement is extremely uncontrolled as in a severely athetoid child, an electronic automatic feeding device such as the Winsford Feeder* in Figure 16-7 can offer more independence for the child. Two motions are required to operate this feeding device. The ball switch is pushed one way to move food onto the spoon and lift it to the mouth. Repetition of the same motion lowers the spoon to the plate. Movement of the

ball switch in the other direction rotates the plate to position the food for scooping. A cup in a holder with flexible plastic straw attached can be positioned for access for the child without upper extremity use. A hand-foot switch option is available to activate the cordless unit. For the severely involved child who cannot use his upper extremities, this device gives some control during feeding.

METHODS TO DEVELOP STUDENT-WORK SKILLS

Methods to develop student-work skills are related to goal numbers 3 to 5 of the occupational behavior approach.

The occupational therapist can assist the student who has cerebral palsy. Communication is one area in which the occupational therapist can work with the

---

*Winsford Feeder, Winsford Products, Inc., 1979 Remington-Harborton Rd., Pennington, NJ 08534.

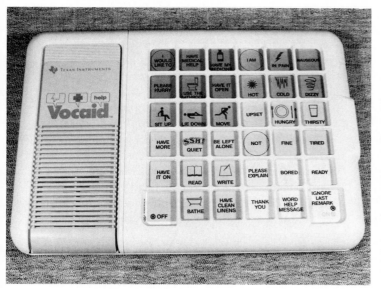

FIGURE 16-8

Vocaid communication device.

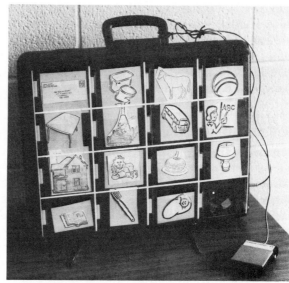

FIGURE 16-9

Zygo communication device.

teacher and speech and language pathologist to improve the child's ability to relate to others. To improve written communication, the adaptation of writing tools such as crayons and pencils can help the child who has poor grasp. The occupational therapist may suggest the use of a large crayon or a pencil with a built-up handle if fine grasp is inadequate. A grease pencil may add just enough friction to allow a child who lacks tonal control to be able to write. To stabilize written work, the use of clipboards and magnets on a metal deck–table top may be suggested.[116]

Communication aids such as language boards with symbols on them to express needs are usually incorporated into lapboards; often the occupational therapist assists the speech pathologist in their use with a child. Electronic aids, such as the Vocaid communication device* (Figure 16-8), use cards with symbols and words, letters, and games. When the appropriate space on the card is touched, this activates an electronic voice. A child with less upper extremity control could use a Zygo† communication device (Figure 16-9). Only depressing a lever is required for a Zygo Board, whereas a Vocaid device has a small intricate board. Phillpot[81] described the successful use of a helmet with a stick extending from the front for severely involved children with cerebral palsy who have appropriate head control. The helmet stick can assist the child with poor upper extremity control in using communication boards and devices, for typing, playing games, turning pages, and operating teaching machines. To assist the child with

cerebral palsy in controlling the environment through adapted means, the occupational therapist may work with rehabilitation engineers to devise an environmental control system that would allow the child to electronically turn on and off lights, radios, tape recorders, and perform other similar environmental manipulations (Chapter 18).

School equipment can often be adapted to increase the functioning of children with cerebral palsy. For example, a child may need to work on a desk top that tilts to specified angles. Adapted equipment for school-related activities of daily living is another area of concern for occupational therapists. Modifications for toilets, methods for handwashing, lunch room management, and wheelchair adaptations to increase mobility around the school environment are but a few examples.[116]

Effective work skills and habits should be stressed for the school-aged child. Responsibility and organization of school materials are important for the child in a wheelchair. School materials may be kept in a bag attached to the chair that the child is responsible to keep neat, organized, and fully equipped. Punctuality, following directions, and social skills, such as eye contact, are important work habits that can be incorporated in occupational therapy activities. Also, responsibility for the repair and maintenance of equipment should be emphasized throughout occupational therapy for children who have the cognitive ability.[116]

Craft activities such as woodworking can establish work habits and maintain functional movement gained through previous neurological treatment. Children need to develop responsibility for the self, including asking for help when needed. In addition, the ability to work

---

*Vocaid, Texas Instruments, Inc., Dallas, TX.
†Zygo Board, Zygo Industries, P.O. Box 1008, Portland, OR 97207.

without constant approval and to accept failure are important work skills and habits that can be promoted through crafts.[116] Children with cerebral palsy often become accustomed to waiting for an activity to be brought to them. Active exploratory behavior in the environment to the maximal extent possible can be incorporated into craft activities. Motivation to work, persistence in a task, and pride in the finished product are all work-oriented factors that need to be established early. Homemaking activities for both sexes help prepare the child for a measure of independence or possibly total independent living. The occupational therapist can counsel parents about appropriate home chores that the child can be held responsible to perform. In later schooling, such as the junior high level, functional gains in the motor, cognitive, and social-emotional areas can be used in schoolwork tasks such as helping with mail, cleaning tables in the lunchroom, or tutoring younger children.

A METHOD FOR MAINTAINING WORK, PLAY, AND SELF-CARE

A method for maintaining work, play, and self-care relates to goal number 4 of the occupational behavior goals.

The results of an activity configuration[74] can indicate to the therapist how the child's life is organized. As part of the play history, Takata[103] recommended recording the weekday and weekend schedule. After analysis of time spent in self-care (including meals and rest), work (school-related activities and household chores), and play, the occupational therapist can suggest changes in the daily schedules to the parents. As Takata noted, the younger child should have a large percentage of play time. More time will be devoted to the student (work) role as the child gets older. Often the time spent in "therapies" and in self-care tasks is quite extensive. Educating the parents about the importance of play to the development of the child's abilities, making suggestions for appropriate play activities, and helping parents to create a play environment are important tasks for the occupational therapist.

Orthopedic treatment

The occupational therapy objectives and treatment methods for the child with cerebral palsy who has undergone upper extremity orthopedic surgery depend on the nature of the procedure and the methods preferred by a particular surgeon. Surgical procedures performed depend on the deformity or problem present and are reviewed by Bleck,[15] Hoffer,[49] Zancolli and Zancolli,[120] and many others.[44,50] The most common surgical procedures described by these orthopedists are transfer of the flexor carpi ulnaris muscle to improve wrist extension; tendon transfers or flexor tendon lengthening of the finger and wrist flexors; and lengthening of the thumb flexor, web release, or intrinsic release to correct the thumb-in-palm deformity (the thumb is in a fixed position in the palm). Thumb extension can also be improved by muscle transfer.

Occupational therapy for the child with cerebral palsy who has had corrective hand surgery is not well-documented. Orthopedists[15,120] have stressed the importance of periodic reassessment by the occupational therapist to document changes following surgery. A proposed program of treatment methods drawn mainly from related literature involving tendon transfer is outlined in the following paragraph. This treatment must be administered according to prescription of the orthopedic surgeon.

1. *Positioning to prevent edema.* Immediately after surgery the occupational therapist needs to assist other professions (for example, nursing) with positioning to maintain elevation of the affected extremity.[110]

2. *Splinting.* After the plaster cast is removed, a protective splint that will immobilize the extremity is devised and applied.[15] After a period of time, the orthopedic physician may prescribe a splint to stabilize the wrist and allow flexion and extension of the fingers.[55]

3. *Adapted techniques and equipment.* The child may need temporary training to perform activities with only one hand, such as tying shoes, opening a jar, or buttoning cuff buttons on the unaffected side. The occupational therapist can suggest ways to perform these activities, such as holding jars and toothpaste tubes between knees to open or using adapted equipment such as jar openers. To stabilize food when eating, the child may require a scoop plate on a nonskid surface. The child can be taught one-handed typing, if able, or given elastic shoelaces to use temporarily. It is likely that a hemiplegic child has already figured out many one-handed techniques on his own. Some children may need permanent adapted equipment if results of surgery are poor or function is not expected to return.

4. *Methods to increase functional movement and strength.* When the orthopedic physician indicates that the child is ready, controlled active motion in all affected joints should be encouraged through exercise and activity. Repetitive functional activities related to self-care, student role, and play can be used to increase strength, to increase endurance, and to integrate actions of transferred muscles into functional movement patterns. Play activities should be at the appropriate developmental level. The occupational therapist can provide a variety of bimanual play, work, and self-care activities to reinforce use of the affected hand as an assistive hand. Games, school-related skills, and self-care activities can aid in adaptation of the affected extremity by offering repetitive purposeful activity.[94] For example, when reaching the play stage of learning to play games

with rules, a boy with spastic hemiplegia who had a wrist flexor transfer to improve wrist extension might build a soapbox "car." The occupational therapist will encourage repetitive bimanual activity by structuring the task appropriately. Pieces of wood could be pegged together, thereby requiring the use of two hands: the affected hand to stabilize while the unaffected hand manipulates a piece of wood onto a peg.

Bobath[18] suggested that sensory impairment in the hemiplegic hand results from lack of sensory experience. Ferreri[37] reported increased sterognosis following a sensory retraining program for spastic adult cerebral palsy patients. Further research is needed to substantiate the effects of sensory experience and stereognosis activities to increase function of the surgically managed upper extremity of children with cerebral palsy.

Biofeedback has been suggested[80,110] in the muscle reeducation of patients with peripheral nerve injury who have received tendon transplants. This technique could be researched with some children with cerebral palsy who are having difficulty in retraining and who have the cognitive capabilities required.

By providing the opportunity to succeed in performance of bimanual activities, occupational therapy promotes the growth of self-esteem and self-confidence in the child with cerebral palsy. If surgery has provided a more cosmetically acceptable arm and hand, this can also affect the psychosocial status of the child and his family in a positive direction. Improvement in hygiene may also increase social acceptability.

Psychosocial treatment

Some specific methods the occupational therapist can use in the treatment of psychosocial dysfunction related to physical disability are interpersonal helping skills, milieu therapy, and the use of groups to achieve treatment objectives. Behavior modification approaches using reinforcement are often used to motivate the child with cerebral palsy and to aid the child with self-control.

One treatment method described by Llorens and Rubin[69] is milieu therapy, which is defined as "the planned manipulation of the environment aimed at producing changes in the personality of the patient" (p. 16). Included as part of the milieu are appropriate attitudes and methods of discipline. Attitudes consist of understanding the child and his problems, acceptance of assets and limitations, support of treatment goals, consistency of management, and a morally nonjudgmental attitude toward the child.

As noted earlier, children with cerebral palsy can be either aggressive or withdrawn. Llorens and Rubin[69] offered guidelines for treatment of the aggressive child. Definition of boundaries with consistent, clear, reasonable limits and purposes; avoidance of unacceptable be-

havior and forbidden objects; and restating limits as necessary are all important guidelines. Intervention techniques for the aggressive child include (1) planned ignoring of unacceptable behavior, (2) controlling by proximity or touch, (3) extra attention and affection, (4) clarification of difficult situations to develop insight, (5) restructuring an activity or situation by removing objects that prompt unacceptable behavior or removing the child from the situation, and (6) directly appealing to the child's sense of responsibility and fairness.

To create a therapeutic milieu for the withdrawn child, Llorens and Rubin[69] suggest the following:

1. Provide the child with a benign setting and easily available protective adults.
2. Reduce stress of competition and expectation beyond the child's level of competence.
3. Provide structure and routine initially. A gradual decrease of such structure may be introduced as the child is able to tolerate it.
4. React in a nonjudgmental manner to behavior and attitudes displayed by the child.
5. Avoid a too-close affectional relationship by personnel initially (p. 22).

A well-organized milieu consisting of (1) appropriate objects for sensorimotor growth and play development, (2) supportive and caring therapists, and (3) a physical environment conducive to producing positive affect will enhance the effectiveness of the neurological, occupational behavior, and orthopedic approaches. The occupational therapist must consider milieu, not only in relation to play and sensorimotor activity, but also from the psychosocial perspective.

CASE STUDY
Case history

1. Demographic data
   Name: Jimmy
   Age: 3 years, 5 months
   Diagnosis: Cerebral palsy, predominantly athetoid
2. Medical history
   Jimmy was born 3 months prematurely and experienced anoxia at birth. He was hospitalized for 2 months after birth and was on a respirator for the first month. He has had two surgerys to correct strabismus. He had seizures until the age of 6 months; these were controlled by medication. He no longer requires seizure medication. General health appears within normal limits at this time.
3. Social and educational history
   Jimmy is from a lower middle class, Caucasian family. The father is employed as a warehouse clerk. The mother is a housewife who occasionally does volunteer work at a church. There is one older female sibling in the family. Up to 25 months of age Jimmy was cared for at home; then he was placed in an early training program for children with developmental disabilities. The parents are concerned about Jimmy's delay in achieving developmental milestones, such as walking, and express interest in being involved in a therapy program for Jimmy.

Jimmy is receiving programming from a multidisciplinary team that includes physical therapy, speech and language therapy, psychological services, special education, and social service.

Assessment

1. Neurological assessment
   Sensorimotor development
   Muscle tone
   Reflex
   Fine motor
   Oral motor
   Sensory integration–perceptual-motor
   Cognitive-adaptive
2. Occupational behavior assessment
   Play history
   Play assessment
   Self-help evaluation
   Activity configuration
3. Psychosocial assessment
   Observation
   Parent and teacher interview

Problem identification

1. Abnormal muscle tone; fluctuating tone in upper extremities and increased extensor tone during activity in the lower extremities
2. Lack of development of righting and equilibrium reactions
3. Delayed gross and fine motor milestones
4. Tactile system disorder
5. Visual-perceptual delays
6. Delayed cognition
7. Delayed progress in play stages
8. Lack of balance between work, play, and self-care
9. Infrequent play interactions with play models
10. Delayed in self-care skills
11. Decreased self-concept and self-esteem
12. Inappropriate adjustment to authority; an aggressive child
13. Lack of socialization skills
14. Decreased coping skills
15. Lack of self-control
16. Decreased performance in life role of preschooler

Treatment goals

1. Provide play and self-care activities and positioning to adjust tone in the extremities
2. Provide play and self-care activities that promote the development of righting and equilibrium reactions and motor milestones
3. Provide stabilization as necessary to carry out work, play, and self-care
4. Provide self-care and play activities that give sensory input to normalize the tactile system
5. Provide play and self-care activities that provide visual perception and cognitive skills
6. Continue sensorimotor play and emphasize symbolic, imaginative play in conjunction with the neurological goals
7. Adjust the balance of work, play, and self-care

8. Increase socialization and preschool skills
9. Assist adjustment to authority through milieu therapy and behavioral methods
10. Increase self-concept, self-esteem, and coping skills through milieu therapy
11. Increase interaction with play models

Precautions related to treatment

1. Falling
2. Sensory overload from too much sensory stimulation
3. Hypertonia from too much tactile stimulation

SUMMARY

A theoretical model was presented to describe current occupational therapy approaches to treatment of children with cerebral palsy. The impact of these approaches, used both separately and in combination, on the overall goal of occupational therapy—adaptation—was explained. Major thrusts of theory and practice from pertinent literature were reviewed and integrated to form the model. Research is needed to demonstrate the effectiveness of this model.

From each of the theoretical approaches, assessments appropriate for the child with cerebral palsy were described. Derived from these assessments, the general goals in each area were stated. The major treatment procedures related to each goal and combination of goals were explained. Treatment that integrates goals and procedures was emphasized. It is only by use of a holistic, but specifically tailored, treatment program that maximal adaptation can be achieved for children with cerebral palsy.

REFERENCES AND SELECTED READINGS

1. Abbot, M.: Present day trends in cerebral palsy, Am. J. Occup. Ther. **4:**53, 1950.
2. Abell, M.K., and others: Movement. In Conner, F.P., Williamson, G.G., and Siep, J.M., editors: Program guide for infants and toddlers with neuromotor and other developmental disabilities, New York, 1978, Teachers College Press.
3. Annual Psycho-social Evaluation, Cerebral Palsy Clinic, Indianapolis, Ind.: In Sample forms for occupational therapy, Rockville, Md., 1980, American Occupational Therapy Association, Inc.
4. Arens, L.J., and others: Cerebral palsy in C.T.—a comparative 12 year retrospective study, South Afr. Med. J. **53:**319, 1978.
5. Ayres, A.J.: Sensory integration and learning disorders, Los Angeles, 1972, Western Psychological Services.
6. Ayres, A.J.: Effects of sensory integrative therapy on the coordination of children with choreoathetoid movements, Am. Occup. Ther. Assoc. **31:**291, 1977.
7. Ayres, A.J.: Sensory integration and the child, Los Angeles, 1979, Western Psychological Services.
8. Ayres, A.J.: Southern California Sensory Integration Tests manual, rev. ed., Los Angeles, 1980, Western Psychological Services.
9. Ayres, A.J.: Aspects of somatomotor adaptive response and praxis. Unpublished paper presented at the Occupational Therapy for Sensory Integrative Dysfunction Conference, University of Cincinnati, June 27, 1981.

10. Ball, T.S., McCrady, R.E., and Hart, A.D.: Automated reinforcement of head posture in two cerebral palsy retarded children, Percept. Mot. Skills **40:**619, 1975.

11. Banks, H.H.: Cerebral palsy. In Lowell, W.W., and Winter, R.B., editors: Pediatric orthopedics, vol. 1, Philadelphia, 1978, J.B. Lippincott Co.

12. Basmajian, J.V.: Biofeedback: principles and practice for clinicians, Baltimore, 1979, The Williams & Wilkins Co.

13. Bax, M.: Management of cerebral palsy, Dev. Med. Child Neurol. **23:**703, 1981. (Editorial.)

14. Bergen, A.F., and Colangelo, C.: Positioning the client with central nervous system deficits: the wheelchair and other adapted equipment, Valhalla, N.Y., 1982, Valhalla Rehabilitation Publications, Ltd.

15. Bleck, E.: Orthopedic management of cerebral palsy, Saunders Monographs in Clinical Orthopedics, vol. II, Philadelphia, 1979, W.B. Saunders Co.

16. Bledsoe, N.P., and Shepherd, J.T.: A study of reliability and validity of a preschool play scale, Am. J. Occup. Ther. **36:**783, 1982.

17. Bobath, B.: The very early treatment of cerebral palsy, Dev. Med. Child Neurol. **9:**373, 1967.

18. Bobath, K.: Neurophysiological basis for the treatment of cerebral palsy, Clinics in Developmental Medicine No. 75, London, 1980, William Heinemann Medical Books, Ltd.

19. Bobath, K., and Bobath, B.: The treatment of cerebral palsy based on the analysis of the patient's motor behavior, Br. J. Phys. Med. **15:**107, 1952.

20. Bobath, K., and Bobath, B.: The facilitation of normal postural reactions and movements in the treatment of cerebral palsy, Physiotherapy **50:**246, 1964.

21. Bobath, K., and Bobath, B.: Cerebral palsy. In Pearson, P.H., and Williams, C.E., editors: Physical therapy services in the developmental disabilities, Springfield, Ill., 1972, Charles C. Thomas, Publisher.

22. Brunnstrom, S.: Movement therapy in hemiplegia, New York, 1970, Harper & Row, Publishers.

23. Carlsen, P.N.: Comparison of the two occupational therapy approaches for treating the young cerebral palsied child, Am. J. Occup. Ther. **29:**267, 1975.

24. Chee, F., Kreutzberg, J., and Clark, D. Semicircular canal stimulation in cerebral palsied children, Phys. Ther. **58:**1071, 1978.

25. Cherry, D.: Review of physical therapy alternatives for reducing muscle contracture, Phys. Ther. **60:**877, 1980.

26. Cherry, D., and Weigand, G.: Plaster drop-out casts as a dynamic means to reduce muscle contractures, Phys. Ther. **61:**1601, 1981.

27. Colarusso, R.P., and Hammill, D.D.: Motor-Free Visual Perception Test, Los Angeles, 1972, Western Psychological Services.

28. Cristella, M.: Comparison of straddling and sitting apparatus for the spastic cerebral palsy child, Am. J. Occup. Ther. **29:**273, 1975.

29. Cruickshank, W.: The problem and its scope. In Cruickshank, W., editor: Cerebral palsy: a developmental disability, ed. 3, Syracuse, 1976, Syracuse University Press.

30. Cruickshank, W., Hallaban, D., and Bice, H.: Personality and behavioral characteristics. In Cruickshank, W., editor: Cerebral palsy: a developmental disability, ed. 3, Syracuse, N.Y., 1976, Syracuse University Press.

31. Denhoff, E.: Medical aspects. In Cruickshank, W., editor: Cerebral palsy: a developmental disability, ed. 3, Syracuse, N.Y., 1976, Syracuse University Press.

32. DiJoseph, L.: Neurophysiologically-based treatment techniques within an O.T. framework, Occupational Therapy Audio Tape/Slide Programs, Buffalo, N.Y., 1981, Communications in Learning, Inc.

33. Epling, C.: Positioning highchair, Am. J. Occup. Ther. **28:**112, 1974.

34. Erhardt, R.: Developmental hand dysfunction, Laurel, Md., 1982, Ramsco Publishing Co.

35. Farber, S.: Neurorehabilitation: a multisensory approach, Philadelphia, 1982, W.B. Saunders Co.

36. Feltham, K.: Personal communication, June 1983.

37. Ferreri, J.: Intensive stereognostic training: effect on spastic cerebral palsied adults, Am. J. Occup. Ther. **16:**141, 1962.

38. Finnie, N.: Handling the young cerebral palsied child at home, New York, 1974, E.P. Dutton & Co., Inc.

39. Fiorentino, M.R.: Reflex testing methods for evaluating C.N.S. development, ed. 2, Springfield, Ill., 1973, Charles C. Thomas, Publisher.

40. Florey, L.: An approach to play and play development, Am. J. Occup. Ther. **25:**275, 1971.

41. Florey, L.: Studies of play: implications for growth, development, and for clinical practice, Am. J. Occup. Ther. **35:**519, 1981.

42. Gardner, M.: Test of Visual-Perceptual Skills (nonmotor), Seattle, 1982, Special Child Publications.

43. Gilfoyle, G., Grady, A., and Moore, J.: Children adapt, Thorofare, N.J., 1981, Charles B. Slack, Inc.

44. Goldner, J.L.: The upper extremity in cerebral palsy. In Samilson, R.L, editor: Orthopedic aspects of cerebral palsy, Clinics in Developmental Medicine, Nos. 52/53, London, 1975, William Heinemann, Medical Books, Ltd.

45. Gralewicz, A.: Play deprivation in multihandicapped children, Am. J. Occup. Ther. **27:**70, 1973.

46. Grayson, E.: Occupational therapy for the cerebral palsied baby, Am. J. Occup. Ther. **6:**64, 1950.

47. Green, W.: Historical notes—the past generation. In Samilson, R.L., editor: Orthopedic aspects of cerebral palsy, Clinics in Developmental Medicine Nos. 52/53, London, 1975, William Heinemann Medical Books, Ltd.

48. Gunn, S.: Play as occupation: implications for the handicapped, Am. J. Occup. Ther. **29:**222, 1975.

49. Hoffer, M.: Cerebral palsy. In Green, D., editor: Operative hand surgery, New York, 1982, Churchill-Livingstone.

50. Hoffer, M., and Koffman, M.: Cerebral palsy. In Nickel, V.L., editor: Orthopedic rehabilitation, New York, 1982, Churchill-Livingstone.

51. Howison, M., Perella, J., and Gordon, P.: Cerebral palsy. In Hopkins, H., and Smith, H., editors: Willard and Spackman's occupational therapy, ed. 5, Philadelphia, 1978, J.B. Lippincott Co.

52. Hyland, J.: Sensory history form. In Abreu, B., editor: Physical disabilities manual, New York, 1981, Raven Press.

53. Imperio, A., Cullinan, T., and Riklan, M.: Characteristics associated with cerebral palsy and dystonia musculorum deformans, Percept. Mot. Skills **48:**1003, 1979.

54. Reference deleted in proofs.

55. Jewel, K.: Personal communication, June, 1983.

56. Jones, M.: Differential diagnosis and the natural history of the cerebral palsied child. In Samilson, R., editor: Orthopedic aspects of cerebral palsy, Clinical Developmental Medicine, Nos. 52/53, 1975, London, William Heinemann Medical Books, Ltd.

57. Kenny, W.: Certain sensory defects in cerebral palsy, Clin. Orthop. **21:**193, 1963.

58. Kester, D.: Prevocational and vocational assessment. In Hopkins, H., and Smith, H. editors: Willard and Spackman's occupational therapy, ed. 5, Philadelphia, 1978, J.B. Lippincott Co.

59. Kielhofner, G., and Burke, J.: The evolution of knowledge and practice in occupational therapy: past, present, and future. In Kielhofner, G., editor: Health through occupation: theory and practice in occupational therapy, Philadelphia, 1983, F.A. Davis Co.

60. King, L.J.: Toward a science of adaptive responses, Am. J. Occup. Ther. **32:**429, 1978.

61. King, T.: Plaster splinting as a means of reducing elbow flexor spasticity: a case study, Am. J. Occup. Ther. **36:**671, 1982.

62. Kiss, R.: Occupational therapy. In Cruickshank, W., editor: Cerebral palsy: a development disability, ed. 3, Syracuse, N.Y., 1976, Syracuse University Press.

63. Kleiman, B., and Bulkley, B.: Some implications of a science of adaptive responses, Am. J. Occup. Ther. **36:**15, 1982.

64. Knox, S.: A play scale. In Reilly, M.: Play as exploratory learning: studies in curiosity behavior, Beverly Hills, Calif., 1974, Sage Publications, Inc.

65. Levine, M.: Cerebral-palsy diagnosis in children over age 1 year—standard criteria, Arch. Phys. Med. Rehabil. **61:**385, 1980.

66. Lewko, J.: Current practices in evaluating motor behavior of disabled children, Am. J. Occup. Ther. **30:**413, 1976.

67. Lindquist, J., Mack, W., and Parham, L.D.: A synthesis of occupational behavior and sensory integration concepts in theory and practice. Part I: theoretical foundations, Am. J. Occup. Ther. **36:**365, 1982.

68. Livingston, D.: Achievement recording for the cerebral palsied, Am. J. Occup. Ther. **4:**66, 1950.

69. Llorens, L., and Rubin, E.: Developing ego functions in disturbed children: occupational therapy in milieu, Detroit, 1967, Wayne State University Press.

70. Matsutsuyu, J.: Occupational behavior—a perspective on work and play, Am. J. Occup. Ther. **15:**291, 1971.

71. Mental Scale, occupational therapy progress notes, Wishard Memorial Hospital, Indiana University Hospitals. In Sample forms for occupational therapy. Rockville, Md., 1980, American Occupational Therapy Association, Inc.

72. Michelman, S.: Play and the deficit child. In Reilly, M., editor: Play as exploratory learning: studies in curiosity behavior, Beverly Hills, Calif., 1974, Sage Publications, Inc.

73. Milani-Comparetti, A., and Gidoni, E.A.: Routine developmental examination in normal and retarded children, Dev. Med. Child Neurol. **9:**631, 1967.

74. Mosey, A.: Activities therapy, New York, 1973, Raven Press.

75. Motor Development Test, Bronson Methodist Hospital, cerebral palsy section, Occupational Therapy Department. In Sample forms for occupational therapy, Rockville, Md., 1980, American Occupational Therapy Association, Inc.

76. Nober, E.H.: Auditory processing. In Cruickshank, W., editor: Cerebral palsy: a developmental disability, ed. 3, Syracuse, N.Y., 1976, Syracuse University Press.

77. Norton, Y.: Neurodevelopment and sensory integration for the profoundly retarded multiply handicapped child, Am. J. Occup. Ther. **29:**93, 1975.

78. Paisley, S.: Occupational therapy treatment for a group of spastic cases; children under twelve years of age, Occup. Ther. Rehabil. **8:**83, 1929.

79. Pezzuti, L.: An exploration of adolescent feminine and occupational behavior, Master's thesis, 1970, University of Southern California.

80. Philips, C.: Hand therapy. In Trombly, C., editor: Occupational therapy for physical dysfunction, ed. 2, Baltimore, 1983, The Williams & Wilkins Co.

81. Phillpot, R.E.: Headstick helmet for cerebral-palsied children, Am. J. Occup. Ther. **25:**291, 1975.

82. Pollack, G.: Assessment of the results of surgery in cerebral palsy. In Samilson, R.L., editor: Orthopedic aspects of cerebral palsy, Clinics in Developmental Medicine Nos. 52/53, London, 1975, William Heinemann Medical Books, Ltd.

83. Price, A.: The issue—neurotherapy and specialization, Am. J. Occup. Ther. **34:**810, 1980.

84. Price, A.: Sensory integration therapy for nonstandardized populations. Unpublished paper presented at the Ohio Occupational Therapy Association Conference, Kent, Ohio, Oct. 15, 1982, Kent State University.

85. Reilly, M.: A psychiatric occupational therapy program as a teaching model, Am. J. Occup. Ther. **20:**61, 1966.

86. Reilly, M.: An explanation of play. In Reilly, M., editor: Play as exploratory learning: studies in curiosity behavior, Beverly Hills, Calif., 1974, Sage Publications, Inc.

87. Richmond, H.: An adaptive chair for the athetoid child, Am. J. Occup. Ther. **18:**260, 1964.

88. Robinson, A.: Play: the arena for acquisition of rules for competent behavior, Am. J. Occup. Ther. **31:**248, 1977.

89. Rodgers, J.: The study of human occupation. In Kielhofner, G., editor: Health through occupation: theory and practice in occupational theory, Philadelphia, 1983, F.A. Davis Co.

90. Rollefson, V.M., and Culver, B.E.: An adjustable fiberglass chair, Am. J. Occup. Ther. **26:**309, 1972.

91. Rood, M.: The use of sensory receptors to activate, facilitate, and inhibit motor responses, autonomic, and somatic in developmental sequence. In Sattely, C., editor: Approaches to the treatment of patients with neuromuscular dysfunction, Dubuque, Iowa, 1962, William C. Brown Co., Publishers.

92. Samilson, R.L., and Perry, J.: The orthopedic assessment in cerebral palsy. In Samilson, R.L., editor: Orthopedic aspects of cerebral palsy, Clinics in Developmental Medicine Nos. 52/53, London, 1975, William Heinemann Medical Books, Ltd.

93. Scherzer, A.L., Mike, V., and Ilson, J.: Physical therapy as a determinant of change in the cerebral palsied infant, Pediatrics, **58:**47, 1976.

94. Schroder, M.: Tendon transplants of the hand and their treatment in occupational therapy: surgical aspects of tendon transplants, Am. J. Occup. Ther. **1:**339, 1947.

95. Sellick, K., and Over, R.: Effects of vestibular stimulation on motor development of cerebral-palsied children, Dev. Med. Child Neurol. **22:**476, 1980.

96. Semans, S., and others: A cerebral palsy assessment chart. In The child with central nervous system deficit, Children's Bureau Publication No. 432, 1965, U.S. Government Printing Office.

97. Shannon, P.D.: The work-play model: a basis for occupational therapy programming in psychiatry, Am. J. Occup. Ther. **24:**215, 1970.

98. Shannon, P.D.: Work-play theory and the occupational therapy process, Am. J. Occup. Ther. **26:**169, 1972.

99. Shearer, A.: A right to love?, London, 1972, The Spastics Society, The National Association for Mental Health.

100. Sussman, M., and Cusick, B.: Preliminary report: the role of shortleg, tone reducing casts as an adjunct to physical therapy of patients with cerebral palsy, John Hopkins Med. J. **145:**112, 1979.

101. Swartz, R., and others: Motivation of children with multiple functional disabilities, JAMA **145:**951, 1951.

102. Takata, N.: The play milieu—a preliminary appraisal, Am. J. Occup. Ther. **25:**281, 1971.

103. Takata, N.: Play as prescription. In Reilly, M., editor: Play as exploratory learning: studies in curiosity behavior, Beverly Hills, Calif., 1974, Sage Publications, Inc.

104. Talbot, M.L., and Junkala, J.: The effects of auditorally augmented feedback on the eye-hand coordination of students with cerebral palsy, Am. J. Occup. Ther. **35:**525, 1981.

105. Teplin, S., Howard, J., and O'Connor, M.: Self-concept of young children with cerebral-palsy, Dev. Med. Child Neurol. **23:**730, 1981.

106. Tizard, T., Paine, R., and Crother, B.: Disturbances of sensation in children with hemiplegia, JAMA **155:**628, 1954.

107. Torok, N., and Perlstein, M.: Vestibular findings in cerebral palsy, Ann. Otol. Rhinol. Laryngol. **71:**51, 1962.

108. Toys adapted to cerebral palsy children, Milwaukee Curative Workshop, Am. J. Occup. Ther. **4:**68, 1950.

109. Trombly, C.A., editor: Occupational therapy for physical dysfunction, ed. 2, Baltimore, 1983, The Williams & Wilkins Co.

110. Trombly, C.A., and Scott, A.D.: Occupational therapy for physical dysfunction, Baltimore, 1977, The Williams & Wilkins Co.

111. Tyler, N., and Kogan, K.: Measuring the effectiveness of occupational therapy in the treatment of cerebral palsy, Am. J. Occup. Ther. **19:**8, 1965.

112. Tyler, N., and Kogan, K.: Reduction of stress between mothers and their handicapped children, Am. J. Occup. Ther. **31:**151, 1977.

113. Tyler, N., Kogan, K., and Turner, P.: Interpersonal components of therapy with young cerebral palsied, Am. J. Occup. Ther. **28:**395, 1974.

114. Uniform terminology for reporting occupational therapy services, rev. ed., Rockville, Md., 1983, American Occupational Therapy Association, Inc.

115. Versluys, H.: Psychosocial adjustment to physical disability. In Trombly, C., editor: Occupational therapy for physical dysfunction, ed. 2, Baltimore, 1983, The Williams & Wilkins Co.

116. Wade, A.S.: Personal communication, December 1982.

117. Waters, J.S.: Body image training doll, Am. J. Occup. Ther. **4:**322, 1968.

118. Weiss, D., and Weiss, L.: The sandwich holder, Am. J. Occup. Ther. **30:**384, 1976.

119. Wright, T., and Nicholson, J.: Physiotherapy for the spastic child: an evaluation, Dev. Med. Child Neurol. **15:**146, 1973.

120. Zancolli, E.A., and Zancolli, E.R: Surgical management of the hemiplegic spastic hand in cerebral palsy, Surg. Clin. North Am. **61:**395, 1981.

17

M. JEANETTE MARTIN

Children with mental retardation

The retarded individual is a person who, by an error in the developmental process or by severe trauma, is unable to perform adaptive living skills well enough to compete with the majority of independent human beings in society. The American Association on Mental Deficiency (AAMD)[7] defines mental retardation:

> Mental retardation refers to significantly subaverage general intellectual functioning existing concurrently with deficits in adaptive behavior and manifested during the developmental period.

The retardation process is an interruption in the person's sensory, motor, or cognitive growth that may occur as early as the first trimester of development. The retarded individual may develop at a slowed rate through the sensorimotor, preoperational, and possibly the concrete stage of development as described by Piaget, but the inability to quickly process cognitive areas of thinking, understanding, and acting based on logical progression will not allow the individual to reach the formal operational stage of development. Mental retardation is a broad diagnostic category and may include the person who is physically and cognitively impaired or one who has as few as one or two deficits in effectively adapting to the social demands of his environment.

The caretakers and the caregivers for the mentally retarded individuals have throughout history attempted to explain these individuals and locate the reasons for their lack of adaptive living skills. The general problem of mental retardation has been explained in a historical vein by various authors.[8,13,15,17] It has been only in the last 150 years that a positive, progressive approach has been taken in caring for the retarded. Before the early 1800s the retarded person was ridiculed, ignored, or sheltered. In the past 50 years the caretaker and the caregiver roles have gradually changed to the roles of trainer, teacher, counselor, or houseparent. Retarded individuals are now expected to learn and develop to the limits of their ability, while society is expected to accept them for the extent of these abilities.

Researchers are gradually redefining the set of causative factors for retardation. It is now evident that the retarded may be clustered into two general and somewhat dissimilar groupings: the clinical-organic causes and the cultural-related causes. However, this division is not clear-cut or simple. There is great impact on both groups by the interactive consequences of prenatal and postnatal nutrition and infections, as well as the effects of postnatal, somatic experiences. Researchers have identified at least 200 types of medical problems associated with mental retardation.[5,11,14] The causes of these problems have been identified, and extensive research efforts have helped to ameliorate many predisposing conditions. For example, early diagnosis of conditions such as phenylketonuria (PKU) can, by the use of medication and special diets, offset severe and profound mental retardation to a large degree. Prenatal and postnatal surgery has been performed to sidestep the effects of hydrocephalus; and surgery has also helped the retarded person with orthopedic problems and other birth defects.

SETTINGS FOR PRACTICE

Any one of the 6 million retarded persons may be found in community agencies, including

1. The neonatal nursery with babies at "high risk" who require specific sensory stimulation, special handling techniques, and parent training
2. The early developmental evaluation and screening programs where cytogenetic screening and family counseling are provided
3. The preschool training centers for at-risk or developmentally delayed children
4. The "developmental home" where the retarded person is housed with a foster family who provides special training and care
5. The schools, either in the special education classes, or as mainstreamed students
6. The sheltered workshop or adult training center
7. The residential institution that may be privately or publicly operated
8. The group home where two or more retarded persons live under the supervision of a houseparent
9. The training apartment or cluster apartment complex where one or more retarded persons live who are visited regularly by a counselor or sponsor
10. The skilled nursing facility that cares for the retarded person requiring physical care on a 24-hour, long-term basis.

The occupational therapist or the certified occupational therapy assistant may serve the retarded population in any one or more of these settings, depending on the needs of the retarded person. The occupational therapist with postgraduate training in handling newborns and training parents can provide direct services in the neonatal nursery and in the early developmental evaluation and screening programs. With experience in consultation and training, the therapist can help develop and monitor individualized programs and refer children to preschool training centers and to developmental homes. The school therapist provides support services to mainstreamed retarded persons (Chapter 24). In sheltered workshops, adult training centers, residential institutions known as state schools, developmental centers or retardation centers, and in skilled nursing facilities certified occupational therapy assistants give much of the daily care and training under the supervision of the occupational therapist. Occasional direct or indirect services from the occupational therapist may be needed in independent living situations such as the group home or cluster apartment complex.

Local chapters of the Association for Retarded Citizens (ARC) and state chapters of the American Association on Mental Deficiency provide information and service opportunities for the occupational therapist. The Association for Retarded Citizens was founded as a parent interest group but has grown to include many important legislative and service functions. The local chapters make a powerful contribution to public education regarding the prevention of birth defects and the location of services when assistance is required.[7]

OCCUPATIONAL THERAPY IN MENTAL RETARDATION SERVICES

Mentally retarded persons will always require some measure of mental or physical assistance from the more capable members of society. Occupational therapy offers appropriate evaluation and habilitative treatment or training to facilitate the development and readiness of retarded persons so that they may master and maintain the use of a range of adaptive living skills.[3]

The general goals of an occupational therapy program in mental retardation facilities include

1. Facilitating development in areas where physical and emotional delays exist
2. Minimizing the disabling effects of a physical handicap
3. Developing attitudes and skills basic to independent functioning

Each retarded person should have the opportunity to develop innate capacities to his full potential. As discussed throughout this text, task occupation is an integral part of normal living. It is an important, natural means through which relationships occur and feelings may be expressed. Purposeful activity is the agent through which human beings learn and develop. Occupational therapy emphasizes coordinated performance of the entire psychomotor system. In physical restoration there is an interdependence between emotions, intellect, and physical functioning. The useful objects constructed while using corrective hand splints; the games played while learning to tolerate longer periods of standing; the completion of a series of sheltered workshop assembly tasks while learning to control the motor patterns appropriate to good eye-hand coordination; or the simple meals cooked while learning independent living skills are all symbols of occupational therapy. Intangible tools of occupational therapy include planning skills, the sharing of tools and equipment, expression of feelings, development of natural relationships, and satisfaction, which is necessary for a healthy self-image. Activity requires involvement. It develops a sense of self as a contributing participant rather than a recipient.

Activity adaptation

To be involved in an activity the retarded person may need special positioning devices attached to the bed or wheelchair. Articles used in performing activities of daily living may be modified to provide the multihandicapped retarded person with the assistance necessary to perform self-care and household or vocational tasks. Testing the retarded person's physical capacities to perform vocational tasks must be accompanied by a critical review of the architectural barriers of the work place.

As treatment of the retarded person progresses, the person assumes more of the responsibility for the direction of treatment under the guidance of the therapist, the parent, or the direct caregiver. The therapist gradually provides less direct care of the retarded person and more indirect care by monitoring skills learned or changes made in the treatment program.

Referral

The retarded person may be referred for occupational therapy by any advocate who is aware of problems and the potential for intervention or assistance. The request for help could originate from the parent, physician, school personnel, hospital staff, social worker, court personnel, volunteer agency, or others. The referral may be as simple as a verbal request, or it may be written in great detail.

Service to the retarded person is considered to be longitudinal in scope, that is, the occupational therapist does not cause an abrupt change or interruption in the person's rhythm of daily life. Instead, intervention is designed to enhance the current life pattern through assessment and treatment that is integral to it. Therefore the occupational therapist will place the retarded person's physical age, developmental level, adaptive living skills, potential, and environmental conditions into perspective when the referral is acknowledged and the person undergoes screening for services.

Screening

The use of a screening tool enables the occupational therapist to determine if the referral is appropriate for services, what those services may be, or whether further assessment is required. The screening tool establishes a general developmental range or capability level in adaptive living skills. Screening tools may be standardized, nonstandardized, or developed in a specific referral location or agency to handle special areas of competency. To obtain basic information, the occupational therapist may use one or more of the following screening tools: (1) Denver Developmental Screening Test (Chapter 9), (2) Milani-Comparetti Neurodevelopmental Screening Examination (Chapter 10), (3) nonstandardized screening tool. Often it may be more appropriate to develop a screening process that uses the operational definitions common to the specific agency (Chapters 9 and 10). On the assumption that it is more informative to have a retarded individual demonstrate his abilities in real situations rather than in office interviews, the occupa-

tional therapy department of the Georgia Retardation Center developed assessment instruments specific to its population and environment (Appendix C). These instruments are a screening tool, tests for ADL (activities of daily living) in food preparation, an outline for occupational therapy evaluations, and an equipment-rehabilitation survey.

If occupational therapy is indicated, the parent, guardian, or court advocate must give written permission to proceed with services. This is done to protect the rights of the retarded person. In many agencies permission to proceed with evaluation and services is covered in the admission agreement, provided that the occupational therapist is a regular staff member. The occupational therapist should inform the retarded person's primary physician when the screening discloses a physical problem. As manager of the retarded person's physical welfare, the primary physician is responsible for directing and documenting changes in physical care.

Assessment

The retarded person benefits from comprehensive assessment that uses the special evaluation tools of each interdisciplinary team member. A more complete picture of the individual's capabilities and splinter skills will emerge so that an effective program can be developed by the team to capitalize on and expand those abilities. The occupational therapist looks at the results of standardized and nonstandardized tests, checklists, observation of performance, and communication from all persons who directly take care of the retarded person to develop a meaningful evaluation. The evaluation team should use a comprehensive developmental behavioral test at this stage. This type of test can serve as a good place to store raw data over a period of time and can serve as a retest vehicle so that change over several years is clearly seen (Appendix C).

VULPE ASSESSMENT BATTERY

The Vulpe Assessment Battery[16] is a useful tool for therapists who are learning to evaluate retarded persons. It was developed for the atypical child and includes developmental assessments, performance analyses, and examples of individual program plans (see Exhibit 17-1, a sample page from the Vulpe battery). This battery covers test items for events from birth to 6 years of age in the adaptive living areas of basic senses and functions; gross and fine motor behaviors; language behaviors; cognitive behaviors; organizational behaviors; activities of daily living; and the behaviors of the caregiver in the person's living environment.

TIME SERIES OBSERVATIONS

Time series observations are effective for baseline evaluation, because the retarded person is in familiar

EXHIBIT 17-1

Performance analysis/developmental assessment

Date: _____   Name: _____   Birthdate: _____

Developmental area: Activities of daily living—feeding

Age	Activity and references	Equipment and directions	Scale score								Comments
			1 *No*	2 *Attention*	3 *Phys. assis.*	4 *Soc./emot. assis.*	5 *Verbal assis.*	6 *Independent*	7 *Transfer*		*Information processing and activity analysis*
3–5 months	5. Anticipation of feeding 2,4,6,11,44,48,50,63 RL–8 AGM–8	Breast or bottle— Present breast or bottle to child. The child shows signs of recognition without stimulation, for example, quieting, reaching, beginning to suck, puckering or opening mouth.									1. Analyse activities considering component parts of each and relationship to: basic senses and function; organization behaviors; cognitive processes and specific concepts; auditory language; gross and fine motor 2. Information processing consider: input; integration; feedback; assimilation; output
	6. Acceptance of pureed solids 2,4,11,44,48	Pureed food, spoon— Observe the child's response when offered pureed food from a spoon. The child opens mouth and removes food from spoon.									
	7. Use of tongue in accepting pureed food 4	Pureed food, spoon— Observe the motion of the child's tongue when accepting pureed food from a spoon. The child moves food around in mouth using tongue to aid swallowing food.									
	8. Swallowing pureed food 4,44,45	Pureed food, spoon— Observe the child's response when accepting pureed food from a spoon. The child swallows food without gagging or choking, and coordinates swallowing with breathing.									

From Vulpe, S.G.: Vulpe Assessment Battery, rev. ed., Downsview, Ontario, Canada, 1977, National Institute on Mental Retardation. With permission of the National Institute on Mental Retardation.

surroundings using media and materials common to her daily routine. From three to five separate observations by the same evaluator of performance of activities of daily living such as dressing, toileting, and self-feeding should provide sufficient data regarding level of competency and problems in physical motor performance and emotional growth.

When evaluating a retarded person who is over the chronological age of 6, the occupational therapist may need to select evaluation tools that focus on a specific area of daily living skills. Dressing, feeding, and toileting assessments are better done by observation over a period of a week or more with documentation of each observation. These pieces of information, with data obtained by other evaluators, can present a true picture of the retarded person's strengths and weaknesses in adaptive living skills.

Behavior during evaluation

Until the retarded person has formed an acceptable level of a relationship with the evaluator, he will tend to have difficulty in testing situations. At the first testing session, the retarded person may be very cooperative or may reject any or all test items. This rejection or defensive reaction is often the result of the person's difficulty in dealing with new situations and sensory experiences. With careful and considerate negotiating,[9] the occupational therapist may gradually break down the barriers of the retarded person's "personal space" and fear. The evaluator often needs to place the test item within the context of the environment and the current behavior of the retarded person. In addition, the individual may need to learn the test item over several sessions before the formal testing. The testing process might be accomplished as quickly as one session, but it usually requires three to five sessions to get acceptable levels of performance. For this reason, it is more expedient to begin assessment by using observation and group interaction before using individual testing. Through observation it is possible to define the usual range of a person's general behavior, whether socially cooperative or maladaptive. Does the person demonstrate stereotypic, self-stimulating, or self-abusive movements in a group situation? Does he take food or toys from another person, or does he share with others?

Team or composite evaluations

In some agencies the baseline evaluation is administered jointly by the professional staff by use of one tool that is limited to the scope of the program activities available at that agency. This type of evaluation is often self-limiting because it does not reflect each retarded person's potential or the possible areas for pro-

gram growth in the agency. Also, it does not allow for indicators of potential future problem areas. When a general performance test such as the AAMD Adaptive Behavior Scale[6] is used as a comprehensive evaluation, or when only parts of such a test are used, a great disservice is done to the retarded person.

Because each person is unique, extensive evaluation into problem areas should be done to pinpoint the exact focus of treatment or training. It benefits the retarded person to be evaluated by specialists in all areas of adaptive living. Two or more professional staff members could conduct assessment in a specialized area to investigate associated problems in depth and to develop a task analysis or a treatment or training program designed for the individual. For example, the occupational therapist and the speech and special education teacher could develop an effective treatment or training program in the agency or school setting for the adaptive feeding area (see Exhibit 11-3).

Program planning

The appropriate format and outline for documentation of information gathered or developed by the occupational therapist is found in the Uniform Terminology for Reporting Occupational Therapy Services[2] and those portions of the Uniform Occupational Therapy Evaluation Checklist[3] that apply. It is recommended that the report format be consistent with headings of specific reporting areas underlined (Appendix C). The evaluator need use only the relevant topics in the report. This type of report format is easy for other mental retardation workers to follow, and it makes possible a quick chart audit (Chapter 11).

In addition to these guidelines, the occupational therapist should report specific program recommendations in the format used by the agency so that they are included in the team recommendations for the treatment or training program. For example, all individualized education programs (IEPs) must be written within 1 month after referral of the child to special education, and annually thereafter. The interdisciplinary program plan (IPP) is used in day and institutional programs for the mentally retarded. The IPP is written by the team for the annual review of a retarded person monitored by an agency. It generally requires a broad view of each area of adaptive living, touching on skills such as body control, communication, self-help, social behaviors, effective use of time, basic knowledge or practical skills, and general health care.

It is for these reasons that the occupational therapist's report should clearly define the timeliness of occupational therapy services and whether these services should be direct or indirect. The IPP should state the specific treatment items, if any, that must be delivered by occupational therapy staff members; list those training skills to be taught by any professional staff; and state the due date for any follow-up evaluation.

Treatment or training

The occupational therapist who provides treatment or training services seldom, if ever, works in isolation with the retarded person. Interdependence of the professional staff strengthens the effectiveness and quality of the training program for the retarded person. The addition of parents and paraprofessional workers aids the day-to-day consistency needed to reinforce and maintain an effective action-oriented program.

In general the educational model is used in the delivery of mental retardation services (Chapter 24). The role of the occupational therapist is supportive. This supporting role is shared by other members of the interdisciplinary program team. The size of this team varies with the type and location of the facility or agency. With contributions of information from as many sources as possible, the team develops a plan of training or treatment activities on behalf of the retarded person. The individually tailored program is a list of adaptive living skills described in tasks with operational definitions written in behavioral terms. Progress or lack of progress is determined after review of the collection of data on the task. When the program goal calls for a treatment or a service to be performed by a staff member directly on or for the retarded person, this is listed as a "staff activity" for the retarded person. The occupational therapist is able to insert monthly reports of progress into each individual's summary of progress report that is compiled each month.

When developing a program of treatment or training for the retarded person, the occupational therapist has many good resources available, including the resource packet on mental retardation developed by the American Occupational Therapy Association's Division of Professional Development.[4] This guide includes the *Standards of Practice for Occupational Therapy Services for the Developmentally Disabled Client* (Appendix A). The occupational therapist can also draw from other guidelines and resource packets such as those for physical disabilities, prevocational evaluation and training, adaptive equipment, and mental health to fully cover the many areas of adaptive living that apply to the retarded person's program.

Adaptive equipment

All of the aids and devices required by the retarded person for adaptive living are grouped under the general heading of adaptive equipment. The standards of the Accreditation Council for Services for Mental Retarda-

tion and Other Developmentally Disabled Persons[1] categorize types of adaptive equipment under a variety of headings, including physical development and health, habilitation, education and training, behavior management, and mobility. These standards assure that the facilities and agencies have the services and programs necessary for providing adequate care and training of the retarded individual. Items of adaptive equipment are categorized by purpose and location of use. For example, a padded and modified helmet could be used either as a protective device or as part of an approved training program.

The standards[1] define types of devices used for restraint, support, or protection as follows:

Restraint A physical or mechanical device that may appear to be a protective device, but is always fully described as a part of an approved program of behavior management. It is employed only when absolutely necessary and to protect the retarded person from injury to himself or others.

Mechanical support A device used to provide support for the achievement of functional body position or proper balance, or a device used for specific medical and surgical treatment. This category includes wheelchairs and any or all modifications to the wheelchairs; rollators and other types of walkers, canes, and crutches; splints, body jackets, and the orthopedic, prescriptive shoes ordered by the physician; and other devices that meet the definition of body support.

During the habilitation, education, and training process, the aids and devices necessary to enable the individual to learn self-help tasks may be considered adaptive equipment. These items include the clothing adapted for dressing training; electronic, environmental control systems; specialized communication devices; specialized devices used in self-feeding, dressing, and other tasks performed as activities of daily living; and the architectural modifications that allow for increased independence in living tasks. Recent technology has opened the door to the use of switches commanded by the slightest touch or movement of air. When connected to toys or aids to daily living, these switches can enable the retarded person with extensive physical handicaps to have some control over his environment. Once aware of the ability to make something happen, the individual may be able to add other tasks or events to increase his level of functional performance.

When a referral for an adapted device is received, it is necessary for the therapist to have a clear understanding of the retarded person's problems, the living situations in which the adapted device is to be used, the number of caregivers to be instructed in the use of the device, and a working knowledge of the sources of supply of a variety of devices. Also, the occupational therapist is expected to have a working acquaintance with federal guidelines and requirements for accessible design in order to request and describe the exact location for placement of adapted equipment. It is up to the therapist to know what items are needed and to be able to write specifications clearly so that the exact item needed is received. The requisition and delivery processes usually take more than a month, so it may be necessary to assemble a temporary device to begin the training procedure.

Once adaptive equipment is obtained, accountability for these items must be considered. Because these items are vital to the retarded person's habilitation program, each must be listed in permanent records as part of the individual's program. Equipment should be inventoried periodically, and its use should be monitored during programming (Appendix C). Unless another person has the responsibility for repair of adaptive devices, this is to be handled by the therapist. Those items of adapted equipment used by the retarded person should be listed prominently in the written program, and all persons working with that student should be aware that the items exist, why and how they are used, and how to maintain them properly. Appropriate photographs make a useful addition to the record.

Discharge

When retarded individuals meet the criteria for change of placement, the persons responsible for their care develop a plan for that change. The group of responsible persons might include the parent, guardian, program planning team, and the court representative or retarded individual. Any changes in placement must be planned before the change date and in sufficient time to allow for adequate preparation. If an individual is now capable of a less restrictive placement, the occupational therapist writes a summary of previous treatment or training, including any recommendations for care that can be handled in the forthcoming placement. Likewise, if the placement is to be to a more restrictive or physically limiting area, appropriate recommendations for care are sent to the receiving area.

MANAGEMENT OF OCCUPATIONAL THERAPY SERVICES

The variety of duties required of the occupational therapist demands the use of a complex but flexible schedule. Priorities may vary from day to day. For example, the retarded person with self-abusive seizure episodes that involve injurious falls will have an immediate need for head-protective or other body-fitting devices to protect against injury. These unexpected events and others will interrupt any set schedule. Generally, though, it is possible to establish a regular and specific period at least every other week to reevaluate individuals before their annual review meetings. The occupational therapist working in or for any agency will also need to designate time each month to prepare progress summaries. Usually the caseload of retarded clients is so varied that it is imperative to reassess all current tasks and decide whether a change in the schedule is needed to accomplish a change in programming. Such recommendations must be presented to and decided by the team because of the complex nature of each individual's schedule.

Behavioral data collection

A clear understanding of the various types and uses for data collection is essential for objective reporting. This collection of data may refer to

1. *Frequency:* a count of the number of times a behavior occurs
2. *Rate:* a count of how often a behavior occurs per unit of time
3. *Durations:* a measure of how long each instance of a behavior lasts
4. *Instantaneous time sampling:* a gross estimate of how much of the time a person is engaged in the behavior, rather than a precise measure of it
5. *Interval recording:* a method in which the observation period is divided into intervals of equal length and continuous observation is maintained (Chapters 7 and 10).

Research

Work in the field of mental retardation lends itself to clinical research. Questions arise about why a particular technique was successful for one individual's training program and not another's, why a retarded person with a particular medical diagnosis responds better to one training technique than another, or why one system of monitoring care provider activities is more successful than another. The answers to these and other questions may be found through the scientific inquiry procedures known as research.[10] This method is set in an orderly process that includes

1. A statement of the question
2. A review of prior research in that area
3. A selection and explanation of the procedure to be used
4. A listing of operational definitions
5. A description of the person or group to be studied
6. A clarification of the method of collecting data
7. The specific procedures for analyzing the data
8. A statement of the hypothesis

9. An objective report of the results of the research methodology

10. The conclusions drawn by the researcher.

Perhaps the most practical and useful research methods for the occupational therapist to use to verify treatment or training with the mentally retarded are the single case design and the time series design.[12] This is not meant to imply that other types of research designs have no value in mental retardation research. In fact, important work has been done by occupational therapists acting as technical assistants to other members of the interdisciplinary team during drug studies, biofeedback studies, and others. A major benefit of interdisciplinary research is the continuing education and role expansion of all interdisciplinary team members. Examples of these efforts may be found in the literature. However, the single case design and the time series design are valuable to the clinician in mental retardation because these models make allowances for individual differences, provide an excellent way to integrate practice and research, and allow the therapist to ask and answer most of the scientifically important questions raised in the clinical environment. In the short term these designs help the therapist to make assessment and treatment decisions. In the long term it appears that the continuity of clinical science depends on the generation of data from on-line clinical work rather than the laboratory. In addition, it is necessary to report only the standard deviation, because it is the measure of the variability of the single subjects. The Office of Professional Research Services of the American Occupational Therapy Foundation is committed to assisting the occupational therapist with research efforts and will provide the names and addresses of nearby research consultants.

Staff development or in-service training

The treatment or training aspect of occupational therapy services does not end with the therapist-student dyad. To maintain the newly acquired skills in his repertoire of adaptive behaviors, the individual needs encouragement and prompting from daily care providers to perform this skill. The providers may be parents, other relatives, teachers and aides, direct care staff, houseparents, other professional staff, or any other persons whose participation is relevant to meeting the needs of an individual.

Instruction of other care providers demands the use of group training methods beyond the basic training methods in the occupational therapy undergraduate curriculum. The instructional analysis and the lesson plan are two teaching methods that produce effective results. *The instructional analysis* contains the (1) in-structional objective, (2) desired learning outcome, and (3) main points of discussion. In addition, a method of recording the names of participants and a method for follow-up or monitoring the skill learned by the caregiver should be included in the instructional analysis. One or more instructional objectives may be developed as a part of the instructional analysis. When writing the instructional objectives, it should be remembered that a therapist's own knowledge of the subject matter limits what can be taught and learned and that participants will have a variety of prior learning experiences in the topic area. The length of time necessary to provide instruction will vary, and the physical surroundings of the instructional setting will affect the learning experience. Each instructional objective should include a clear reference to the needs of the participants; present a simple, limited topic; adjust for the level of learning or understanding of the participant; and have a purpose or value to the participant.

If the occupational therapist develops topic areas by using the same outline for each instructional analysis and develops lesson plans for the instructional analysis, it will be possible to develop future classes with less preparation time. Also, as personnel change, each new care provider receives every part of skill training needed to train the retarded person exactly as his predecessor.

When writing the instructional analysis, include the following:

1. *Topic.* State the general topic area.
2. *Course.* State the specific title.
3. *Time.* State the expected length of instruction.
4. *Objective.* State the skill to be learned.

Then make two columns listing the desired learning outcomes on one side, and list the main points briefly on the other side.

The *lesson plan* is a detailed version of the instructional analysis, and it may contain the following list and procedure:

1. *Topic.* State the general topic area.
2. *Course.* State the specific title.
3. *Time.* State the expected length of instruction.
4. *Objective.* State the skill to be learned.
5. *Materials and equipment.* List all audiovisuals, demonstration items, writing materials, and handout materials.
6. *Presentation.*
   a. Introduce yourself by name and area of expertise.
   b. Establish the interest of the audience by discussing the topic area in general.
   c. Review the specifics and measurable desired learning outcomes with the audience.
   d. Proceed with the narrative portion of the presentation, using audiovisual and other media.
   e. Summarize the points or procedure taught.

7. *Examination.* Present a written test or have each participant demonstrate skill in the topic lesson.
8. *Documentation of training.* Before the audience leaves the classroom area, they should sign a roster for attendance records.
9. *Follow-up.* Develop a procedure for direct supervisors to monitor the application of the new skill in the work setting.

Monitoring programs

When monitoring the treatment or training program, the occupational therapist should write out the program, describing the techniques to be used; consult with the person who will teach the retarded individual for training; demonstrate the techniques; record the training session; and check periodically that the training techniques are used as designed.

CASE STUDY
Occupational therapy evaluation

I. Personal information:
   Todd, born Jan. 27, 1974.
II. Referral information: Referral received on Sept. 1, 1983 from the Butler County Training Center for evaluation and training in preparation for mainstreaming into the local classroom.
III. Personal history
   A. Developmental history: Todd was a very miserable baby before his thoracotomy. After surgery, he often smiled. He began to roll over at 4 years and to push himself around the floor by using his feet at 5 years. He does not sit independently or feed himself. At the age of 7 toilet training was attempted with no success.
   B. Educational history: Todd was kept at home until age 6 when he began attending the training center. He enjoys watching other children play. Because he is severely handicapped, formal testing has not been possible. His expressive communication is limited to head shaking for yes or no and to the sounds "mama" or "papa" when he is calm.
   C. Medical history: Todd is the second of three children. He was placed in an incubator at birth because of respiratory problems. At 8 weeks a thoracotomy was done on his left lung. During this procedure he suffered three cardiac arrests. He has a history of asthmatic attacks and seizures. The primary physician reports that he seems to see and hear. His head control is good; trunk control is poor; the right upper and lower extremities have less function than the left extremities. The right upper extremity is held in flexion pattern. The left upper extremity has severe flexion and ulnar deviation of the wrist. There is a 2-inch shortening of the right lower extremity, and both feet are in minimal varus position. Medical diagnosis on referral is profound psychomotor retardation, cause undetermined.
IV. Skills and performance areas
   A. Independent living: daily living skills and performance

1. Physical daily living skills: Todd requires total assistance.
2. Psychological: Emotional daily living skills; Todd nods his head yes to recognizing his image in a mirror.
3. Play: Todd enjoys all visual and auditory entertainment.
   B. *Sensorimotor skills and performance components*
   1. *Neuromuscular performance components*
      a. *Reflex integration:* The Milani-Comparetti Screening Tool revealed the following personal baseline results:
         (1) Primitive reflexes: 5 months of normal development
         (2) Righting reactions: 7 months of normal development
         (3) Parchute reactions: 4.5 months of normal development
      b. *Range of motion:* Severe spasticity and high diazepam (Valium) dosage precludes accurate measures of passive range of motion. Functional range of motion of upper extremity is not evident because of severe contractures and very poor muscle tone. *(Note: See physical therapy report for arc of passive motion of joints.)*
   2. *Sensory integration*
      a. Sensory awareness: Todd responds appropriately to pinprick, rough surfaces, and soft surfaces on extremities.
      b. Visual: Spatial awareness was not tested.
   3. *Cognitive skill and performance components*
      a. Todd responds with head nod or shaking when direct questions are posed. This communication method does not allow for problem solving.
      b. His attention span is average for his physical age.
   4. *Psychosocial skills and performance components*
      a. Self-management: Todd flings out his arms or legs to get attention from passerby.
      b. Group interaction: Todd watches other children and staff.
   5. *Therapeutic adaptation:* Todd uses a standard wheelchair in junior size.

Proposed direct or indirect client needs from occupational therapy

(Note: Inform the primary physician of your recommendations.)
   I. Positioning for functioning and therapeutic goals
      A. Bed or mat
      B. Wheelchair adaptations
      C. Classroom environment
      D. Home environment
   II. Communication orthosis—head wand
      A. Fitting and training
   III. Activities of daily living skills
      A. Adapt toileting devices for home and for school.
      B. Adapt bathing devices for home.
      C. Assess oral motor skills and develop training program.
      D. Refer dental hygiene to his dentist.
   IV. Body control
      A. Develop program of relaxation techniques.

B. In conjunction with the physical therapist or the therapeutic recreation staff, develop general physical conditioning program to be used at school.

V. In-service training: Train home and school personnel who work with Todd in each of the techniques he has learned and in the proper use of his special aids and devices. Include copies of his home program in his occupational therapy department client record.

VI. Follow-through: If Todd is not under the care of the school occupational therapist, set up a follow-up visit within 1 year.

SUMMARY

The mentally retarded person has significantly subaverage general intellectual function that exists concurrently with deficits in adaptive behavior. Occupational therapy can make an important contribution to the development of the retarded person where physical and emotional delays exist; can aid in minimizing the disabling effects of a physical handicap; and can provide treatment or training to develop attitudes and skills basic to independent function. As an active member of the treatment team, the occupational therapist provides the evaluation, habilitative treatment or training and follow-up of the retarded person so that she will be able to master and maintain adaptive living skills.

REFERENCES

1. Accreditation Council for Services for Mental Retardation and Other Developmentally Disabled persons: Standards for services for developmentally disabled individuals, Washington, D.C., 1981, ACMRDD.
2. American Occupational Therapy Association, Inc., AOTA Commission on Practice: Uniform terminology for reporting occupational therapy services, Rockville, Md., 1979.
3. American Occupational Therapy Association, Inc., AOTA Commission on Practice: Uniform occupational therapy evaluation checklist, Rockville, Md., 1981.
4. American Occupational Therapy Association, Inc., Division of Professional Development: Mental retardation, Resource packet, Rockville, Md., 1981.
5. Buda, F.B.: The neurology of developmental disabilities, Springfield, Ill., 1981, Charles C Thomas, Publisher.
6. Fogelman, C.J., editor: AAMD Adaptive Behavior Scale, rev. ed., Washington, D.C., 1974, American Association on Mental Deficiency.
7. Grossman, H.J., editor: Classification in mental retardation, Washington, D.C., 1983, American Association on Mental Deficiency.
8. Halpern, A.S.: Mental retardation. In Stolov, W.C., editor: Handbook of severe disability, Washington, D.C., 1981, U.S. Department of Education, Rehabilitation Services Administration.
9. Huss, A.M.: Touch with care or a caring touch, Am. J. Occup. Ther. **31**(1):11, 1977.
10. Jantzen, A.C.: Research: the practical approach for occupational therapy, Laurel, Md., 1981, Ramsco Publishing Co.
11. Koch, R.: Bio-medical problems in mental retardation . . . a review. Unpublished paper presented at the National Prevention Showcase and Forum, Atlanta, Sept. 15-17, 1982, President's Committee on Mental Retardation.
12. Payton, O.D.: Research: The validation of clinical practice, Philadelphia, 1971, F.A. Davis Co.
13. Scheerenberger, R.C.: A history of mental retardation, Baltimore, 1982, Brooks Publishing Co.
14. Scheiner, A.P., and Abroms, I.F.: The practical management of the developmentally disabled child, St. Louis, 1980, The C.V. Mosby Co.
15. Sebelist, R.M.: Mental retardation. In Hopkins, H.L., and Smith, J.D., editors: Willard and Spackman's occupational therapy, ed. 5, Philadelphia, 1978, J.B. Lippincott Co.
16. Vulpe, S.G.: Vulpe Assessment Battery, rev. ed., Downsview, Ontario, Canada, 1977, National Institute on Mental Retardation.
17. Wright, N.: Total rehabilitation, Boston, 1981, Little, Brown and Co.

SUGGESTED READINGS

Books

Bergen, A.: Selected equipment for pediatric rehabilitation, Valhalla, N.Y., 1975, Blythedale Children's Hospital.

Bernstein, G.S., Ziarnik, J.P., and Rudreed, E.H.: Behavioral habilitation through proactive programming, Baltimore, 1982, Brooks Publishing Co.

Copeland, M., Ford, L., and Salon, N.: Occupational therapy for mentally retarded children, Baltimore, 1976, University Park Press.

Finnie, N.: Handling the young cerebral palsied child at home, New York, 1970, E.P. Dutton & Co., Inc.

Frank, J.: Resource guide to protective aids, Washington, D.C., 1979, George Washington University.

High, E.C., editor: Resource guide to habilitative techniques and aids for cerebral palsied persons of all ages, Washington, D.C., 1979, George Washington University.

Hofmann, R.: How to build special furniture and equipment for handicapped children, Springfield, Ill., 1970, Charles C Thomas, Publisher.

Macey, P.: Mobilizing multiply handicapped children, Lawrence, Kan., 1974, University of Kansas.

Morris, S.E.: Program guidelines for children with feeding problems, Edison, N.J., 1977, Childcraft Education Corp.

Robinalt, I.: Functional aids for the multiply handicapped, Hagerstown, Md., 1973, Harper & Row, Publishers.

U.S. Architectural and Transportation Barriers Compliance Board: A guidebook to: the minimum federal guidelines and requirements for accessible design, Washington, D.C., 1981, U.S. Government Printing Office.

Articles

Berdslee, G.R.: Fieldwork experience in mental retardation, Am. J. Occup. Ther. **30:**656, 1976.

Bonadonna, P.: Effects of a vestibular stimulation program on stereotypic rocking behavior, Am. J. Occup. Ther. **35:**775, 1981.

Bright, T., Bittick, K., and Fleeman, B.: Reduction of self-injurious behavior using sensory integrative techniques, Am. J. Occup. Ther. **35:**167, 1981.

Clark, F.A., and others: A comparison of operant and sensory integrative methods of developmental parameters in profoundly retarded adults, Am. J. Occup. Ther. **32:**86, 1978.

DeMars, P.: Training adult retardates for private enterprise, Am. J. Occup. Ther. **29:**39, 1975.

Ford, L.: Teaching dressing skills to a severely retarded child, Am. J. Occup. Ther. **29:**87, 1975.

Goldman, L.: Behavioral skills for employment of the intellectually handicapped, Am. J. Occup. Ther. **29:**539, 1975.

Hurff, J. Gaming technique: an assessment and training tool for individuals with learning deficits, Am. J. Occup. Ther. **35:**728, 1981.

Kantner, R., Kantner, B., and Clark, D.: Vestibular stimulation effect on language development in mentally retarded, Am. J. Occup. Ther. **36:**36, 1982.

Kielhofner, G.: The temporal dimension in the lives of retarded adults: a problem of interaction and intervention, Am. J. Occup. Ther. **33:**161, 1979.

Kielhofner, G., and Miyake, S.: The therapeutic use of games with mentally retarded adults, Am. J. Occup. Ther. **35:**375, 1981.

Kielhofner, G., and Takata, N.: A study of mentally retarded persons: applied research in occupational therapy, Am. J. Occup. Ther. **34:**252, 1980.

Ling-Fong Zee-Chen, E., and Hardman, M.: Postrotary nystagmus response in children with Down's syndrome, Am. J. Occup. Ther. **37:**260, 1983.

Mann, W., and Sobsey, R.: Feeding program for the institutionalized mentally retarded, Am. J. Occup. Ther. **29:**397, 1975.

McCracken, A.: Tactile function of educable mentally retarded children, Am. J. Occup. Ther. **29:**397, 1975.

McCracken, A.: Drool control and tongue thrust therapy for the mentally retarded, Am. J. Occup. Ther. **32:**79, 1978.

Norton, Y.: Neurodevelopment and sensory integration for the profoundly retarded multiply handicapped child, Am. J Occup. Ther. **29:**93, 1975.

Resman, M.: Effect of sensory stimulation on eye contact in a profoundly retarded adult, Am. J. Occup. Ther. **35:**3, 1981.

Shuer, J., Clark, F., and Azen, S.: Vestibular function in mildly mentally retarded adults, Am. J. Occup. Ther. **34:**664, 1980.

Weber, N.: Chaining strategies for teaching sequenced motor tasks to mentally retarded adults, Am. J. Occup. Ther. **32:**385, 1978.

Webster, P.: Occupational role development in the young adult with mild mental retardation, Am. J. Occup. Ther. **34:**13, 1980.

Weeks, Z.: Effects of the vestibular system on human development. Part 2: effects of vestibular stimulation on mentally retarded, emotionally disturbed and learning–disabled individuals, Am. J. Occup. Ther. **33:**450, 1979.

Wehman, P., and Marchant, J.: Improving free play skills of severely retarded children, Am. J. Occup. Ther. **32:**100, 1978.

White, J.: Stimulus box for the profoundly mentally retarded, Am. J. Occup. Ther. **30:**167, 1976.

18

FROMA JACOBSON-SADACCA

Children with communicative impairment

COMMUNICATION

Communicative interaction is a basic task of daily living. People who cannot speak or make themselves easily understood by others are frequently assumed to be less competent and less intelligent than others. In the story of Snow White, the nonspeaking seventh dwarf, Dopey, symbolizes society's amused tolerance of its nonarticulating members. The assumption that people who cannot talk also cannot think or feel represents an attitude that health professionals and educators must constantly combat in the general public.

One of the best defenses is a system of communication that is tailored to the individual's abilities and disabilities. Each system may include elements of written and oral interactions, gestures, facial expressions, and body language. Occupational therapists, with their commitment to building competence in tasks of daily living and with their skills in activity adaptation and positioning, are among the critical personnel who can help develop communication systems for nonspeaking persons. This chapter introduces the concept of augmentative communication and discusses the occupational therapist's roles and functions in programs for children with motor speech impairment.

Incidence of oral-motor impairment of speech

It is difficult to establish the number of persons classified as nonoral because of large differences in survey methods and findings. Two 1978 surveys, however, placed the number between 200,000 and 1,000,000.[4,6] Nonoral, in this instance, simply means without speech. The population estimate cited is increased by those persons who are temporarily unable to express themselves verbally or in writing because of acute pathological conditions or injuries.

Classrooms for children with special needs include many youngsters who are labeled "unable to test" because of communication impairment associated with physical or developmental disabilities. The primary diagnoses for these children include cerebral palsy, postcerebral vascular accident, developmental delay, organic brain syndrome, head trauma, spinal cord injury, arthritis, muscular dystrophy, multiple sclerosis, and laryngectomy. Without communication skills, clients must rely on family and professional team members to meet their needs and organize resources to allow achievement of maximal function and independence. This implies that the level of independence achieved will not depend on one's own capacities, but instead will depend on the cababilities of others.

In a study performed in Canada by rehabilitation engineers and reported by LeBlanc,[5] physically handicapped individuals were asked to rank their needs. Communication was accorded the highest priority, with activities, mobility, and ambulation following in order.

Augmentative communication

Imagine sharing information with a colleague, conversing at a party, conducting a transaction at a grocery store, or lecturing to a class. One relies primarily on oral speech for self-expression. However, careful review of these presentations indicates that hands, gestures, body language, eye gaze, pauses, audiovisual equipment, and writing are used to augment the oral messages. These combined components of communication are called *total, adaptive,* or *augmentative communication.* Augmentative communication incorporates all those systems that are used in addition to oral speech to improve understanding of the speaker's message. This can include mechanical systems for nonoral communication that have been designed for persons with physical speech impairment.

The following are examples of children who can be assisted by augmentative communication systems:

1. The child with cerebral palsy whose loss or impairment of motor function includes the ability to reliably produce intelligible expressive speech. Traditional speech therapy may be ineffective. Augmentative communication, including eye gaze, vocalizations, gestures, body language, manual signing, communication boards, and electronic aids, may allow more language development. Functional interaction can then replace frustration.

2. The child with other neurological or developmental deficits whose attempts at speech can range from complete silence to babbling, with varying degrees of word production and comprehension. The prognosis for the development of functional oral speech may be guarded, yet it is desirable that the child have the advantage of communication within physical and cognitive limitations.

3. The child whose speech has been affected by trauma. This child faces additional problems. The child has had speech and is suddenly deprived of it; she may be frustrated in many previously accomplished daily life activities. Loss of control and interaction often disrupts the rehabilitation process. An augmentative communication system in such cases might be temporary, allowing the child to communicate while in the hospital. An alternative system may ultimately be indicated.

In the past children with such handicaps have had to rely on "yes-no" indications and "20 questions" routines to make their wishes known. Augmentative systems help these children not only immediately and mechanically but also developmentally. It has been observed clinically that removing the pressure to produce oral speech in fact facilitates its development.

Augmentative communication aids range from very simple ones made in the therapy clinic to the very elaborate, comprehensive systems that are microprocessor or computer controlled. An example of the clinician-made aid is a simple picture board and some type of pointer that is used by the child to indicate the picture showing the desired message.

CLINICIAN-MADE SYSTEMS

Clinician-made systems continue to be quite effective for many children and are recommended in addition to more complex electronic systems. Such aids are reliable and multifunctional. Creativity is employed in developing a communication board that is meaningful to both the speaker and listeners. Objects, miniatures, photographs, pictures, line drawings, symbols, words, letters, and a combination thereof may be used. These representations can be mounted to a vest, belt, apron, pants, or multisurfaced board. Miniboards as well as books can be used.

ELECTRONIC EDUCATIONAL AIDS

Electronic educational aids were introduced in England approximately 20 years ago and allowed even severely physically handicapped children to have appropriate learning experiences. The Possum Basic Skill Set* allows children to match items. By hitting a switch, the child moves a light on the board from one selection to another. A correct answer is rewarded with a musical response. The machine gives a negative reinforcement for errors and keeps track of the mistakes. Simple exercises can include object matching, whereas more complex tasks might address such skills as reading comprehension. The manufacturer has also developed an expanded keyboard for adapted direct selection typing. A scanning system for permanent hard copy could be easily accessed by use of input switches.

Many other systems have been developed since this early start, including nonoral communication systems, educational aids, and environmental controls. The technology continues to expand rapidly so that many kinds of aids are available to nonverbal children who are physically handicapped or developmentally delayed. Each system must be selected according to the motor, perceptual, receptive, and expressive needs of the child communicator, with consideration of the persons who will be receiving the messages.

Typically, when one envisions a language board, the image is of a piece of cardboard with words arranged in a noun-verb-noun format. This thinking has been expanded to meet the level of the child who uses the sys-

---

*From Possum Controls, Ltd., Middlegreen Trading Estate, Middlegreen Rd., Langley, Slough, Berks SL3 6DF; New York office: Twelfth Floor, 105 Madison Ave., New York, NY., 10016.

tem. Again, creativity is the key. Some clinician-made communication boards may be designed in the format of a clear acrylic eye scanner or as shadow boxes, books, folders, flip-top address books, leg chaps, communication handkerchiefs, or vests.

Developmentally, children become familiar with objects long before they are able to read and use the written word. The typical progression of recognition begins with the object itself and proceeds to the miniature, photograph, color picture, line drawing, and, most sophisticated, the word or symbol system. The word should always accompany the item symbol.

SYMBOL SYSTEMS

Some children are not able to read and thus rely on other symbol systems. Three examples of symbolic representation include Bliss, rebus, and Picsyms.

1. *Bliss symbols* were created by Charles Bliss of Australia as a visual graphic system. The symbols are adapted from basic geometric shapes[1,2] (Figure 18-1, *A*).
2. *Rebus* is the Latin word for thing. Instead of using a spelled word, a meaning can be represented by a thing.[3] (Figure 18-1, *B*).
3. *Picsyms** is a picture symbol system and is based on easily recognized line drawings of familiar objects. This system allows nonspeaking preschoolers to "send" messages by choosing a series of symbols. (Figure 18-1, *C*).

---

*Developed in 1981 by Faith Carlson, Meyer Children's Rehabilitation Unit, Nebraska Medical Center, Omaha.

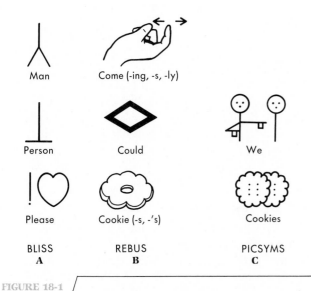

Man Come (-ing, -s, -ly)

Person Could We

Please Cookie (-s, -'s) Cookies

BLISS REBUS PICSYMS
A   **B**   **C**

FIGURE 18-1

Symbol systems. **A**, Bliss. **B**, Rebus. **C**, Picsyms.

Classification of aids

An augmentative communication system is designed for the individual according to two main considerations: (1) how the child can best indicate what is to be said and (2) how the message is to be expressed. Therefore aids are commonly classified by (1) the type of input, or selection mode required (direct selection, scanning, or encoding) and (2) the type of display mode (output) that is generated, such as visual display, permanent written copy, synthesized speech, video display, and combinations.

DIRECT SELECTION MODE

Severely handicapped children must have a means of selecting messages that is physically achievable by them. Direct selection, as the name implies, requires the child to specifically select one picture, photograph, object, phrase, word, or letter from an established grouping. Selection is generally accomplished by touching with a finger, fist, hand, elbow, foot, headstick, tongue, or nose—whatever the child can use most reliably with the best energy efficiency and the least fatigue.

Examples of direct selection modes include the typewriter keyboard and picture board. A direct selection mode allows the user to plan and select voluntarily. This mode is relatively fast, simple, and straightforward for those who have appropriate motor control and range of motion. It is easy for the child to learn to use a direct selection mode, and messages are easily understood by the listener.

SCANNING MODE

The display of the scanning mode device looks very similar to the direct selection board, but it is used in a different way. Because the child may not have the necessary skills to use a board independently, the listener points at different options until the desired areas are reached. Possible communications have been arranged in rows or matrices, and the listener assists the client by "narrowing in" on the correct item.

To illustrate, imagine the typewriter keyboard. After establishing the client's ability to indicate a yes-no response, the listener points to two halves of the keyboard and asks, "Is your message in this half or in this half? Is it in this half?" "Yes" or "no" is then indicated by the child using the prearranged response. Through the process of elimination, the listener may then proceed along the rows of keys on the selected half until the desired message is revealed. This method resembles the twenty questions approach, but it is more systematic. Disadvantages of the scanning mode are that messages are limited by the capacity of the system, the methodology is relatively slow, the user must see the display, and the listener is required to be actively involved. However, since minimal motor response is required from the speaker, this mode is more reliable and

FIGURE 18-2

Coding matrix and board. **A,** Matrix. **B,** Board.

less fatiguing than others. It is usable by even the most severely involved person. Often external switches are used by the speaker to operate a scanning electronic device.

ENCODING MODE

The encoding mode requires the communicator to use a predetermined code for message selection and the listener to scan down and across a matrix to determine the intended message (Figure 18-2). This presentation mode would be used by a person whose range of motion is too limited to access a larger board, but who has adequate cognitive ability to remember codes. A large board, with the matrix of coded messages, would be placed in an area that is visually convenient to both the speaker and listener. The small coding board would be placed within easy motor access of the communicator. The child may then directly select an area on the horizontal and vertical axes. For example, in the illustration, 1-A would mean "yes." To indicate "I need help," the child would point to 4-A, 7-C, 5-B, 5-B, 4-B, and 6-A.

Encoding is a form of scanning, but it is usually faster than that method. It requires more motor response than scanning and less than direct selection. Therefore it could be less reliable and more fatiguing. It is also more abstract and symbolic than scanning.

OUTPUT MODE

With an output mode, the message can be presented by visual display, permanent written copy (paper printout), speech output, video presentation, and a combination of these. This is a matter for individualized choice. Some systems can be incorporated into a lapboard, others cannot.

Elements of visual display output may include lights and a pointing apparatus. It may be large and easy to read, or small and compact. There may be interchangeable overlays for flexibility. Some visual displays have the capacities to chain and remember information.

Permanent written copy may be produced on strip printers, calculator tape, typing paper, and computer printouts. These systems are most appropriate for academic use, correspondence, permanent copy, or community interaction.

Aids with speech output produce verbal communications in the form of a recorded voice, synthesized speech, or digitized speech. The client chooses from speech, text, or speech sounds (phonemes) to generate instantaneous speech. Because of the verbal nature of the output, this system can be used most effectively in groups. Memory and capacity of the systems can vary from unit to unit, ranging from 10 words to thousands of sound components.

Portable and stationary microcomputers have become invaluable as communication and education aids. Children with severe motor involvement can use adapted equipment to access the computer and its software.

• • •

As augmentative communication systems become increasingly sophisticated, both in specialization and versatility, one aid can often generate more than one type of output. It is also recognized that more than one system may be necessary to meet all the needs of a child in his different functional environments, to provide for communication, education, and environmental control and interaction.

Therapeutic considerations

FUNCTIONAL COMMUNITY INTERACTION

In contrast to the emphasis of speech and language specialists on language arts, occupational therapists address communication as an activity of daily living. The occupational therapist evaluates communication skills in all life roles and teaches the child to extend these skills beyond the therapy environment to the classroom, play group, Brownie troop, or wherever the child goes. This multienvironment approach generates the term *functional community interaction.* It implies that the individual will be able to interact in all environments of people, both handicapped and able-bodied. Any communication system must be adapted to the child's needs so that the system itself does not limit independence.

Ideally, a specialized communication system should be available to the child for all those postures that are assumed daily, such as prone and supine positions, wheelchair sitting, possibly ambulating, sidelying, and unsupported sitting. Adaptation and flexibility in the choice of systems are important if maximal communication potential is to be reached.

PSYCHOSOCIAL CONCERNS

Therapists will be especially concerned about children's self-images: specifically, how they feel about using the chosen systems. Ideally, children contribute to the decisions concerning the system of choice for them, but lack of speech frequently precludes their making life role decisions. How children accept the devices and how they present themselves to others will affect how others respond to them. This same sensitivity to self-image should be extended to any adaptive aid or position, including splints, headsticks, mobile arm supports, or other devices that are used as interfaces with the communication system.

A closely related issue that is often ignored by professionals is nonverbal communication. What message does the child receive when others

- "Do for" the child, rather than letting the child perform the task independently?
- Finish a sentence for the child?
- Pretend to understand attempts at oral speech because of limited time?
- Ignore attention-getting efforts to avoid the time-consuming interactions?
- Choose a toy for the child, thereby preventing the development of decision-making processes?
- Pour ketchup on hot dogs and thus presume the child's preference?
- Talk for the child in her presence?

Perhaps the greatest insult is in not asking the child to communicate. Therapists must consider how much this noncommunication affects the child's other developmental processes: gross motor, fine motor, psychosocial, and adaptive. Sensitivity to the feelings of the child nurtures the interpersonal relationships that are crucial to building a communication system and process.

TEAM CONCEPT

Interdisciplinary team involvement is important in the initial choice of aids and in the direct training of children to use the augmentative systems for functional community interaction. Team composition is variable but often includes the child, family, certain friends, occupational therapist, physical therapist, educators, speech and language specialist, psychologist, social worker, child advocate, nurse, caretaker, physician, and even fund-raisers. These specialists must know the limitations as well as strengths of their disciplines and personalities and offer interventions ranked by priorities of need to best serve the child. A transdisciplinary approach is essential because of the nature of daily communication needs.

In the emerging field of augmentative communication, the speech and language specialist works with language, using the augmentative system for communication, language development, and syntax. The teacher strengthens the educational program by incorporating newly developed communication skills into classroom activities. The role of the occupational therapist is less well-defined at present, although therapists have traditionally instructed children in typing with and without adaptations.

ROLE OF OCCUPATIONAL THERAPY

The occupational therapist is the key person to bridge the space between the child and the communication device. This is done by organizing that space so that the child has access to the device in a consistently reliable manner, by solving problems of position, making adaptations, choosing interfaces, identifying perceptual and motor assets and liabilities, and using reflex patterns. The skills of the occupational therapist can enhance the child's functional access to whatever device the communication specialist deems linguistically appropriate.

Assessment

Occupational therapists evaluate each child to determine

- Organization of space to make access to equipment easier
- Positions required during the child's typical day
- Visual perception assets and liabilities, including visual tracking, figure-ground discrimination, object performance concepts, spatial relationships, and visual perception of position in space
- Suitable switches and other interfaces, keyboard styles, positioning, placement of switch, and placement of aid
- Most reliable motor responses in a variety of positions
- Potential social, educational, and vocational opportunities that will be made more practical by development of communication skills
- Reaction to types of systems under consideration, including reactions of family members and peer group

The occupational therapist collaborates with the child and the team to select systems that will work for the child. This criterion far surpasses the search for a system that the child can work. As part of the assessment the therapist can also gather base information from the primary multidisciplinary team and the family group regarding

- Medical aspects that may affect positioning
- Pending medical procedures
- Adaptive aids presently used, as well as information about aids that were previously used and why discarded
- Visual and auditory acuity
- Reliable motor responses used in other activities and with other equipment
- Independence in self-maintenance activities
- Activities performed in a typical day, including participation and positioning
- Child and family goals and priorities

A critical goal within the motor function portion of the evaluation is the identification of an appropriate, reliable, volitional, and controlled movement pattern that will not interfere with the child's concentration on communication. It is advisable to look at all the positions assumed by the child in a typical day, including the optimal and typical, and consider how the typical can be improved. Creativity is the key to finding more than one position and movement pattern that will allow access to the system. The reliable motion may be, for example, direct selection with one finger, or oral sucking and puffing, or chin depression or thigh abduction. With an adolescent it may be advisable to look at reflex patterns to consider how these might be used initially to gain access to a system.

During this search many factors must be considered. Important motor components include reflex patterns, overflow, possibility of triggering seizure activity, level of fatigue, range of motion, as well as strength and endurance. Ability to learn new tasks, attention span and attention to the task during the motor response, and probability of success are significant cognitive factors. The need for interfacing adaptive equipment must be considered. And finally, the therapist must focus on such emotional factors as the child's reactions to stress and fatigue, motivation, eye contact during interaction, and, perhaps most important, the child's feelings about using this position and motor response.

In cooperation with the speech and language specialist, who has also evaluated the child and suggested a suitable system, the occupational therapist determines the specific interfaces for that system. The therapist may be able to use a commercially available switch quite well with the child's reliable responses or may need to fabricate a makeshift switch for the evaluation and begin the design for a custom switch. Multisensory feedback, such as tactile, visual, and auditory, must be considered. For the direct selector, the occupational therapist is able to suggest size of menu (number of available items for selection), size of input areas, placement of different areas, and required pressure to obtain an output. To choose a switch for scanning or encoding, the switch placement, pressure for output, need for visual pursuit, and safety precautions must be considered.

Visual perception and cognitive factors must also be evaluated, including figure-ground, position in space and spatial relationships, and visual sequencing ability. Important task components include following directions, making eye contact, taking turns, relating cause and effect, visual memory, visual matching, categorizing information, and visual midline crossing (Exhibit 18-1).

A final step in the initial occupational therapy assessment is to determine the spatial relationships between the child, interfaces, system, and output modes. These relationships will be different for each position that the child assumes during the day. Options for portable, semiportable, or stationary systems must be considered. Semiportable systems include those that may be lightweight but require several pieces of equipment and interfaces and assistance for assembly and transportation.

EXHIBIT 18-1

Skills to be assessed when planning augmentative communication systems

Motor
Midline crossing
Range of motion
Eye-hand coordination
Strength
Speed-accuracy-control
Time-energy saving
Reliability of response of

Activities of daily living
Independence using communication
Communication to enhance social,
    educational, vocational opportunities
Communication via phone
Communication for emergency
Communication for pleasure
One-to-one communication
Group interaction
Communication to order products

Visual perception
Spatial relationships
Position in space
Figure-ground
Visual tracking
Directionality
Ability to follow directions
Eye contact
Symbol permanence
Cause-and-effect relationships
Timing
Sequencing
Spelling
Reading
Word recognition
Decision making
Problem solving
Visual-auditory memory

Visual pursuit
Visual-auditory discrimination
Attention span
Attention to task
Risk taking
Information categorization
Information finding
Visual matching
Motor planning

EXHIBIT 18-2

Activities that facilitate access to augmentative communication systems

Switch control
Battery-operated toys
Electric trains
Freddy the Frog (Fisher Price)
Oscar the Grouch (Fisher Price)
Monster Dash (Prentke Romich)
Prentke Romich Toy Modifications
Votrax Research Handi Toy
Wall switch for a room light
Remote control television
Garage door opener
Shower
Outside sprinkler system
Garbage disposal
Blue Bird (Fisher Price)
Jumping Jack (Fisher Price)
Molly Moo Cow (Fisher Price)
Ring a Bell bicycle crib toy
Ring a Bell fire engine crib toy
Musical crib toy
Juggler crib toy
Crib aquarium
Surprise boxes
Jack-in-the-box
Pass the nuts
Mattel Tuff-Stuff wordwriter, calculator, letters
Mattel See 'n Say
Battery-operated remote-controlled animals
Push-button telephones
Coleco Good Puppy
Perceptual motor facilitators
Pioneer board
Mechanical pointing boards

Cause and effect
Jack-in-the-Box (variety of)
Surprise box (variety of)
Sesame Street House (Child Guidance)
Push-and-Go toys (Tomy)
Egg timer (Playskool; Fisher Price)
Building blocks (variety of)
Pop beads
Cash register (Fisher Price)

Risk taking
Table games
Monster Dash (Prentke Romich)
Candy Land
Chutes and Ladders
Hungry, Hungry Hippos
Possum Basic Skill Set
Old Maid (card game)
Go Fish (card game)
Imitation activities
Pass the Nuts (Tomy)

Pointing
Table games
Push button telephones
Telephone truck (Tonka Toddler)
Operator Telephone (Fisher Price)
Finger painting
Little Maestro (Creative Playthings)
Imitation of postures
Mirror play
Clay
"Show me" activities
Melody Mike (Child Guidance)
Tactile stimulation activities or cards
Little Professor (Texas Instruments)
Speak and Spell (Texas Instruments)
Calculator games
Typing
Bubbles
Active range of motion

Perception
Possum Basic Skill Set
Concentration (card game)
Imitation of postures
Gross motor directionality activities
Figure-ground cards or activities
Dot-to-dot games
Puzzles (visual matching, word, symbol)
Two-to-four step sequencing activities
Visual matching cards
Lotto (commercial or clinician-made)
Domino games
Lincoln logs (Playskool)
Peg bus and racing car (Creative Playthings)
Shape sorting toys (variety of)
Systems 80 (Borg-Warner)
Potato head type game
Bristle blocks (Playskool)
Bubbles
Size discrimination activities
Categorization (by color, size, shape, and so on)
Color pegs
Developmental learning materials
Self-care activities
Sequencing cards
Tipsy Tea Cups (Child Guidance)
Blockhead (Saalfield)
"What would you do if?"
Simon (Milton Bradley)

The last component of the assessment requires the sensitivity of the entire team. As was discussed previously, severely physically handicapped children have generally not had the opportunities for development that more normal children experience. They have probably never crawled around a kitchen pulling everything out of cabinets, nor knocked over a lamp with a toy. They may never even have been given the chance to choose what they will wear, watch on television, give as a gift, or put on their hot dogs. Family constellations develop, often quite comfortably, wherein the child becomes the recipient of the action, the thing rather than the person. When evaluating children for communication systems, we ask them to make decisions and be involved in a cause-and-effect activity. We respect them as persons who have a lot to say, and we may be preparing them to say what others are not ready to hear. Much more is happening to them than simply spending time with a variety of systems. The first taste of autonomy may be unsettling for both the family and the child. The team must be sensitive to hints from the family and the child's home team. Their suggestions are important to continued successful use of communication systems and skills.

Treatment activities

Successful operation of an augmentative communication system is dependent on many variables. The most obvious are motor access to the equipment and the development of receptive and expressive language skills. The lists in Exhibit 18-1 suggest other areas to be considered throughout the assessment-training-reassessment process. Activities chosen to facilitate these skills and functional components, individualized to the child and devices, should improve the child's successful operation of the augmentative communication system.

The occupational therapist has traditionally used activities to facilitate functional performance. Exhibit 18-2 provides a list of recommended activities that will enhance the basic task components of perceptual-motor access to augmentative communication systems. In theory the best response will be obtained through activities such as these, in addition to or instead of drill on the actual system. Obviously this effect is most likely to occur if the selected activities are appropriate to the system and to the skills of the particular child.

CASE STUDY

Jane is 4 years, 2 months old. She was brought to Bayshore Rehabilitation Center, an agency offering transdisciplinary evaluation and treatment by specialists in nursing, occupational therapy, physical therapy, speech therapy.

Medical diagnosis: Cerebral palsy. Evaluation 1 year ago described "severe developmental delays and severe spastic quadriplegia, probably resulting from a hypoxic episode at 3 weeks of age." She has no history of seizures. Additional medical information shows normal hearing in at least one ear with history of chronic ear infections and bilateral myringotomies. She has reduced visual abilities because of cortical problems.

Functional status: Jane is dependent in all activities of daily living and self-care.:

Mobility: She is able to roll and crawl on the floor, but is otherwise dependent.

Dressing: Dependent

Eating: Manages food in her mouth

Self-feeding: Dependent, but does indicate food preference by pointing to food choice or verbalizing "more"

Hygiene: Dependent, but makes motor response to the verbal cue, "Give me your hand."

Communication: Inconsistent

Previous adaptive equipment: Prone board and Bobath ball. The ball is still used occasionally, but the board was discarded because the mother understood the doctor to say it was no longer needed. Pillows should be used to position her in the standing position.

Present aids: Wheelchair, eyeglasses, corner chair, and mobility aids.

Reliable motor responses (described by family and transdisciplinary team): Head response yes-no; eye pointing; left and right direct selection is more reliable right of midline area; right joystick; and right rocker switch. Jane's tendency not to cooperate during structured testing situations affected communication and performance to potential during the assessment. She sometimes avoided looking at objects or pictures indicated by therapists.

Reason for referral: It appeared to the transdisciplinary team at Jane's preschool that she exhibits the entry level readiness skills for enhancement of her present communication modes.

Current communication: Communication methods currently used at home include some verbalization (for example, "sick" and "yeah"), kicking her feet, rolling over to an adult for help, crying, and jabbering. When asked, "Jane, do you want to eat or drink?" she kicks her feet and may verbalize. When responding to a directive, "Are you wet? Come over here," she rolls over to the questionner, crying to express the need to be changed or fed. She has no way to indicate needs. In other environments, including preschool, she interacts by choosing between food or two toys and expresses needs by vocalizing, crying, or smiling.

Spontaneous communications included during the assessment process were occasional word approximations and the perseverative repitition of "ice cream" after she identified a picture of an ice cream cone. She also babbled reduplicated syllables, which also may have been word approximations.

Communication need: Specific needs for Jane include a communication system or combination of systems that will allow her to participate more independently in her educational environment and facilitate and augment her oral speech. Immediate needs include means to make choices and indicate her desires.

Equipment introduced: Zygo 16, joystick, Prentke-Romich Training Aid with rocker switch, Apple 2 + computer with disk drive, Echo 2 Voice Synthesizer, video display, and Unicorn membrane keyboard.

Assessment environment: Jane was seen by the transdisciplinary team in multistage assessment at the center. The team members also know Jane through the traditional therapy program at her preschool. The overall atmosphere, therefore, was relaxed and supportive. Jane attempted most tasks and activities asked of her.

Positioning: Jane shows the following movement patterns that may present difficulty in using the special equipment: increased muscle tone in either total flexion or extensor patterns, although Jane has enough control to operate simple switches. Head control is fair and more consistent when she is motivated. No problems with retention of any primitive reflexes. Jane's most functional position is in the corner chair with the lapboard and with switch or board placement at midline. Other recommendations: attach a dowel to her tray for her to hold with her left hand so as to decrease associated movements when she uses her right hand.

Motor response and visual perception: Jane successfully accesses the communication systems while sitting in her corner chair using both scanning and direct selection. For scanning, she used her right arm to approach the joystick and one-way rocker switch. With her head in midline, both the switch and reinforcement are placed in midline to maximize potential for success. Areas on a large membrane keyboard were approached with both the right and left hand, with total access to the interface. When presented with a small keyboard requiring direct selection (3½ inches), Jane exhibited increased tone and drooling. Jane wears corrective eyeglasses and appears to have some visual perception deficits related to the use of augmentative aids. More specifically, she does not appear to cross midline, does not regard materials placed left of midline, has difficulty attending to the task, and shows deficits with visual tracking.

Communication-interaction: Using a membrane keyboard with colored drawings of objects found in a purse, therapists demonstrated naming items in the purse. The keyboard was positioned at midline on the tray of the corner chair in which Jane was sitting. Each item was named by pressing the appropriate picture on the keyboard that activated the computer voice and an identical picture on the video screen. The purse was opened wide, and all items in the purse were visible. As each item was named, it was taken from the purse and given to Jane or placed on the pictured item on the keyboard. She smiled while she watched the demonstration. She did not raise her eyes to look at the video screen, nor did she look toward the pictures on the membrane keyboard. Her gaze moved primarily in the lower quadrant of the board. When encouraged to press pictures to get items in the purse, she pressed mirror and keys, the two pictures closest to her right hand. Some assistance was necessary to help her reach the "keys" picture.

Summary of findings: This child was seen for assessment and showed functional potential to be most effective in her corner chair. Reliable motor responses included scanning, using a rocker switch or joystick approached at the right and placed in midline, and direct selection with bilateral upper extremity access. Visual perception assets and liabilities that could affect success within a program or system are probably related to her motor status and developmental level. These are (1) difficulties with attention to task, (2) midline crossing, (3) regard for the full visual field, and (4) visual tracking.

Important indications of communicative interaction are Jane's ability to indicate choices by touching her choice, her attempts to say words, and head nodding for "yes" and "no." At present she tends to choose items on her right side more frequently than those on her left, her word approximations are often unintelligible, and her head-nodding responses are not reliable. However, Jane is steadily improving in all three areas.

Professional recommendations: Based on these findings, the transdisciplinary team made the following recommendations. Because Jane presently responds to objects as stimuli, a progression to photographs seems appropriate. This would encourage her to indicate choices. Direct selection appears to be an appropriate motor response, although a scanning aid might be incorporated into her program to facilitate cause and effect and visual tracking.

Jane's present functional performance and the clinical judgment of this team suggest the probability that she will become a more reliable verbal communicator. Thus efforts should be directed toward the implementation of systems and programs to facilitate her oral speech. Electronic aids would be more directive as educational motivators.

Jane would be more functional in her daily activities if she used systems that encourage verbalization and allow her to participate more independently in her academic readiness program. Clinician-made and commercially available aids that meet these criteria are Zygo 16, using a one-way rocker switch; Communicator, using a one-way rocker switch; Magic Wand Speaking Reader by Texas Instruments; Prentke-Romich Training Aid; Systems 80 with five-way rocker switch or scanning interface; Apple 2 + 48K computer with disk drive monitor membrane keyboard; and Echo 2 Voice Synthesizer.

Short-term therapy recommendations: Team intervention will be necessary in the development and training of these systems to facilitate more successful interaction. Direct therapy training at the center includes developmental-cognitive and play-work activities, including the communication systems and task components. This will take place in the center within a peer group and, as appropriate, within Jane's community interactions. At the appropriate time, equipment will be made available to Jane on a temporary basis. When it has been demonstrated that these systems help Jane to be more functional and assume appropriate life roles, third-party funding will be sought.

Immediate short-term goals for Jane, with assistance from either the therapy team at Jane's preschool or the transdisciplinary team at the center, are as follows:

1. At lunch time Jane will progress from her present stage of pointing to actual food to indicate preference to the stage of pointing to photographs. Long-term goals will expand this to other categories and line drawings.
2. To improve her visual perception, Jane will use the training aid and light scanners.
3. Activities to improve her motor reliability and energy efficiency are recommended.
4. Jane showed interest and success with a joystick. This motor control system might suggest potential for a motorized mobility system.

SUMMARY

Communication is an important activity of daily living, but verbal communication may be beyond the capacity of many children who have physical handicaps, developmental delays, or emotional disorders. Augmentative communication is a skill that is readily used by the typical verbal youngster, but it must be carefully and appropriately integrated into the developmental day and life roles of the nonspeaking child. Technological advances are such that even the most severely physically handicapped child may use an augmentative communication system through knowledgeable choice of motor access, selection mode, and output possibilities.

Multidisciplinary team intervention is indicated for the selection and training of an appropriate system, by use of assessment-training-reassessment model. In efforts to avoid the "dusty device syndrome," careful attention must be directed to positioning, linguistic skills, cognition, motor assets, motivation, expressive and receptive language development, perception, and psychosocial aspects. The occupational therapist is concerned with a traditional evaluation and treatment model directed toward the concept of communication as an activity of daily life. The therapist analyzes the components of related tasks, systems, and program designs and implements an activity program with the child to develop communication skills for functional community interaction.

Indeed, it is through my expressive language as author and your receptive language as reader that I have been able to convey my message to you. I have used an input mode of direct selection on a typewriter and have given you, the reader, permanent, readable, copy (output) in the form of this chapter: a true example of augmentative communication.

REFERENCES

1. Bliss, C.K.: Semantography, Sydney, Australia, 1965, Semantography Publications.
2. Bliss, C.K., and McNaughton, S.: The book to the film, "Mr. symbol man," Sydney, Australia, 1975, Semantography Publications.
3. Clark, C.D., Davies, C.O., and Woodcock, R.W.: Standard rebus glossary, Circle Pines, Minn., 1974, ARS, American Guidance Service, Inc.
4. Firing, M.: The physically impaired population of the United States, San Francisco, 1978, Firing and Associates.
5. LeBlanc, M.: personal communication, 1983.
6. Rehabilitation engineering, a plan for continued progress—II, Richmond, Va., 1978, Rehabilitation Engineering Center, University of Virginia.

SUGGESTED READINGS

Beukelman, D.R., and Yorkstown, K.A.: Communication system for the severely disarthric speaker with an intact language system, J. Speech Hear. Disord. **42:**265, 1977.

Computers and the disabled, Byte: The Small Systems Journal, Sept., 1982.

Copeland, K.: Aides for the severely handicapped, New York, 1974, Grune & Stratton, Inc.

Fountain Valley School District, Title IV-C ESEA: Non oral communication, Fountain Valley, Calif., 1980, California State Department of Education.

Hagan, C., Porter, W., and Brink, J.: Nonverbal communication: an alternative mode of communication for the child with severe cerebral palsy, J. Speech Hear. Disord. **38:**448, 1973.

McDonald, E.T.: Conventional symbols of English, In Vanderheiden, G., and Grilley, K., editors: Nonvocal communication techniques and aids for the severely physically handicapped, Baltimore, 1976, University Park Press.

Proceedings of the Johns Hopkins first national search for applications of personal computing to aid the handicapped, Baltimore, 1981, IEEE Computer Society.

Van Bruns-Connolly, S., and Shane, H.C.: Communication boards: help for the child unable to talk, Except. Parent, p. F19, April, 1978.

Vanderheiden, G.: Nonvocal communication resource book, Baltimore, 1978, University Park Press.

Vanderheiden, G., and Grilley, K.: Nonvocal communication techniques and aids for the severely physically handicapped, Baltimore, 1975, University Park Press.

Vanderheiden, R.C., and Harris-Vanderheiden, D.H.: Communication techniques and aides for the nonvocal severely handicapped. In Lloyd, L., editor: Communication assessment and intervention strategies, Baltimore, 1976, University Park Press.

Vickers, B.: Nonoral communication systems project: 1964-1973, Iowa City, Iowa, 1974, Campus Stores.

19

FLORENCE CLARK
ZOE MAILLOUX
DIANE PARHAM

Sensory integration and children with learning disabilities

I n the 1940s, if a child had normal measured intelligence but could not learn in a circumscribed area of academics (for example, reading), he was simply called an underachiever or, in extreme cases, labeled emotionally disturbed. Sometimes the child as well as the parents were referred for psychotherapy. In the 1950s, a child with this problem was more typically labeled as having minimal brain damage or minimal brain dysfunction, and parents were no longer regarded as contributors to the problem. Educationally handicapped or *learning disabled* are the terms most likely to be used to classify these children today, terms that circumvent the implication of brain damage or dysfunction. Why the periodic changes in the labels attached to these children? Are they merely capricious, or do they reflect some systematic historical trend in how this dysfunction and its origins are viewed? Is it important that the entry-level pediatric occupational therapist be aware of the forces that contributed to these developments?

Today the field of learning disabilities is described as lacking consensus on the basic issues of definition, assessment, and programming.[155] Eminent researchers, Kirk and Kirk,[94] recently called it nebulous and without a unified body of theory and practice. Wiederholt,[164] in a now often cited historical review on the history of the education of learning disabled children, identified controversies over definition, territorial rights of respective health and educational professions, and the lack of studies establishing the effectiveness of programs as major problems confronting the field.

Entry-level therapists must understand the history of the learning disabilities field. As they begin their practice in this area, they will be entering a field that has been plagued with uncertainties and controversies.[87] Therapists will be asked to clarify what they mean by a learning disability, to describe what their role is in the remediation of this problem, and to present data that give support to their practice. The basic assumptions therapists make about the nature of learning disabilities may be challenged by educators or physicians with a different orientation, and therapists must be prepared to address their concerns.

This chapter prepares the entry-level therapist to face and manage such conflict; it is naive to expect to enter this field and avoid the controversies. Facing conflict and managing it requires a broad view of the field and an understanding of the sources of its uncertainties and controversies. Knowledge of the ways in which the disciplines of occupational therapy and education interface with other professions involved in the management of learning disabilities must also be part of the entry-level therapist's preparation. In the first part of this chapter the field of learning disabilities in general is discussed. In the second part the focus is narrowed to occupational therapy intervention with learning disabled children. Sensory integrative procedures are used widely with this group of children, thus this chapter devotes considerable attention to them. In addition, how the occupational behavior approach might be used with such children is discussed. In the final section of this chapter there is an attempt to sort out the similarities and differences between sensory integrative, perceptual-motor, and sensorimotor approaches to treatment. The intent is that, after reading this chapter, the entry-level therapist will be prepared to communicate, with clarity, to the educators, speech pathologists, physicians, and other professionals about the role of occupational therapy in the treatment of the learning disabled child.

A discussion of educational and medical perspectives on learning disabilities should begin with a definition of this condition. Unfortunately, consensus on the definition of this term does not exist within the discipline of special education, much less across disciplines. At this point, much uncertainty exists surrounding the notions on the nature of this disorder. Despite the difficulties inherent in defining the term, learning disabled children can usually be readily recognized,[114] and educators seem to believe it to be a viable classification.[155] The presentation of the existing, and controversial, definitions of learning disabilities will be deferred until after the reader is provided with a historical perspective on the education of these children who seem to defy definition but who are apparently identifiable.

A HISTORICAL PERSPECTIVE ON THE EDUCATION AND IDENTIFICATION OF LEARNING DISABLED CHILDREN

The education and identification of some children as learning disabled was spawned by three forces: (1) the results of brain localization studies on adult brain damaged patients, (2) the inference that children with specific learning problems and normal intelligence had brain damage or brain dysfunction that interfered with learning, and (3) the federal legislation in the 1960s and 1970s that mandated educational service delivery to these children. The following analysis of these forces and their effects is based largely on Wiederholt.[164]

Results of brain localization studies: foundation phase

A number of nineteenth century physicians studied the specific effects of circumscribed lesions of the brain. Wiederholt[164] considered these physicians to have laid the foundation for the identification of learning disabilities in children. He called the period in which they worked, from about 1802 to 1933, the foundation phase. These physicians were interested in the disorders of spoken language, written language, and perceptual-motor processes that were the functional correlates of (associated with) specific brain lesions.

In the foundation phase, knowledge about the site of brain lesions and their concomitant effects was acquired through postmortem studies of the brains of pa-

tients who had demonstrated specific learning problems. For example, based on autopsy studies, Broca in the 1860s argued that a lesion to the third frontal convolution resulted in aphasia.[134] Later in 1926 Head[80] extended many of Broca's theories.

Other physicians focused on description of the brain structures implicated in disorders of written, rather than spoken, language.[82,118] Word blindness was defined by Hinshelwood[82] as "a condition in which, with normal vision and therefore seeing the letters and words distinctly, an individual is no longer able to interpret written or printed language." Based on the autopsy of a patient with this condition, Hinshelwood believed the brain's left angular gyrus to be implicated in the condition. He went a step further in that he believed that some children were born with "congenital word blindness," and he suggested a method involving three steps for teaching them to read. Twenty years later Orton[119] questioned many of Hinshelwood's views and presented a theory on alexia (the inability to read) that placed great emphasis on the dominance of one hemisphere over the other for adequacy of reading functions. Orton[120] believed that roughly 10% of school-aged children had reading disabilities because of poorly established dominance.

A third group, made up of psychologists and physicians who conducted research during this period, studied the perceptual-motor disturbances that were associated with brain lesions. Goldstein[74] proposed that, in addition to the specific learning disabilities that seemed to arise from circumscribed areas of brain injury, general manifestations of brain damage were also obvious. He described the behaviors of brain-injured adults as disordered, inattentive, and emotionally explosive. In the 1940s Strauss, a psychiatrist, and Werner, a psychologist, studied the characteristics of brain-injured children who were, in addition, mentally retarded.[143,146,162] In particular, they were interested in determining whether these children would be symptomatically similar to the brain-damaged adults described by Goldstein. Strauss and Lehtinen[145] reported that, like their adult counterparts, these children had perceptual disturbances, but the children were less able to compensate because they were born with the damage, and they had never possessed intact perceptual abilities. These children with brain damage and retardation were described as uncontrolled, erratic, inhibited, and socially less acceptable than normal children.

Whether they studied disorders of spoken language, disorders of written language, or disorders in perception, the physicians and psychologists who worked during the foundation phase contributed to the overall conceptualization of learning disabilities. First, their studies led to the belief that specific learning disabilities, for example, language or reading problems, were associated with lesions of circumscribed areas of the brain.

Second, their studies suggested that more general behavioral problems, such as distractibility, could also be associated with brain damage in both adults and retarded children. Third, they provided descriptions of clinical cases in which the manifestations of brain injuries seemed to be congenitally acquired rather than secondary to a postnatal insult.

Interventions based on inference of brain damage: transition phase

Wiederholt[164] proposed that in the period from around 1930 to 1960 the education of handicapped children was in a transition phase. In 1955 Strauss and Kephart[144] emphasized the need for professionals to work with the brain-injured child of normal intelligence. Here the conceptual leap was made that children without known brain injury did, nevertheless, possess minimal brain damage. These children were described as having problems in learning, poorly coordinated perceptions, lack of purposeful behavior, distractibility, disinhibition, and perseveration. This cluster of symptoms was called the "Strauss syndrome."[144]

Whereas physicians had been the leaders in the foundation phase, psychologists and educators were the primary contributors to the field during the transition phase. In this phase, programs for educating the child with disorders of spoken language, disorders of written language, and perceptual-motor disturbances were developed. The programs were based on models of brain processing and the assumption that learning disorders were reflections of a dysfunction in, or damage to, the brain. The knowledge of brain functioning that had been an end product of the earlier autopsy research was now translated into intervention models. It was assumed with these models that by aiming at better efficiency in brain processes, learning disabilities could be remedied. Assessment procedures were developed to identify the dysfunctional brain processes, and corresponding intervention programs were designed to change them. Because the intervention programs focused on changing the processes underlying academic learning, they collectively are referred to as process-oriented approaches.

Models of auditory-language processing were constructed by Osgood[121,122] and Wepman and others[161] and were used to guide the development of the Illinois Test of Psycholinguistic Abilities (ITPA),[95] which today, despite criticisms, is widely used in the learning disabilities field.[69] In this test the child is assessed in his receptive, associative, and expressive language functions at the automatic and representational levels. Both the auditory and visual channels are tested. Educational programs are then developed for teaching these abilities.[109] These process-oriented programs are today referred to as the psycholinguistic approach.

A second approach to developing interventions for learning disabled children was also based on the assumption that these children's brains were not processing information adequately. However, this approach presumed, in an additive manner, that the more sensory systems that were called on during a learning activity, the better would be the learning. Called multisensory teaching strategies, they emphasized kinesthetic, auditory, and visual reinforcement during learning tasks.[58,59] For example, a child would be required to say the word *circle* as she drew a circle on the blackboard.

Finally, a third type of intervention was developed in this period and, like those just described, it assumed that learning disabilities were consequent to brain dysfunction. These programs involved an initial assessment on a perceptual-motor test and then training in specific skills,[63,64,89] such as walking a balance beam, performing angels in the snow, or tracing dot-to-dot designs. Although a number of perceptual-motor training programs were developed and subtly differed from one another in some ways, all were based on the assumptions that (1) motor learning provided a foundation for symbolic learning, (2) motor development unfolded hierarchically, (3) unsatisfactory motor development would interfere with academic learning, and (4) remediation of motor deficits should contribute to better coping with traditional academics.[40]

Legislation and studies on treatment effectiveness in the 1960s and 1970s: integration phase

The 1960s ushered in what Weiderholt[164] described as an integration phase. Most of the contributions in this period were from the field of education. Educators, motivated by federal mandates and incentives, began to establish educational programs for children with learning disabilities and test the effectiveness of the process-oriented models that had been developed in the transition period.

FEDERAL LEGISLATION

The federal government was highly instrumental in the 1960s in making services available to children identified as learning disabled. Gearheart[69] provided an excellent review of this legislation. Public Law 89-10, the Elementary and Secondary Education Act of 1965, provided significant monies for local educational programs. Gearheart[69] believes that these programs probably involved children who today would be called learning disabled, since they addressed, in part, children with reading problems and neurological impairment. He qualifies his statement by pointing out that this law did not explicitly fund programs for the learning disabled child.

Public Law 91-230, the Education of the Handicapped Act, contained a title (Title VI) that addressed the educational needs of the handicapped child. Learning disabled children were *not* included in the definition of handicapped under this law. However, under Part G, the government was authorized to allocate grants to fund research, training, and model programs for learning disabled children. Gearheart[69] singles this out as the first piece of federal legislation that treated learning disabilities as a distinct handicapping condition. In 1969 only 12 states had passed legislation for funding programs for learning disabled children. By 1974 all 50 states had programs, although various terms were used to designate this group of children, such as educationally handicapped, neurologically impaired, and learning disabled. Through grants awarded under Public Law 91-230, Education of the Handicapped Act, Title VI, Part 6, Child Service Demonstration Projects (CSDP's) proliferated, and learning disabilities were established as a subcategory of special education.

Finally, in 1975 under Public Law 94-142, the Education for All Handicapped Children Act, funding was explicitly provided specifically for the education of learning disabled as well as children with other handicapping conditions. Importantly, under this law occupational therapy was mandated as a related service that should be provided to the learning disabled child, as well as to children with other handicapping conditions, when this service will improve the child's ability to benefit from special education.

STUDYING THE EFFECTIVENESS OF INTERVENTION

Not only did educational programs proliferate for the learning disabled child in the integration phase, but also many educators engaged in research on the effectiveness of existing programmatic approaches. Studies were conducted on the effectiveness of the educational systems that had been developed during the transition phase.[54,77,105,116,147] In the 1970s this issue came to a head. The perceptual-motor and psycholinguistic approaches were called process-oriented, or ability, models because the intervention was focused on remediating a particular ability (for example, visual sequencing), rather than on skill development in tasks more directly identifiable as academics. In process-oriented approaches the child is given a diagnostic test that identifies the processes in which there is dysfunction. Remediation is focused on the process, rather than on the area of academic skill in which the child is deficient.

Process-oriented models are contrasted with task analysis models that are aimed directly at skill development in specific academic tasks. The tasks are analyzed into components based on complexity, and the child is theoretically taught to master simple tasks before more complex ones. The emphasis is on component skills, rather than on terminal behaviors. Through incremental gains the child is moved from where he is to where he should be.

In 1974 Ysseldyke and Salvia[168] published a study in which they analyzed the predictive efficiency of the most frequently used instruments for measuring abilities. Based on this analysis, they concluded that ability models were essentially nonvalidated. Another study, published by Hammill and Larsen,[77] also provided data that failed to support the validity of ability models. They reviewed 37 studies in which remediation followed from a diagnosis based on the Illinois Test of Psycholinguistic Abilities,[95] and they computed percentages to estimate the net effect of all the programs. Hammill and Larsen concluded that the effectiveness of the psycholinguistic training programs had not been conclusively demonstrated.[77]

In 1977 Vellutino and others[156] provided a lengthy critique on conceptual and empirical grounds of the perceptual-deficit hypothesis of learning disabilities. They argued that data did not support the basic premise that visual perceptual disturbances contributed to reading disabilities and that the effectiveness of the programs had not been established. They then recommended task analysis for intervention with learning disabled children that emphasized behavioral rather than psychoneurological processes.

Current models of the contributors to learning disabilities

It is misleading to suggest that the entire field of special education rejected psychoneurological approaches in the integration phase. Eminent special educators such as Frostig and Maslow[65] and Cruickshank[49] tenaciously continued to endorse the position that the knowledge of the status of brain functioning is central to remediation for these children. Others argued that neurological considerations are probably relevant for some but not all learning disabilities.[86,104]

In the late 1970s the literature did not reflect a total rejection of the idea that brain dysfunction was implicated in learning disabilities. Papers published in the integration phase did raise questions about the validity of the treatment approaches that had been generated from nineteenth century conceptualizations of brain processes. New explanations of learning disabilities appeared, based on more current ideas on how the brain processes information, matures, or attends to relevant stimuli. Alternative explanations for the presence of learning disabilities emerged as well. Four of these perspectives will now be briefly presented. Familiarity with these models enables entry-level therapists to bring to their practice a broadened view on current thinking about learning disabilities.

THE ATTENTIONAL DEFICIT HYPOTHESIS

In the attentional deficit hypothesis, learning disabilities are seen as being related to deficient attentional mechanisms. While reading, a child must focus her attention on words on the page; during a classroom lecture, the instructor's words must be attended to; working a problem in geometry requires sustained concentration on the task demands. Children who have difficulty directing their attention to relevant stimuli will have problems with learning.

Harris[78] defined attention as "the presence of those behaviors which have become associated with adaptation to classroom environments and yield correct or learned responses to pertinent, task relevant stimuli or stimulus dimensions." Mirsky[110] defined it as "a focusing of consciousness or awareness on some part of the multitude of stimuli from the environment; usually on the basis of learning or training." Kinsbourne and Caplan[92] considered a type of learning disability, called a cognitive-style disorder, to be a problem with attention. These perspectives reflect the current interest in the field of learning disabilities in linking problems with attention to disorders in learning.

The attentional deficit hypothesis of learning disabilities suggests that learning disabled children may be unable to filter relevant from irrelevant information. Such impairment may result in problems with selective attention or the ability to attend to only relevant stimuli. In extreme cases the child may appear to be distractible. Selective attention has been found to be age-related.[76,100] With increased age, children become more efficient at blocking out irrelevant stimuli. Research suggests that children with dyslexia acquire selective attention in the same developmental progression as do normal children, but they seem to do so at a slower rate.[152]

Other researchers have linked learning disabilities to problems with attention.[60,85,135] In a particularly interesting study Shields[136] measured the average evoked responses (AERs) of learning disabled children to visual stimuli. In this procedure, as the children looked at the stimuli, very small changes in EEG patterns were recorded and electronically averaged. Results suggested that learning disabled children may need to focus more attention on tasks than do nonlearning disabled children. Fuller[66] also compared the brain wave activity of learning disabled and normal children. He found that the learning disabled children, when they were engaged in school-related tasks, showed immature patterns of brain activity. Other studies have suggested that learning disabled children spend more time attending to irrelevant stimuli.[52,111]

The studies that support the attentional deficit hypothesis implicate brain dysfunction in learning disabilities. After all, the brain regulates attention. Intervention strategies that have been developed in accord with the position have *not*, however, been similar to the process training systems that were developed in the transition phase. For example, in accepting the position that at least some learning disabilities may result from attentional deficits, Keogh and Margolis[88] suggest that teachers make their task expectations clear and explicit and encourage students to review available responses before acting. These procedures are not reminiscent of either perceptual-motor training or psycholinguistic interventions. They are based on the assumption that some learning disabled children act on inappropriate information in the presence of adequate perceptions. Keogh and Margolis[88] believe these children may be responding too quickly or giving insufficient attention to stimuli.

INFORMATION-PROCESSING MODELS

The advent of the computer has had its impact on psychology, particularly on how this discipline conceptualizes human information processing. Information-processing models of brain functioning liken the brain to a computer. Farnham-Diggory[56] presented a perspective on learning disabilities that employs an information-processing model. According to Farnham-Diggory, computer models of information-processing mechanisms tend to consist of certain components (Figure 19-1).

Feature detectors register minute pieces of sensory information, feature buffers store the information, and a feature synthesizer integrates it with whatever information is applied to it from a working memory. Pro-

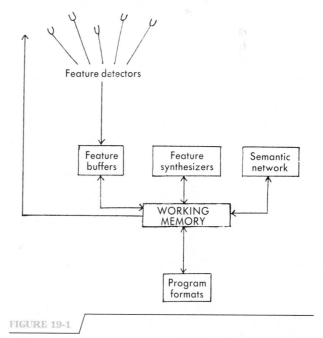

FIGURE 19-1

Schematic flowchart of human information-processing system.

From Farnham-Diggory, S.: Learning disabilities: a psychological perspective, Cambridge, Mass., 1978, Harvard University Press.

grams stored in the system guide how the information will be acted on and what responses will be made. The semantic network consists of memories of interconnected concepts. Information acquires meaning when it is interpreted in relation to the semantic network. The example of reading the word *by* illustrates the functioning of the system: visual feature detectors would register minute visual elements, and a feature synthesizer would enable the child to recognize the letters *b* and *y*; a program directs the child to combine *b* and *y* to form *by*; the child reads *by*, and the meaning he attributes to this word is acquired through reference to his semantic memory. Information-processing models do not describe the actual anatomical areas of the brain that perform these functions, but since the brain is the organ that processes information in humans, the approach implies that information-processing problems may be secondary in some instances to brain dysfunction.

Information-processing models like the one just described generate interesting theoretical explanations for the presence of learning disabilities. Farnham-Diggory[56] suggested that the type of learning disability to emerge may be contingent on the component in the system where breakdown occurs or on the availability of programs. Some children may have perfectly intact components, but they simply never have learned the strategies that enhance learning. Other children may be victims of faulty processing in any one or several of the components. The former group seems less likely to have a brain dysfunction than the latter. The information-processing model, then, suggests that some but not all learning disabilities could be neurologically related.

A number of studies have been conducted to determine at which points, as information flows through the system, a learning disability may emerge. Stanley and Hall[142] suggested that dyslexics compared to normal readers seemed to retain information in the sensory buffer for longer periods of time and retrieve information less efficiently. Farnham-Diggory[56] interpreted this study to suggest that the feature detector in the dyslexics was sluggish in clearing itself out, and the feature synthesizer was slower in synthesizing information. Dyslexics seem to retrieve and react to letters more slowly than normal readers; visual images (with the exception of digits) seem to linger for longer periods of time in their memories.[140,141,142] Farnham-Diggory[56] proposed that, if information persists in the buffer, it may interfere with the registration of new information. She suggested the net effect of this may be a blurring of details. It seems logical to assume that washing away of detail could result in a reading problem.

Other research suggests that children with dyslexia or other learning disabilities may have an insufficient supply of programs or strategies for acting on information available to them. Verbal rehearsal is an example of a program that maximizes learning. In essence, the program consists of repeating silently or aloud new information to enhance its storage in memory. Learning disabled children have been shown to be deficient in the use of this program.[148,152,153] They also seem to have trouble retrieving verbal labels into working memory.[139] A child having difficulty retrieving verbal labels (that is, she perceives a word but searches and searches for the auditory-linguistic label that she should attach to it) may not have time to verbally rehearse. Finally, Farnham-Diggory and Gregg[57] provided convincing data suggesting that learning disabled children may be more susceptible to fatigue than normal children during information processing.

There is an emerging trend for information-processing models to be used to guide educational intervention with the learning disabled child. One group of researchers has developed a series of computer-type programs for the teaching of various mental activities associated with academics.[96] Meichenbaum[107] developed an elaborate system for teaching children to be more effective in cognitive strategies, or in information-processing terms, in the use of programs. In this approach the children are taught to assess the demands of the task and use cognitive rehearsal to guide performance. A paper by Abikoff[4] reviewed the development of information-processing interventions.

THE COGNITIVE DELAY HYPOTHESIS

A group of researchers and theoreticians endorse the position that some so-called learning disabilities are actually nothing more than manifestations of immaturity.[5,47] In this perspective, learning disabilities are explained on the basis of timing. Proponents believe that the vast majority of learning disabilities would be eliminated if educational demands were tailored to the developmental, rather than the chronological, age of the child.[5]

To some extent the cognitive delay hypothesis overlaps with the information-processing and attentional deficit models of learning disabilities. Attentional mechanisms and information-processing strategies have been shown to be age dependent and acquired at a later chronological age in children with alleged learning disabilities.[34,66,76,136,153] Perhaps poor school adjustment is simply due to the child's unreadiness in his ability to focus attention on relevant stimuli or due to expecting the child to master academic skills for which he has not yet developed sufficient cognitive strategies.

Acceptance of the position that underachievement is a manifestation of delayed maturity leads to specific guidelines for intervention. Ames[5] recommends that the label *learning disabled* not be used. Instead, she suggests that school officials make a simple adjustment in grade assignment. Placement of the child in a grade with chronologically younger children in which he can meet the task demands eliminates the need for any special program. A counterposition might be that the child be retained in a class with children his age but that he be provided with a program that might accelerate maturation.

THE HEMISPHERIC DYSFUNCTION OR INADEQUATE CEREBRAL SPECIALIZATION HYPOTHESIS

In brief, the hemispheric dysfunction or inadequate cerebral specialization view suggests that learning disabilities may emerge when one cerebral hemisphere is not sufficiently specialized for a function or when, in the presence of adequate specialization, one hemisphere is dysfunctional. The position assumes that adequate hemispheric specialization and functioning is a requirement for effective learning. Research suggests that the left hemisphere specializes (becomes dominant) in verbal functions, tasks requiring sequencing, and abstract thinking.[38,68,117] In contrast, the right hemisphere assumes dominance for visual spatial tasks, intuition, and holistic thought.[117] A task such as reading, which requires attaching a verbal meaning to a visual symbol, involves the functioning and communication between the two hemispheres.[56]

A number of studies have been published linking either hemispheric dysfunction or inadequate specialization to learning disabilities.[45] It should be mentioned, however, that after reviewing the literature in this area, Kinsbourne and Hiscock[93] concluded that it was impossible to reach a consensus on the contribution of cerebral specialization to learning.

The definitional quandary: characteristics of the child with learning disabilities

The history of the education of learning disabled children has had its impact on the terms used as labels for the condition. Learning disabilities were first identified as concomitants of brain damage. When children without known lesions had the characteristics of brain-damaged persons, an inference was made that they too had brain damage, or dysfunction, of a minimal nature. The term minimal brain damage, or dysfunction, was coined and loosely used to classify a variety of children who to one extent or another had learning problems, were hyperactive, had perceptual problems, perseverated, and were clumsy. Generally, children labeled with these terms possesed measured intelligence within the normative range.

Minimal brain damage and minimal brain dysfunction, both popular terms in labeling these children in the 1950s, make certain assumptions about the precise nature of the condition. The first term, minimal brain damage, implies that these children have a lesion, that is, a site of pathology, in the brain. This term might be considered pejorative by both the child and his parents when no hard evidence can be produced indicating anatomic damage to the brain. The term minimal brain dysfunction is more nebulous, softer, and perhaps less offensive. This term does not imply that the child's brain is literally damaged. Rather, it suggests that an area of the brain may not be functioning adequately. Although the latter term is less objectionable to parents than the first, some still found it unacceptable.[69]

In 1963 Dr. Samuel Kirk, at a conference sponsored by the Fund for Perceptually Handicapped Children, argued that the term minimal brain dysfunction was of little use in educational settings because it did not lead to classroom management strategies.[69] He then went on to say that he was recently using the term learning disabilities to describe children with disorders in speech, language, reading, and associated communication skills who were neither blind, deaf, nor mentally retarded. He pointed out that this definition had the advantage of avoiding the difficulties inherent in trying to establish with certainty brain dysfunction.

Definitions that have been used at the federal level have, in essence, been in accord with Kirk's ideas. Under Public Law 94-142, specific learning disability is defined as

> A disorder in one or more of the basic psychological processes involved in understanding or in using language, spoken or written, which may manifest itself in an imperfect ability to listen, think, speak, read, write, spell or to do mathematical calculation. The term includes such conditions as perceptual handicaps, brain injury, minimal brain dysfunction, dyslexia, and developmental aphasia. The term does not include children who have learning problems which are primarily the result of visual, hearing, or motor handicaps, of mental retardation, or of environmental, cultural or economic disadvantages.[69]

Gearheart[69] points out that although this definition was accepted on a federal level, it was not accepted without controversy in the field of special education. He suggests that the definition was written into federal law because it was the least unacceptable among several alternatives. Criticisms leveled against the definition have been that it does not sufficiently emphasize the neurophysiological nature of the disorder[48,49] and that it is not sufficiently usable.[164] Standardized tests are not available that reliably differentiate learning disabled from emotionally disturbed children or children who underachieve because of educational deprivation.[164] So much controversy still exists regarding an acceptable definition of learning disabilities that the January 1983 issue of the *Journal of Learning Disabilities* featured articles on the topic written by a set of experts.[87,114,133] In addition, data from a survey published in this issue revealed that Child Service Demonstration Centers (the federally funded educational model programs for learning disabled children) failed to comply with the federal definition of learning disabilities.[104]

However, in another study a national sample of experts in the field of learning disabilities indicated that they believed that learning disabilities were clinically identifiable, either by one particular symptom or by a cluster of symptoms.[155] Entry-level therapists need to be provided with a sense of what the criteria used in the diagnosis of learning disabilities by educators are. Several examples are presented.

Chalfant and King[44] suggested the following five characteristics as being necessary to the diagnosis of learning disabilities: (1) problems in school learning, (2) uneven performance across several school-related tasks, (3) physiological correlates, (4) impaired basic psychological processes, and (5) exclusion from other categories. In the previously mentioned national study of the Child Service Demonstration Centers, low achievement, language difficulties, perceptual deficits, a discrepancy between ability and achievement, and failure in the mainstream were the most frequently cited criteria for diagnosing children as having learning disabilities.[104]

Widely used textbooks in the field of learning disabilities may be considered reflective of the views held by the proverbial average special educator. Gearheart[70] lists a severe discrepancy between academic achievement and ability and learning in a specific area (for example, oral expression and written expression) as being central to identification. He then lists the following eight other characteristics.[70] It should be noted that some of these characteristics are contradictory, but this is reasonable since Gearheart makes the point that not all the symptoms must be present in a single child.

1. *Hyperactivity.* Restlessness; the quality of being unable to sit still. Excessive movement that may interfere with the ability to selectively attend to stimuli. The child is in perpetual motion.

2. *Hypoactivity.* The opposite of hyperactivity; listlessness; sluggishness. Gearheart states that this characteristic is not as common as hyperactivity.

3. *Inattention.* The inability to focus attention on any one task for any sustained length of time.

4. *Overattention.* The inability to break a focus after having been concentrating on an activity for a sustained length of time. Gearheart links overattention to figure-ground ability. Rather than directing the attention to the significant elements in a picture, the child will focus on the background.

5. *Lack of coordination.* The inability to move the muscles in a smooth manner. Gearheart points out that although some learning disabled children do not have problems with coordination, many do. At a young age, the signs of poor coordination may be poor or slow achievement of developmental milestones. For example,

the child may have difficulty throwing a ball, skipping or running. The child may be clumsy and trip frequently.

6. *Perceptual disorders.* Gearheart lists problems in visual, auditory, tactile, proprioceptive, and vestibular perception as those most commonly seen. He believes that problems in olfactory and gustatory perception to be less likely to be associated with a learning disability, but he does not document his statement. Gearheart points out that visual-spatial problems may interfere with accurate copying of letters. He suggests that these children may have difficulty distinguishing the ringing of a phone from that of a doorbell. If a sensory acuity deficit is ruled out, perceptual disorders may be present.

7. *Perseveration.* These children may repeat actions persistently in several behavioral domains. Perseveration of verbal responses, but especially in writing and copying, may be noted.

8. *Memory disorders.* Problems may be with either visual or auditory memory or both. The child may be unable to remember a sequence of objects he has just seen or repeat several letters he has just heard. Children with these problems may forget the words in the beginning of a sentence before they read those at the end.

INCIDENCE AND TYPICAL PRACTICE SETTINGS OF OCCUPATIONAL THERAPISTS

Before the 1960s, occupational therapists working in school settings provided services nearly exclusively to orthopedically handicapped children.[72] The trend now is for most pediatric occupational therapists who work in school settings to treat learning disabled children, as well as orthopedically handicapped children. From 1973 to 1978 the numbers of occupational therapists working in the schools nearly tripled.[72] In 1977, 14% of registered occupational therapists were employed in school settings, second only to those working in acute care hospitals (22.3%).[167] The major impetus leading to increased numbers of therapists working in the schools was Public Law 94-142 and related legislation, which designated occupational therapy as a related service to which handicapped students are entitled if beneficial to the child's learning.[123]

However, nearly one third of those children who are considered to be severely learning disabled in the sixth grade are considered to be behavior disordered in secondary schools.[133] This statistic suggests that occupational therapists may be called on to treat children with the primary diagnosis of emotional disturbance who also have learning disabilities. These children may be inpatients or outpatients in mental health facilities. Occupational therapy intervention for learning disabled children, then, may be provided in either school or hospital settings. Private practices and clinics provide other alternatives.

The incidence of learning disabilities is difficult to estimate because of the problems inherent in defining the condition and the fact that a child's primary diagnosis may change to emotional disturbance when adolescence is reached. Estimates range from 1% to 20% to 30% of the school-aged population.[164]

Treating learning disabled children in educational settings

Gearheart[69] states that, in accord with the mandates of Public Law 94-142, learning disabled children in educational settings will spend most of their school day in the least restrictive environment (Chapters 1, 2, and 24). Whenever possible, and when it will not interfere with educational achievement, these children will be kept in the regular classroom. While most learning disabled children are provided with extra assistance in a resource room, a minority may require assignment on a full-time basis in a self-contained classroom. Gearheart[70] points out that it is only those who are hyperactive and have severe learning problems who will need this structure.

Because occupational therapy is designated as a related service under Public Law 94-142, it may be part of a child's educational plan when it can be shown that it is needed to maximize educational attainment. In general, the occupational therapist will be involved in identification of dysfunctional areas, implementation of planned programs, integration of occupational therapy concepts into classroom curricula, and documentation of student progress.[72] Implementation of specific therapy procedures will usually occur outside the child's classroom in a setting that is equipped with therapy media.

Treating learning disabled children in medical settings

Learning disabled children are sometimes diagnosed by physicians. Hospitals may have neurological clinics through which the learning disabled child may be provided with occupational therapy. In medical settings such children are likely to be given the diagnosis of hyperactivity syndrome, attention deficit disorder, minimal brain damage, minimal brain dysfunction, minimal cerebral dysfunction, or minor cerebral dysfunction. Learning disabilities is an educational, rather than a medical, term. In the American Psychiatric Association's[4] *Diagnostic and Statistical Manual of Mental Disorders* it is recommended that physicians use the term attention deficit disorder for children showing

short attention spans and distractibility. The manual also includes the diagnoses of other specific learning difficulties, specific reading retardation, specific arithmetical retardation, developmental speech or language disorders, and mixed developmental disorders. In a medical setting any of these labels may be used to refer to the child who, in an educational setting, would fall under the umbrella term, learning disabled.

As already pointed out, some occupational therapists will be expected to treat children with learning disabilities in mental health facilities. These children in all likelihood will have emotional and behavioral disturbances as their primary problems. Their learning disabilities will be viewed as of secondary concern. In these settings the occupational therapist will usually function as a member of an interdisciplinary mental health team. Typically, he or she will provide treatment in a clinic that is equipped with the necessary media. Patients may be treated in groups or on an individual basis.

Treating the learning disabled child in private practice settings

Occupational therapists may provide therapy to learning disabled children in private practices. While private practice offers the therapist an opportunity for a great deal of autonomous decision making, it usually results in a decreased amount of interdisciplinary contact as well. A concomitant danger is that the therapist may work in isolation, setting goals or using methods that are in conflict with those of other professionals who work with the child. The deeper insights into a child's behavior that spring from interdisciplinary communication may be curtailed. Therefore it is in the best interests of the child that the occupational therapist in private practice make special efforts to establish contact and form ongoing lines of communication with the other professionals who serve the child.

Other professionals involved in service delivery to the learning disabled child

In both medical and educational settings, occupational therapists will need to communicate with other professionals involved in service delivery to the learning disabled child. An interdisciplinary perspective on the historical development of the field has been provided in previous sections of this chapter. This orientation will not only deepen the entry-level therapist's knowledge of the field, but will also enhance the therapist's ability to communicate with professionals in other disciplines who also provide services to the learning disabled child. The evaluations and treatment approaches used by those professional groups with whom the entry-level therapist working in this area will be likely to interface are briefly described here.

EDUCATORS

As indicated so far, educators have played a central role in the learning disabilities field. Educators focus on academic performance and classroom social adjustment. They will use achievement and cognitive tests to compare the child's academic performance to age and grade expectancies. The Wide Range Achievement Test (WRAT)[83] is an example of a commonly used educational evaluation. Educational approaches for the learning disabled vary widely depending on the setting. Process-oriented methods and task analysis are often used to facilitate learning and reduce the effects of specific learning deficits.

PHYSICIANS

Pediatricians, neurologists, and psychiatrists are often consulted in the evaluation of a learning disabled child. As medical specialists concerned with amelioration of disease processes, physicians will usually evaluate the child for possible pathology within the central nervous system. Electroencephalograms, blood and urine analysis, and neurological testing may be used to help uncover dysfunction that may be contributing to a learning disorder. For children with attention deficit disorders, medications such as methylphenidate (Ritalin) or pemoline (Cylert) may be prescribed. Some physicians may also make recommendations regarding the child's diet and a general health maintenance program.

PSYCHOLOGISTS

Psychologists are generally on both educational- and hospital-based teams. They often administer educational and psychological tests to determine the child's strengths and weaknesses. Depending on the setting, a psychologist may be involved in various aspects of intervention with the learning disabled child. Psychologists may be involved in counseling programs, behavior management, and educational placement. In addition, they may provide programs aimed at enhancing overall social and emotional adjustment.

AUDIOLOGISTS

The audiologist examines the integrity of the ear and related structures and conducts assessments to determine whether hearing is impaired. When necessary, hearing aids may be prescribed to reduce learning deficits related to the hearing impairment.

SPEECH PATHOLOGISTS

Speech pathologists assess general language ability. With a learning disabled child, they may present data on whether a language or speech problem is associated with the learning problem. The Illinois Test of Psycholinguistic Abilitites[95] is an example of a language test often administered. Intervention may include activities and exercises to improve articulation, comprehension, expression, and overall language development.

OPTOMETRISTS

Optometrists are licensed specialists who measure the range and power of vision, examine the eye, and prescribe corrective lenses. They may prescribe orthoptics, which are exercises to improve oculomotor functions.

ADAPTIVE PHYSICAL EDUCATORS

Adaptive physical education teachers are specially trained to provide physical education programs for handicapped children. Evaluations such as the Bruininks-Oseretsky Test of Motor Proficiency[41] may be used to evaluate motor functions such as strength and coordination. Perceptual-motor programs aimed at developing specific motor skills are commonly integrated into the school system by adaptive physical educators to enhance physical conditioning and skill development.

OCCUPATIONAL THERAPY AND THE TREATMENT OF THE LEARNING DISABLED CHILD

Occupational therapists are concerned with the role performance of the learning disabled child. The student role requires competence in learning and in the organization of the customary daily round of activities in which one must engage to support learning. A learning problem can result from a child's brain's inability to organize sensory input or from the child's inefficiency in organizing his behavior and concentrating on learning tasks. A type of neural irregularity may be associated with difficulty in developing habits that support academic achievement, such as automatic use of verbal rehearsal, or the discipline required to do homework and study. The child may be unable to manage daily activities in ways that optimize student role performance.

Most often the occupational therapist has treated the learning disabled child by using sensory integrative procedures that aim to improve efficiency of neural processing. While research has shown that a sensory integrative approach can benefit some learning disabled children,[18,23,27] it is not appropriate for all. The occupational behavior frame of reference, which can be interpreted to subsume the use of sensory integrative procedures,[101,128] provides a global perspective that expands the focus of occupational therapy from the neurobiological to the sociocultural and environmental dimensions.

Most of this chapter goes into detail on the use of

sensory integrative procedures with learning disabled children. Initially, however, a brief coverage of the occupational behavior frame of reference in relation to the child who is considered to be learning disabled is provided. The inclusion of this section reflects the conviction that occupational behavior is a broad conceptual framework that can guide occupational therapy with learning disabled children, regardless of whether or not sensory integrative procedures are applied.

The occupational behavior frame of reference and the child with a learning disability

The occupational behavior approach (Chapter 3) has special relevance for the child with learning disabilities. Takata,[151] in the introduction to a series of articles on occupational behavior in pediatrics, states that the movement of pediatric occupational therapy practice from hospitals to schools requires an expansion of occupational therapy approaches beyond those derived from sensory integrative theory. In the occupational behavior approach, as Takata describes it, the focus is on how effectively the individual occupies particular life roles in the family, in school, and in the community. Children and youth in need of health care are seen not as individuals with categorical disabilities, such as cerebral palsy, or learning disabilities, or mental retardation, but as individuals who are required to meet specific expectations associated with particular roles. This assumption, when applied to the child with learning disabilities, translates into a concern for how well the child is performing in a student role. In using the occupational behavior approach with the learning disabled child, the therapist might address the following questions.

1. How does the child play? Is play encouraged or discouraged by her parents or by the home environment? Does the child's play support the building of skills that are required for success in the student role?[61,131,149]

2. How is the child proceeding in the occupational choice process? Is he in the fantasy, tentative, or realistic stage? Will his learning disability render his occupational choices unrealistic?[158]

3. How does the child's home environment encourage or discourage success in the student role? Does it contain elements that suggest a valuing of school-related competencies? Is it conducive to an organized approach to studying and mastery of school requirements? What are the attitudes of the family toward the skills that support academic achievement and school social adjustment? Is the home environment one that would generate in the child a desire to do well in school?[33]

4. What kind of habits has the child developed? Does she effectively organize her behavior into routines that are consistent with task requirements, both in the home and in the school setting? To what extent does someone else organize her activity?[90,91]

5. What are the unspoken demands of the home and school environment? Is the child expected to perform beyond his current levels of skill? What are the requirements of the child's role as student?[33]

These questions were generated from the occupational behavior perspective that was originated by Reilly[128] and that since has been extended in the writing of numerous other therapists. Kielhofner and Burke[90] and Kielhofner, Burke, and Igi[91] have synthesized many of the ideas presented in these papers. In brief, these writers suggested that central to the occupational behavior perspective is the idea that skills are consolidated by the child into habits and internalized roles. Habits are defined as automatic routines that provide consistency in daily life. When habits fail, conscious decision making (or volition) must be employed. Habits undergo transformations as the child matures. For example, on entry to school, the first grade child will apply habits learned at home to the new setting. If she had had the pattern of hanging her coat up when she entered her home, she would be likely to adapt and use this habit in the new school setting. Similarly, if she had learned to maintain a neat work space during projects at home, it is unlikely she would be messy in task performance in kindergarten.

Internalized roles were defined by Kielhofner and Burke[90] as a personal sense of the complete set of behaviors required in occupying a position in a social group. The role of student encompasses behaviors that support both academic achievement and social adjustment in the classroom. It is conceivable that a child labeled as learning disabled might possess the habits that could support competency in the student role, but he simply is oblivious to what is required of him. He may misread the expectations his teachers and peers have of him. For example, he may think that being overattentive is a desirable trait, and his enactment of this characteristic might interfere with learning. More commonly, though, the breakdown of role performance of the learning disabled child would seem to be a result of insufficient or inappropriate skills and habits that organize behavior, rather than of a misconstruing of role expectations.

Thus far the discussion of the role dysfunction of the learning disabled child has focused on the role of student. This focus is consistent with a major tenet of the occupational behavior frame of reference that treats the occupational role as an entity distinct from familial and sexual roles. Occupational roles are defined by Kielhofner and Burke[90] as "the productive roles that determine the bulk of daily routines and thus organize most of the behavior within the system." For the school-aged child, the role of student meets the specifications of this definition. At the same time, it is permissible for the therapist using this approach to address familial and sexual roles, especially in relation to how they influence occupational role performance.

Following assessment of the learning disabled child, which addresses the questions previously listed and which may use some of the instruments described by Florey,[62] a treatment program is developed. Because the aim in this section is simply to provide the reader with a sense of how the occupational behavior perspective could be used with a learning disabled child, no attempt is made here to provide specific information on this approach. Instead, a sketch of what form the treatment might take is presented.

The occupational behavior frame of reference holds that skills are learned and mastered within the context of play. If a learning disabled child had a specific writing disability, for example, and was clumsy in her execution, the occupational therapist might provide a pressureless environment in which the child could use play experiences to improve coordination. In this arena the child would be free to explore the properties of writing implements and of her own body as she uses them. The therapist might consult with the child's parents, providing guidance on how play experiences at home could be constructed and encouraged to support writing proficiency.

If the child was found not to have developed sufficient interests to eventually support an optimal occupational choice, and was at the age when this is expected, the therapist might use the therapy situation for exploration of interests. The therapist might involve the child in activities he had never engaged in before and encourage him to appraise how satisfying such an experience was. The therapist additionally might try to familiarize the child with potential occupations with which his learning disability would not interfere.

A third goal of therapy might be to make recommendations for how the home environment might be altered to support the child's student role performance. If the child was found to be distractible, a minimally stimulating and isolated area of the house could be designated as a study area for the child. A proper work space could be designed or constructed and supplies could be purchased (presuming the family had sufficient funds); lighting could be assessed and altered if it was found to be less than optimum. The child's daily habits could be addressed. If she lacked organization, the therapist could work with her on organization and sequencing of simple daily tasks. If her parents have not provided opportunities for the child to organize her own behavior, the therapist could encourage them to do so.

Finally, within the clinic situation the child could be presented with environmental challenges matched to his level of skill so that he could experience a sense of success. Media such as art, games, and play chosen to be in accord with the child's readiness would be used. While participating in these activities, the therapist could note whether there is improvement in the child's ability to selectively attend to relevant stimuli and improvement in his work habits, organization of behavior, risk-taking, and decision making.

The emergence and use of sensory integrative procedures

Sensory integrative procedures are widely used in occupational therapy practice with children with learning disabilites. The guidelines for the use of these procedures were derived from principles of sensory integrative theory as developed and described by Ayres[19,28] (Chapter 3). For the entry-level therapist to comprehend the place of this approach within the practice of occupational therapy and how it is specifically used with the learning disabled child, the knowledge of the forces that contributed to its evolution is essential. The entry-level therapist needs to be provided with an overview of how the applications of sensory integrative theory were developed and underwent change. A perspective is also needed on the current use of these procedures with learning disabled children.

Before the development of sensory integrative theory, occupational therapists had traditionally been concerned with the relationship of childhood occupation to disability. Occupations, in this context, refer to the purposeful, culturally defined, and self-directed activities children engage in during their customary daily round of activities.[165] Occupational therapists also had a long history of addressing the disorders of language, movement, and perception that followed brain injury. Sensory integrative procedures, when they emerged, were a logical and natural extension of past practice.

THE TRADITIONAL FOCUS ON CHILDHOOD OCCUPATION

In the 1940s and 1950s pediatric occupational therapy was described by physicians as an essential medically related profession that contributed to the well-being of the hospitalized child.[36,126,129] Occupational therapists were described as being concerned with the play and daily life activities (occupations) of the child. In this period Allessandrini[2] extolled the virtues of play, arguing that it was a serious undertaking for children, which should not be confused with diversion or ill use of time.

The tradition of using play as a treatment medium has been continued through the development of the occupational behavior frame of reference.* However, the

---

*References 51, 61, 62, 108, 131, 149, and 150.

idea that culturally defined self-directed and purposeful activity should be used as a treatment medium was also retained in the applications of sensory integrative theory to practice. Treatment in this approach would be directed toward improvement in the organization of behavior through self-directed, purposeful, and pleasurable activity, which in addition was chosen for its organizing effects on the brain.

INTEREST IN DISORDERS OF SYMBOLIC FUNCTION FOLLOWING BRAIN INJURY

Occupational therapists, before the emergence of sensory integrative theory, had had an interest in disorders of symbolic functions following brain injury. Their experience in the area made them a natural choice among the available professions for treating learning disabled children. In the early 1950s two papers were published that addressed the relationship of occupational therapy to aphasia.[71,125] Palmer and Berko[125] reviewed the classic works on brain localization and aphasia (for example, studies by Broca) and described Goldstein's ideas on the characteristics of brain-damaged adults. Giden, Eno, and Bosley[71] described how aphasia and the other disturbances associated with brain injury affected performance of workshop activities such as weaving. They suggested that with aphasia patients therapists should deemphasize perfection and allow success, and therapists should start with familiar activities and select those that would prepare the patient for future role performance.

McDaniel[106] reiterated many of the ideas originally presented by Giden, Eno, and Bosley. In her paper the aphasia-related disorders were reviewed with descriptions of both the language-related (for example, sensory aphasia and motor aphasia) and the nonlanguage-related disturbances (for example, loss of attention, concentration, perseverance, and poor organizational abilities). McDaniel[106] recommended that occupational therapists provide speech reeducation programs when speech therapists were not available. When they were, she suggested that occupational therapists reinforce speech acquisition within the context of purposeful activity.

The fact that occupational therapists had had a tradition of working with aphasic adults and children before the 1960s when sensory integrative theory was developed probably influenced how that theory would be conceptualized. The publications previously cited[71,106] presented two principles that would be retained in sensory integrative theory. First, they suggested that within the context of occupation (or purposeful activity) language acquisition might be indirectly enhanced. Second, they suggested that engagement in activity could be graded in accord with severity of brain dysfunction.

USE OF SENSORY STIMULATION TO EVOKE COORDINATED MOTOR RESPONSES

Occupational therapists had traditionally practiced in hospital settings with patients who had neuromuscular problems secondary to brain damage (for example, cerebral vascular accident or cerebral palsy). Uncoordinated movement patterns, abnormal muscle tone, and the presence of abnormal reflexes interfered with performance of functional and purposeful activities. It became clear to therapists in the 1950s and 1960s that increased normalization of motor performance was a prerequisite to the achievement of self-care and other skills.

In this period a number of treatment approaches were described in the literature in which neurophysiological principles, emphasizing sensory stimulation, were employed to promote better execution of movement patterns. These approaches are called sensorimotor because all of them emphasized the relationship between sensation and the motor response. Principles of these approaches would be incorporated in sensory integrative theory when it emerged. However, in its concern with occupation, self-directed activity, symbolic functions, and the capacity of the individual to organize his own behavior, sensory integrative theory would depart from these approaches and become a distinct entity.

In the 1950s and 1960s publications by Mysak and Fiorentino,[115] Ayres,[8] and Voss[157] were representative of the sensorimotor approach. Procedures described tended to be specific to particular muscle groups and were based on detailed and precise descriptions of neurophysiological principles derived from laboratory studies on lower animals. Concepts in neurophysiology, such as summation, irradiation, and inhibition, were defined and inferences were made as to how these concepts could be employed in treatment to foster more normal movement patterns in patients with brain lesions. The proprioceptive and tactile base of movement was given strong emphasis.

The sensorimotor approaches armed occupational therapists with numerous techniques based on sound physiological principles for improving patient neuromuscular responses. The notion that sensory input could improve motor responses would become a major principle of sensory integrative theory.

CONCERN WITH PERCEPTION AND THE ORGANIZATION OF BEHAVIOR

Occupational therapists have had a tradition of being concerned with how brain-damaged and mentally ill patients could learn to better organize their behavior, perceive their environments accurately, and exercise sufficient concentration on a task to complete it successfully. They have been particularly concerned with how occupation could be used to promote these capacities. In 1949 Ayres[6] presented principles of grading activities in accord with organic reactions of the brain to electroshock (a treatment that is used in mental health facilities for depressed patients). She suggested that activities be selected that psychodynamically matched the affective state of the client. Postelectroshock patients were described as having "confused and clouded sensorium,"[6] progressive memory loss, impaired coordination, and an inability to perform abstract reasoning or use their imaginations. The ways in which numerous craft activities (occupations) could be adapted to promote organized behavior in these patients were then detailed.

Engagement in purposeful activity required patients to be able to accurately perceive the tools and other objects in their environment, sequence their actions to accomplish a goal, and execute the appropriate motor responses. In 1954 Robinault[130] argued that the role of occupational therapy needed to be broadened with the child with cerebral palsy. She suggested it should include the teaching of colors, shapes, and size discrimination. She regarded the focus on the mechanics of grasp and release and on self-care skills as necessary but not sufficient for the rehabilitation of these children.

In the same year Ayres[7] published a paper in which she discussed how principles of ontogeny could be used for developing arm and hand functions. In a paper published in 1958, which was influenced by the ideas of Rood,[132] Hebb,[81] and Strauss and Kephart,[144] Ayres[9] further elaborated on her ideas on the interface between occupational therapy and visual-motor functions, that is, eye-hand coordination. Ayres defined perception as "the use of sensations, rather than raw sensations in themselves."[9] The perceptual process was defined as being concerned with how the sources of sensation were integrated for use. In contrast to it, Ayres described the motor process as entailing ideation of the task to be performed (ideational motor planning). Principles and procedures for training visual-motor functions involving primarily tabletop activities, such as puzzles and pegboards, were then described.

Occupational therapy's concern with perceptual functions was also reflected in an article by Troyer[154] who presented many ideas on how therapists could use activity to enhance perceptual-motor functions. Troyer maintained that integration of the sensory and motor systems was required for the development of precise, coordinated, active, and perceptive individuals.

The emergence of sensory integrative theory and its research base for practice

Sensory integrative theory has been developed over the course of more than 20 years: 1960 to the present. The theory addresses how humans develop the capacity to organize sensation for the purpose of accomplishing self-directed, meaningful activity. It continues to undergo modification. Support for its validity is found in neurobehavioral studies (generally conducted on animals), in studies on child development, and in research on children with learning disabilities, as well as on those with other disabling conditions. In this section some key principles of the theory that provide the foundation for treatment and how these principles influenced the practice that would follow them are presented. Next, the steps in the research process, which Ayres took in developing the theory, are reviewed. Knowledge of the latter lessens the potential for misuse of the theory, its procedures, and its instruments. A grasp of the research base of this theory is also essential for those therapists who may be called on to justify its use in practice, for example, in testifying at an educational placement hearing.

BASIC PRINCIPLES OF SENSORY INTEGRATIVE THEORY

Sensory integrative theory in this text is being defined as the concepts presented by Ayres.[19,28,29] We do not consider this theory to be within the same category as the sensorimotor theories that have primarily addressed the eliciting of coordinated motor responses, that is, neuromuscular function.[37,132,157] At the same time, we acknowledge, and so did Ayres, that some of the principles of the sensorimotor approaches were incorporated into the building of sensory integrative theory. The use of sensory integrative procedures is sometimes referred to as sensory integrative therapy. We discourage the use of this term, because it implies separateness from occupational therapy. Sensory integrative procedures are designed to be used within the context of occupational therapy.

Sensory integrative theory is complex, and mastery of it requires extensive reading of the neurobiological literature, a solid preparation in neurophysiology and neuroanatomy, and study of Ayres' original writings. We distinguish between the theory, which refers to selected concepts and principles related to central nervous system functioning and development, and the treatment procedures that follow it.

Central to the theory is an explanation of how children develop the capacity to organize their own behavior. Ayres[28] pointed out that the newborn hears, sees, and feels sensations from his body; however, he is unable to judge distances or attach meanings to the sounds he hears. As the ability to organize sensation and behavior develops, the child may become better able to focus attention on relevant stimuli, remain organized for longer spans of time, and execute a customary daily round of activities in a manner that supports an occupational role. This process of organizing sensory information in the brain to make adaptive responses is what Ayres called sensory integration.[19]

The application of sensory integrative theory to practice can be summarized through explication of the following principles that are drawn from Ayres.[19,28,29]

1. *Controlled sensory input can be used to elicit an adaptive response.* Ayres defines an adaptive response as "an appropriate action in which the individual responds successfully to some environmental demand."[28] It implies dealing with the environment in a "creative and useful way."[28] An example of an adaptive response in an infant is observed when she sucks competently. Rocking a hobby horse constitutes an adaptive response in the toddler (in which she must coordinate trunk flexion and extension). For the older child it may be ice skating. Adaptive responses require the child to organize sensation, accurately judge the requirements of the situation, and execute the response competently. Whenever a child experiences the type and amount of sensory stimulation that challenges but does not overwhelm the central nervous system, the evincing of an adaptive response is potentiated (Figure 19-2).

2. *An adaptive response contributes to the development of sensory integration.* Each time a child is able to successfully meet a challenge from the environment, the ability to organize sensory input to meet environmental demands increases. Ayres[19] believes that motor activity is a powerful organizer of sensory input. As adaptive responses are emitted, the nervous system uses its knowledge of the results of past actions to guide the organization of sensory information for future use.

3. *The more inner-directed a child's activities, the greater the potential of the activities for improving neural organization.* This principle assumes that children possess an inborn motivational force toward sensory integration, which Ayres calls "inner drive."[19,28] The child is seen as naturally attracted to activities that require and bring about brain organization of sensory input. For example, it can be speculated that an 18-month-old whose nervous system may be overwhelmed by the vestibular input provided by swinging would shy away from this activity. On the other hand, possibly because of an increased capacity to organize sensation of this type, 3- and 4-year-olds will seek out those activities that incorporate swinging. Therapy that makes use of this inner drive capitalizes on the inherent capacity of the child to seek out those activities that will bring about brain organization (Figure 19-3).

4. *More mature and complex patterns of behavior are composed of consolidations of more primitive behaviors.* Ayres believes that children meld previously learned functions together for the creation of more mature adaptive responses. Emission of increasingly mature adaptive responses is a product of practice of each sensory and motor element. Underlying the changes in behavioral complexity are parallel advances in neural organization. As brain stem processing of sensory input becomes more efficient, higher cortical functions are freed to develop more fully.

5. *Better organization of adaptive responses will enhance the child's general behavioral organization.* While some adaptive responses are simple unitary acts, others require more complex sequencing and timing of motor activities. The child must figure out how to order and time a set of motor responses to achieve a goal (Figure 19-4). In essence, the child must program her actions. Ayres reasons that engagement in this process may en-

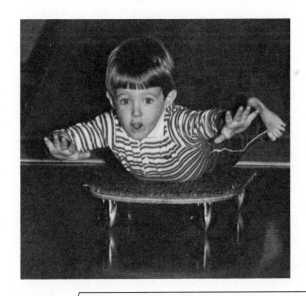

FIGURE 19-2

Adaptive response elicited by linear vestibular stimulation.
Photograph by Dooley Brown.

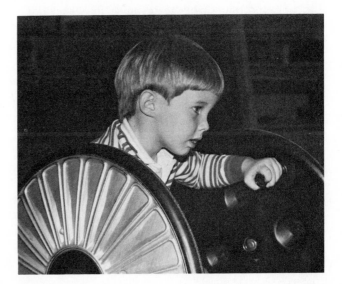

FIGURE 19-3

This child's expression reflects inner direction, suggesting that this activity requiring motor planning will promote neural organization.
Photograph by Dooley Brown.

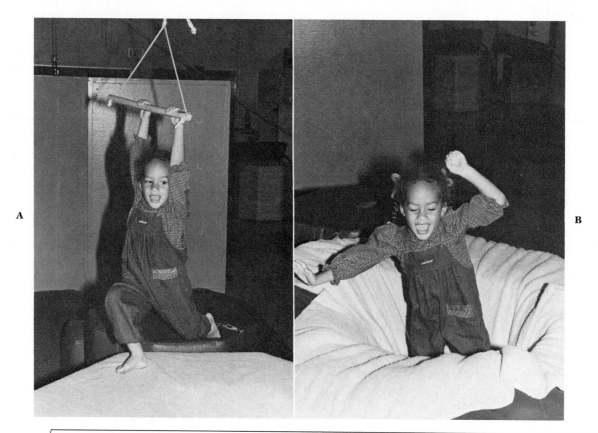

FIGURE 19-4

Activity requiring sequencing and timing. **A,** Child must push off and grasp the trapeze. **B,** Child then must time the release of her hands and her jump into the blanket.

Photograph by Dooley Brown.

hance the child's general programming capacity.[29] For example, an improvement in this general capacity may lead to being better able to organize the usual daily round of activities or the steps required to accomplish a school-related task.

6. *Registration of meaningful sensory input is necessary before an adaptive response can be made.* During the course of a day, individuals notice some but not all of the stimuli in their environments. The stimuli that are noticed influence the motor responses that are made. If a child is oblivious to many of the stimuli in the environment, her repertoire of adaptive responses will be limited, and her potential for developing more complex behaviors will thus be thwarted. On the other hand, some children seem to register sensory input excessively. These children may be bombarded by input to such a degree that they have difficulty extracting meaning from sensation or focusing on a goal-directed task.

• • •

These principles provide the foundation on which treatment is based. Discussion of treatment will be deferred until after an overview of the steps Ayres took in the construction of the theory is provided.

THE EMPIRICAL BASE OF AN EVOLVING THEORY

Instrument construction. In the late 1950s and early 1960s, based on review of the literature in development, neurobiology, psychology, education, and clinical experience, Ayres formulated hypotheses about which psychoneurological functions might be implicated in learning disabilities. She then constructed the precursors of the 18 tests that are now called the Southern California Sensory Integration Tests (SCSIT).[20] Each test was presumed to be a measure of a psychoneurological process that contributed to the capacity to learn and had set administration and scoring procedures. The tests were given to large groups of normal children, and tables of normative data were prepared. These tables indicated the average performance of children without dysfunction and within specific age groups. The tests measured aspects of visual and tactile perception and certain motor functions.

Typology. Ayres was interested in using these tests diagnostically with children who had already been labeled as having learning problems. An assumption she made was that there were probably many different kinds of learning problems, each of which might be associated with dysfunction in a particular neural substrate. She conceived of the Southern California Sensory Integration Tests as tests that would allow for the differential diagnosis of the neural substrates that contributed to learning problems.

Before the Southern California Sensory Integration Tests could be used in this way, a classification system (typology) of neural systems related to learning needed to be constructed. Ayres used a procedure called factor analysis to develop the typology. In this procedure, sets of test scores are grouped according to their associations. Ayres interpreted the clusters that emerged from the factor analytic studies she conducted on learning disabled children as being representative of several neural substrates contributing to learning.[19]

The factor analytic studies Ayres conducted are summarized in Table 19-1. In 1965 Ayres[13] administered the precursors of the Southern California Sensory Integration Tests to 100 children suspected of having perceptual-motor handicaps (note that this term was used as a synonym for learning disabled in the 1960s) and to 50 normal children. Ayres was interested in determining whether the neural systems (factors) measured by these tests would differ in the two groups of children. Four of the factors—which she called tactile defensiveness, perceptual dysfunction form position in two dimensional space, deficit of bilateral integration, and apraxia—emerged only in the dysfunctional group of children. These neural systems were interpreted to represent dysfunction rather than a developmental process. The fifth factor, called figure-ground perception, emerged in both groups and was interpreted as being related to a developmental process.

This study was especially important in that it suggested that perceptual-motor problems were associated with neural processes involving integration of input from more than one sensory modality. The dysfunctional children did not appear from the data to have unimodal sensory disturbances (for example, a discrete problem in visual perception). Each factor (neural system) that emerged was contributed to by at least two sensory systems. It appeared that neural substrates concerned with intersensory integration contributed to learning disabilities. This idea became a major tenet of sensory integrative theory.

In 1966 Ayres[14,15] performed the next two factor analytic studies. In the first of these, the precursors of the Southern California Sensory Integration Tests were given to 92 children, 10% of whom had possible central nervous system dysfunctions. In the second study the tests were given to 64 adopted children, ages 4 to 8, who were within the normative range on the Gesell Developmental Schedules. This study suggested that normal children did not vary in the same way as did dysfunctional children in their performances on the Southern California Sensory Integration Tests. These findings

reinforced the idea that the neural systems being measured on the tests in the dysfunctional group were representative of dysfunction rather than a developmental progression. These data found support for the idea that learning disabilities were related to brain dysfunction.

In 1969 Ayres[16] conducted another major factor analytic study. In this study the neural syndromes were further defined by their extent of relationship to auditory-language functions. Ayres gave the 36 educationally handicapped (another popular term synonymous with the term learning disabled) children the Southern California Sensory Integration Tests along with the Illinois Test of Psycholinguistic Abilities. The factor structure (interpreted as neural syndromes) that emerged was relatively consistent with that found in the prior factor analytic study in which dysfunctional children made up the sample. The results suggested that the typology that had emerged could be used for diagnosing types of neural dysfunction in children with learning disabilities.

In 1972 Ayres[21] conducted a factor analysis of scores on 48 tests (including the Southern California Sensory Integration Tests and the Illinois Test of Psycholinguistic Abilities) obtained by 148 educationally handicapped children. Ayres published another paper in which she used statistical procedures (the computation of regression equations) to determine which tests were predictive of the six factors that had been isolated in the study published in 1972.[17] (Note that these two studies seem to have been published out of sequence.) The factors that emerged were labeled form and space perception, auditory-language functions, postural and bilateral integration, praxis, and functions of the left side of the body. These studies found additional support for the notion that the tests were measuring particular neural substrates related to learning that could be used to classify types of dysfunction in learning disabled children.

In 1977 Ayres[24] reported the findings on another major factor analysis. The subjects were 128 educationally handicapped children. Results suggested the Southern California Sensory Integration Tests, along with auditory-language tests, were measuring five major domains: somatosensory processing and motor planning, auditory-language functions, postural ocular responses, eye-hand coordination, and postrotary nystagmus. Importantly, in this study, the results on the Southern California Postrotary Nystagmus Test (SCPNT)[22] were included. This test was a measure of the duration of reflexive to-and-fro movements of the eyes that are induced by rotation about the body axis. Results of this test were interpreted as an index of the status of some aspects of vestibular function.

It is apparent that when the Southern California Sensory Integration Tests were given to different samples of children, their factor structure remained fairly

TABLE 19-1   Purpose, hypotheses, design, results, and contributions of Ayres' factor analytic and regression studies

Year	Purpose	Instruments	Hypothesis	Design	Subjects	Results	Contribution to theory
1965	Identify relationships among sensory perception, motor performance, laterality in normal and children with perceptual problems Establish construct and discriminant validity	Early versions of the Southern California Sensory Integration Tests, (SCSIT), additional perceptual-motor and laterality tests, also freedom from hyperactivity and tactile defensiveness	Test results would identify factors for children with and without dysfunction Normal and dysfunctional children will demonstrate different factors	Thirty-three tests Two behavioral parameters Analysis of difference between group means Q- and R-technique factor analysis	N = 100 dysfunctional N = 50 normal Dysfunctional children had learning or behavioral disorders	Tests discriminated between normal and dysfunctional groups Five patterns detected: Apraxia Dysfunction form and space perception Deficit bilateral integration Visual figure-ground perception Tactile defensiveness	Established discriminant validity of early versions of test Most children demonstrated more than one factor, therefore factors related Sensory integration-clusters were not by sensory systems Praxis and tactile functions linked Tactile defensiveness, hyperactivity, distractibility linked Cognitive aspects deemphasized Eye-hand agreement not discriminative Empirical support for syndromes
1966a	Explore perceptual-motor function relationships in a normal sample and compare with prior studies Establish construct validity	Frostig tests, early versions of the SCSIT Also freedom from hyperactivity and tactile defensiveness	That factors would emerge	Seventeen tests Two behavioral parameters R-technique factor analysis (simplified matrix)	N = 92 Formed normal distribution, 10% abnormal, three with mild CP	Praxis accounted for most variance: Motor planning, kinesthesia, tactile functions, motor accuracy, bilateral coordination Visual perception factor: Ayres Space Test, Frostig	More support for praxis syndrome Visual component without motor element Perceptual-motor functions correlate as a whole in normative sample Kinesthesia closer to tactile than visual perception as in prior study

Year	Purpose	Tests/Procedures	Hypothesis	Sample	Analysis	Results	Comments
1964b	Provide an understanding of whether syndromes represent dysfunction or developmental lag. Establish construct validity	Nearly the same as 1966a	That variation in perceptual-motor abilities would be small in a group of normal children	N = 64 Adopted, all normal on Gesell	Sixteen tests. Two behavioral parameters. R-technique factor analysis	Visual motor ability accounted for most variation. Praxis and tactile perception were least variable. Hyperactivity, distractibility, tactile defensiveness factor. Factors weak because of lack of variance in performance of normal children	Suggested that low scores in praxis and tactile perception represent developmental deviation, not delay. Little systematic variation when tests given to normal children. Tactile defensiveness-hyperactivity may have a maturational component
1969	To provide an in-depth analysis of dysfunctional patterns in children with learning handicaps. Establish construct validity	Sixty-four tests and observations: SCSIT, psycholinguistic, intelligence, auditory, postural-ocular reactions, academic achievement	Brain functions involve several levels and will cluster accordingly	N = 36 Educationally handicapped children	Q-technique factor analysis	Five factors identified: Auditory language, sequencing. Postural and bilateral integration. Right hemisphere dysfunction. Apraxia. Tactile defensiveness	Hints to left hemisphere dysfunction
1971	To identify predictors of severity of sensory integrative syndromes	Forty-eight tests and observations: SCSIT, psycholinguistic, intelligence, eye-hand usage, postural responses	That predictive equations would emerge	N = 140 Educationally handicapped	Ten-step regression equations for each syndrome calculated	Presence of more than one type of disorder was the norm. Prone extension best predictor of postural-bilateral integration. Imitation of postures best predictor of praxis	Somatosensory and praxis linked again. Elucidated best predictors of syndromes. As many children may have apraxia as have postural and bilateral coordination problems

Continued.

Adapted from Ayres, A.J.: Percep. Mot. Skills **20**:335, 1965; Ayres, A.J.: Am. J. Occup. Ther. **20**(2):68, 1966; Ayres, A.J.: Am. J. Occup. Ther. **20**(6):288, 1966; Ayres, A.J.:J. Learn. Disabil. **2**(3):44, 1969; Ayres, A.J.: Am. J. Occup. Ther. **25**(7):329, 1971; Ayres, A.J.: Am. J. Occup. Ther. **26**(1):13, 1972; Ayres, A.J.: Am. J. Occup. Ther. **31**(6):362, 1977.

TABLE 19-1, cont'd   **Purpose, hypotheses, design, results, and contributions of Ayres' factor analytic and regression studies**

Year	Purpose	Instruments	Hypothesis	Design	Subjects	Results	Contribution to theory
1972	To further analyze and refine factors Establish construct validity	Same as above	That similar factors as previously would emerge	R-technique factor analysis	N = 148 Educationally handicapped	Six factors identified: Form and space perception Auditory language Postural occular Motor planning Reading-spelling and IQ Hyperactivity, tactile perception	Further confirmed left hemisphere dysfunction Reconfirmed syndromes found in other samples of learning disabled children
1977	To further analyze interrelationships (add Southern California Postrotary Nystagmus Test [SCPNT]) so that differential diagnosis can be further refined	SCSIT SCPNT, postural-ocular and lateralization measures, dichotic listening, Illinois Test of Psycholinguistic Abilities (ITPA), intelligence, academic achievement Flowers-Costello (auditory)	That clusters would continue to be refined	Series of R-technique factor analyses (not all measures entered each time)	N = 128 Learning disabled	Five major domains identified: Somatosensory-motor planning Auditory-language Postural-ocular Eye-hand coordination Postrotary nystagmus	Further elucidated nature of interhemispheric integration Role of vestibular system clarified

consistent. Table 19-2 provides a perspective on which of the factors (neural systems) were isolated most consistently. It can be seen that the apraxia factor emerged in nearly all the studies in which dysfunctional children made up the sample. Deficits in form and space perception were more varied, and the configuration and patterns of the clusters suggested that there were at least two kinds of visual perceptual problems. The first seemed to be related to somatosensory processing, the second to functions associated with the right hemisphere. Deficits in postural and bilateral integration emerged relatively consistently and in later studies[23,27] were linked to vestibular dysfunction. Finally, auditory-language dysfunctions seemed to bifurcate in the same way that visual spatial perception had. One type seemed to be related to the left hemisphere and did not seem to be related to sensory integrative processes. The second type was found in association with vestibular dysfunction and poor bilateral integration. In nearly every study a strong association between tactile defensiveness and hyperactivity was found.

Results across these studies were synthesized, and a typology was adopted for diagnosing types of sensory integrative dysfunction on the basis of the Southern California Sensory Integration Tests and Southern California Postrotary Nystagmus Test scores; results of clinical observations of neuromuscular responses; and information, when available, from auditory-language tests. The following is the typology in current use:

1. Vestibular bilateral integration dysfunction
2. Dyspraxia
3. Left hemisphere dysfunction
4. Right hemisphere dysfunction
5. Generalized dysfunction

Detailed descriptions of these neural systems are presented in a subsequent section of this chapter. It should be noted that the factor structure of the tests suggested that the various neural systems were interrelated. It could also be interpreted hierarchically with some factors hypothesized to be substrates for others. The factor structure was found to make sense in relation to neurobiological theory. (See Ayres[19,20] for the interpretation of these factors.) This finding helped to validate that the tests were measuring neurophysiological function. The complexity of the factor structure and its dependence on both scores on standardized tests and on clinical observations suggested that clinical experience, familiarity with tests and measurement theory, and knowledge of sensory integration research and theory were requirements for sound interpretation of the Southern California Sensory Integration Tests. These tests could not be mastered at the undergraduate level.

Experimentation. The development of the typology enabled experienced therapists proficient in the administration and interpretation of the Southern California Sensory Integration Tests to provisionally and differentially diagnose the type of neural dysfunctions that might be present in children with learning disabilities. However, the ultimate test of the theory's validity rested on whether it could be demonstrated to possess predictive validity. Evidence was needed that, once children were diagnosed as having a sensory integrative dysfunction and were then treated in accord with the specific type of dysfunction identified (such as dyspraxia or vestibular bilateral integration dysfunction), the treatment was effective in remediating learning problems. Such studies could provide further evidence that sensory integration was a contributor to some types of learning disabilities and that inferences made to treatment based on the theory were sound.

Ayres[18,27] conducted two studies that addressed these issues. In the first study she tested 148 learning disabled children on the Southern California Sensory Integration Tests to identify those in the group who had the type of learning disabilities for which sensory integrative procedures had been designed. The selection process resulted in the constitution of two groups. One group was made up of children judged to have a generalized sensory integrative dysfunction. The second group consisted of 24 subjects considered to have discrete auditory-language problems. In each group one-half of the subjects received sensory integrative procedures along with their usual special education program (the experimental subjects). The remainder received equivalent time in special education (control group). The children in both experimental groups received 25 to 40 minutes of sensory integrative procedures daily over a 5- to 6-month period.

All the children had been pretested on achievement tests. Following the intervention they were retested on these measures. Results indicated that, within the group with generalized dysfunction, the children who had received sensory integrative procedures, on the average, had made greater gains in reading and in overall academic achievement than those who had not received therapy. In the group with discrete auditory-language disorders, those who had received the sensory integrative procedures improved more, on the average, in reading than the control group. An additional but important finding was that both experimental groups seemed to make greater gains than their matched control groups in language acquisition.

This study was important because it provided tentative evidence that, for those children who on the basis of being tested on the Southern California Sensory Integration Tests and on the basis of clinical impressions of an occupational therapist could be diagnosed as being very good candidates for sensory integrative procedures, the procedures did seem to enhance academic achievement and auditory-language functions. It is essential that therapists be aware that this study did not provide evidence that sensory integrative procedures were ap-

TABLE 19-2   **Factors identified in studies by Ayres (1965-1977)**

Date of study	Apraxia	Deficit in form and space perception	Deficit in postural and bilateral integration	Deficit in auditory and language functions	Tactile defensiveness	Miscellaneous
1965: 100 dysfunctional, 50 normal	Tactile tests Motor planning (imitation of posture, motor accuracy, MAC, Grommet) Eye pursuits	Frostig tests Kinesthesia Manual form perception Ayres' space test	Right–left discrimination Avoidance crossing midline Rhythmic activities	Not tested	Poor tactile perception Hyperactive-distractible behavior Tactile defensiveness	Figure-ground a separate factor Eye-hand agreement not related to perceptual-motor dysfunction
1966a: Normal distribution of Gesell developmental quotients	Accounted for most variance Motor planning Tactile and kinesthesia Motor accuracy Figure-ground Frostig tests	Figure-ground Frostig spatial relations Ayres' space test		Not tested	Low association of tactile defensiveness with praxis factor	Identified two main factors in normal sample: General perceptual-motor (somatosensory and motor) Visual perception
1966b: Only normal children		Frostig tests Ayres' space test Motor accuracy Figure-ground	Integration two sides of body and tactile perception	Not tested		Tactile defensiveness and hyperactivity—may be a maturational factor involved Visual-motor ability accounted for most variation in normal children Poor motor planning–tactile perception not seen in normal children

1969: Educationally handicapped children	Tactile Motor planning	Most Southern California Sensory Integration Tests (SCSIT) visual tests not included in analysis Possible right hemisphere dysfunction: eye movement deficits, better right- than left-sided function	Bilateral integration Postural reactions Reading and language problems	Possible left hemisphere dysfunction: Auditory-language Reading achievement Auditory and visual-motor sequencing	Tactile defensiveness and hyperactivity—loaded together but not a separate factor	
1972: Educationally handicapped children	Motor planning Hyperactivity Tactile defensiveness (more emphasis on motor than tactile)	Position in space Illinois Test of Psycholinguistic Abilities visual closure Space visualization Design copying Tactile tests	Poor ocular control Excessive residual primitive postural responses Relatively good left-hand coordination	Auditory language Intelligence	Hyperactivity-distractibility Tactile perception	Reading-spelling load together Motor accuracy highly associated with all parameters
1977: Learning disabled children	*Analysis 5:* Imitation of postures Composite tactile Kinesthesia	*Analysis 3:* Four SCSIT visual tests Manual form Perception	*Analysis 5:* Prone extension Composite postural Flexion posture Composite tactile Kinesthesia	*Analysis 5:* Composite language (ITPA) Dichotic listening Flowers-Costello (auditory)	Not measured	Visual tests have strong cognitive component (loaded with IQ on Analysis 2) Space Visualization Contralateral Use (SVCU) score associated with lateralization indices Motor accuracy loaded separately on all

Adapted from Ayres, A.J.: Percep. Mot. Skills **20**:335, 1965; Ayres, A.J.: Am. J. Occup. Ther. **20**(2):68, 1966; Ayres, A.J.: Am. J. Occup. Ther. **20**(6):288, 1966; Ayres, A.J.: J. Learn. Disabil. **2**(3):44, 1969; Ayres, A.J.: Am. J. Occup. Ther. **26**(1):13, 1972; Ayres, A.J.: Am. J. Occup. Ther. **31**(6):362, 1977.

propriate for all learning disabled children. The children who made up the samples were selected from among the general population of learning disabled children because they could be diagnosed as having the type of dysfunctions that were thought to be most responsive to sensory integrative procedures. Also, the study did not suggest that perceptual-motor or sensorimotor programs or other facsimiles of these sorts of programs were effective in lessening academic problems. The treatment program that the experimental groups received had the unique features of the sensory approach described by Ayres,[19] and may have only borne a slight resemblance to these other types of programs.

In 1974 Ayres was awarded a grant by the Center for the Study of Sensory Integrative Dysfunction and the Valentine-Kline Foundation for further study of the effects of sensory integrative procedures on learning disabled children. In this study[23,27] she was especially interested in identifying which learning disabled children would, and which would not, benefit academically from sensory integrative procedures. (It should be noted that this study had numerous other facets that cannot be covered in an introductory chapter of this kind.) In the one facet of the study that addressed the relationship of sensory integrative procedures to academic achievement, 46 learning disabled children received sensory integrative procedures for 6 months. A control group remained in class receiving equivalent time in special education. When the average differences in change in pretest and posttest scores between the groups were compared, no significant differences were found. However, when only the children with depressed nystagmus who had received the sensory integrative procedures were compared with those with depressed nystagmus who had not, significant results emerged. In this analysis it was found that a greater number (among those learning disabled children with depressed nystagmus) who had received the sensory integrative procedures gained more academically than those who had only been exposed to special education. This study was of much importance because it helped to pinpoint which learning disabled children were the best candidates for sensory integrative procedures. The results suggested that not all learning disabled children should be provided with the procedures. Children with depressed postrotary nystagmus and other signs of vestibular dysfunction were identified as those most apt to benefit from the procedures.

• • •

In summary, these studies suggested that sensory integrative procedures were effective in enhancing academic learning in some learning disabled children. They also provided evidence that, since all learning disabled children did not benefit from the procedures, an evaluation process before the recommendation for therapy was essential.

The studies had the net effect of tempering enthusiasm for the approach. It seemed that the procedures benefited some subgroups of the learning disabled population. Since in the studies sensory integrative procedures were provided to children who were also receiving special education, the studies implied that sensory integrative procedures were a supplement to, and not a substitute for, special education.

Several criticisms can be made of these studies. Perhaps the most obvious one is that the control group children did not appear to receive equal time in individualized attention as did the children in the experimental groups. This argument assumes that within their regular special education program the children were not routinely provided with equivalent individualized attention from classroom, itinerant, or resource room teachers. However, even if the experimental children did receive more individualized attention than the control groups, it is unlikely that the results could be adequately explained on the basis of attention alone. The difficulty in attributing the findings to an effect of attention centers on the fact that some (the children with depressed duration of nystagmus and other signs of vestibular dysfunction) but not all of the children in the experimental group seemed to benefit from the procedures. The possibility that children with attenuated nystagmus are more responsive to individualized attention than other learning disabled children is unlikely and strains the argument.

A second criticism that can be made of the studies is that they were conducted by the originator of the theory. Studies of the validity of a theory are more powerful when they are conducted by independent investigators. A number of studies have been conducted by independent investigators on the effectiveness of sensory integrative procedures,* but all except one of these were on children without learning disabilities. One of these studies, however, deserves special mention because it was on children who were later identified as having reading failures. White[163] identified 21 children out of 124 when they entered first grade as at-risk for reading failure. Approximately one half of the children were given the Southern California Sensory Integration Tests and then treated in accord with their diagnoses with the procedures recommended by Ayres[19] (experimental group). Each child received 48 half-hour treatment periods (over a 6-month period). At the end of the year, White reported the experimental group had attained a significantly higher reading level than the control children. Moreover, this difference persisted 1 and 2 years later.

---

*References 46, 50, 75, 102, 112, 123, 124, and 163.

A third type of criticism has been leveled, not against these studies on sensory integrative procedures, per se, but against perceptual-motor programs and their facsimiles. The problem is that the writers who take this stand do not distinguish between sensory integrative procedures and the programs that resemble them, and they use the term sensory integration loosely. For example, Kinsbourne and Caplan,[92] a physician and a psychologist respectively, in providing guidelines for parents on how to choose remedial programs, advise them to avoid "speculative methods." They define speculative methods as "any procedure that relates hypothetically, rather than logically, to educational good." Multisensory approaches and physical education approaches "purporting to accelerate brain maturation (as opposed to raise morale)" are listed as examples of speculative approaches. Similarly, Reid and Hresko[127] state that "poor performances on perceptual, perceptual-motor, and sensory integrative tasks are characteristic of learning disabled children." But, they maintain, their significance is not clear and their relevance to intervention not validated. These authors make no reference to Ayres' studies or writings because they loosely use the term sensory integration in their statements. Their comments, however, might be inappropriately generalized to sensory integrative procedures. Other authors[39,98,137] have specifically criticized the approach described by Ayres. That is why it is suggested that therapists using the procedures be familiar with these papers. Therapists must "have a handle" on the research base that has both tentatively justified and delineated the use of sensory integrative procedures. They should be able to anticipate criticisms they will need to respond to in practice through familiarity with these publications. Each therapist has a responsibility of being a research consumer who can defend his or her practice with empirical support.

Inferences for intervention. Sensory integrative procedures have undergone modification throughout the past 20 years they have been in use. In another section of this chapter these procedures are described as they are currently used. As part of this discussion of the empirical base of the use of sensory integrative procedures, an overview of the ways in which the research brought about changes in practice is presented.

As already mentioned, from 1958 through 1960, Ayres recommended perceptual-motor training progressions with a heavy emphasis on practice of tabletop tasks. The early 1960s were marked by a shift to an emphasis on tactile stimulation and away from cognitive processes. In her Eleanor Clark Slagle Lecture, Ayres[11] described the factors (referred to in this chapter as neural systems or syndromes) that had been isolated in her factor analytic study[13] (discussed in the section on typology).

This study suggested that the factors were related to neural substrates that processed intersensory information. In her Slagle lecture Ayres[11] suggested that tactile functions were especially important to treatment. She also recommended that treatment should focus on sensorimotor behavior, rather than on cognitive processes. The same general line of thought was apparent in a paper Ayres published on body scheme in 1961.[10] In this paper a case study was presented that described therapy procedures that relied heavily on cognitive processes. However, tactile and proprioceptive stimulation to enhance motor planning was also described as part of the program, reflecting Ayres' shifting emphasis on what should constitute therapy.

Just as tactile stimulation had been emphasized in the 1960s, in the 1970s greater attention was given to the vestibular system. The series of factor analytic studies that had been published up through this period had suggested that the neural substrates (factors) could be interpreted hierarchically. For example, the neural systems that seemed to be concerned with vestibular and tactile integration were interpreted as subserving more complex functions such as reading, visual perception, and language. Moreover, because some of the more important structures in the nervous system that were known to integrate sensory information were located in the brain stem, the inference was made that improvement in efficiency of neural processing at this level might enhance higher cortical functions. The result of this line of thought was that in the 1970s treatment relied heavily on procedures thought to enhance brain stem integration of sensory input. Major integrating mechanisms in the brain stem were found to be closely tied to vestibular mechanisms. As a logical development, treatment in this period came to emphasize provision of vestibular stimulation.

In her 1972 and now classic book, Ayres[19] listed numerous activities that she hypothesized would improve the efficiency of neural integration at a brain stem level. The procedures incorporated provision of tactile, proprioceptive, and especially vestibular input. Use of the net hammock, platform swing, inner tube, and scooter boards was described and has since become a symbol of the approach, although such equipment is not always used by therapists in accord with the principles of sensory integrative theory.

Therapy was described as relying even less on cognitive processes than it had in the 1960s.[19] Moreover, the concept of self-direction emerged as being critical to the treatment process. Ayres described therapy as providing the child with opportunities to organize his or her own behavior. The therapist's challenge is to draw out the child's inner drive and to provide a blend of freedom and structure that will promote exploration (Figure 19-5).

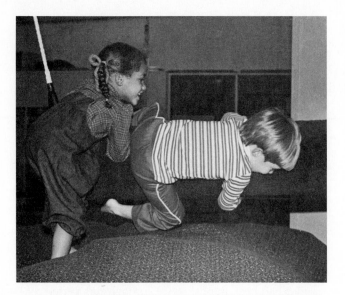

FIGURE 19-5

This activity, providing potent vestibular stimulation, also taps the children's inner drives.

Photograph by Dooley Brown.

In the late 1970s Ayres conducted the major effectiveness study that had implicated the vestibular system in the type of learning disabilities that were responsive to sensory integrative procedures.[26,27] The finding led to even greater emphasis being placed on the provision of many types of vestibular stimulation varying in intensity, directionality, and speed. Concomitant with this evolving focus was a decrease in the emphasis placed on reflex integration and on tactile input, although procedures addressing these were still used intermittently as part of the overall therapy program. Sensory integrative procedures had evolved to the point that they no longer resembled the perceptual-motor systems that had been developed in the 1960s. The procedures required an elaborate array of equipment and overhead beams permitting suspension. They also required highly trained therapists who could tailor the therapy situation so that it drew forth the child's self-direction, yet demanded more complex adaptive responses than the child had previously performed.

Treating the learning disabled child with a sensory integrative dysfunction: current practice

Entry-level therapists should not expect to be able to provide sensory integrative procedures upon graduation. The correct use of these techniques requires a great deal of professional skill and a blend of science and art. Science has generated the knowledge base in neurobehavioral science that provides a foundation for use of the procedures. Science has also furnished the data that tentatively suggest that the procedures are ef-

fective in promoting gains in children who have a variety of handicapping conditions.*

However, the provision of sensory integrative procedures also requires considerable artfulness. The therapist must make judgments about whether this approach should be initially recommended for the child. As much as possible, the therapist will use objective data from an evaluation procedure, but some subjectivity may need to enter into this decision. Throughout the treatment sessions the therapist will need to make judgments based on the child's characteristics and history, the equipment available in the treatment setting, relevant theories and facts, and past clinical experience. For each child, and during each moment of the therapy session, procedures are highly individualized in accord with the practical wisdom of the therapist and his or her knowledge of sensory integrative theory.

Although there are limited data to suggest that these procedures are effective in promoting developmental gains in mentally retarded, autistic, and aphasic children,[31,42,46] this discussion will be confined to their application with learning disabled children. The therapeutic process begins with assessment, with a consequent decision on whether the child should be recommended for therapy. If the child is recommended, treatment is initiated. In this section an overview of the assessment process and guidelines for provision of sensory integrative procedures is presented. The purpose is simply to expose the reader to some of the central considerations that must be addressed in using these procedures. Competence in provision of the sensory integrative procedures is accrued over time through the interplay of advanced study and experience.

ASSESSMENT

An appropriate initial assessment, as well as a means for determining progress, is essential in all areas of clinical practice. Although this process creates a professional challenge for all therapists striving to provide quality care, several unique factors arise when the potential use of sensory integrative procedures is anticipated. Sensory integrative dysfunctions are not directly observable. Their presence is inferred from meaningful clusters of poor performance on a great number of tests and on clinical observations of neuromuscular performance and behavioral organization.

The diagnoses children are given on the basis of this evaluation procedure are not incontrovertible. They represent provisional hypotheses (tentative assumptions) about the nature of the contributors to the child's learning disorder. The correctness of the diagnosis is tested in the therapy situation. If the hypothesis is correct, then the procedures should produce certain predictable effects. The act, then, of arriving at a diagnosis is per-

---

*References 26, 46, 50, 102, 112, 123, and 163.

formed to guide intervention. It is essential that treatment effects (or the correctness of the hypothesis) be carefully documented.

Because sensory integrative theory purports that sensory integrative processes can affect many aspects of the child, in addition to his academic performance, evaluation and documentation of change should be multifaceted. No single test can provide information of sufficient magnitude to infer the presence of a sensory integrative disorder. Many tests must be used. Change, as a consequence of therapy, may occur in language acquisition, play, self-esteem, self-care, attention to relevant stimuli, or any aspect of the child's role performance. Both the complexity of diagnosis and the wide range of possible treatment effects must be considered in evaluating the child for a sensory integrative dysfunction.

The diagnosis the therapist gives the child will not rest exclusively on the results of the Southern California Integration Tests. Also considered are the child's history and presenting problems, as well as observations of the child's neuromuscular status and behavioral organization. Observations of the following will usually be included: eye pursuits; oral praxis; equilibrium reactions; postural responses; the ability to assume total body patterns, such as prone extension and supine flexion; the presence of choreoathetosis; cocontraction; fine coordination; smoothness of movement; eye and hand usage; organization of behavior; spontaneous language; expression and comprehension; clinical motor planning ability; gravitational security; and emotional lability. In some instances the dichotic listening test[25] (Chapters 9, 10, and 11) is also used to assess cerebral dominance for auditory language functions.

Finally, results of testing conducted by professionals from other disciplines, such as psychology and speech pathology, may be considered in the formulation of an overall diagnosis. In particular, measures of intelligence and auditory-language performance are helpful in rounding out a final impression of what neural processes may be contributing to the child's learning problems.

Documentation of the effects of sensory integrative procedures also requires the use of a variety of tests. Since sensory integrative theory suggests that the purpose of therapy is to enhance the child's capacity to develop and learn through more efficient neural processing,[19] changes are not expected before at least 6 months of intervention. The common expectation of weekly or monthly formal progress reports is often not necessary.

Another problem with documentation is that the areas in which the child is expected to improve are not the same as those emphasized directly in the activities employed in therapy. Treatment provides a situation in which the child can receive and respond to meaningful sensory input and environmental challenges involving motor planning, ideation, and problem solving. However, the areas in which parents and teachers initially perceive problems are also those in which changes, as a consequence of therapy, are likely to take place. These areas encompass physical, academic, social, and emotional development. Informal and nonstandardized observations by the child's parents, teachers, and other significant persons outside the therapy environment can buttress the therapist's impressions of the child's progress.

In addition, standardized tests must be used to tease out actual treatment gains from maturational effects. A number of standardized tests have been found to be clinically useful for documenting change. The Bruininks-Oseretsky Test of Motor Proficiency[41] is designed for children 4½ years to 14½ years and measures perceptual and motor functioning. It is especially helpful because the areas tested are not specifically addressed in therapy but nevertheless do seem to depend on efficient sensory processing for performance to meet age expectations. The Developmental Test of Visual Motor Integration[35] is designed for children 2 years to 15 years and measures visual perception and eye-hand coordination in the form of a design copying test. This test helps provide information on change for the same reason as the above test. An additional test for measuring visual motor integration is the Primary Visual Motor Test by Haworth.[79]

Language scores are especially helpful for documenting change since (1) a large number of children diagnosed as presenting sensory integrative dysfunctions demonstrate speech and language disorders and (2) the language domain may be one of the systems most likely to benefit from the implementation of sensory integrative procedures. Some evaluations that have language items can be administered by the occupational therapist with practice; others should be administered only by qualified speech and language specialists. Tests that are sometimes used include the following: (1) the Peabody Picture Vocabulary Tests,[53] (2) the Expressive One Word Picture Vocabulary Test,[67] (3) the Test for Auditory Comprehension of Language,[42], (4) the Carrow Elicited Language Inventory,[43] (5) the Weiss Comprehensive Articulation Test,[160] and (6) the Sentence Repetition Test.[138]

In addition, academic tests may be useful in measuring the effectiveness of therapy, depending on the child's problems. The Wide Range Achievement Test by Jastak and Jastak[83] or the Woodcock-Johnson Psycho-educational Battery[166] may be appropriate. Evaluations of activities of daily living, self-esteem, and student role performance may also be helpful in the assessment of behavioral changes.

Although specific gains may not be documentable on a short-term basis, careful and frequent informal notetaking can be an essential element of demonstrating measurable progress or lack thereof. Documentation of individual therapy sessions should emphasize the child's response to activities, rather than the activities themselves. Videotapes are particularly helpful in carefully analyzing a child's behavior before treatment is instituted and at subsequent intervals. Progress notes may include information on the child's ability to organize behavior, complexity of motor planning, tendency to seek various types of sensory stimulation, relationship to space, communication skills during therapy, and emotional response to therapy.[30]

DIFFERENTIAL DIAGNOSIS

As was earlier mentioned, there are complexities involved in labeling children as learning disabled. Learning disabled is a catchall term in which children with various characteristics are subsumed. Not all children with learning disabilities will present clinical pictures suggestive of the presence of a sensory integrative dysfunction. Those who do not should not be recommended for the procedures. The evaluation process previously described enables the therapist to generate a hypothesis about the contributors to a child's learning disability. The impressions generated by this process guide the therapist's decisions on what procedures to recommend. Overdiagnosis of children and overenthusiasm for the approach must be counteracted by a sound understanding of the proper use of the tests and knowledge of the data that suggest which types of learning disabled children are most apt to benefit from the procedures.

SENSORY INTEGRATIVE DYSFUNCTIONS

Several types of sensory integrative dysfunctions were identified in Ayres' factor analytic studies (Table 19-2). All seem to involve, at least in part, brain stem integration of sensory information. The following syndrome descriptions rely heavily on Ayres.[19,20,28,29]

Vestibular bilateral integration dysfunction. In Ayres' earlier book,[19] vestibular bilateral integration dysfunction was called postural bilateral integrative dysfunction. Children hypothesized to have this disorder usually are the least affected among the learning disabled children.[23] They tend to have above average measured intelligence, are quite healthy, but have difficulty with reading or other tasks related to learning. These children may dislike sports and do poorly in them. They may be poorly coordinated, especially in tasks requiring the two hands to work together.[28]

In clinical observations, the therapist may detect that the child's two eyes do not seem to be working together properly. A jerk may be noticed as the child's eyes cross their midline. The child may not show a clear preference for one hand, although he is well beyond the age at which hand dominance should have been established. In the prone position the child may be unable to simultaneously raise her arms, hands, heels, and thighs (in what is called the prone extension posture). On the Southern California Postrotary Nystagmus Test the induced postrotary nystagmus may be found to be depressed in duration relative to that of other children her age.[22] This constellation of problems suggests inefficiency in vestibular processing.[28]

It is posited in sensory integrative theory that the vestibular system has a considerable influence on postural tone, ocular pursuits, the coordination of input from the two body sides, the establishment of laterality, language function, and visual-perception. Ayres[28] describes the developmental progression of a vestibular-bilateral integrative disorder as follows. In early childhood the child may experience problems mastering directionality (he may turn to the left when asked to turn to the right). In middle childhood he may have difficulty learning to dance (which requires smooth rhythmical movement) or learning to play the piano (which requires the two hands to work together with precision). At this age the child may also be identified as having a reading disability.[28]

This cluster of problems is seen in sensory integrative theory as related to inefficiency in vestibular processing.[28] It is thought that these children begin to cognitively compensate for their poorly functioning vestibular systems. For example, to point to the left hand on a command to do so, they will think longer and harder than children normally do. This compensation is then proposed to interfere with adequate establishment of hemispheric dominance for auditory language functions, visual-spatial perception, or both. In other words, both hemispheres may have to deal with the same functions, rather than specializing. Without adequate hemispheric specialization, neither visual-spatial nor auditory-language functions may be done well. Moreover, activities such as reading, which require both visual perception and auditory language skills, may be impaired because the two hemispheres are thought, when this syndrome is present, to not communicate adequately. Research has suggested that children hypothesized to have this dysfunction are among the best responders to sensory integrative procedures.[23] In therapy these children typically seek out intense and rapid vestibular stimulation.

Developmental dyspraxia. In her earlier writings Ayres[19,20,21] used the term apraxia to refer to developmental dyspraxia. In a more recent book, Ayres[28] stated that the term apraxia is used when the individual is unable to motor plan. She believes the term dyspraxia is better suited for the child who can formulate motor plans but who is slow and inefficient in doing so. Learning disabled children who have problems in motor planning almost invariably fall into the latter category.

Children with developmental dyspraxia were described by Ayres[28] as having a problem in the "bridge between the intellect and muscles." She defines developmental dyspraxia as an "inefficiency or inability to carry out an unusual, nonlearned movement when there is potentially adequate motor reasoning and conceptual capacity to do so."[29] These children have no problems in executing motor activities that they have practiced in the past. The breakdown in their performance occurs when they attempt to execute nonhabitual motor acts.[28,29]

Ayres[29] believes that there are several types of dyspraxia. The first, which she calls somatosensory apraxia, consistently emerged in the factor analyses (Table 19-2). The single best indicator of this type of dyspraxia is the score of the Imitation of Postures Test[17] in which the child is required to quickly snap into a posture the examiner assumes. Children hypothesized to have the disorder generally do poorly on tests of somatosensory perception. In these instances the dyspraxia is viewed as an end product of poor tactile perception and consequent to poor development of a body scheme (defined as mental representation of the body stored in the brain).[10] In other instances the vestibular system may also be implicated.[28]

Ayres[28] does not describe children with somatosensory dyspraxia as having problems with smoothness of movement, although their postural responses may be deficient. Centrally programmed movements such as walking that seem to be wired into the nervous system are also adequate in these children. What these children lack is a well-developed repertoire of skills.

The second type of dyspraxia with which Ayres[29] has been concerned is called constructional dyspraxia. Children with this condition seem to have difficulty combining objects to build a new structure. Ayres[29] believes that constructional praxis requires the organization of spatial information as well as an ideational component. The building of structures requires the child to analyze the requirements of the task and construct in her mind a scheme to accomplish it. This sort of ideation, Ayres[29] maintains, requires imagining what must be done to accomplish an end (Figure 19-6).

Ayres[29] points out that children must use ideation while involved in sensory integrative procedures. They must conjure up an idea for how to play on a piece of equipment. Some children, she points out, will be unable to formulate an original plan. Their play on the equipment will be restricted to imitation of the play activities in which they see other children engage.[29]

Ayres[29] gives the example of an activity she frequently uses in therapy. In this activity the child must

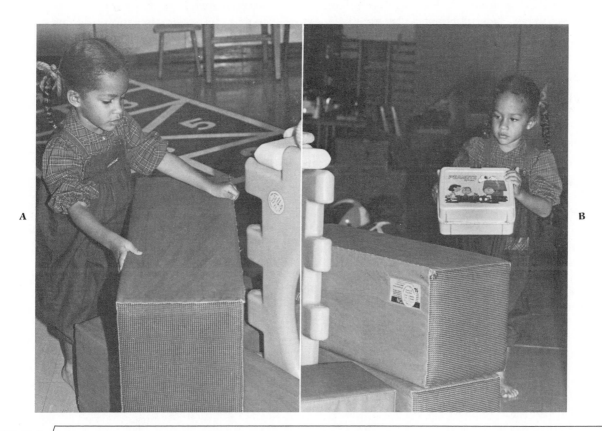

FIGURE 19-6

Activity requiring constructional praxis. **A,** This child must organize spatial information as she combines objects to build a house. **B,** On completing the activity, the child uses fantasy as she plans to have lunch in the house.

Photograph by Dooley Brown.

propel himself with a trapeze off the top of a ramp, swing, and then drop into a pillow. He must time his release on the trapeze at the instant he is over the pillow. Children with problems in sequencing and timing tend to find this type of activity difficult. Finally, Ayres[29] suggests that some dyspraxic children may have difficulty initiating activities or persevering in them once they have started (Figure 19-4).

Dyspraxia is frequently associated with distractibility and hyperactivity.[21] Dyspraxic children are considered to be good responders to sensory integrative procedures.[31]

Generalized dysfunction. Children who, on the basis of results from the Southern California Sensory Integration Tests, are classified as having generalized dysfunction, are thought of as having severe sensory integrative dysfunctions. In their cases, academic learning is probably restricted by many factors, only one of which may be related to their sensory integrative dysfunction. When learning problems are a result of a complex interplay of factors, it is doubtful that provision of sensory integrative procedures would appreciably enhance academic learning. These children are not considered to be prime candidates for sensory integrative procedures. However, a child with generalized dysfunction may benefit from a sensory integrative approach in terms of general adaptive behavior, if a disorder in modulation of sensory input (discussed later) is also present.

DYSFUNCTIONS FOR WHICH SENSORY INTEGRATIVE PROCEDURES ARE NOT RECOMMENDED

Ayres[30] points out that many children in classes for the learning disabled appear to have other nervous system irregularities that could severely interfere with learning. These children, like those hypothesized to have a vestibular bilateral integration dysfunction, are likely to score poorly on the Southern California Sensory Integration Tests. Because of the type, severity, and complexity of the nervous system disorders, provision of sensory integrative procedures is likely to make little difference in their academic achievement.[30] Therapists who fail to recognize this situation may inappropriately select clients for treatment. They may be overenthusiastic in their recommendations, make unrealistic predictions about the outcomes that are expected from therapy, and generate criticism.

Left hemisphere and right hemisphere dysfunctions were detected by Ayres' factor analytic studies, but experimental data suggested that children with these diagnoses did not benefit academically from sensory integrative procedures.[23] The reader is reminded that occupational behavior concepts may provide a viable basis for occupational therapy treatment.

Left hemisphere dysfunction. As previously mentioned, data exist suggesting that some learning disabled children may have a dysfunction in processing information in the left hemisphere.[45] A sensory integrative evaluation can provide tentative evidence of the presence of this kind of a dysfunction and assist in the diagnosis. Most right-handed individuals demonstrate left-sided dominance for auditory language function.[25] The diagnosis of left hemisphere dysfunction is suggested when a child demonstrates poor auditory-language skills and a pattern of poorer right-handed performance than left-handed performance in the presence of normal sensory integrative functions. These children do not tend to show hyperactivity, distractibility, or poor postural responses. Postrotary nystagmus is usually prolonged or within normative expectations. It is hypothesized that these children are underachieving because of left hemisphere inefficiency. Data suggest that they do well in traditional special education programs and are not among the best responders to sensory integrative procedures.[27]

Right hemisphere dysfunction. Results of a sensory integrative evaluation may assist in the diagnosis of a right hemisphere dysfunction. Children hypothesized to have this dysfunction may show discrete visual-spatial perceptual problems without other evidence suggestive of a sensory integrative dysfunction. Usually in right-handed persons the right hemisphere specializes in visual-spatial tasks. If this side of the brain is not processing information optimally, visual-spatial perception may be compromised. Children who are hypothesized to have this dysfunction are thought to demonstrate adequate postural responses, unimpaired auditory-language functions, better right- than left-hand performance, and underuse or disregard of the left hand. This dysfunction seems to be one of the less frequently made diagnoses, and only a few children with this diagnosis were included in Ayres' effectiveness studies.[18,23,27] In general, children hypothesized to have this type of dysfunction are not recommended for sensory integrative procedures.

DISORDERS IN MODULATION OF SENSORY INPUT

In addition to the types of dysfunction reviewed earlier, Ayres has described disturbances in modulation of sensory input that may appear along with a sensory integrative dysfunction or in isolation. In contrast to the typology of syndromes, which is quantitatively grounded in test scores, the notion of sensory modulation addresses the more qualitative aspects of sensory processing, which are closely related to the emotions. Specifically, hyperresponsivity to motion and to touch fall within this category.

Two types of hyperreactive vestibular responses are

described by Ayres.[28] The first, gravitational insecurity, is defined as intense anxiety and distress in response to movement or to a change in head position. Ayres[28] suggests that the child may experience a sensation of falling when in a stable, but threatening position. Typically, the child prefers to be in secure contact with a firm ground and thus may avoid activities that involve jumping, climbing, swinging, and other forms of active or passive movement. Ambulation tends to be slow and overly cautious. This condition is thought to be associated with inadequate inhibition of vestibular input.[28] The second type of vestibular hyperresponsivity, intolerance to movement, is described as an aversive reaction to rapid spinning and circular movement. For these children, movement is unpleasant but not threatening. They may readily approach movement activities, unlike the gravitationally insecure, but react to vestibular stimulation with excessive nausea and discomfort.

Tactile defensiveness has been associated with vestibular dysfunction as well as with dyspraxia. Defined as an aversive reaction to touch, it was repeatedly linked with hyperactivity and distractibility in Ayres' factor analysis (Table 19-2). Like gravitational insecurity, it is thought to involve oversensitivity to sensory input. The reader is referred to Ayres[12,19] for a lengthy discussion of the hypothesized neural substrates of this disorder.

Little research has directly addressed the effects of therapy on tactile defensiveness or gravitational insecurity. Ayres and Tickle[32] found that vestibular and tactile hypersensitivity were among the strongest predictors of a good response to therapy in a group of autistic children. Informal case reports have suggested that significant improvement in adaptive behavior results when sensory integrative procedures are employed with children who are hypersensitive to touch and movement. Further research in this important area is warranted.

OTHER CONSIDERATIONS IN DIAGNOSING THE PRESENCE OF A SENSORY INTEGRATIVE DISORDER

Results of a sensory integration evaluation on some learning disabled children do not permit interpretation in accord with the typology presented earlier. Rather than strain to force a diagnosis, it is recommended that the therapist use alternative models for interpretation as presented in the Southern California Sensory Integration Tests Manual.[20] Therapists need to be cautious in diagnosing children. As a rule, learning disabled children who do not fit the available interpretation models probably should not be recommended for therapy. If the data are suggestive but do not clearly indicate a sensory integrative dysfunction, therapy could be provided on a trial basis with an extensive reevaluation after 6 months.

EXHIBIT 19-1

Goals of therapy using sensory integrative procedures

Increase in the frequency or duration of adaptive responses to sensory input.
Development of increasingly more complex adaptive responses.
Increase in self-confidence and self esteem.
Improvement in cognitive skills, language acquisition, or academic achievement.
Improvement in daily living and personal-social skills.

Adapted from Ayres, A.J.: Sensory integration and learning disorders, Los Angeles, 1972, Western Psychological Services; Ayres, A.J.: Sensory integration and the child, Los Angeles, 1979, Western Psychological Services; Ayres, A.J.: Aspects of the somatomotor adaptive response and praxis. Audiotape, Pasadena, Calif., 1981, Center for the Study of Sensory Integrative Dysfunction.

Goals and objectives of treatment

The specific objectives of sensory integrative procedures will vary according to the kind of dysfunction that is diagnosed and the individual differences that make each child unique. In short, objectives are individualized for each patient. However, it is possible to list some general goals from which specific objectives can be derived (Exhibit 19-1). While these goals usually apply to most children involved with sensory integrative procedures, they may not all be appropriate for each child. Furthermore, specific objectives generated toward the same goal may vary substantially from one child to another.

INCREASE IN THE FREQUENCY OR DURATION OF ADAPTIVE RESPONSES TO SENSORY INPUT

Increase in the frequency or duration of adaptive responses to sensory input is dependent on the therapeutic application of controlled sensory input. During provision of sensory integrative procedures, the therapist constantly monitors the child's responses to be certain that the stimulation is organizing rather than disorganizing, integrating rather than overwhelming. Sensory input is considered to be optimal when it is neither overstimulating nor understimulating.[28] The therapist "reads" the child's autonomic nervous system responses (for example, skin color, breathing rate), as well as changes in behavioral organization, and makes judgments about whether the child's responses are adaptive (Figure 19-7). Contingent on this ongoing appraisal is the modification of the therapeutic activity. Manipulation of the sensory environment in this way enables the child to produce adaptive responses more frequently and sustain them for longer periods of time than might otherwise be possible.

Stimulation generally is not confined to one sensory modality. The activities that are used provide natural combinations of proprioceptive, vestibular, and tactile stimulation. Sensory integrative procedures, to be appropriate, must provide the right combination of stimulation in accord with the status of the child's nervous system (Figure 19-8). The availability of attractive suspended equipment that can be used for rich provision of vestibular stimulation is essential.

With sensory integrative procedures, active stimulation is usually preferred over passive stimulation, although in some instances passive applications may be used.[28] Passive application of vestibular stimulation, in particular, is more likely to be used in severely involved children who appear to have difficulties with sensory registration. Even with these children, active stimulation is encouraged whenever possible, since it is more likely to engage the child's inner drive and lead to more complex adaptive responses. Ayres[29] suggests that sensory registration can be further enhanced in treatment by simplifying the environment so that there are only a few choice pieces of equipment to which the child might attend.

It should be kept in mind that Ayres' definition of an adaptive response encompasses a broad range of behaviors. Ayres described it as a purposeful goal-directed response through which motions achieve functional meaning.[19] Recently Ayres coined the term somatomotor adaptive response to mean a motor response that is dependent on integration of vestibular and tactile information.[29] Examples would include equilibrium reactions, protective responses, or lying prone with neck and hips extended to ride successfully on a scooter board. Adaptive responses can vary in complexity, quality, and effectiveness.[29] They may entail sequences of behaviors, such as going down a ramp prone on a scooter board and then knocking down an inflated toy, or single motor patterns, such as sitting on a scooter board and maintaining an upright posture for a sustained period of time[29] (Figure 19-9).

Successful repetition of a new adaptive response provides evidence that the child's nervous system is consolidating new strategies for dealing with sensory information. Similarly, when a child sustains an adaptive response for a longer period of time than ever before, a measure of the internal process of sensory integration is provided. An example is the child who initially was unable to sustain a flexed body position to stay on a swinging suspended bolster for more than a few seconds but who now is able to enjoy a 5-minute ride.

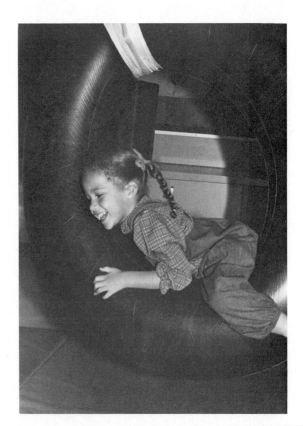

FIGURE 19-8

Many children place their cheeks on the inner tube, maximizing tactile stimulation (touch-pressure) to the face as they receive vestibular stimulation

Photograph by Dooley Brown.

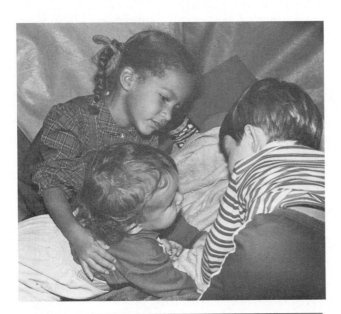

FIGURE 19-7

The comforting effects of the tactile stimulation these children are receiving are reflected in their facial expressions.

Photograph by Dooley Brown.

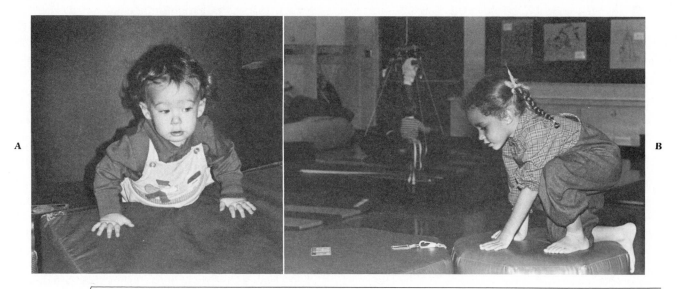

FIGURE 19-9

Adaptive responses varying in complexity. **A,** Weight bearing on hands on a stable surface in preparation for climbing, a simple adaptive response. **B,** Weight bearing on hands on an unstable surface, a more complex adaptive response.

Photograph by Dooley Brown

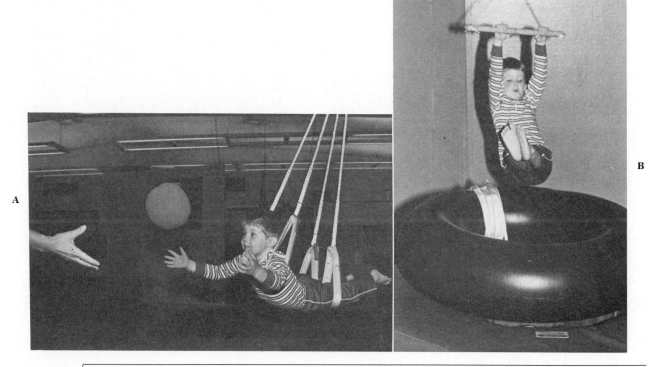

FIGURE 19-10

This child demonstrates two complex adaptive responses elicited through sensory integrative procedures. **A,** Prone extension pattern as child swings in suspended "helicopter" and attempts to catch a ball. **B,** Hip flexion as child clears his legs in preparation for a jump requiring timing into the inner tube.

Photograph by Dooley Brown.

DEVELOPMENT OF INCREASINGLY MORE COMPLEX ADAPTIVE RESPONSES

Not only are adaptive responses expected to occur with greater frequency and duration, they also are expected to become more complex in organization. This goal is based on the assumption that the types of stimulation provided are thought to promote more efficient brain stem organization of multisensory input. It is posited that better neural organization at this level will enhance the child's ability to make judgments about what is in the environment, what can be done with objects, and what specific actions need to be taken to accomplish a goal[29] (Figure 19-10).

Ayres[29] believes that repeating activities is acceptable during the period when the child is perfecting the response; however, development of more complex abilities occurs only when tasks become slightly more challenging than any the child has successfully accomplished before. The therapist uses activity analysis, assessment information, ongoing observations, and knowledge of child development to guide the arrangement of the therapeutic environment so that it will engage the child's inner drive and draw forth more complex interactions with the equipment. For responses to be adaptive, however, they must be successful. Ayres defines therapy as a combination of challenge and success[29] (Figure 19-11).

Minimally involved children are eager to explore sensory integrative equipment and will initiate more complex variations of an activity within a single session.

For more involved children, the adaptive responses usually will be less complex, will require more repetition, and will advance more slowly. The task of the therapist in such cases is to simplify the challenge so the child can succeed, then gradually change the activity by altering its components on a fine gradient of complexity. Ayres[29] suggests requiring an adaptive response of only a few body parts, rather than the total body, as one means of simplifying the challenge. Ayres also suggests that activities which involve movement patterns that are centrally programmed in the nervous system, such as walking and sitting, and do not require planning will be less demanding than those which involve the assumption of unusual positions.[29] A short-term objective for a very gravitationally insecure and dyspraxic child, for example, might be to walk up a large inclined ramp without physical assistance from the therapist.

Other children in the therapy environment can be of help in eliciting more complex adaptive responses from a particular child, since they can serve as models of a variety of activity options. It should be noted, however, that sensory integrative procedures are provided

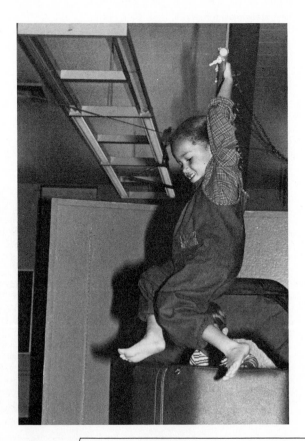

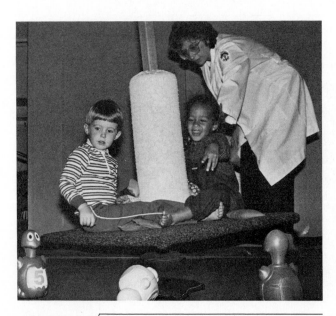

FIGURE 19-11

After successfully knocking down a turtle with a beanbag while riding the flexor swing, this girl's facial expression shows the characteristic signs of pleasure associated with success.

Photograph by Dooley Brown.

FIGURE 19-12

Successful accomplishment of adaptive responses are thought to enhance self-confidence and self-esteem.

Photograph by Dooley Brown.

dyadically (that is, with a one-to-one child-therapist ratio) in an optimal situation. If other children are present, each should be with his or her own therapist. When other children are not present, the therapist may model activities.

INCREASE IN SELF-CONFIDENCE AND SELF-ESTEEM

Ayres[28] claims that adaptive responses promote self-actualization by allowing the child to experience accomplishment of a task that previously could not have been mastered. When a child is responding adaptively to demands in the environment, she will appear creative, efficient, and satisfied. Therapy will be fun, and the child will be emotionally involved[28] (Figure 19-12).

From the outset, the therapeutic procedures generally are directed by the child, not the therapist. An assumption of the treatment approach is that children will seek out the stimulation they need to organize their nervous systems.[19] The therapist assists the child in responding adaptively to it. Ayres stated that the adaptive response cannot be imposed on the child by the therapist; it can only be generated within the child. The child wants to accomplish an act and attempts it. The child initiates and emits the response while the therapist helps to ensure success. The child is following an inner drive, while the therapist encourages and lures the child into pursuing those activities that may enhance nervous system development. Ayres emphasizes that therapy at its best involves a self-directed child.[19]

Therapists can promote self-direction of the child first, by structuring the environment so the possible adaptive responses are not beyond the child's capacity and second, by making assistance available so the child will succeed[29] (Figure 19-13). Knowledge of normal development guides the therapist's decision on how to manipulate the environment or offer assistance. Although, in principle, it is suggested that treatment should follow a developmental sequence, Ayres[19] maintains that it is best to allow the child to guide treatment, provided the procedures do not become nontherapeutic. The course of treatment, then, needs not to invariably follow a strict developmental progression.

The final outcome of therapy that encourages successful self-directed experiences is a child who perceives herself as a competent actor in the world. Therapy entails involvement in challenging activities that are achievable and guided by the child.[29] It is expected that engagement in such activities will promote feelings of mastery as well as a sense of personal control that resides within the self.[28] The resulting gains in positive self-concept can be critical to the emotional development of learning disabled children who often are characterized as having low self-esteem.[103]

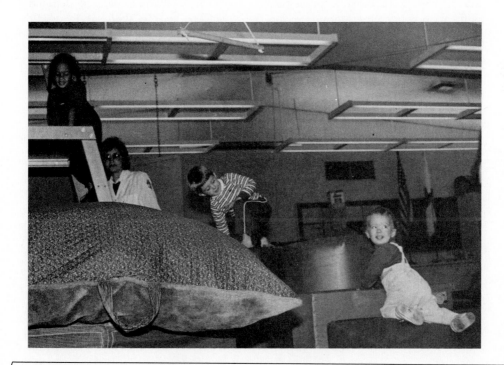

FIGURE 19-13

Therapists can promote self-direction by structuring the environment in accordance with the child's abilities.
Photograph by Dooley Brown.

Behavioral changes over time can provide an index of gains in self-confidence and self-esteem. For example, a child whose initial approach to the physical environment was inhibited, constricted, or fearful may demonstrate exploratory and risk-taking behaviors with growing frequency. A child who originally reacted to difficult tasks with destructive actions or self-denigrating remarks may show a decrease in those behaviors along with an increasing willingness to tackle potentially threatening activities.

IMPROVEMENT IN COGNITIVE SKILLS, LANGUAGE ACQUISITION, OR ACADEMIC ACHIEVEMENT

Research discussed earlier in this chapter provides tentative evidence that provision of sensory integrative procedures to some types of learning disabled children is associated with enhancement in language and cognitive abilities and increased proficiency in some academic skills.[18,23,27] In treatment, however, the therapeutic techniques do not directly address these functions. Rather, gains in these areas are seen as eventual outcomes of enhancement of sensory registration, sensory integration, and general programming capacity. Practice of specific visuomotor skills (for example, tabletop activities) or academic tasks are not customarily included in the treatment context.

Recently Ayres[29] speculated that programming of motor actions during sensory integrative procedures may provide a pathway to better programming of language and cognitive functions. She proposed that to ac-

complish an unfamiliar purposeful activity the child must first generate an idea of what is to be accomplished. Next, a "program" must be formulated for how to accomplish the act. Finally, execution of the task will involve sequencing of motor activities.[29]

Specific procedures have been developed by Ayres that are aimed at promoting ideation, sequencing, and programming.[29] Activities requiring these components are a particularly important treatment of a child with dyspraxia. Ayres[29] believes that programming functions can be encouraged through the use of verbal behaviors, such as counting or singing, to regulate motor output (Figure 19-4).

IMPROVEMENT IN DAILY LIVING AND PERSONAL-SOCIAL SKILLS

Sensory integrative procedures encourage the child to organize his own activity. The child must generate ideas about what is to be done with a piece of equipment and then program the actions needed to accomplish a goal. In what Ayres calls the "optimum for growth situation,"[19] the child will go on to execute the acts and experience the consequences of planning. Ayres hypothesizes that, with improvement in programming of action, a general programming ability will be enhanced. The outcome of this will be a child who is better able to organize behavior, daily routine, and self-care and who is better able to focus attention on relevant tasks that support role demands.[28] As competency develops in life skills, it is usually accompanied by growth in self-esteem. Often the child will begin to in-

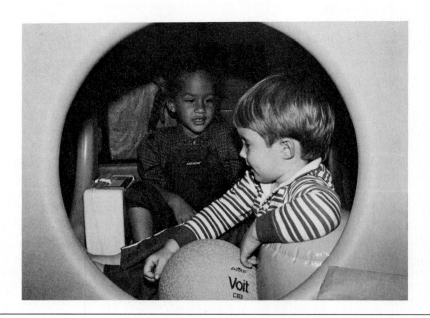

FIGURE 19-14

After engagement in sensory integrative activities, these children show comfort in peer interaction in a house they constructed. Photograph by Dooley Brown.

teract with peers and adults in more effective and enjoyable ways as a function of greater self-confidence and emotional self-control.

Therapy may help the child who is overly sensitive to touch or movement to deal with these sensations in a more adaptive manner. As a result, the child is enabled to approach the world with greater security. Not only are daily living skills improved, but relationships with others are more likely to be entered with greater physical comfort. The child will be better able to enjoy social interaction without the interference of distrust in her own reactions to ongoing sensation (Figure 19-14).

Other treatment considerations

ROLE OF THE THERAPIST

The therapist cannot employ a cookbook approach in providing sensory integrative procedures. It is inappropriate to enter the therapy situation with a list of activities the child eventually will be required to do. The therapist's judgments on what should be encouraged in a given treatment session depend on the capacity to imagine what the child is experiencing and the ingenuity to figure out how to help the child accomplish the task successfully[29] (Figure 19-15). The therapist learns with experience to "read" the child's responses and to anticipate the possible outcomes of the child's behavior. This ability is called artful vigilance by the authors. Within the therapy context, the therapist must learn how to establish rapport with the child and create a sense of safety in the child. A relationship with these

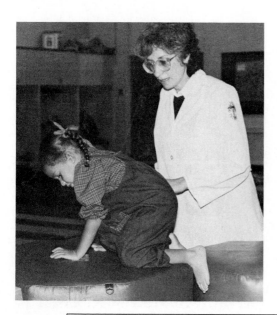

FIGURE 19-15

The therapist must be able to imagine what the child is experiencing.

Photograph by Dooley Brown.

characteristics fosters the child's inner urge to explore his environment. The therapist must also decide on a style of interaction with the child. While some children will do better with little and unadorned verbal communication, others may need the therapist to be more verbal, emotive, and enthusiastic.

The central role of the therapist providing sensory integrative procedures is to arrange an environment that is conducive to the child's organization of her own behavior.[29] Ayres believes that preparation of the remedial environment is one of the most demanding requirements of the therapist.[28]

Although, in general, the therapist guides while the child directs the therapy, it should be noted that this is not invariably the case. In instances in which a child shows little or no evidence of an evocable inner drive, the therapist may need to impose a therapeutic procedure.[29]

CHARACTERISTICS OF THE ENVIRONMENT

The availability of a wide range of equipment and a suspension system from which to hang and arrange it is absolutely essential. Just as ultrasound therapy cannot be accomplished without ultrasound equipment, sensory integrative procedures cannot be provided without the appropriate facility and equipment. Ayres[19,28] described the equipment required for sensory integrative procedures.

The clinic setting should provide for accessibility of equipment. It helps if equipment not in use can be hung on pegs within arm's reach of the therapist. Ideally, a number of swivel hooks should be available and secured in the beams that support the ceiling. When it is within the child's capacity, he can assist in rearrangements of the environment during the therapy session.

The treatment area should be designed to allow for subdivisions of space. Movable partitions make possible the blocking off of areas for individualized therapy. This same space can be enlarged by opening the partitions, and it can be used for activities requiring considerable excursion or for tandem therapy in which more than one child, each with his or her own therapist, receive therapy together.

THE FLOW OF THE THERAPY SESSION

Therapy sessions should have a flow. One activity should follow another in natural succession. Sessions do not consist of the therapist's asking the child to do one and then another preplanned activity. As much as possible, the child should be encouraged to be self-directed. The optimal therapy situation is one in which a balance is achieved between the therapist's structure, and the child's freedom.[19] But the child's self-direction can become chaotic without the structuring provided by the therapist.

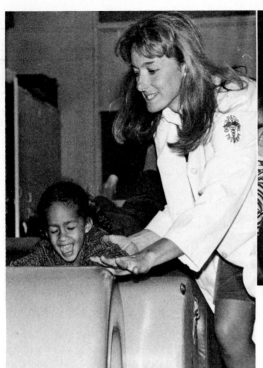
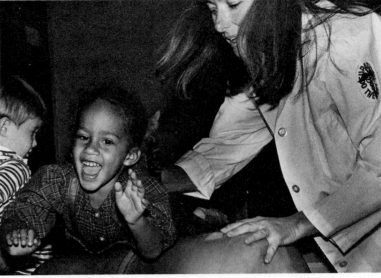

The therapist promotes self-direction in the child by making assistance available as the session flows.

Photograph by Dooley Brown.

The therapist's artful vigilance enables the creation of the balance of structure and freedom that is essential in the therapy environment (Figure 19-16). The therapist attends to the child's behavior, interprets the adaptiveness of her actions, and anticipates the next event, helping the child whenever necessary. Such help may include adding suspended handles the child can grasp, lowering equipment, or providing a cushion into which the child already swinging can jump.[29]

A well-developed ability to analyze therapeutic activities in relation to individual client needs allows the therapist to create a treatment milieu that falls midway between rigidity and chaos. The flow of the therapy situation is contingent on the proficiency of the therapist in making judgments about when to provide structure versus when to allow the child's self-direction to prevail. The choice of an activity to be used within the therapy context results from interaction of the child with the therapist. The therapist brings to this situation impressions of the child's capabilities, impressions that are formed through the results of formal evaluation and past experience in treating the child. The child similarly brings a conception of his own capabilities. Both therapist and child have some knowledge of the activity options in the environment, although the therapist's knowledge in this area will be far more comprehensive and substantive than the child's. Knowledge in these two areas will influence the child's motivation toward particular activities. The therapist, observing the child's self-direction toward a particular activity, makes a decision on whether it is challenging and achievable by the child, with or without the therapist's assistance. If

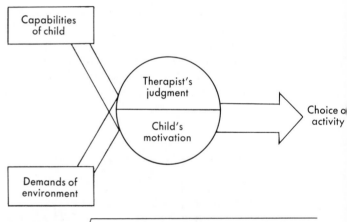

The process of activity analysis during sensory integrative procedures.

it is, the child's self-direction will determine the choice of activity; if not, another activity may be encouraged by the therapist. A therapy session consists of recurrences of this process, with the choice of each new activity resulting from interaction of child and therapist. A thread of continuity links activities and imbues the session with the qualities of spontaneity and flow (Figure 19-17).

DIFFERENTIAL TREATMENT BASED ON DIAGNOSIS

In general, children diagnosed with a vestibular bilateral integration problem will seek out great amounts of potent vestibular stimulation and will put forth

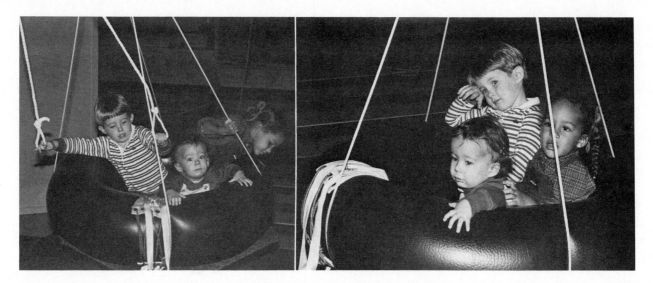

FIGURE 19-18

The change in affect demonstrated in these children alerts the therapist that the activity is overwhelming.
Photograph by Dooley Brown.

much effort to make responses reflecting increased adaptive capacity. The types of vestibular stimulation they seek may vary in direction, acceleration, and potency. A child may vary her position on a piece of equipment so that a variety of vestibular receptors can be stimulated. Such a child may spend as much as three-fourths of a therapy session involved in the reception of intense vestibular stimulation.

Children with gravitational insecurity or intolerance to movement will not seek out vestibular stimulation. They will want to keep their feet touching the floor. Therapy for these children begins with activities that involve minimal vestibular stimulation while their feet are anchored firmly to the floor. The stimulation is provided in positions in which the head is upright. Security can be furthered by the therapist's holding the child or doing an activity with him. Providing a helmet and bringing attention to the mats and pillows that are under the child may decrease the threat of movement.

A child with dyspraxia typically seeks out vestibular stimulation, but not as much as the child who is diagnosed as having a vestibular bilateral integration dysfunction. Frequently these children are distractible. Providing limited equipment can enhance the flow of the therapy session. There should be more emphasis on ideation and programming of action and on the quality of adaptive responses. For example, a child with dyspraxia may be encouraged to set up an obstacle course and figure out what to do in navigating through it. Because such a child sometimes self-directs toward repetitive activites, she may need to be gently pushed on to new activities. Verbal regulation such as singing or counting can assist such a child in making adaptive responses.[29] Climbing activities may be especilly beneficial, as well as activities involving initiating, timing, and sequencing.[29]

Provision of tactile and vibratory stimulation is usually appropriate for children with poor somatosensory processing. It is also central to the treatment of tactile defensiveness. Generally, tactile stimulation is not imposed but is made available to the child through the provision of a variety of brushes, napped fabrics, and other textured objects that can be applied to the skin. Carpeted equipment can effectively provide tactile stimulation in an activity so that attention can be directed to the activity and not to the tactile input, per se. Fuzzy blankets, sheepskins, or cloths with which the therapist can unobtrusively line or pad surfaces are also helpful.

INDIVIDUAL DIFFERENCES

Each child brings to the therapy session unique differences that change over time.[113] Individual differences in children exist in their physical attributes and in their behavioral and emotional styles. For example, one child may be emotive while another is apathetic; one may be sociable and another shy. Therapists will also have individual differences in their approaches to children. Because sensory integrative procedures are influenced by the individual differences of the child and therapist, a description of the activities that were used in a therapy session is only a partial presentation of the therapeutic process. Indeed, two children may participate in identical activities, but the qualitative aspects of their treatment experience may be diametrically opposite. One child may have experienced success and freedom, the other failure and coercion.

PRECAUTIONS

Sensory integrative procedures should not be administered by occupational therapists with limited clinical experience. Ayres[19] warns that the provision of tactile, and especially vestibular, stimulation can have deleterious effects on the nervous system. There is the danger that the child may experience sensory overload signaled by flushing, blanching, or perspiring. Overinhibition of brain stem mechanisms can result in cyanosis or depressed respiratory functions. Finally, Ayres[19] points out that there is a risk of accident when children who are unskilled and lacking in judgment and accurate perceptions are encouraged to respond to environmental challenges. The provision of sufficient mats, equipment that is kept in a good state of repair, and an artfully vigilant therapist all lessen the risks involved (Figure 19-18).

CASE STUDY

This case study that illustrates the use of sensory integrative procedures was selected because the subject was one of the best responders to therapy. Few other children, even though they may be recommended for therapy, will do as well. As a child with a vestibular bilateral integrative dysfunction, the subject could be identified as a child with the characteristics for which sensory integrative procedures seem to be most effective. It may be that such a child responds best to therapy because there is little other central nervous system impairment.

Tammy, an 8-year-old white female, was referred to occupational therapy by an educational psychologist on staff at the public school she was attending. At that time Tammy was having academic difficulties, and her mother reported that she was distractible, frustrated, and often discouraged. In addition, she seemed to be having visual perception problems. An occupational therapist certified in the administration and interpretation of the Southern California Sensory Integration Tests evaluated Tammy on these tests and on a variety of neuromuscular responses considered to be related to learning to make a decision as to whether Tammy should be recommended for sensory integrative procedures.

The results of the evaluation suggested the presence of a vestibular bilateral integration dysfunction. This impression was supported by the findings of depressed postrotary nystagmus, low muscle tone, inadequate equilibrium reactions, poor balance, difficulty with assumption of the prone extension posture, and irregular eye pursuits. In addition, Tammy demonstrated tactile defensiveness. Scores on the tests measuring visual perception supported Tammy's mother's report of an apparent problem in this domain. The type of vestibular deficit Tammy displayed had been associated with learning disabilities in Ayres' research and was considered to be a possible contributor to Tammy's academic problems. The processing of vestibular input is proposed to be crucial in sensory integrative theory to many aspects of development because of the numerous neurological associations between this system and other parts of the nervous system. Inefficient processing in the vestibular system was thought to be related to Tammy's distractibility, decreased attention, poor organization of behavior, and difficulty interacting with peers.

Tammy received eight 1-hour sessions of occupational therapy per week from Jan. 28 to Aug. 31 (7 months). Because there was reason to believe that the type of sensory integrative dysfunction Tammy seemed to have would be responsive to sensory integrative procedures, and because the dysfunction seemed to contribute to her underachievement, the school district agreed to finance the therapy. Therapy was aimed at providing Tammy with the opportunity to receive vestibular and tactile input in a manner that allowed her to self-direct the sessions and elicit adaptive responses. Tammy proved to be very self-directed within the nonthreatening milieu of the one-to-one therapy sessions. She demonstrated a strong tendency to seek out the type of stimulation that the therapist had hypothesized had not been efficiently processed by Tammy's nervous system before the intervention (vestibular and tactile input). In general, Tammy selected the activities she would engage in during therapy, while the therapist helped to make the tasks both challenging and achievable.

Progress notes recorded during the 8-month period reflected the changes in Tammy that seemed to be a consequence of therapy. In the first month the therapist wrote that Tammy appeared to be "highly motivated but moved without planning," that "she experimented with all the equipment" and seemed to enjoy "self-directed vestibular input," and that she interchanged her right and left hands when throwing objects. Tammy was described as being unable to throw with sufficient force to reach a target. In these in-

TABLE 19-3	**Tammy's test results**		
Test	*January*	*April*	*June*
Slosson oral reading	3.4 grade	3.7 grade	3.7 grade
Beery visual-motor	6 years, 7 months	6 years, 7 months	8 years, 8 months
Wide Range Achievement Test (WRAT)			
reading	3.6 grade	4.1 grade	4.2 grade
WRAT spelling	2.6 grade	3.5 grade	3.9 grade
WRAT arithmetic	3.5 grade	3.9 grade	4.1 grade

stances, the therapist reported, Tammy would become upset.

Four months after therapy had been initiated the progress notes reflected an increase in Tammy's ability to engage in creative play. Improved ability to monitor her own activity was also noted. For example, Tammy was reported to frequently enjoy rolling inside a blue hollow ball, but before rolling she would say, "I need to get organized." Soon after Tammy began to develop better social interactions with other clients who were receiving therapy. A note written at the seventh month of treatment read, "As usual, directs activities pretty much by self," although it should be noted that in the course of time in which sensory integrative procedures were used with Tammy, there were times when she would express boredom. The last note read, "Tammy brought a vase of flowers for the therapists and appeared sad to leave. She did a lot of gymnastic-type tricks using the glider, swing, stacked inner tubes, and trapeze and rings to flip and hang upside down. . . . She explored the clinic as though saying farewell. Hugged all therapists—definitely hated to leave."

To assess Tammy's academic and visual-perceptual progress, several standardized tests were administered. These were given in January before intervention, in April (3 months after the initiation of therapy), and in June (5 months after therapy began). The results are in Table 19-3. Samples of Tammy's

handwriting before intervention and after are shown in Figure 19-19. It can be seen that considerable progress in this area was made.

Gains made by Tammy in other domains, for example, behaviorally, in peer interaction, and role performance, are difficult to quantify. Comments made by Tammy's mother provide qualitative data that suggest improvements. A year after therapy had been instituted Tammy's mother was interviewed. She stated that "Tammy used to have few friends. She now seems so much happier, interacts very well, and has many friends. What I really notice is how much better her self-concept seems to be and how much more confidence she has." She also said that she was appreciative of an "improvement in the quality of Tammy's life."

In the posttreatment interview, Tammy's mother also commented on her impressions of Tammy's progress. She said, "One year ago Tammy hardly ever did well on any of her academics. This year she is doing fabulously."

It is cases such as Tammy that lead therapists to become overly enthusiastic. Few children are expected to respond as well. Tammy's case is an example of a child with a certain type of learning disorder who seems to benefit in morale, academic performance, and social interaction from engagement in sensory integrative activities.

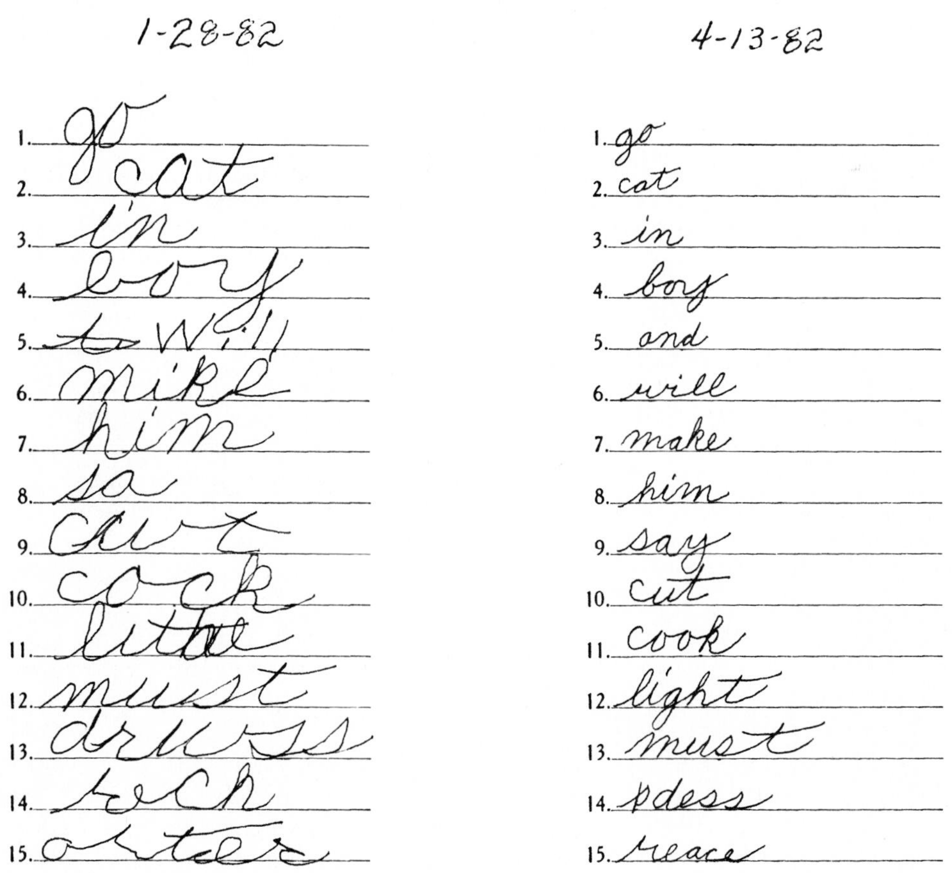

FIGURE 19-19

Tammy's handwriting samples before and after intervention.

DISTINCTIONS BETWEEN SENSORY INTEGRATIVE AND OTHER NEUROPHYSIOLOGICAL APPROACHES IN OCCUPATIONAL THERAPY

Ayres[19] states that "theoretical models, like children, follow a developmental sequence." Although sensory integrative theory and its procedures incorporate some of the principles of perceptual-motor and sensorimotor approaches, in its present state the sensory integrative approach should be treated as a distinct and separate treatment approach not to be confused with the other two types of programs. In the discipline of occupational therapy the terms cognitive perceptual-motor, sensorimotor, sensory-motor-sensory, sensory integration, and multisensory have been used to refer to a variety of neurophysiological approaches to treatment or to processes in the brain.[19,55,73,99] Ayres chose to use the term sensory integration to refer to the theory and procedures she developed, and she provides a sound rationale for doing so. She prefers sensory integration because it emphasizes an organizational process occurring in the brain. Other terms, such as sensorimotor, in contrast focus on the relationship of sensation to specific motor responses. We suggest that sensory integration be strictly used to refer to the theory and treatment that Ayres originated.

Our position may differ from that presented by other therapists. For example, Weeks[159] subsumed the sensory integrative approach developed by Ayres under the general category of sensorimotor integration approaches. Weeks used the term sensorimotor integration in referring to "the multisensory treatment approach, except in discussion of underlying sensory integrative processing or of tests and approaches labeled sensory integration by their developers." However, because Weeks covered the sensory integration approach under the broader category of sensorimotor integration, there is blurring of the distinctions between a variety of approaches.

Farber[55] listed Ayres' approach as one of several sensorimotor integrative treatment approaches. To add to the confusion, the American Occupational Therapy Association[3] listed the term sensory integration under sensorimotor components of occupational therapy treatment and then defined the terms as referring to skill and performance, rather than to neural organization.

In contrast, Ayres' use of the term sensory integration downplays emphasis on the motor response. Instead, it stresses the brain's organization of information (sensory input). In prior sections of this chapter we have stressed that sensory integrative procedures are used to help the child develop a more efficient general organizational capacity. Enhancement of this ability is seen as contributing to the creation of a child who is more creative and better able to adapt to environmental demands, more proficient in organizing behavior and in performing daily activities, and better able to approach and succeed in academic tasks. The concern is more on how well the child uses his brain to organize information, than on how sensation can be used to produce more normal motor responses.

A distinction should also be made between Ayres' use of the term adaptive response and use of that term by other occupational therapists. Farber,[55] for example, uses adaptive response to refer to a specific neuromuscular response that the therapist attempts to bring about in the client through application of a particular hands-on technique. Developmentally appropriate techniques are repeatedly applied until the desired adaptive response is obtained. Ayres,[28] on the other hand, uses adaptive response to refer to a behavioral response that originates in and is controlled by the client in conjunction with therapist manipulation of the environment. The specific adaptive responses that the child will emit often cannot be predicted beforehand, because they arise spontaneously within the child during interaction with the equipment. A therapy session using sensory integrative procedures might elicit adaptive responses at varying levels of complexity, although over many sessions the complexity of overall responses would increase. An adaptive response at a specific developmental level would not be demanded before progression to higher levels is allowed.

Sensorimotor approaches

The treatment approaches that we would choose to classify as sensorimotor are those that are strictly concerned with how sensation and neurophysiological principles can be employed to effect the neuromuscular motor response, per se. The procedures described by Bobath and Bobath,[37] Rood,[132] and Kabat and Knott[84] fall within this category. In their pure form, these approaches are generally used with children and adults suffering from neuromuscular disorders (for example, cerebral palsy or cerebral vascular accidents). They are characterized by hands-on procedures in which the therapist applies pressure or other types of sensation, or otherwise handles the patient so that motor responses reflect more normal movement patterns or tone.

Ayres acknowledges that concepts from the sensorimotor approach have been incorporated into some sensory integrative procedures.[19] The concept of applying sensory stimulation to enhance motor responses originated with Kabat and Knott.[84] Ayres credits Rood[132] with first having elucidated the therapeutic role of tactile and vestibular stimulation. A uniqueness of sensory integrative procedures is that they emphasize potent vestibular stimulation, the type that is provided by swinging in net hammocks and on swings. Sensory integrative procedures also depart from the sensorimotor approaches in that the goals of therapy go well beyond the promoting of a more normal neuromuscular response. Sensory integrative procedures are directed toward the evincing of broadly defined adaptive responses, thereby encouraging the child to organize her own behavior.

Perceptual-motor programs

Another category of neurophysiological approaches is called perceptual-motor programs or systems. As was previously discussed, the characteristics of these programs originated primarily in the field of education. Here the differences between the characteristics of these programs and those of the sensory integrative approach are addressed (Table 19-4).

Perceptual-motor programs are more cognitively oriented than the sensory integration approach. They may ask the child to focus attention on coordinated execution of specific motor acts, often with verbal guidance. For example, they may require the child to practice specific visuomotor activities, such as drawing a circle, while the child or therapist says the word *circle*. With sensory integrative procedures, gross motor activities are heavily used to elicit adaptive responses automatically, and verbalizations are deemphasized.

In perceptual-motor programs the child is required to follow a predetermined sequence of activities. A lesson plan may be used to outline how the session will proceed. The child may be instructed to move on from one activity station to the next and perform certain skills at each. As was previously illustrated, the choice of activities that will be used in a sensory integration treatment session cannot be predetermined. It results from an ongoing interplay of child self-direction and therapist judgment. The status of the child's nervous system through the course of the therapy session is central in how treatment will flow. The therapeutic situation must be flexible yet simultaneously provide the child with a sense of organization.

Repetitive activity is seen as of value in perceptual programs because, through practice, skills are mastered. In the sensory integrative approach, while repetition may be allowed at times, the emphasis is on exploration and creativity. The child's opportunities to generate ideas about what can be done with a piece of equipment is considered as important as the perfecting of particular skills.

Perceptual-motor programs tend to be more program-centered, while the sensory integration approach is primarily child-centered. In the former a logically developed sequence of activities may be prescribed that makes developmental and neurophysiological sense. The program guidelines determine the lesson plan. In the sensory integrative approach the child is given considerable say in what activities will be done. The therapist assists in making the activities achievable by the child. Knowledge of developmental sequence may guide the therapist in doing this, but a predetermined developmental sequence is not imposed.

The two types of programs also differ in the role of the teacher or therapist. In perceptual-motor programs the teacher may command, expect, or instruct the child to do certain tasks. In the sensory integrative approach the therapist assists the child in organizing his own behavior.[29] This is accomplished through a variety of techniques, including making available the appropriate equipment, adapting the equipment in accord with the child's needs through activity analysis, asking the child to participate in the arrangement of the equipment, and, of course, allowing the child to choose activities.

Perceptual-motor programs lend themselves to group activity because they clearly map out predetermined sequences of tasks. The use of lesson plans and adult direction makes management of groups feasible. Self-direction of the child, which is so important in a sensory integrative approach, can lead to chaos if permitted in groups. Careful monitoring of autonomic and behavioral responses to sensory stimulation and structuring of the environment to meet individual needs also would be impossible if one therapist were in charge of a group of children. Sensory integrative procedures, then, are best carried out in a one-to-one situation.

Two other characteristics distinguish sensory integrative and perceptual-motor programs. First, an essential feature of sensory integrative procedures is the elaborate array of suspended equipment that can be used to provide potent and varied types of vestibular stimulation. Perceptual-motor programs typically do not involve this. Tabletop activities and gross motor skills involving jumping, balancing, laterality, or coordination are usually described as characteristics of these programs. Second, perceptual-motor programs usually fo-

TABLE 19-4	Comparison of perceptual-motor and sensory integrative programs
Perceptual-motor	*Sensory integrative*
Cognitive orientation	Noncognitive emphasis
Predetermined sequence	Flexible sequence
Repetitive drill	Exploration and creativity
Program-centered	Child-centered
Adult-directed	Adult-guided
Group program	Dyadic interaction
Teach specific skills	Improve brain processing
Suspended equipment optional	Suspended equipment mandatory

cus on the teaching of specific skills rather than on the enhancement of brain processing.

Knickerbocker's holistic approach

Knickerbocker[97] described yet another occupational therapy treatment approach that is neurophysiologically based. She cites Ayres as the inspiration for her program, which is designed specifically for learning disabled children. Examination of this program shows that some aspects closely resemble Ayres' sensory integrative procedures, while others clearly fall into the perceptual-motor realm. A unique element of parent involvement is added as well.

Knickerbocker[97] divides her treatment program into two major content areas, or phases. Phase I is characterized by sensory stimulation and gross motor acitivities using equipment that is associated with Ayres's work, such as the scooter board, carpeted barrel, and suspended equipment. Furthermore, a child-oriented, exploratory process that closely parallels the classic sensory integrative approach is described for this phase. Phase II, however, is made up of tabletop activities and laterality training tasks, many of which have been traditionally used in perceptual-motor programs. Here the therapist assumes a more didactic role, and specific sequences of training activities are delineated. These activities are cognitive in nature, ranging from the sequencing of toys, blocks, and words, to verbally directed handwriting training.

While Knickerbocker does advocate one-to-one therapy that is individualized and sensitive to child cues, the overall structure of her approach appears to be program centered rather than child centered. A series of eight developmental program plans are spelled out, with certain lower level tasks identified as "precise prerequisites" for higher ones. Flexibility in the use of the program plans is emphasized, yet their specificity may lead therapists to focus attention more on predetermined program structure than on individual child characteristics and motivation.

The systematic combination of sensory integrative and perceptual-motor techniques makes Knickerbocker's approach an attractive alternative for therapists faced with the task of treating children for whom a "pure" sensory integrative approach may not be appropriate. Some cautions are in order, however. Quantitative reports on the efficacy of Knickerbocker's program have not been published. Moreover, the striking resemblance of Phase II activities to process-oriented special education techniques may lead to conflict between therapists using the program and educators who may reject it as being invalid on the grounds that process approaches do not generalize to academic success.

SUMMARY

Clarification has been made of the differences between sensorimotor, sensory integrative, and perceptual-motor programs because of the widespread confusion in the profession regarding the use of these terms. We urge occupational therapists to apply the criteria we have suggested for classifying interventions and for generalizing the results of treatment studies that employ neurophysiological approaches. For example, we do not believe that the findings on the effectiveness of a particular perceptual-motor program can be generalized to sensory integrative procedures or vice versa. Ayres' effectiveness studies,[23,26] should not be used to justify programs that only remotely resemble her methods of treatment. The reader is warned that programs called sensory integrative therapy in the literature may not constitute sensory integrative programs according to our criteria.

REFERENCES

1. Abikoff, H.: Cognitive training interventions in children: review of a new approach, J. Learn. Disabil. **12**(2):65, 1979.
2. Allessandrini, N.A.: Play—a child's world, Am. J. Occup. Ther. **3**(1):9, 1949.
3. American Occupational Therapy Association: Uniform terminology for reporting occupational therapy services, Rockville, Md., 1979, American Occupational Therapy Association, Inc.
4. American Psychiatric Association: Diagnostic and statistical manual of mental disorders, ed. 3, DSM-III, Washington, D.C., 1980.
5. Ames, L.B.: Learning disability: truth or trap, J. Learn. Disabil. **16**(1):19, 1983.
6. Ayres, A.J.: An analysis of crafts in the treatment of electroshock patients, Am. J. Occup. Ther. **3**(4):195, 1949.
7. Ayres, A.J.: Ontogenetic principles in the development of arm and hand functions, Am. J. Occup. Ther. **8**(3):95, 1954.
8. Ayres, A.J.: Proprioceptive facilitation elicited through the upper extremities. Part 1: background, Am. J. Occup. Ther. **9**(1):1, 1955.
9. Ayres, A.J.: The visual-motor function, Am. J. Occup. Ther. **12**(3):130, 1958.
10. Ayres, A.J.: Development of body scheme in children, Am. J. Occup. Ther. **15**(3):99, 1961.
11. Ayres, A.J.: The Eleanor Clark Slagle Lecture, The development of perceptual-motor abilities: a theoretical basis for treatment of dysfunction, Am. J. Occup. Ther. **17**(6):221, 1963.
12. Ayres, A.J.: Tactile functions: their relation to hyperactive and perceptual motor behavior, Am. J. Occup. Ther. **18**(1):6, 1964.
13. Ayres, A.J.: Patterns of perceptual-motor dysfunction in children: a factor analytic study, Percep. Mot. Skills **20**:335, 1965.
14. Ayres, A.J.: Interrelationships among perceptual-motor functions in children, Am. J. Occup. Ther. **20**(2):68, 1966.
15. Ayres, A.J.: Interrelations among perceptual-motor abilities in a group of normal children, Am. J. Occup. Ther. **20**(6):288, 1966.
16. Ayres, A.J.: Deficits in sensory integration in educationally handicapped children, J. Learn. Disabil. **2**(3):44, 1969.
17. Ayres, A.J.: Characteristics of types of sensory integrative dysfunction, Am. J. Occup. Ther. **25**(7):329, 1971.
18. Ayres, A.J.: Improving academic scores through sensory integration, J. Learn. Disabil. **5**:338, 1972.

19. Ayres, A.J.: Sensory integration and learning disorders, Los Angeles, 1972, Western Psychological Services.

20. Ayres, A.J.: Southern California Sensory Integration Tests, Los Angeles, 1972, Western Psychological Services.

21. Ayres, A.J.: Types of sensory integrative dysfunction among disabled learners, Am. J. Occup. Ther. **26**(1):13, 1972.

22. Ayres, A.J.: Southern California Postrotary Nystagmus Test, Los Angeles, 1975, Western Psychological Services.

23. Ayres, A.J.: The effect of sensory integrative therapy on learning disabled children: the final report of a research project, Los Angeles, 1976, Center for the Study of Sensory Integrative Dysfunction.

24. Ayres, A.J.: Cluster analyses of measures of sensory integration, Am. J. Occup. Ther. **31**(6):362, 1977.

25. Ayres, A.J.: Dichotic listening performance in learning-disabled children, Am. J. Occup. Ther. **31**(7):441, 1977.

26. Ayres, A.J.: Effect of sensory integrative therapy on the coordination of children with choreoathetoid movements, Am. J. Occup. Ther. **31**(5):291, 1977.

27. Ayres, A.J.: Learning disabilities and the vestibular system, J. Learn. Disabil. **11**(1):18, 1978.

28. Ayres, A.J.: Sensory integration and the child, Los Angeles, 1979, Western Psychological Services.

29. Ayres, A.J.: Aspects of the somatomotor adaptive response and praxis. Audiotape, Pasadena, Calif. 1981, Center for the Study of Sensory Integrative Dysfunction.

30. Ayres, A.J.: Personal communication, Feb. 15, 1983.

31. Ayres, A.J., and Mailloux, Z.: Influence of sensory integration procedures on language development, Am. J. Occup. Ther. **35**(6):383, 1981.

32. Ayres, A.J., and Tickle, L.: Hyperresponsivity to touch and vestibular stimuli as a predictor of positive response to sensory integration procedures in autistic children, Am. J. Occup. Ther. **34**:375, 1980.

33. Barris, R.: Environmental interactions: an extension of the model of occupation, Am. J. Occup. Ther. **36**(10):637, 1982.

34. Bauer, R.H.: Memory processes in children with learning disabilities: evidence for deficient rehearsal, J. Exp. Child Psychol. **24**:415, 1977.

35. Beery, K.: Developmental Test of Visual Motor Integration, Chicago, 1967, Follett Publishing Co.

36. Berko, M.J.: Mental evaluation of the aphasic child, Am. J. Occup.Ther. **5**(6):241, 1951.

37. Bobath, K., and Bobath, B.: The facilitation of normal postural reactions and movements in the treatment of cerebral palsy, Physiotherapy **50**:246, 1964.

38. Bogen, J.E.: The other side of the brain: an appositional. In Ornstein, R.E., editor: The nature of human consciousness, San Francisco, 1973, W.H. Freeman and Co., Publishers.

39. Boucher, S.: Ayres' sensory integration and learning disorders: a question of theory and practice, Aust. J. Ment. Retard. **5**:41, 1978.

40. Bruininks, R.H.: Physical and motor development of retarded persons: In Ellis, N.R., editor: International review of research in mental retardation, vol. 7, New York, 1974, Academic Press, Inc.

41. Bruininks, R.: Bruininks-Oseretsky Test of Motor Proficiency, Circle Pines, Minn., 1978, American Guidance Service.

42. Carrow, E.: Test for Auditory Comprehension of Language, Austin, Tex., 1973, Learning Concepts.

43. Carrow, E.: Carrow Elicited Language Inventory, Austin, Tex., 1974, Learning Concepts.

44. Chalfant, J., and King, F.: An approach to operationalizing the definition of learning disabilities, J. Learn. Disabil. **9**(4):228, 1976.

45. Clark, F.A.: Right and left hemisphere specialization: implications for the laterality and hemispheric dysfunction hypothesis of learning disabilities. In Tyler, N.B., editor: Sensory integration

topics: faculty reviews, Pasadena, Calif., 1980, The Center for the Study of Sensory Integrative Dysfunction.

46. Clark, F.A., and others: A comparison of operant and sensory integration methods on vocalizations and other developmental parameters in profoundly retarded adults, Am. J. Occup. Ther. **32**:86, 1978.

47. Critchley, M.: The dyslexic child, ed. 2, Springfield, Ill., 1970, Charles C Thomas, Publisher.

48. Cruickshank, W.: Concepts in learning disabilities, vol. 2, Syracuse, N.Y., 1981, Syracuse University Press.

49. Cruickshank, W.: Learning disabilities: a neurophysiological dysfunction, J. Learn. Disabil. **16**(1):27, 1983.

50. DePauw, K.P.: Enhancing the sensory integration of aphasic students, J. Learn. Disabil. **11**(3):142, 1978.

51. deRenne-Stephan, C.: Imitation: a mechanism of play behavior, Am. J. Occup. Ther. **34**(2):95, 1980.

52. Doyle, R.B., Anderson, R.P., and Halcomb, C.G.: Attention deficits and the effects of visual distraction, J. Learn. Disabil. **9**:48, 1976.

53. Dunn, L.M., and Smith, J.O.: The Peabody Picture Vocabulary Tests, Circle Pines, Minn., 1966, American Guidance Service.

54. Ensminger, E.E.: The effects of a classroom language development program on psycholinguistic abilities and intellectual functioning of slow learning and borderline retarded children, Doctoral dissertation, 1966, University of Kansas.

55. Farber, S.D.: A multisensory approach to neurorehabilitation. In Farber, S.D., editor: Neurorehabilitation: a multisensory approach, Philadelphia, 1982, W.B. Saunders Co.

56. Farnham-Diggory, S.: Learning disabilities: a psychological perspective, Cambridge, Mass. 1978, Harvard University Press.

57. Farnham-Diggory, S., and Greggg, L.W.: Short term memory functions in young readers, J. Exp. Child Psychol. **19**:279, 1975.

58. Fernald, G.M.: Remedial techniques in basic school subjects, New York, 1943, McGraw-Hill Book Co.

59. Fernald, G.M., and Keller, H.: One effect of kinesthetic factors in the development of word recognition in the case of nonreaders. J. Educ. Res. **4**:355, 1921.

60. Firestone, B.: Auditory reaction time of reading disabled children on three processing tasks, Doctoral dissertation, 1976, University of Southern California.

61. Florey, L.L.: An approach to play and play development, Am. J. Occup. Ther. **25**:275, 1971.

62. Florey, L.L.: Studies of play: implications for growth, development, and for clinical practice, Am. J. Occup. Ther. **35**(8):519, 1981.

63. Frostig, M., and Horne, D.: The Frostig program for the development of visual perception, Chicago, 1964, Follett Publishing Co.

64. Frostig, M., Lefever, D.W., and Whittlesey, J.R.B.: A developmental test of visual perception for evaluating normal and neurologically handicapped children, Percept. Mot. Skills **12**:383, 1961.

65. Frostig, M., and Maslow, P.: Neuropsychological contributions to education, J. Learn. Disabil. **12**(8):538, 1979.

66. Fuller, P.W.: Attention to the EEG alpha rhythm in learning disabled children, J. Learn. Disabil. **11**:303, 1978.

67. Gardner, M.: Expressive One Word Picture Vocabulary Test, Norato, Calif., 1979, Gardner, Morrison Academic Therapy Publications.

68. Gazzaniga, M.S., Bogen, J.E., and Sperry, R.W.: Dyspraxia following division of the cerebral commissures, Arch. Neurol. **16**:606, 1967.

69. Gearheart, B.: Learning disabilities educational strategies, ed. 2, St. Louis, 1977, The C.V. Mosby Co.

70. Gearheart, B.: Learning disabilities educational strategies, ed. 3, St. Louis, 1981, The C.V. Mosby Co.

71. Giden, F.M., Eno, M.L.: and Bosley, E.C.: The occupational therapist discusses aphasia, Am. J. Occup. Ther. **4**(4):160, 1950.

72. Gilfoyle, E., editor: Training: occupational therapy educational management in schools (a competency-based educational program), vol. 3, mod. 1-8, Rockville, Md., 1979-1980, American Occupational Therapy Association, Inc.

73. Gilfoyle, E., and Grady, A: Posture and movement. In Hopkins, H., and Smith, H., editors: Willard and Spackman's occupational therapy, Philadelphia, 1978, J.B. Lippincott Co.

74. Goldstein, K.: The organism, New York, 1939, American Book Co.

75. Grimwood, L.M., and Rutherford, E.M.: Sensory integrative therapy as an intervention procedure with grade one "at risk" readers—a three year study, Except. Child. **27**:52, 1980.

76. Hagen, J.W.: The effect of distraction on selective attention, Child Dev. **38**:685, 1967.

77. Hammill, D.D., and Larsen, S.C.: The efficacy of psycholinguistic training, Except. Child. **41**:5, 1974.

78. Harris, L.P.: Attention and learning disordered children: a review of theory and remediation, J. Learn. Disabil. **9**:100, 1976.

79. Haworth, M.: The Primary Visual Motor Test, New York, 1970, Grune & Stratton, Inc.

80. Head, H.: Aphasia and kindred disorders of speech, vols. I, II, London, 1926, Cambridge University Press.

81. Hebb, D.O.: Organization of behavior, New York, 1949, John Wiley & Sons, Inc.

82. Hinshelwood, J.: Congenital word blindness, London, 1917, Lewis.

83. Jastak, S.R., and Jastak, S.W.B.: Wide Range Achievement Test, rev. ed., Wilmington, Del., 1976, Guidance Associations of Delaware.

84. Kabat, H., and Knott, M.: Principles of neuromuscular reeducation, Phys. Ther. Rev. **28**:107, 1948.

85. Katz, P., and Deutsch, M.: Relation of auditory-visual shifting to regard achievement, Percept. Mot. Skills **17**:327, 1963.

86. Keogh, B.K.: Marker variables: a search for compatibility and generalizability in the field of learning disabilities, Learn. Disabil. Q. **3**(3):8, 1978.

87. Keogh, B.K.: Classification, compliance, and confusion, J. Learn. Disabil. **16**(1):25, 1983.

88. Keogh, B.K., and Margolis, J.: Learn to labor and to wait: attentional problems of children with learning disorders, J. Learn. Disabil. **9**(5):276, 1976.

89. Kephart, N.C.: The slow learner in the classroom, Columbus, Ohio, 1971, Charles E. Merrill Publishing Co.

90. Kielhofner, G., and Burke, J.: A model of human occupation. Part 1: conceptual framework and content, Am. J. Occup. Ther. **34**(9):572, 1980.

91. Kielhofner, G., Burke, J., and Igi, C.: A model of human occupation. Part 4: assessment and intervention, Am. J. Occup. Ther. **34**:777, 1980.

92. Kinsbourne, M., and Caplan, P.J.: Children's learning and attention problems, Boston, 1979, Little, Brown and Co.

93. Kinsbourne, M., and Hiscock, M.: Cerebral lateralization and cognitive development. In Chall, J.S., and Mirsky, A.E., editors: Education and the brain: the seventy-seventh yearbook of the National Society for the Study of Education (part 2), Chicago, 1978, University of Chicago Press.

94. Kirk, S.A., and Kirk, W.D.: On defining learning disabilities, J. Learn. Disabil. **16**(1):20, 1983.

95. Kirk, S.A., McCarthy, J.J., and Kirk, W.D.: Examiner's manual: Illinois Test of Psycholinguistic Abilities, rev. ed., Urbana, Ill., 1968, University of Illinois Press.

96. Klahr, D., and Wallace, J.G.: Cognitive development: an information processing view, Hillsdale, N.J., 1976, Lawrence Erlbaum Associates, Publishers.

97. Knickerbocker, B.M.: A holistic approach to the treatment of learning disorders, Thorofare, N.J., 1980, Charles B. Slack, Inc.

98. Leher, R.J.: An open letter to an occupational therapist, J. Learn. Disabil. **14**:3, 1981.

99. Llorens, L.A., and others: The effects of cognitive perceptual-motor training approach on children with behavior maladjustment, Am. J. Occup. Ther. **23**(6):502, 1969.

100. Maccoby, E.E.: Selective auditory attention in children. In Lippsitt, L.P., and Spiker, C.C., editors: Advances in child development and behavior, vol. 3, New York, 1967, Academic Press.

101. Mack, W., Lindquist, J., and Parham, D.: A synthesis of occupational behavior and sensory integration concepts in theory and practice. Part I: theoretical foundations, Am. J. Occup. Ther. **36**(7):365, 1982.

102. Magrun, W.M., and others: Effects of vestibular stimulation on spontaneous use of verbal language in developmentally delayed children, Am. J. Occup. Ther. **35**:101, 1982.

103. Mailloux, Z.: The relationship between self-esteem and praxis, visual motor integration and student role performace in learning disabled children, Masters thesis, 1980, University of Southern California.

104. Mann, L., and others: L.D. or not L.D., that was the question: a retrospective analysis of child service demonstration centers in compliance with the federal definition of learning disabilities, J. Learn. Disabil. **16**(1):14, 1983.

105. McConnell, F., Horton, D.B., and Smith B.R.: Sensory-perceptual and language training to prevent school learning disabilities in culturally deprived preschool children, Nashville, Tenn., 1972, the Bill Wilkerson Hearing and Speech Center. Final report, project no. 5-0682, grant no. OE6-32-52-7900-5025, USOE Bureau of Research.

106. McDaniel, M.: The role of the occupational therapist in the reeducation of aphasia patients, part III, Am. J. Occup. Ther. **8**(2):63, 1955.

107. Meichenbaum, D.: Cognitive-behavior modification: an integrative approach, New York, 1977, Plenum Publishing Corp.

108. Michelman, S.: The importance of creative play, Am. J. Occup. Ther. **25**:285, 1971.

109. Minskoff, E., Wiseman, D.E., and Minskoff, J.G.: The MWM program for developing language abilities, Ridgefield, N.J., 1972, Educational Associates.

110. Mirsky, A.F.: Attention: a neurophysiological perspective. In Mirsky, A.F., editor: Education and the brain: the seventy-seventh yearbook of the National Society for the Study of Education, part II, Chicago, 1978, University of Chicago Press.

111. Mondani, M.S., and Tutko, T.A.: Relationship of academic underachievement to incidental learning, J. Consult. Clin. Psychol. **33**:558, 1969.

112. Montgomery, P., and Richter, E.: Effect on sensory integrative therapy on the neuromotor development of retarded children, Phys. Ther. **57**:799, 1977.

113. Moore, J.: Individual differences and the art of therapy, Am. J. Occup. Ther. **31**(10):663, 1977.

114. Myklebust, H.R.: Toward a sience of learning disabilities, J. Learn. Disabil. **16**(1):17, 1983.

115. Mysak, E.D., and Fiorentino, M.R.: Neurophysiological conditions in occupational therapy for the cerebral palsied, Am. J. Occup. Ther. **15**(3):112, 1961.

116. O'Donnell, D.A., and Eisenson, J.: Delacato training for reading achievement and visual-motor integration, J. Learn. Disabil. **2**:441, 1969.

117. Ornstein, R.E.: Right and left thinking, Psychol. Today **6**:87, 1973.

118. Orton, S.T.: Word blindness in school children, Arch. Neurol. Psychiatr. **14**:581, 1925.

119. Orton, S.T.: Reading, writing and speech problems in children, New York, 1937, W.W. Norton and Co., Inc.

120. Orton, S.T.: A neurological explanation of the reading disability, Educ. Rec. **20**:58, 1939.

121. Osgood, C.E.: Method and theory in experimental psychology, New York, 1953, Oxford University Press, Inc.

122. Osgood, C.E.: Motivational dynamics of language behavior. In Jones, M.R., editor: Nebraska symposium on motivation, Lincoln, Neb., 1957, University of Nebraska Press.

123. Ottenbacher, K.: Occupational therapy and special education: some issues and concerns related to Public Law 94-142, Am. J. Occup. Ther. **36**(2):81, 1982.

124. Ottenbacher, K.: Sensory integration therapy: affect or effect, Am. J. Occup. Ther. **36**(9):571, 1982.

125. Palmer, M.F., and Berko, F.: The education of the aphasic child, Am. J. Occup. Ther. **6**(6):241, 1952.

126. Poncher, H.G., and Richmond, J.B.: Occupational therapy in pediatrics, Am. J. Occup. Ther. **1**(5):276, 1947.

127. Reid, D.K., and Hresko, W.P.: A cognitive approach to learning disabilities, New York, 1981, McGraw-Hill Book Co.

128. Reilly, M.: The educational process, Am. J. Occup. Ther. **23**(4):299, 1969.

129. Richmond, J.B., and Lis, E.F.: Occupational therapy in pediatrics, Am. J. Occup. Ther. **3**(4):185, 1949.

130. Robinault, I.P.: Perception technics for the preschool cerebral palsied, Am. J. Occup. Ther. **8**(1):3, 1954.

131. Robinson, A.: Play: the arena for acquisition of rules for competent behavior, Am. J. Occup. Ther. **31**:248, 1977.

132. Rood, M.S.: Neurophysiologic reactions as a basis for physical therapy, Phys. Ther. Rev. **34**:444, 1954.

133. Sabatino, D.A.: The house that Jack built, J. Learn. Disabil. **16**(1):26, 1983.

134. Schuell, H., Jenkins, J.J., and Jimenez-Pablon, E.: Aphasia in adults, New York, 1964, Harper & Row, Publishers.

135. Senf, G.M., and Feshbach, S.: Development of bisensory memory in culturally deprived, dyslexic, and normal readers, J. Educ. Psychol. **61**:461, 1970.

136. Shields, D.T.: Brain responses to stimuli in disorders of information processing, J. Learn. Disabil. **6**:501, 1976.

137. Sieben, R.L.: Controversial treatments for learning disorders, Acad. Ther. **13**(2):138, 1977.

138. Spreen, O., and Benton, A.: Sentence Repetition Test, Victoria, Canada, 1977, Neuropsychology Laboratory, University of Victoria.

139. Spring, C., and Capps, C.: Encoding speed, rehearsal, and probed recall of dyslexic boys, J. Educ. Psychol. **66**:780, 1974.

140. Stanley, G.: The processing of digits by children with specific reading disability (dyslexia), Br. J. Educ. Psychol. **46**:81, 1976.

141. Stanley, G., and Hall, R.: Short-term visual information processing in dyslexics, Child Dev. **44**:841, 1972.

142. Stanley, G., and Hall, R.: A comparison of dyslexics and normals in recalling letter arrays after brief presentation, Br. J. Educ. Psychol. **43**:301, 1973.

143. Strauss, A.A.: Diagnosis and education of the cripple-brained, deficient child, Except. Child. **9**:163, 1943.

144. Strauss, A.A., and Kephart, N.C.: Psychopathology and education of the brain-injured child, New York, 1955, Grune & Stratton, Inc.

145. Strauss, A.A., and Lehtinen, L.E.: Psychopathology and education of the brain-injured child, New York, 1947, Grune & Stratton, Inc.

146. Strauss, A.A., and Werner, H.: Disorders of conceptual thinking in the brain-injured child, J. Nerv. Ment. Dis. **96**:153, 1942.

147. Sullivan, J.: The effects of Kephart's perceptual motor training program on a reading clinic sample, J. Learn. Disabil. **5**:545, 1972.

148. Swanson, H.L.: Nonverbal visual short-term memory as a function of age and dimensionality in learning disabled children, Child Dev. **48**:51, 1977.

149. Takata, N.: The play history, Am. J. Occup. Ther. **23**:314, 1969.

150. Takata, N.: Play as a prescription, In Reilly, M., editor, Play as exploratory learning: studies in curiosity behavior, Beverly Hills, Calif., 1974, Sage Publications, Inc.

151. Takata, N.: Introduction to a series: occupational behavior research for pediatric practice, Am. J. Occup. Ther. **34**(1):11, 1980.

152. Tarver, S.G., and others: The development of visual selective attention and verbal rehearsal in learning disabled boys, J. Learn. Disabil. **8**:26, 1977.

153. Torgesen, J., and Goldman, T.: Verbal rehearsal and short term memory in reading-disabled children, Child Dev. **48**:56, 1977.

154. Troyer, B.L.: Sensorimotor integration: a basis for planning occupational therapy, Am. J. Occup. Ther. **15**(2):51, 1961.

155. Tucker, J., Stevens, L., and Ysseldyke, J.E.: Learning disabilities: the experts speak out, J. Learn. Disabil. **16**(1):7, 1983.

156. Vellutino, F., and others: Has the perceptual deficit hypothesis led us astray? J. Learn. Disabil. **10**(6):375, 1977.

157. Voss, D.E.: Proprioceptive neuromuscular facilitation: applications of patterns and techniques in occupational therapy, Am. J. Occup. Ther. **13**(4):191, 1959.

158. Webster, P.: Occupational role development in the young adult with mild mental retardation, Am. J. Occup. Ther. **34**(1):13, 1980.

159. Weeks, Z.R.: Sensorimotor integration theory and the multisensory approach. In Farber, S.D., editor: Neurorehabilitation: a multisensory approach, Philadelphia, 1982, W.B. Saunders Co.

160. Weiss, C.: Weiss comprehensive articulation test, Boston, 1978, Boston Teaching Resources.

161. Wepman, J.M., and others: Studies in aphasia: background and theoretical formulations, J. Speech Hear. Disord. **25**:323, 1960.

162. Werner, H.: Comparative psychology of mental development, New York, 1948, International Universities Press.

163. White, M.: A first grade intervention program for children "at risk" for reading failure, J. Learn. Disabil. **12**:230, 1979.

164. Wiederholt, J.L.: Historical perspectives on the education of the learning disabled. In Mann, L., and Sabatino, D.A., editors: The second review of special education, Philadelphia, 1974, JSE Press.

165. Wolf, R., and others: The structure of research in occupational therapy, Unpublished manuscript, 1983, University of Southern California.

166. Woodcock, R.W., and Johnson, M.B.: Woodcock-Johnson psycho-educational battery, New York, 1978, Teaching Resources.

167. Yerxa, E.J.: Preface. In Gilfoyle, E. editor: Training: occupational therapy educational management in schools (a competency-based educational program), vol. 3, mod. 5, Rockville, Md., 1979-1980, American Occupational Therapy Association, Inc.

168. Ysseldyke, J., and Salvia, J.: Diagnostic-prescriptive teaching: two models, Except. Child. **11**:181, 1974.

JANET H. JOHNSON

Children with physical and orthopedic disabilities

SCOPE OF THE PROBLEM

This chapter is the result of a sharing of experiences from work with children who have physical and orthopedic disabilities. The disabilities involved are described according to the presenting problem or diagnosis, and they are reviewed and classified according to the difficulties displayed when children perform activities. Assessment procedures, treatment objectives, and intervention techniques are also presented.

We know that learning and development are complicated processes. The mind and the body are not isolated from each other in the acquisition of skills, but depend on the interaction of the various aspects of the whole organism. The inability of one system to function adequately may impede the development of abilities in another area or interfere with the growth process as a whole. Therefore the physically handicapped child often has developmental problems other than those related specifically to his or her physical disability. For example, a child who cannot move about and cannot manage his body to learn how it relates to the space around him may have difficulty with form and space concepts, directionality, and other perceptual concepts. The child with a physical disability may also exhibit learning problems, mental retardation, or emotional or behavioral difficulties that interfere with a full life. It must be noted that this chapter speaks primarily to problems resulting from physical disability. Reference to other chapters and resources is needed to design treatment intervention that incorporates goals related to addi-

tional problem areas.[12] The occupational therapist must consider the breadth of skills needed by the child that will enable her to enjoy a satisfying life as a child and as an adult.

Presenting problems or diagnoses of children with physical disabilities

Children with physical disabilities that limit their ability to function normally can often be classified by a diagnosis or a syndrome, and they generally have conditions with a medical orientation. The diagnoses most seen are neurological and orthopedic problems and collagen diseases (Chapter 6). Specific examples are cerebral palsy, myelomeningocele, muscular dystrophies and atrophies, traumatic injuries, orthopedic abnormalities and defects such as absence or loss of limb, dwarfism, osteogenesis imperfecta, and rheumatoid diseases. Other less prevalent neuromuscular or orthopedic diseases and syndromes usually exhibit symptoms of weakness, limited joint range of motion, or incoordination, as do the other conditions.

General medical and surgical conditions that limit physical functioning may also be included here (Chapter 6). Examples of this group are children with congenital heart defects, anemias and leukemias, cystic fibrosis, diabetes, and kidney disease. In these cases children are limited in their ability to participate in activities by decreased energy, pain restriction, and certain medications or medical treatments. Occupational therapists may facilitate normalizing growth and development experiences for these children, recommend activities within their energy limitations, or suggest simplification techniques for performing activities.

Although there is some reticence in labeling and categorizing children, a classification such as a diagnosis can simplify communication among those persons working with a child. For example, when discussing a 10-year-old child with muscular dystrophy of the Duchenne type, trained professionals are immediately aware of the common symptoms that this disease exhibits in a child of this age, such as the increasing weakness, the need for braces or a wheelchair, and the tightness seen in certain muscle groups. The time that this knowledge and awareness saves in communication can be significant. However, the danger in categorizing children by diagnosis is the possibility of viewing a child as a medical entity and not perceiving the individual needs and abilities that should be considered in planning and implementing treatment. Such stereotyping should be avoided.

For the purpose of treatment planning and implementation, children with physical disabilities are grouped according to major symptoms that impede function, and not by diagnosis. The causes of the limited function may result from neurological dysfunction, including loss of sensation or musculoskeletal problems. The major symptoms that impede function are

1. Muscular weakness
2. Limited joint range of motion
3. Incoordination

Other services involved

Children with physical and orthopedic disabilities often have a variety of problems that require intervention beyond that which is provided by the family, through public education, or through routine medical care. For these children to develop into adults, having the freedom to contribute to their own and to society's well-being, the child and his parents may need the services of several kinds of trained professionals, such as physicians, nurses, social workers, dietitians, occupational and physical therapists, teachers, and other special educational personnel. Also included are people not specifically trained but involved in the child's care, such as babysitters, bus drivers, and extended family members.

Each profession brings a specific orientation and frame of reference to serve the child and her family. As unique as each profession is, remarkable similarities are seen in the educational programs and in the development of each speciality service. Because of these similarities, there is much overlap of skills and flexibility in the approach to service delivery. An example of this is the person who teaches the fracture patient how to bathe and dress himself: in one setting the occupational therapist fills this role and in another setting the nurse may do so. This overlap can result in some confusion in role definition, but it can also provide common reference points for child care workers.

Medical and educational services are costly. They are often inaccessible or strained to their limits because of cost, geography, or lack of available trained personnel. Therefore service personnel are increasingly finding it necessary and often desirable to teach the child and the parents to take a greater part in their health care and maintenance. This participation in self-care is evident in prevention, treatment, and habilitation. The health professional must educate clients to be active participants in their health and development. For the child who is not yet able to assume this responsibility, particularly the young child, it is the parent who must do so. The parents or primary caretakers are the most significant coordinators of the child's health care and development. To ignore the parent or caretaker in treatment planning and intervention is to limit the scope of treatment (Chapter 8).

Special characteristics of children with physical and orthopedic problems relevant to occupational therapy

VARIETY OF DIAGNOSES

Children with physical disabilities fall into several diagnostic categories. With the exception of cerebral palsy, myelomeningocele, and possibly muscular dystrophy, the number of children with any one diagnosis that one therapist may treat is small. However, the variety of diagnoses within the patient population is great. For this reason the therapist working with these children continually must refer to published references[4,18] and other professionals and participate in continuing education for information regarding the classical medical picture of those conditions not frequently seen.

PROGNOSIS AND CHANGE

Children with physical and orthopedic disabilities often demonstrate minimal and slow medical change. In many children the symptoms of the condition are present from birth, such as myelomeningocele and orthopedic defects. Others evidence a progressively debilitating condition that does not improve, as in muscular dystrophy or atrophy. Although the occupational therapist can do little to change the medical picture of a child's disease, the therapist can be of great assistance in preventing further disabilities, such as contractures, and in helping the child to compensate for lack of strength, limited joint range of motion, and incoordination. Thus the therapist may enable the child to engage in activities that are useful and meaningful to her.

EQUIPMENT

To perform many activities, children with physical disabilities often need to use adaptive appliances and equipment. Some need braces or splints, wheelchairs, prostheses, personal care equipment, standing tables, feeding equipment, and so on. The occupational therapist may fabricate, order, or maintain some of these; the therapist may teach the child to use the equipment in some cases as is appropriate to the occupational therapy goals. The therapist must be aware of the equipped artificial and extended parts of the child's body when considering the child's skills and limitations, for the child is often incomplete without them and may incorporate them into his body image.

TYPICAL TREATMENT SETTINGS

Although children with physical disabilities are seen in general hospitals, physician's offices, and home health agencies, the majority are treated by occupational therapists in settings specifically designed for child care and development. Children's hospitals are frequently the center of medical care for these children. Clinics oriented to specific disabilities may follow the child medically. Because of laws that require all children to attend school in the least restrictive setting and because of laws requiring related services to enable this participation, physically handicapped children in this country are seen, treated, and referred to other settings by occupational therapists working in the public schools.

ASSESSMENT PROCEDURES

In any assessment the occupational therapist is attempting to discover what the client can do and how she does it, and what the client cannot do and why she is unable to do so. Once this procedure has been completed, the therapist is more equipped to determine if intervention will help the client accomplish more and what treatment procedures are appropriate to make this happen.

By definition, a child with a physical disability is unable to perform expected or desired activities because of limitations imposed by her body. The occupational therapist determines which activities of self-maintenance, play, and work the child is unable to perform and what limitations her body is imposing. These limitations most often are a result of muscle weakness, lack of functional range of joint motion, or excessive incoordination.

Assessment of task performance

The nature of the physical disability is often expressed in terms of the problems encountered in performing activities. Therefore many occupational therapy assessment procedures used in working with the child with a physical disability are performance oriented. They evaluate or check the child's ability to perform specific tasks. Typical assessments are

1. Checklists on daily living skills of feeding, dressing, and hygiene
2. Evaluations related to skills needed to function in a particular setting, such as a classroom skills checklist, a prevocational skills checklist, and a homemaking skills checklist
3. Growth and developmental skill evaluations

When the therapist administers these evaluations, or checklists, the child's response in following directions to perform a specific activity is observed. The therapist determines whether the child can perform the activity and how closely the child's response meets the criteria of the test item. For example, when evaluating a child's ability to independently remove his coat, the therapist is not only observing whether the child can take off his coat, but is also observing and judging the quality of the action: Is the coat removed in a reasonable period of time? Does the child use an unusual or adapted method to accomplish the task? Does he need assistance? If so, what kind of help does he need?

Most checklists incorporate some means to record the quality of the child's response. This may be a comments section that is located by each test item, or following a section or area tested, or at the end of the form. Another method for grading the response is to use a letter or number that represents typical degrees of activity accomplishment. For example, one could use a number from 0 to 3, instead of a checkmark, when recording responses: *zero* could indicate that the child could not accomplish the activity; *one* could indicate difficult accomplishment only with assistance; *two* could indicate task accomplishment without assistance, but with difficulty or taking an excessive amount of time; and *3* could indicate that the child accomplished the activity independently and with ease.

Although information from a recorded history or from interviews can be used to note a child's abilities, the primary method for an occupational therapist to gather assessment information is by observing the child's actual performance of the activity. During the assessment the therapist gains information that goes beyond the specific skills being evaluated. Causes of nonperformance can be observed, solutions to problems can be generated, and methods for treatment may be suggested.

EXAMPLES OF TASK PERFORMANCE ASSESSMENTS

1. *Activities of daily living skills.* Lists of skills needed to perform self-maintenance activities are often compiled in a way to group together the skills needed

for one type of self-care. For example, feeding, dressing, and grooming-hygiene are listed separately. The sections of the evaluation may also follow a developmental sequence or a simple-to-complex sequence. The following are examples of checklists of activities of daily living skills:

- Activities of Daily Living[1]*
- Student Check List[24]*
- "Life Works Tasks"[16]
- Callier-Azusa Scale self-help section[23]
- Learning Accomplishment Profile self-help section[18]
- *Portage Guide to Early Education*—Evaluation of fine motor and self skills[5]

2. *School-related physical skills.* There are certain physical skills that a child needs to function in a school setting, aside from the daily living skills previously mentioned. To work with a child, school personnel need to know which of these necessary skills a child can do and which ones must be taught or compensated for in order for the child to take advantage of the educational curriculum. Examples of evaluations of school-related physical skills are as follows:

- Bruininks-Oseretsky Test of Motor Proficiency[6]
- Fine Motor Skill Evaluation[10]*
- Evaluation of Upper Extremity Function[9]*
- Learning Accomplishment Profile[20] sections on fine and gross motor skills
- Southern California Sensory Integration Tests[2] information related to motor planning and motor accuracy

3. *Play skills.* The child uses play as a developmental tool as well as for enjoyment. Physical manipulation of objects is a large part of play. Information regarding these physical skills can be gathered by observing free play, as well as by administering structured evaluation procedures. Examples of assessments of physical skills used in play are as follows:

- Bayley Scales of Infant Development[3]
- Bruininks-Oseretsky Test of Motor Proficiency[6]
- Fine Motor Skill Evaluation[10]*
- Denver Developmental Screening Test[11]
- Learning Accomplishment Profile[20]
- *Portage Guide to Early Education*[5]

Assessment of physical limitations and abilities

In addition to the documentation of specific task performance, there is frequently a need to determine causes for the difficulties encountered by the child or her caretakers. Weakness, limited range of joint motion,

and incoordination are the areas most appropriate to assess to determine a measurable level of physical ability or performance. Sensory testing is performed to determine if there is a loss in the tactile or temperature senses, proprioception, or stereognosis.[22] These evaluations give specific information on a particular physical ability, help to focus and set priorities among treatment goals, and give measurable criteria to assess changes in abilities that result from treatment or from the disease process. These changes may not be evident by looking solely at the child's ability to perform a task.

EXAMPLES OF ASSESSMENTS OF PHYSICAL LIMITATIONS

1. *Measurement of muscle strength.* Muscle tests are used to determine the extent and degree of muscular weakness. The results of the tests provide a basis for planning therapeutic intervention, and in conjunction with periodic retesting, they can be used in evaluating the effect of these procedures. Examples of references related to the measurement of muscle strength are the following:

- Daniels and Worthington's[7] manual muscle tests
- Trombly and Scott's[25] manual muscle tests
- Kellor and others'[14] manual muscle tests
- Kendall, Kendall, and Wadsworth's[15] manual muscle tests
- Hand and pinch strength measurement with a dynamometer[12,26]

2. *Measurements of range of joint motion.* Evaluation of the extent of joint range limitation is necessary before treatment. Remeasurement will document the effectiveness following treatment intervention. References related to measuring range of motion are the following:

- Trombly and Scott's[25] goniometric measurement, outline and palm prints, measurement from x-rays, and functional range of motion tests
- Smith's[21] goniometric measurement

3. *Measurements of coordination.* Examples of measurements of coordination are the following:

- Bruininks-Oseretsky Test of Motor Proficiency[6]
- DeHaven, Mordock, and Loykovich's[8] tests involving speed and smooth movements
- Jebsen's[13] hand function test
- Minnesota Rate of Manipulation Test[17]
- Trombly and Scott's[25] specific tasks for manipulating buttons, scissors, and so on

The more specific the assessment tool, the more specific the information will be regarding areas needing remediation, and the more specifically treatment goals can be stated. Treatment objectives are determined from assessment information, including (1) the reason for referral, (2) information from others about the child, (3) developmental guidelines, and (4) the results of specific assessment procedures.

---

*For further information see Chapters 9 and 11.

TREATMENT OBJECTIVES

In the transition from assessment to treatment lies much of the *art* of therapy. The therapist first gathers information about the specific child or children; weighs that information with the classical medical picture of a disability and his or her knowledge of growth and development and what children do in health; balances all this information with a knowledge and feeling about the needs or expectations of the child, the family, the school, or environmental setting; and finally determines a direction for treatment intervention. This process is scientifically based in classical occupational therapy theory, but it is determined by sound clinical judgment, experience, and creativity in actuality.

The following points are considered in determining treatment objectives: (1) the child's present level of functioning, which is learned from assessments; (2) the child's expected level of performance according to his age or developmental sequence; (3) the environmental expectations or demands from the child's family or school; and (4) the resources available to implement the child's treatment goals.

Objectives for treatment are derived directly from information gathered from assessment results. It is the assessment that describes the areas of strength and the areas needing remediation. Assessments define what limitations a child with a physical disability has and what activities are affected as a result of those limitations. The limitations of a physically disabled child have been identified as weakness, limited range of motion, and excessive incoordination. Typical treatment objectives therefore follow.

Improve or maintain muscle strength and endurance

Muscle weakness may result from the disease process itself, as in muscular dystrophy, or from limited activity because of the difficulties or pain encountered in movement, such as in juvenile rheumatoid arthritis. A medical knowledge of the disease process and prognosis will help determine if it is appropriate to work toward improved muscle strength. Compensation for weakness may be a concurrent or alternative goal. In evaluating a child's ability to perform specific tasks, the therapist may note that the child may have difficulty moving about and using his body to manipulate objects as tools. If assessments show muscle weakness to be a limitation in task performance, improving muscle strength is typically a treatment goal in occupational therapy.

Improve or maintain joint range of motion

Limited range of motion can be observed in task performance. The child may be unable to reach in various directions or to parts of her body and to hold and manipulate objects needed to perform tasks. Assessment of functional range of motion or joint measurement can determine if the joint range is within normal limits.

Range of motion can be affected by muscle weakness or paralysis, as in myelomeningocele. It may be influenced by joint disturbances, as in juvenile rheumatoid arthritis in which range is limited because of pain and changes in the joint structure. Range of motion is also affected by fixed orthopedic disturbances, as in arthrogryposis, or by missing or foreshortened limbs, as seen in phocomelia. In cases where the range is not fixed and where stress on the joint through activity is not contraindicated, the occupational therapist typically may determine that a treatment goal to increase joint range of motion is appropriate. Prevention of contractures might also be a goal when an increase in range is unlikely and when the limited range could progress to a fixed contracture.

Improve the ability to control movements

Incoordination can result from various neuromuscular disease processes or from trauma. It can also occur in children with sequentially progressive but delayed neuromuscular development, often resulting from a lack of experience in doing activities because they are handicapped. For example, a kindergarten child with a disability, such as osteogenesis imperfecta, may have a great deal of difficulty cutting with scissors. It is common to discover that this may be the first experience for the child in using scissors. It is also common to find an improvement in the child's eye-hand coordination and in his accuracy of scissor use after participating in graded, sequential tasks using scissors. The occupational therapist may design treatment to improve the child's speed and accuracy of movement or to teach compensatory methods for activities affected by incoordination.

Compensate for deficit skills resulting from muscle weakness, limited range of motion, or incoordination

If the therapist finds it inappropriate or unfeasible for the child to strengthen muscles, improve joint range, or improve coordination because of medical contraindications such as pain, sensory loss,[22] or limited prognosis, goals may focus on the child's learning specific skills in a variety of ways that allow him greater participation in activities. These goals are stated in terms of specific behaviors. Some examples of compensatory goal statements follow:

1. The child will improve self-maintenance skills.
   a. The child will feed himself independently (using adapted utensils and dishes as necessary).
   b. The child will remove loose-fitting clothing having no fastenings (buttons, snaps, and so on) within a period of one-half hour.
   c. The child will go to the bathroom unassisted (the therapist should note the height of toilet grab bars and type of clothing required for independence).
2. The child will increase her ability to engage in play and leisure time activities.
   a. Using weighted markers, the child will take turns with classmates when playing a board game.
   b. Given three choices of a toy for independent play, the child will make a choice and engage in appropriate play for 10 minutes.
   c. Given a nine-hole pegboard and corresponding pegs in two colors, the child will insert pegs to play tic-tac-toe with the therapist or another child.
3. The child will perform school-related physical skills.
   a. The child will sit at a desk or table that is positioned to enable performance of classroom assignments.
   b. The child will print legibly using a pencil holder and primary paper secured to the work surface.
   c. Using adapted equipment (head pointer and keymask on a typewriter), the child will copy a short paragraph from the blackboard.

The therapist may determine several treatment goals resulting from observations, history, and formal assessments of the child. These goals and reasons for the goals must be communicated to others. While treatment intervention usually addresses more than one goal statement, there is a limit to the number of goals that can be carried out at any one time. Therefore the therapist must determine treatment priorities by considering the most important skills a child needs to be able to do at a particular time or place. Parents, teachers, physicians, and others may guide the therapist in this determination, and the policies of the setting may set some treatment parameters, but it is the occupational therapist's responsibility to accept or consider these suggestions in view of his or her professional knowledge of what is within the scope of the profession and what is appropriate and important for a particular child.

Within any of these goal areas, the therapist must further define the treatment objectives so that they are workable, measurable, and more easily communicated. The more specifically and clearly the goal is stated, the more clearly it will be understood by the child and oth-

ers. Specific behaviors are also more clearly measured as to change. Small improvements can be observed, measured, and reported so that child, parent, therapist, and others can see whether treatment is having an effect and its extent.

TREATMENT MODALITIES

Children with physical disabilities are limited by their bodies in their capability to perform activities. As was said previously, some of these activities can be enhanced by improving the body's potential to perform the activity, such as by strengthening muscles, controlling coordination, or increasing range of joint motion. However, if methods designed to increase the physical function of a child are ineffective or inappropriate, adaptive or compensatory methods to achieve a skill are used.

Corrective modalities

Whenever possible, techniques are employed to enhance a child's ability to control and use his body. By so doing, the improved skills can be generalized and used in a variety of activities. For example, increased hand strength can help the child play with Lego blocks, manage buttons, hold a glass and spoon, write a school assignment, model clay, or construct a model airplane. Increasing the child's hand strength is more effective than teaching the child how to perform any one of these skills by compensating for hand weakness.

IMPROVING MUSCLE STRENGTH

During assessment, measurement and recording of strength are done. This information is necessary to understand the degree of weakness and to determine if there is a change in strength following treatment.

Participation in activities designed to strengthen particular muscles or muscle groups is the key element in the occupational therapy process. In selecting activities to improve muscle strength, two criteria must be considered. One simple consideration is whether the chosen activity requires the contraction of the muscles in question and whether substitution by other muscle groups is occurring. A second factor in activity selection is that the activity should be graded for resistance, for the length of time, or for the number of repetitions the child does the activity. The activity should be set at a low enough level to ensure muscle contraction, but at a high enough level to allow the upper limits of strength or endurance to be reached or measured within a treatment session. A child can operate a video game with an electronic device that requires pronation and supination of the wrist to activate and direct the video action. Resistance can be added to the electronic switch to require more muscle strength. The time or physical tolerance of operating the switch and the score earned can be measured and increased as the limits of strength of wrist pronation and supination are reached.

Periodically during the course of treatment, muscle strength should be remeasured to determine changes in strength and to note when a plateau or level of no change is reached. At this time it is worth noting any changes in functional abilities that may be occurring during the period of treatment intervention. During periods of reevaluation, determination must be made of whether to continue treatment intervention, to monitor strength levels, or to discontinue therapy.

INCREASING JOINT RANGE OF MOTION

A measurement of the joint range before treatment is essential to provide a baseline against which to judge the effectiveness of treatment and changes in function. Because the cause of limited range of motion can be a result of muscle weakness as well as a result of orthopedic disturbances, it is wise to measure both active and passive range of motion. A discrepancy between the two may indicate muscle weakness, and treatment goals and methods would be determined based on that factor.

Treatment methods for a child having limited joint range of motion fall into three areas: (1) active participation in activities requiring movement to the maximal range possible, (2) splinting a joint in a desired position to prevent contractures and deformities, and (3) administering passive stretching to specified joints.

Participation in activities is the one method that requires the interest and motivation of the child. As such, there is more likelihood for carryover of the responses used in therapy to other tasks throughout the day. Because of these adaptive and assimilated behaviors, activity is the primary method used in maintaining or improving joint range. There are three suggestions in using activities for children with this treatment objective: (1) the activity must require as great a joint movement as possible (lacing a sewing card having a long lace would encourage more movement of elbow and shoulder and therefore greater range than using a short string or lace); (2) the placement of the child or the activity can facilitate maximal joint range by requiring the child to reach (a child removing pegs and placing them in a box in front of her but at a distance requiring maximal elbow extension would be using a wider range in her elbow than if the box receiving the pegs was placed close to the pegboard); and (3) the therapist will need to watch for substitute movement that avoids the desired joint movement (in a reaching activity such as picking up puzzle pieces placed at the extreme range of elbow extension, a child may lean with his trunk to reach the object rather than extend his elbow as therapeutically desired).

When contractures are progressing and activity is unable to counteract the effect, it may be necessary to splint a body part to prevent fixed joint limitations from occurring. The splint may be rigid or movable and may be worn for various lengths of time as determined by the therapist and the child's physician.

Occasionally a therapist may find that the only way to keep a joint mobile is through passive range of motion. This can be accomplished through the child's participation in activities such as using a bilateral sander to increase elbow extension or holding a hoop with both hands while being pulled on a wheeled toy such as a scooter board to increase shoulder flexion. Seating a child with her knees extended or standing her with support can help counteract the effect of sitting long periods of time in a wheelchair with her legs flexed. Direct manipulation by the therapist is also employed to maintain or improve joint range. In such cases, the therapist is cautioned to move the joint carefully to, and just beyond, the known passive range, being mindful of the child's diagnosis and its contraindications.

As in all treatment intervention, remeasurement of the joint range at periodic intervals is necessary to see if the range has changed and to what degree. At times of reevaluation, treatment objectives can be altered or eliminated according to the results of reassessment.

IMPROVING COORDINATION

Although children with coordination problems may be treated by being taught compensatory skills, rather than by attempting to change the motor coordination itself, there are some methods that are designed to enable these children to control their excessive or uncontrolled movements. One such method is the

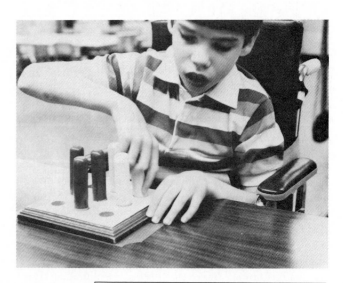

FIGURE 20-1

Tic-tac-toe is played by inserting 1-inch pegs in a nine-hole pegboard.

Photograph by Darin Derstine.

grading of activities to increase the required accuracy of response. An example is the designing of activities by use of 1-inch, ½-inch, ¼-inch, or ⅛-inch pegs and corresponding pegboards. As the child is able to accurately and relatively quickly insert the 1-inch pegs in the board, activities are designed that use the next smaller size pegs (Figure 20-1). Another example is teaching the child to write by using primary lined paper and progressing to narrow-lined, loose-leaf notebook paper.

Analogous to the increase in accuracy is the grading of activities to increase the speed of performance. The child playing the commercial game SIMON can move from level 1 to level 2 or 3 as he responds within the programmed time allotted at each level. Speed can also be graded into activities for the child learning to use the typewriter or the computer in the school setting. Better coordination is thus the increase in speed and accuracy in the performance of activities.

The task of improving coordination does not belong solely to occupational therapy. Indeed, both physical education and physical therapy find this is one of the primary objectives within their professions. The occupational therapist can resolve this apparent overlap in roles by focusing on therapeutic efforts and activities in the major areas of childhood performance relevant to occupational therapy: self-maintenance activities, play and leisure time activities, and schoolwork and prevocational activities (Chapters 12 to 14).

Compensatory methods

When attempts to improve muscle strength, joint range of motion, or coordination are unsuccessful or inappropriate, goals may focus instead on the child's learning to perform specific skills in whatever manner allows him to function as independently as possible. In such cases some adaptation or change in the skill is needed. The task is analyzed into its component parts (1) to teach the sequential parts of the skill, (2) to simplify or change the method of performing the skill, or (3) to teach the skill through the use of adaptive equipment or supplies.

There are some key factors to consider in compensatory skill accomplishment. The use of lighter weight objects and energy-saving devices, often electronic, help to compensate for muscle weakness. Devices to improve reach can be used to accomplish a task by compensating for limited range of motion (Figure 20-2). The performance of coordinated movements can be helped by providing stability, for example, using weights, weighted objects, or nonslippery surfaces (Figure 20-3).

When a particular skill cannot be performed by the child following corrective therapeutic procedures or by teaching, simplifying, or adapting the activity itself, then specific adaptive equipment may be necessary for the most efficient or independent performance of an activity (Figure 20-4). An occupational therapist may teach a child with muscle weakness to write by using an electric typewriter (Figure 20-5), show a child in a full arm cast how to use a card holder to play cards, or teach him how to use a rocker-knife to cut food into bite-size pieces. To make a decision to use a piece of adaptive equipment, the therapist must consider the importance of the skill to be enhanced by the equipment (Figure 20-6), the acceptance of the equipment by the child and her family (Figure 20-7), and the cost or effort involved (Figures 20-8 and 20-9).

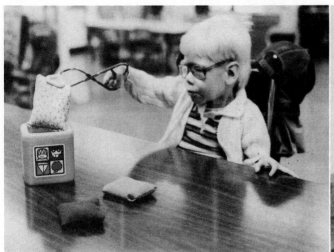
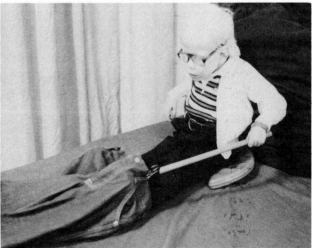

FIGURE 20-2

"Reachers" can extend the reach when range of motion is limited.

Photograph by Darin Derstine.

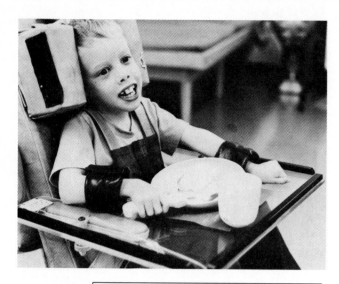

FIGURE 20-3

Stability to control incoordination is achieved by weights, weighted cup and utensils, and a nonslippery surface.

Photograph by Darin Derstine.

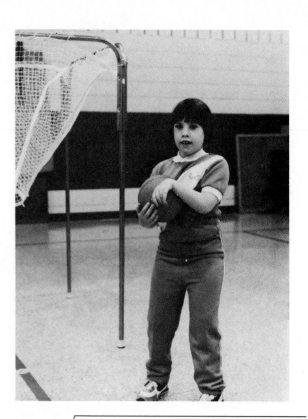

FIGURE 20-4

Stylish clothing with elastic and Velcro fasteners (see Figure 12-8, **B**) eliminates the need to button, zip, snap, and tie and enables many children to be independent in dressing and toileting.

Photograph by Darin Derstine.

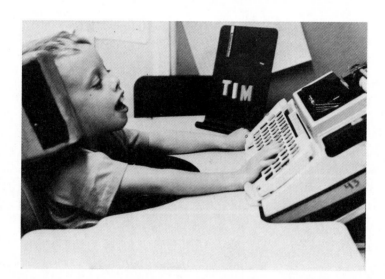

FIGURE 20-5

This child is learning to type on an electric typewriter with a key mask to help control incoordinated movements. A raised desk stabilizes his arms.

Photograph by Darin Derstine.

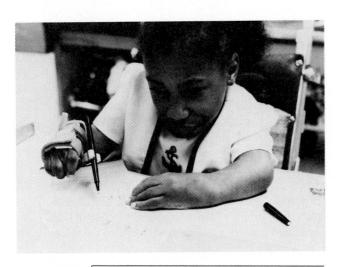

FIGURE 20-6

By using a splint with a pencil holder, this child who has no grasp is able to write.

Photograph by Darin Derstine.

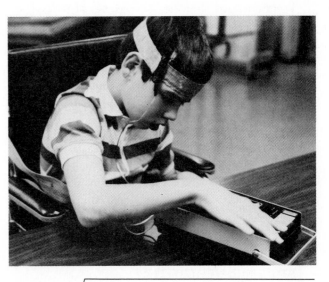

FIGURE 20-7

A mercury gravity switch is attached to a headband and activates the tape recorder when the child's head is held erect.

Photograph by Darin Derstine.

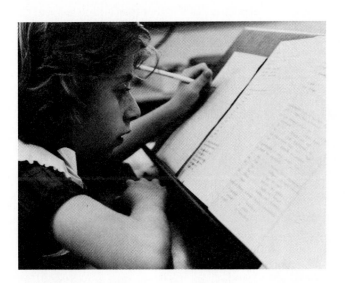

FIGURE 20-8

After surgical decompression of Arnold-Chiari malformation, this child benefits from a raised writing surface to avoid stress on the cervical spine.

Photograph by Darin Derstine.

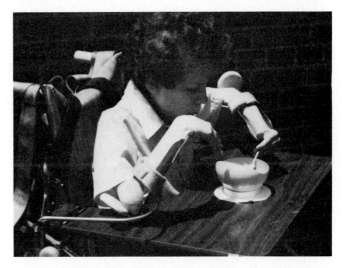

FIGURE 20-9

A balance forearm orthosis can compensate for weak shoulder and elbow musculature to enable independence in self-feeding.

Photograph by Kathy Campbell.

Techniques and materials

The following suggestions should be considered when working with children with physical and orthopedic disabilities.

LEVEL OF ACTIVITY

Recommended activities should be at a level of complexity that is low enough to allow the child to perform and high enough for the child to improve skill competence. The areas to consider in determining the level of activity are the child's (1) age level, (2) interest level, and (3) physical ability level. An example of an activity used to improve bilateral coordination is stringing beads. A young child in preschool or kindergarten finds random stringing of 1-inch wooden beads to be interesting and within his ability level. A teenage girl is interested in jewelry and has the physical and conceptual ability to string small beads in complex patterns to make a necklace. The interest level can range from stringing one color and shape beads to complex patterns of beading to decorate clothing or make Indian costumes.

SEQUENCE OF ACTIVITY

For the child's abilities to improve, the activities must be sequentially graded to greater levels of difficulty, requiring increased strength, greater range of motion, or more refined coordination. In the example of stringing beads to improve coordination, certain materials may be selected to make the task physically easier: use beads with large holes; use pipe cleaners or thick, rigid elastic; or extend the length of the rigid tip of the string by dipping it in nail polish or wrapping the string with tape. The materials selected can also require increased coordination for the task: reduce the size of the bead and the size of the bead hole; use a needle and thread instead of a thicker string; or introduce other skill requirements such as twisting a shaped bead to a certain position on a wire or string.

VARIETY AND REPETITION OF ACTIVITIES

Repetition of a skill is necessary to master it; however, a variety of activities is necessary to motivate the child to perform this repetition. Variety is also important to enable the child to generalize the use of the newly developed skill in more than one way. It is a challenge to select a variety of activities that are at the appropriate age, interest, and ability level for a child.

In the bead stringing example, additional examples for activities requiring inserting an object in a defined hole or space are stringing "tribeads" on a pipe cleaner and twisting to form a holiday wreath for a tree decoration; inserting punched notebook paper in a ring notebook; lacing a wallet having prepunched holes with a cord; placing vegetables on skewers for shish kebab; or placing washers and nuts on bolts. As activities become more complicated, additional skill requirements are often needed to perform the activity, such as perceptual skills of sequencing and positioning or conceptual skills related to following directions.

ADAPTIVE EQUIPMENT

Adaptive equipment may be necessary to perform a skill independently or efficiently. When selecting the most appropriate piece of equipment, the therapist must have a clear understanding of the particular skill that needs to be enhanced and have an awareness of available equipment designed to help perform that skill. If the equipment is not available or cannot be purchased commercially, it may need to be specifically designed and constructed to fit an individual child with a specific skill requirement. It is important for the therapist to have a knowledge of available resources in the community, such as medical equipment houses; carpenters or other skilled craftsmen; biomechanical, electrical, and structural engineers; funding sources, both public and private; and other therapists with experience in this area. The reader is referred to Robinault[19] and several companies* for examples of adaptive equipment.

COMMUNICATION AND REFERRAL

The multiplicity of problems presented by a child with a physical or orthopedic disability results in a variety of people being involved in his care and development. Therefore much of the therapist's time is spent in efforts with the family and other professionals to help solve the problems a child is experiencing.

Preparation for adulthood

The skills needed to enjoy a satisfying adulthood are many and varied. Social, emotional, and cognitive skills, as well as physical skills, are needed to participate in activities of self-maintenance, leisure, and work. Although the occupational therapist working with children having a physical disability will typically focus treatment on whatever physical skills are needed for maximal independence and satisfaction, goals to enhance social and emotional skills are also considered. Through training, education, and experience the occupational therapist appreciates the breadth of the skills needed in adulthood and reflects this appreciation in

---

*Abbey Medical, 13782 Crenshaw Blvd., Gardena, Calif. 90249; Everest and Jennings, Inc., 1803 Pontus Ave., Los Angeles, Calif. 90025; and Fred Sammons, Inc., Box 32, Brookfield, Ill. 60513.

treatment, planning, and implementation. Priorities for each child may vary, but goals related to prevocational, sensory-motor, and social-emotional skill development are considered to enable the child to participate as fully as possible as an adult.

CASE STUDY

Billy is a newly enrolled 10-year-old in a class for orthopedically handicapped children. All children in this setting receive occupational therapy services. He has been medically diagnosed as having muscular dystrophy of the Duchenne type.

Planned assessments for Billy include the Activities of Daily Living checklist, the classroom-related skills checklist, and observation and notations regarding play and leisure skills.

Billy ambulates by wheelchair. He can push his wheelchair for short distances, but he fatigues quickly. Although he appears to have good coordination when writing, cutting, or turning the pages of a book, he does not reach for objects and cannot elevate his arm. He cannot lift his school textbooks, carry his school lunch, or open his carton of milk. When he eats, he lowers his head to his hand or to the spoon, rather than lift the spoon to his mouth. He eats very little. Endurance is a problem in all motor activities. Billy talks a lot to classmates and to the teacher. He seems intent or serious when interacting with his classmates. Occasionally during recess a shouting interchange with a classmate is heard. According to bulletin board displays, Billy is one of the best students in the class, having read the most books and reaching the highest rung on the math ladder.

Results of assessments indicate that Billy needs assistance in dressing and hygiene, but he has the ability to feed himself with a spoon or fork once the food is cut and prepared. He is able to write and use scissors to cut paper. His grasp, pinch, and release are functional, but weak. Functional active range is within normal limits in his hands and wrists, but limited in proximal muscle groups. This limits his reach to perform activities. He appears to have some difficulty interacting with his classmates.

The physical findings correlate with the classical medical picture and demonstrate that the underlying cause of the skill deficits is muscle weakness. To record the present level of strength, the Manual Muscle Test was administered.

Treatment goals

1. Billy will participate in the school curriculum as appropriate to his abilities, using adapted methods or equipment as necessary for functioning.
   a. Billy will sit with his spine as straight as possible, using adaptations to the wheelchair and desk as necessary.
   b. Billy will write classroom assignments with his desk elevated to rest his arms by working short periods of time or using an electric typewriter to reduce fatigue.
   c. Billy will gather materials needed for schoolwork. The therapist will suggest placement and materials to facilitate independence (for example, use of desk organizers to reach materials and lightweight materials when possible).

2. Billy will participate in his self-care as much as possible, using adaptive equipment when necessary.
   a. Billy will use a balance forearm orthosis to enable lifting an eating utensil to his mouth.
   b. When possible, Billy will choose foods that he can manage himself that require no cutting and that have no packages or cartons to open.
   c. Given the appropriate height sink and placement of soap within his reach, Billy will wash his hands independently at school.
   d. Billy will remove a large coat by pulling the cuffs with his opposite hand or with his teeth and shaking out his arm, and will hang the coat on a hook placed within his reach.

3. Billy will participate in play and leisure time activities at school.
   a. Billy will play games within his ability level with classmates (board games, word games), adapting when necessary to participate (for example, scorekeeper, cheerleader).
   b. Billy will participate in individually chosen leisure activities (art, crafts, reading).

4. The therapist will facilitate acceptance of the disease when appropriate.
   a. Refer to agencies or professionals for financial, emotional, or medical assistance, when requested by parents.
   b. Suggest materials and methods to help in Billy's care at home (for example, adaptive clothing or methods of dressing if there are contractures, and leisure time activities for home).

5. The therapist will monitor upper extremity strength by administering muscle tests periodically.

Therapeutic prognosis

Muscular dystrophy is a progressively debilitating disease process evidenced by increasingly weakened muscle strength. The probability of contractures occurring is high, and recurring respiratory problems cause increased threats to life. As Billy becomes weaker, he will benefit from participating in a variety of activities requiring progressively less strength: manipulating objects may need to be replaced by electronically operated equipment for vocational or leisure tasks. Eventually passive activities of viewing and listening at his level of interest will be required. Building interests early and adapting activities to meet these interests in treatment intervention help ensure a full, although short, life.

Billy's parents and caretakers need to be informed about the disease process and about methods and adaptive equipment to help in Billy's care. They need to be shown how their home treatment programs can delay the effects of the disease, such as the development of contractures, and they need to be informed about programs and assistance available to them (for example, the Muscular Dystrophy Association).

SUMMARY

Children with physical and orthopedic disabilities often have problems of development that are separate from, although stemming from, their physical disability. Therapists must design treatment programs that take the child's developmental status into account as well as the presenting physical problem. Both corrective and compensatory treatment methods were presented in this chapter. Methods of assessment and treatment objectives were also discussed.

REFERENCES

1. Activities of daily living, Columbus, Ohio, 1982, Colerain School. (Unpublished evaluation form now in use.)
2. Ayres, A.J.: Southern California Sensory Integration Tests, Los Angeles, 1973, Western Psychological Services.
3. Bayley, N.: Bayley Scales of Infant Development, New York, 1969, Psychological Corporation.
4. Bleck, E.E., and Nagel, D.A.: Physically handicapped children: a medical atlas for teachers, ed. 2, New York, 1982, Grune & Stratton, Inc.
5. Bluma, S.M., and others: Portage guide to early education, Portage, Wisc., 1976, Cooperative Educational Service Agency 12.
6. Bruininks, R.H.: Bruininks-Oseretsky Test of Motor Proficiency, Circle Pines, Minn., 1978, American Guidance Service.
7. Daniels, L., and Worthingham, C.: Muscle testing—techniques of manual examination, ed. 4, Philadelphia, 1980, W.B. Saunders Co.
8. DeHaven, E.G., Mordock, J.B., and Loykovich, J.M.: Evaluation of coordination deficits in children with minimal cerebral dysfunction, Phys. Ther. **49:**153, 1969.
9. Evaluation of upper extremity function—occupational therapy, Columbus, Ohio, 1982, Colerain School. (Unpublished evaluation form now in use.)
10. Fine motor skill evaluation—occupational therapy, Columbus, Ohio, 1980, Colerain School. (Unpublished evaluation form now in use.)
11. Frankenburg, W.K., and Dobbs, J.B.: The Denver Developmental Screening Test, Denver, 1969, LADOCA Project & Publishing Foundation, Inc.
12. Hopkins, H.L., and Smith, H.D., editors: Willard and Spackman's occupational therapy, ed. 5, Philadelphia, 1978, J.B. Lippincott Co.
13. Jebsen, R.: An objective and standardized test of hand function, Arch. Phys. Med. Rehabil. **50:**311, 1969.
14. Kellor, M., and others: Hand strength and dexterity, Am. J. Occup. Ther. **25:**77, 1971.
15. Kendall, H.O., Kendall, F.P., and Wadsworth, G.E.: Muscles testing and function, ed. 2, Baltimore, 1971, The Williams & Wilkins Co.
16. Malick, M., and Sherry, B.: Life works tasks. In Hopkins, H.L., and Smith, H.D., editors: Willard and Spackman's occupational therapy, ed. 5, Philadelphia, 1978, J.B. Lippincott Co.
17. Minnesota Rate of Manipulation Test, Circle Pines, Minn., 1969, American Guidance Service, Inc.
18. Nelson, W.E., and others, editors: Textbook of pediatrics, ed. 11, Philadelphia, 1979, W.B. Saunders Co.
19. Robinault, I., editor: Functional aids for the multiply handicapped, Hagerstown, Md., 1973, Harper & Row, Publishers.
20. Sanford, A.R.: Learning Accomplishment Profile, Chapel Hill, N.C., 1974, Chapel Hill Training-Outreach Project.
21. Smith, H.: Specific evaluation procedures. In Hopkins, H.L., and Smith, H.D., editors: Willard and Spackman's occupational therapy, ed. 5, Philadelphia, 1978, J.B. Lippincott Co.
22. Smith, H.: Sensory testing. In Hopkins, H.L. and Smith, H.D., editors: Willard and Spackman's occupational therapy, ed. 6, Philadelphia, 1983, J.B. Lippincott Co.
23. Stillman, R.; Callier-Azusa Scale, Dallas, Tex., 1975, Callier Center for Communication Disorders.
24. Student check list—activities of daily living skills, Columbus, Ohio, 1980, Colerain School (Unpublished evaluation form now in use.)
25. Trombly, C.A., and Scott, A.D.: Occupational therapy for physical dysfunction, Baltimore, 1977, The Williams & Wilkins Co.
26. Weiss, M.W., and Flatt, A.E.: A pilot study of 198 normal children: pinch strength and hand size in the growing hand, Am. J. Occup. Ther. **25:**10, 1971.

21

CHRISTINE BOSONETTO DOANE

Children with severe burns

SCOPE OF THE PROBLEM

"Each year approximately 745,000 children are burned; 40% of these children are burned severely enough to require hospitalization".[17] This is a startling fact when one realizes that in most cases, and even with the best medical help and rehabilitation, the child is left with physical and emotional scars.

Burns in children are usually caused by thermal sources, such as fire or hot water. Certain electrical burns (microstomia) caused by biting an electric cord are also a serious problem. Other causes of burns include sunburn, chemicals, frostbite, and radiation.

On the basis of age, children between 1 and 3 years old are most frequently burned by hot water scald. Children between 3 and 14 years old are most frequently burned by clothing fires. Teenagers are categorized along with adults and are most frequently burned in house or industrial fires.[29]

Burns are life-threatening or major if (1) they cover more than 10% of the total body surface, (2) the child is under age 4, (3) the child has a history of illness or disability, (4) the burns involve the hands, face, or perineum, (5) the child has respiratory or other problems, or (6) if the burn is electrical.[1,5,10] A patient with a major burn should be hospitalized where lifesaving efforts can be made.

Skin and burn classification

Recall the anatomy of the skin. The skin is composed of layers of epidermis and dermis; and it hosts blood vessels, hair follicles, glands, and nerve cells. Since skin is also the body's largest protective organ, its destruction creates a vulnerability to infection, a loss of body fluids, temperature deregulation, and sensory loss.[3,10]

One of the oldest ways of classifying burns is according to degree. A first degree burn is usually referred to as a minor burn. It can produce redness, slight edema, and soreness; however, blisters do not appear, and it only involves the epidermis.

A second degree burn has blisters and can be superficial or deep with some dermal necrosis. Enough dermis is left, however, to provide for epithelialization. A second degree burn is the most painful, because most of the sensory nerve endings remain effective.

A full thickness burn is also referred to as a third degree burn. Some physicians classify burns further as fourth and fifth degree. Most authors, however, agree that a full thickness burn has the following characteristics: (1) sensation is absent; (2) the burned area is leathery; (3) the color of the burn is usually white or black—if red, it does not blanch with pressure; and (4) the epidermis is completely destroyed, and the dermis is for the most part destroyed. Underlying muscles and tendons can be seriously affected.[1,3,5,10,26]

When the dermis is destroyed, the skin is unable to regenerate; therefore grafting is necessary to cover those body areas that are exposed to infection. Types of skin grafts include (1) autografts, (2) heterografts or xenografts, and (3) homografts. Autografts, which are made of the patient's own skin, are usually grafted from the buttocks or thighs, but can be taken from almost any unburned compatible area. A dermatome is the instrument used to skive the desired thickness of skin from the donor site. Autografts have a high success rate and are considered permanent coverage. Heterografts, or xenografts, are made of pigskin and are used as a temporary cover only. In deep second degree wounds this type of temporary cover allows reepithelialization to take place. Homografts made of cadaver skin are also temporary.[10,12,26]

Whenever full thickness burns occur, the effects of scar tissue must be addressed. Scar tissue is different from normal epithelial tissue, not only in its appearance, but also in the way it grows. Normal skin collagen is laid down in neat organized patterns. After a third degree burn, the collagen becomes more profuse, and the pattern becomes very disorganized; the body loses its ability to reproduce normal skin, and hypertrophic scars result. Scar tissue does not have normal elasticity, but it is contractile. This is thought to be the result of myofibroblasts found in the collagen. Lamberty and Whitaker[18] state,

> Fibroblasts contain contractile elements in their cytoplasm similar in appearance to the striations seen in smooth muscle. They also appear to be responsible for, and possibly the main factors in, burn scar contracture.

If patients who have sustained full thickness burns are not appropriately treated, splinted, positioned, and exercised, the unmanaged growth of scar tissue can result in grotesque and serious disfigurement. This deformity in turn causes equally serious limitations in functional performance, including range of motion, strength, dexterity, and activities of daily living.

GENERAL ROLE OF OCCUPATIONAL THERAPY INTERVENTION

The specific professional role of occupational therapy to be demonstrated depends on the policies, the participating physicians, and the history of the institution in which therapy is to be provided. It is important to note that there are slight to significant differences in burn care procedures and methodology. Some general guidelines, however, can be discussed to present the basics of burn care in pediatrics. Hospitals with burn units or beds allocated to burn care would have the greatest opportunity for occupational therapy intervention. However, smaller hospitals that treat less severe burns or see burn patients for joint scar contractures on an outpatient basis have significant need for an occupational therapist as well.

The role of the occupational therapist with the burned child covers the following aspects[14,16,25]:

1. To assist in the prevention of deformity, contracture, and hypertrophic scar formation
2. To provide appropriate and carefully selected treatment tecniques and therapeutic activities for range of motion, strength, functional coordination, and developmental skills
3. To enable the child to return to as independent

a life-style as possible and as is appropriate for the child's age
4. To provide psychosocial therapeutic intervention for the patient's emotional well-being

This role is also translated into services as follows: basic splinting; progressive splinting; exercise through purposeful activities, including educational, avocational, and leisure tasks; activities of daily living, such as hygiene, feeding self, dressing, and playing; provision of adaptive equipment; maintaining development abilities as possible; alleviating anxiety; providing opportunities to express underlying emotions and feelings; enhancing self-esteem and self-image; and assisting patients and families with reintegration into society.

Treatment of the burned child presents a very special challenge to the occupational therapist. Most areas of academic learning and practical experience are applied and used daily. Although certain procedures have routine or sequential criteria, it is most usual with burn patients that diversity, creativity, adaptation, and a dynamic challenge are the order of the day. Occupational therapists, therefore, must be prepared to (1) extend themselves beyond the routine and expected, (2) be flexible, (3) be able to deal with significant amounts of human suffering, (4) demonstrate sincerely caring and empathic attitudes, and (5) be willing to attain specialized or additional training to guarantee competence.

Although the team approach is emphasized in most health care areas, it is vitally important to note that burn care *must* be handled by a team.[11,15] The occupational therapist should regularly confer with team members to ensure a unified and consistent progressive treatment methodology with each patient. Burn team members should include the physician, nurse, occupational therapist, physical therapist, and social worker. Additional team members may include the psychologist or psychiatrist, teacher, recreational therapist, vocational counselor for teenagers, and religious leaders.

SPLINTING AND POSITIONING

Splinting, as provided by the occupational therapist, should be a part of the patient's care as early as possible. When the patient is brought to the emergency room, lifesaving efforts are the first priority. However, the occupational therapist may be called to fit the patient with splints in the emergency room or in the intensive care unit.

Malick[21-24] and Willis[35-38] are well-known occupational therapists who are considered respected authorities regarding various aspects of splinting and burn care. Many of the splint designs initially introduced by them remain the most suitable. Both therapists are well-published, and anyone working with burn patients should read their contributions.

The basic splinting rules apply to the burned child. However, extra care must be taken to avoid inappropriate pressure when desensitization is a problem, and infection must be controlled. The general rules of all splint designs include (1) meeting the exact custom needs of the patient, (2) keeping the design simple, (3) providing for easy application and removal, (4) providing for easy cleaning, (5) avoiding any inappropriate pressure, and (6) considering future adjustability.

Most burn specialists agree that splinting a hand with major burns is necessary to prevent contractures and deformities. Positioning the hand is important to maintain a balance between the flexor and extensor tendons. In dorsal third degree burns, permanent damage, including slipping or permanent lesion of the extensor mechanism, is a serious concern. The resulting boutonnière deformity consists of metacarpophalangeal (MP) hyperextension, proximal interphalangeal (PIP) flexion, and distal interphalangeal (DIP) hyperextension.

The burned hand of a child over 4 years old should be splinted in the same position most often used with an adult: wrist neutral to 30 degrees of hyperextension; metacarpophalangeal joints at 45 to 60 degrees of flexion; and proximal interphalangeal and distal interphalangeal joints at 0 degree or full extension (Figure 21-1). Children under 4 years of age may be splinted in a neutral flat pan position. Some therapists prefer to splint the metacarpophalangeal joints at 90 degrees of flexion and the wrist with dorsal burns at 15 degrees of flexion. Other areas splinted early in the course of treatment include the axillas, neck, elbows, knees, and feet.

Axillary splints are used to prevent bands of scars from forming and holding the upper extremity closely adducted to the body (Figure 21-2). Of the splints used, however, axillary splints present the most difficulties. For example, if a patient is not receiving sufficient nutrition, a subclavicular central venous pressure (CVP) line may be inserted for parenteral hyperalimentation. This is the intravenous method of giving high concentrations of nutrient supplements. Placing an upper extremity at 90 degrees or higher with an axillary splint

may cut off the flow of the central venous pressure line when it is on the same side of the body. This problem must be worked out with the physician and nursing staff. Hyperalimentation should take priority over splinting, but often a temporary compromise abducted position of 70 to 80 degrees can be attained.

Axillary splints are also difficult to secure comfortably. Patients seem to complain more about abduction of the shoulder (as a constant position) than any position in which they are placed. One of the reasons may be that it limits their functional ability more than any other position. Hand splints can at least be adapted to hold an eating utensil, but nothing much can be done to assist self-care when both arms are fixed in an over head position. Once patients begin to ambulate, the axillary splint may require additional closures to secure it in the proper position. Because of patient's movement and his size and weight, the splint will have a tendency to slip.

Elbow and knee splints can be made in the simplest form or can be designed to look like a sophisticated brace. The use of a bivalve or two-piece splint is preferred (Figures 21-3 to 21-5). One reason is that using a one-surface splint does not provide sufficient support for an active child. The bivalve splint also provides gentle initial pressure to the anterior surface where scar hypertrophy often creates flexion contractures.

Anterior neck conformers (Figure 21-6) have been described extensively. The most dramatic demonstrations of their ability to prevent and correct deformity are presented by Larson and others[19] and Willis.[37] Neck scars can be so extensive as to eliminate a recognizable neck, creating a triangular shape between the head and shoulders. Even if the face was not burned, neck scars can create sufficient pull on the facial skin to grossly disfigure the facial features and produce a monsterlike appearance.[9] Standard pillows that increase neck flexion

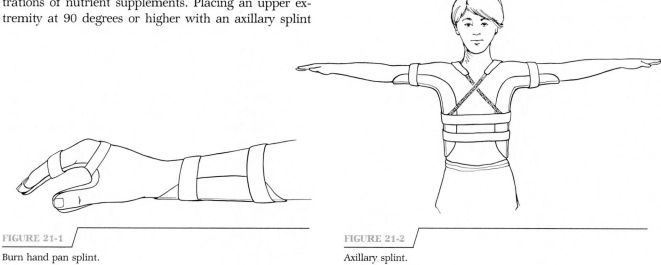

FIGURE 21-1

Burn hand pan splint.

FIGURE 21-2

Axillary splint.

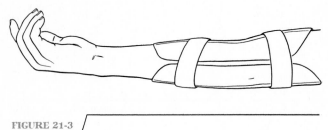

FIGURE 21-3

Bivalve elbow splint.

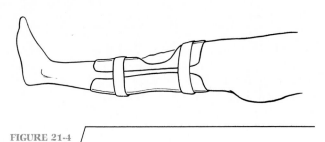

FIGURE 21-4

Bivalve knee splint with open patella.

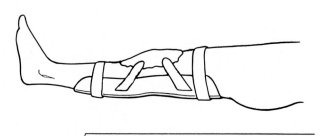

FIGURE 21-5

Posterior knee splint with padded knee support.

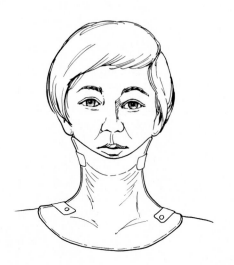

FIGURE 21-6

Neck conformer.

EXHIBIT 21-1

General guidelines for splint positioning

Splints or special devices should provide the following positioning:

   Neck: 0 degree or neutral

   Shoulders: 90 to 150 degrees of abduction (if possible, include external rotation)

   Elbow: Neutral with 5 to 10 degrees of flexion to avoid bony blocks

   Wrist: Neutral with 30 degrees of hyperextension

   Metacarpophalangeal: 45 to 60 degrees of flexion

   Proximal interphalangeal and distal interphalangeal joints: 0 degree or full extension (except with children under 4 years old)

   Knees: Neutral, but avoid hyperextension

   Ankles: 70 to 90 degrees of dorsiflexion

should never be used. However, neck rolls that encourage neck extension are helpful. Precautions must be taken if the patient has any respiratory problems.

Microstomia, or unusually small mouth, frequently results from scarring around the lips and commissures of the mouth.[6,32] Although there are a few variations on the microstomia splint, the prefabricated Microstomia Prevention Appliance (MPA)* has been found to adapt to most patients' needs for a device to stretch the mouth opening and reduce perioral contractures. Both the small and large sizes are adaptable and stretch the mouth between 2.2 and 4 cm. Specially fabricated mouth splints are necessary when an extra large size is needed. This is rare in children.

If patients are left to position themselves, they tend to assume the "position of comfort."[29] This is basically flexion throughout with slight abduction and internal rotation of the shoulders. It becomes obvious, therefore, that splinting is very important to prevent contractures and deformities in those positions. Exhibit 21-1 provides general guidelines for positioning splints to achieve maximal benefit.

It cannot be emphasized enough that all splints should be worn continuously except for exercise periods, dressing changes, whirlpool treatments, or short-term activity of daily living tasks. Otherwise, splinting benefits are seriously compromised.

The therapist may also be called into surgery to make specific splints following grafting. The purpose of splinting at that time is to maximize proper positioning immediately and before the patient can become tense

*M.P.A., Inc., R.R. 1, Box 176, Iowa City, Iowa 52240.

Checklist of points necessary to ensure adequate communication between all persons regarding splints

1. Purpose of the splint
2. Proper application
   a. Exact placement
   b. Closures (straps, gauze, Ace wraps)
3. Amount of time splint should be worn
4. Specific details on proper cleaning procedures per hospital's infection control policies
5. Special precautions
   a. Edema
   b. Pressure areas
   c. Growth factor
   d. Patient's complaints of pain, discomfort, or decreased sensation directly related to the splint or its closures

Splinting and pressure device supplies

Basic splinting supplies
Orthoplast: Plain or perforated
Plastizote: Plain and perforated ¼ and ⅛ inch
Scissors
Heat gun
Method for heating water (stove or electric fry pan)
Velcro regular and self-adhesive hook and pile, 1 and 1½ inches
Velfoam, 2 and 6 inches
Rivets, small, medium, large, and extra large
Hole punch
Hammer
Velcro glue
Carbona
Webbing, 1, 1½, and 2 inches
Reston foam (for nonburned surfaces only)
Stockinette
Gauze
Moleskin
Vinyl

More complete splint supplies and pressure device supplies
K-Splint
Polyfoam
Hexaplast
Uvex
Plaster strips and loose plaster
Alginate material
Drill
Screw drivers
Petroleum jelly
Ultracare sheeting
Files
Sandpaper
Utility knife
Steel wool
Motto tool
D' rings
Elastic for strips
Anvil
Vise and pliers
Wire
Silastic Medical Grade Elastomer (#382)
Dow Corning Medical Fluid (#360)

or fearful of increased pain. If the therapist is notified ahead of time that a splint must be fabricated in surgery, he or she should make every effort to be totally prepared to avoid any unnecessary time under anesthesia for the patient. The therapist should communicate with the operating room supervisor to have a clear understanding of all operating room dressing and infection control procedures. The operating room supervisor should be made aware of the therapist's needs, for example, an electrical outlet for heat, approved extension cord, or working surface near the patient. The surgeon who requests that the splint be provided in surgery may prefer that as much of the splint as possible be prefabricated on the patient long before surgery. In this way only final adjustments need to be made in surgery, thereby eliminating extended anesthesia time.

Persons removing or reapplying splints, including physicians, nurses, physical therapists, other occupational therapists, recreational therapists, parents, and sitters, should demonstrate an understanding of appropriate application, positioning, removal, and care of the splints and devices. They should also be provided with careful instruction concerning the hospital's and physician's specific infection control policies. See Exhibit 21-2 for a helpful checklist of important factors to be communicated between all persons involved in the child's care.

Various splinting materials can be used. A few that are easy to use include the Orthoplast, K-splint, Polyform, Aquaplast, Hexaplast, and Plastizote. A list of basic and more complete splinting supplies is provided in Exhibit 21-3. For complete information on materials and on splinting details, refer to Malick.[21,22]

More complicated methods of positioning that have been successfully used include skeletal suspension, skeletal traction, and surgical procedures involving skeletal pinning or insertion of Kirschner wires. Evans and others[8] give excellent reference with photographs in their article, *Prevention and Correction of Deformity After Severe Burns.*

Patients are positioned by their physicians within the more complex traction techniques. The therapist working with these patients must be sure that any treatment techniques that are used do not disrupt the suspension or traction.

The patient's mobility is significantly deterred by positioning through traction. This in turn creates a need for the therapist to provide the patient with additional self-help aids to enhance independent functioning. Depending on the parts of the body that are immobilized or limited, the therapist can adapt equipment to meet the patient's needs. Ideas to keep in mind include the use of reachers, prism glasses, rocker knives, built-up handles, utility clips on splints, devices for hanging frequently needed items from a traction bar, and mirrors to see around corners or down the hall.

DRESSINGS

Dressings in burn care cover exposed areas to prevent infection and to promote healing. The splint must be congruent in this relationship as well. Splints are usually applied with the dressings, and adequate allowances must be made for required dressing space. If the splint is fabricated before full edema occurs (approximately 24 hours after injury), then the size of the splint should allow for increase in hand and forearm width.

Two commonly used methods of medical treatments involve applying dressings to wound areas that have been debrided of eschar. Eschar is the scablike material or the dead skin that contains bacteria and must be removed. One treatment method requires frequent dressing changes with close infection monitoring, whirlpool treatments, additional debridement, continuous exercise, and opportunities for splint adjustments. The other method involves one surgical debridement, applications of dressing, and possibly splints at that point, followed by application of bulky dressings or a wrap over the extremities. These dressings stay in place for whatever number of days is decided on by the physician unless obvious infection occurs. Skin grafting can also immediately follow surgical debridement.

In both methods it is important that the splints be positioned properly. These are usually held in place with Kerlex or Flexinet. If additional supports or closures are required to hold the splint in place, Velcro straps wrapped in plastic or Ace wrap can be used. Special attention must be given to the possibility of inappropriate pressure in such cases. In the first method the therapist should check the splint fit after each dressing change.

In some hospitals the dressing changes are carried out by occupational therapists, physical therapists, and nurses. In other hospitals each specific area is designated to a professional group, that is, physical therapists will do whirlpools, nurses will apply dressings, and occupational therapists will apply splints.

Innovations in scar reduction

Some of the latest innovations in burn care procedures used by occupational therapists involve the use of specific pressure to avoid or decrease burn scar hypertrophy. Rivers[27,30] is credited with the clear plastic face mask procedure that has been shown to significantly reduce hypertrophy of burn scars. The cellulose acetate butyrate (Uvex) transparent mask is unlike its predecessors made from opaque materials, such as Orthoplast, Polyform, and K-splint. Uvex is totally clear and therefore provides the therapist and physician with visual demonstration of pressure by specific blanching. Although the material is more difficult to work with and requires fabrication of both negative and positive molds, the end result is worth the effort. For specifics on the use of this procedure, refer to Rivers.[27] The procedure has proved helpful in clinical practice. The following is a general overview of the Rivers procedure.

Since the clear plastic Uvex requires a high temperature for fabrication, a mold must be made of the patient's face. Alginate material (a dental impression compound) is used to make an exact impression, or negative mold. This procedure can be difficult with small children who cannot be expected to cooperate. If the child is going to surgery for grafting, the therapist can arrange to make an alginate mold while the child is under anesthesia. The exact steps in taking an impression must be discussed not only with the surgeon but also with the anesthesiologist before making the mold. This is of utmost importance in that the endotracheal tube used for anesthesia and the airway must be protected from becoming dislodged when the impression compound is lifted off. Every effort should be made to take an impression while the child is already under anesthesia for another surgical procedure. If it is determined by the physician that the patient, such as an older teenager, can be cooperative while awake, then straws can be placed in the patient's nose or mouth for an airway, and the procedure can be continued as just described. Care must be taken to reassure an awake patient in order to prevent the fear or panic that can result in aspiration of the alginate material.

Alginate is easily mixed with water until a frosting-like consistency is attained. This is then applied directly to the impression area, which can be prepared with a thin layer of petroleum jelly to provide easy lift off. Once the compound is set, it should be reinforced with plaster strips. When the plaster strips harden, the impression material is removed as a unit with the plaster strips.

The impression is then filled with plaster of paris. After the plaster is set, the alginate is removed. The plaster mold is refined (filed, sanded, wiped, and smoothed down) to remove burrs and approximately ⅛ inch of the plaster that corresponds to the hypertrophic scars. The clear plastic is then heated in a conventional oven and immediately shaped over the plaster mold. Uvex has different properties from those of conventional splinting materials. Therefore the therapist should become familiar with these by practicing with the material before making the first mask for a patient. Once the plastic is molded, typical elastic and Velcro closures can be used to secure the face mask.

Uvex and this procedure can be used on burn scar areas other than the face. Certainly, taking the initial impression becomes an easy task when precautions regarding respiration are not a concern.

Another material that is used more widely than Uvex in providing pressure is Dow Corning's Silastic Medical Elastomer #382. Elastomer is not clear. However, because it is applied in a thick liquid state and hardens to a firm rubbery material, exact specific contact is made with all tissue. Elastomer is easy to use.[24] It can be thinned, reinforced with other materials such as gauze for strength, and used to line splints made with perforated Orthoplast or Plastizote.[2,9] Elastomer hardens quickly after the catalyst has been added, and the patient has a conformer following one fabrication session. Elastomer is most often used in conjunction with Jobst garments. Jobst garments are elastic pressure gradient garments carefully and specifically measured and custom-made to provide 25 mm Hg pressure to burn scar areas.[19] According to Lamberty and Whitaker,[18]

> Controlled pressure of greater than 25 mm Hg induces realignment of collagen whorls, increases tissue Pco_2 and decreases tissue O vascularity and edema. It is significant that 25 mm Hg is the capillary pressure and it may be that pressure controls the hypertrophic scar by producing a relative ischaemia.

Jobst garments are used internationally with great success. Jobst representatives are available in most major cities and should be contacted for specific information on the appropriate use of their garments.*

Jobst garments stretch over concave areas and therefore cannot provide adequate pressure to these areas (that is, around the clavicles, sides of the nose, chest, and ears). However, by inserting Elastomer conformers, these areas can be provided with appropriate pressure. Malick and Carr[24] give an excellent account of Elastomer uses, fabrication, and results. Although Elastomer is easy to use, the therapist should thoroughly experiment with the material before applying it to a patient. Elastomer must be refabricated during progress made in reduced scar hypertrophy until a totally flat and subtle effect is attained.

Both the Uvex mold and the Silastic Medical Elastomer #382 should be worn continuously (for 20 out of 24 hours per day) until scar growth has been exhausted. They should be removed for brief periods of time (three to four times per day) for cleaning and also to facilitate activities of daily living (that is, the face mask can be removed during meals and at bath time).

SELF-CARE

Basic self-care independence should be started as soon as the physician decides that it is medically safe to do so. A child who is old enough to eat independently and who is receiving nutrition by mouth should be given every opportunity to succeed in this task with a minimum of physical assistance. The occupational therapist should assess the child's abilities and limitations and provide adaptive techniques and devices immediately, before dependent habits are developed.

Examples of self-help feeding devices for children include built-up handles on utensils; handles and trays covered with Dycem (a nonslip material); large hooklike handles on cups; utensil clips on hand splints, if the patient is not ready for active modified grasp; extra long reusable straws; plate guards; and extra long-handled or curved utensils. *Modified grasp* refers to the ideal position for the burned hand of metacarpophalangeal flexion with proximal interphalangeal and distal interphalangeal extension, with the thumb in opposition.

It is important to note that patients should be encouraged to relinquish devices as soon as possible to maximize their independent behavior and function. Children who are encouraged early to take an active part in their own care display not only less dependent behavior, but also less dependent attitudes overall.

One way to include children in the treatment process is to have them participate in removing their dressings. Their involvement during dressing changes also reduces their anxiety and fear of pain inflicted by others.

With such strong emphasis on early maximal, appropriate independence, the therapist must be very careful not to diminish the child's need for warm human relationships. Providing support, encouragment with positive reinforcement, attention, and companionship should not be confused with assistance. Independence should never result in loneliness.

Often family members and special significant others stay with children receiving specialized burn care. In such situations these individuals can provide the appropriate positive and loving reinforcement for independent behavior, while at the same time providing the physical attention and closeness so often missing. The occupational therapist should be instrumental in educating the family in how to provide the appropriate necessary support.

---

*Jobst garments, Box 653, Toledo, Ohio 43694.

Independent programs

Independent programs are made up of activities and exercises to be carried out when the therapist is not present. These include both bedside-inhospital programs and postdischarge-home programs. Both are absolutely necessary for the child to derive full benefit from rehabilitation. Burn care is a 24 hour a day procedure. Long after wound closure takes place, burn scars continue to grow. It is mandatory that patients demonstrate their understanding of home programs or independent bedside programs. Written diagrams and posted instructions are very helpful; however, with actual demonstration by the patient, understanding can be documented. This in turn demonstrates quality assurance.

The occupational therapist can be one of the most valuable assets to the patient in planning independent programs. Here the application of activity analysis becomes very important. Hobbies, interests, games, sports, and other leisure activities can be adapted or introduced to make what seems like the never-ending exercises not only bearable but even a little fun.

When the child is ready for discharge, it is very helpful for the parents and responsible persons to have a clearly written out home program to ensure that the patient is receiving all necessary aspects of treatment while reassuring the parents that they are carrying out the program properly.[7]

Such a home program can be developed into a nicely printed or packaged booklet. Some issues that should be covered in home program instructions include skin care, precautions, use of Jobst garments, exercises and positioning, splint care and wear, nutrition, emotional readjustment, and who to call in case of problems or questions, with a list of the burn team and hospital phone numbers.[7]

THERAPEUTIC ACTIVITIES

Therapeutic activities that are intended to increase children's physical function include all the play, developmental, and educational tasks that are used with orthopedically or neurologically involved children. The difference, of course, is in the adaptation of such activities. If the child does not have hand burns, the therapist can use activities with near normal motion for the child. When the hands are involved, the appropriate burn position must be maintained during acute healing. The child should not make a fist until it is determined that the extensor mechanism will not be damaged in the process. One exercise that is frequently used is referred to as "tabletops and curls." This is carried out simply by first assuming metacarpophalangeal flexion with proximal interphalangeal and distal interphalan-

geal extension. This is the tabletop. Then the patient assumes the opposite position of metacarpophalangeal extension with proximal interphalangeal and distal interphalangeal flexion. This is the curl. In this way all joints are exercised, but a fist is never made.

Active range of motion is most important in burn care. Splints can be removed for these exercises four to five times per day. Needless to say, it is much easier to attain maximal cooperation from children when play is involved, particularly where some discomfort is unavoidable.

DEVELOPMENTAL ASPECTS

It is difficult to accurately assess developmental level when a child is hospitalized for acute burn care. Initially the child may be too ill, and mobility may be seriously restricted. Also, the therapist can expect anxiety and imposed life-style restrictions to cause a certain amount of regression in the child's level of performance and behavior. This would make standardized testing results invalid in predicting performance outside the hospital environment. Modified, adapted, or partial developmental assessments can, however, be very helpful to the therapist in planning for therapeutic exercise activities that the child needs during the progressive healing stages. The development assessment tools and techniques, and the therapeutic activities that have been presented in all the other chapters of this book, apply to this discussion.

Since the child learns through experiential sensory motor input, including tactile, visual, auditory, proprioceptive, and kinesthetic stimuli, immobilization and confinement can lead to delays in the normal development pattern. The occupational therapist's ability to apply and adapt knowledge of normal neuromotor and psychosocial development to daily living skills and daily exercise tasks will more often result in the patient's being motivated to actively and appropriately participate in, and benefit from, the treatment plan. By using occupational therapy treatment techniques during long hospitalizations, development delays and emotional problems can at least be partially avoided.

PSYCHOLOGICAL ASPECTS

From a psychological standpoint, the burned child experiences feelings that include fear, anxiety, loss and separation, distorted body image, guilt, anger, and depression.[33,34] In a study conducted at the University of Michigan Burn Center, researchers found that the children who were burned before age 11 had the lowest self-esteem. Self-esteem is a long-term treatment problem. Bowden[4] found that patients with low self-esteem spent more days in the hospital and more days in bed after discharge. Occupational therapists have a distinct advantage from training in psychiatry as well as physical disabilities. Providing the child with appropriate channels for self-expression in addition to support and reassurance can begin in the very initial phases of treatment. Passive activities should be initiated early, such as storytelling (bibliotherapy)[33] or specially made talking books that can be played during times when a therapist is not available and the child feels fearful. Subject matter should be carefully selected to provide positive results. Fairy tales with characters such as the Big Bad Wolf can increase the anxiety the small child is already experiencing, whereas stories with positive characters such as the Smurfs or Care Bears can be uplifting and supportive. Talking books and special tape recordings are also useful in special care areas where television sets cannot be operated in conjunction with monitoring equipment.

Relaxation techniques can also be used with children. Children enjoy fantasy, and therefore imagery is easily used both for relaxation and for self-expression. The therapist must be careful to understand the proper use of such techniques to attain positive results.[31]

Often the burned child has other problems. Therefore his history is very important. The therapist should talk to the parents or guardian and establish a workable rapport. The social worker can provide a great deal of assistance with respect to history, family problems, financial concerns, and support systems.

• • •

Children who are developmentally delayed, emotionally disturbed, or physically handicapped present additional challenges to the burn team. During the acute phase these problems may not be apparent without a good history from a responsible party.

In cases of child abuse the parents may not be emotionally able to give an accurate history because of fear or guilt. The burn team members must be aware of specific warning signs of child abuse. Any suspicious cases should be reported to the government agency concerned with child welfare. This is usually the Department of Social Services.

Some of the warning signs include several small burn areas or scars the size of a cigarette tip, unexplained bruises, a history of repeated visits to the emergency room, or a history of accidents or broken bones. Certain burn patterns are indicative of possible abuse as well, for example, burns of the buttocks, feet, and perineum when the backs of knees and anterior hip areas are not burned. This occurs when a child is placed in a tub of hot water. The child reflexes into a protective position by flexing the knees and hips. Burn team members should learn to listen to the child's version of his home life and observe the burned child's behavior.

REINTEGRATION INTO SOCIETY

Part of the therapist's responsibility should include assisting the patient to reenter society. With infants and very small children this of course primarily involves educating parents and significant others in the child's immediate world. With older children this education needs to be taken further to assist the child in making the first difficult transitions.

The occupational therapist may go to the child's school ahead of time with samples of devices, splints, and Jobst garments the burned student will be using and wearing in school. Providing educational information and allowing classmates to try on and experience feeling these garments, splints, or devices can provide an immediate acceptance of the student by peers.

Field trips to shopping centers and public malls can be a part of the occupational therapy treatment plan. The occupational therapist's attitude and presence during the first such excursions can provide reassurance to the child and family and furthermore may mean that such trips will be made much sooner and without anxiety when the child is discharged.[13]

BURN PREVENTION

Since burns are most often accidents caused by human error, educational burn prevention programs are valuable. The participation of the occupational therapist as well as other burn team members in burn prevention programs is becoming more and more routine. The occupational therapist has an excellent opportunity to help the community by becoming involved in these programs.

The burn team members are seen by people in the community as professionals and experts with a great deal of credibility. This credibility, along with that provided by the fire department, can leave a lasting impression on an audience.

Fire departments have had burn prevention programs for years. They work closely with hospitals that treat burn victims, and they welcome working with the hospital burn team on prevention programs. They voluntarily give speeches at PTA meetings, show burn prevention audiovisual materials to school children, and provide ideas for burn prevention activities to teachers and parents. An excellent resource is *Project Burn Prevention: A Guide to Activities for Children 4 to 7.*[28]

Luther and Price,[20] in *Burns and their Psychological Effects on Children*, present an epidemiological example of appropriate education for the community in burn prevention. They take into account that all three interacting factors—the host (or child), the environment (or kitchen), and the agent (or hot water)—must be dealt with, or the educational process is incomplete.

SUMMARY

It is the occupational therapist's professional responsibility to provide the burned child with every possible benefit that can be derived from occupational therapy intervention. To meet standards of excellence in providing the service, the therapist is usually required to attain additional knowledge and training in this specialty area.

When working with the burned child, particular emphasis is placed on splinting, positioning, special devices for scar reduction, and increased self-help performance. The therapist should also exhibit expertise and versatility in adapting play activities that will incorporate exercise programs. These activities should provide the patient with a psychological outlet, as well as serve as a basis of support.

The therapist's responsibility does not stop when the patient is discharged from inpatient status in the hospital. Burn patients are often followed for years. The outpatient program can be started immediately after discharge with frequent visits for therapy and pressure device follow-up. As the patient progresses, visits become less frequent. The therapist must keep in mind that long-term follow-up is important with children, who will experience changes through growth, both physically and emotionally.

The challenge for the occupational therapist and other health care specialists increases as more people survive serious burns each year. Approximately 50% more people survive burns than they did 10 years ago. This survival rate refers to the seriously burned population and therefore implies a greater need for health care specialists to work with this population. Medically, scientifically, and practically we are much more knowledgeable with respect to services we can offer to provide burn survivors with a life-style that is significantly more desirable and certainly more normal.

REFERENCES

1. Abston, S.: Burns in children, Ciba Clin. Symp. **28:**1, 1976.
2. Alston, D.W., and others: Materials for pressure inserts in the control of hypertrophic scar tissue, J. Burn Care Rehabil. **2:**40, 1981.
3. Bailey, W.: Pediatric burns, Miami, 1979, Symposia Specialists, Inc.
4. Bowden, M.L., and others: Self esteem of severely burned patients, Arch. Phys. Med. Rehabil. **61:**449, 1980.
5. Camacho-Martinez, F.: Evaluation and complete overview of the burned patient, J. Dermatol. Surg. Oncol. **6:**10, 1980.
6. Clark, W.R., and McDade, G.O.: Miscrostomia in burn victims: a new appliance for prevention and treatment and literature review, J. Burn Care Rehabil. **1:**33, 1980.
7. Doane, C.B., and Fannon, M.M.: Home care guide for burn patients, Atlanta, 1980, St. Joseph's Hospital.
8. Evans, E.B., and others: Prevention and correction of deformity after severe burns, Surg. Clin. North Am. **50:**1361, 1970.
9. Feldman, A.E., and Mac Millan, B.G.: Burn injury in children: declining need for reconstructive surgery as related to use of neck orthoses, Arch. Phys. Med. Rehabil. **61:**441, 1980.
10. Feller, I, and Jones, C.A.: Nursing the burned patient, Ann Arbor, Mich., 1974, Press of Braun–Brumfield, Inc.
11. Feller, I., and others: Care of the burned patient: (post graduate course materials), Ann Arbor, Mich., 1976, University of Michigan Burn Center.
12. Gordon, M.: The burn team and you, Phoenix, 1978, The Burn Treatment Skin Bank.
13. Granite, U.: Multidisciplinary discharge and rehabilitation planning for burn patients, Qual. Rev. Bull. **5:**30, 1979.
14. Hand rehabilitation center procedure manual and teaching syllabus, Loma Linda, Calif., 1980, Department of Occupational Therapy, Loma Linda University.
15. Heimbach, D., and Engrov, L.: Advances in burn care, West. J. Med. **134:**274, 1981.
16. Kamil-Miller, L.: Occupational therapy treatment with burn patients: a learning module, Ann Arbor, Mich., Occupational Therapy Division, University of Michigan Medical Center.
17. Kibbee, E.: Life after severe burns in children, J. Burn Care Rehabil. **2:**44, 1981.
18. Lamberty, B.G., and Whitaker, J.: Prevention and correction of hypertrophic scarring in post-burn deformity, Physio-therapy **67:**2, 1981.
19. Larson, D.L., and others: The prevention and correction of burn scar contracture and hypertrophy, Galveston, 1973, Shrivers Burns Institute.

20. Luther, S.L., and Price, J.H.: Burns and their psychological effects on children, J. Sch. Health **51:**419, 1981.
21. Malick, M.H.: Manual on static hand splinting, Pittsburgh, 1972, Harmarville Rehabilitation Center.
22. Malick, M.H.: Manual on dynamic hand splinting with thermoplastic materials, Pittsburgh, 1974, Harmarville Rehabilitation Center.
23. Malick, M.H.: Management of the severely burned hand, Br. J. Occup. Ther. **38:**76, 1975.
24. Malick, M.H., and Carr, J.A.: Flexible elastomer molds in burn scar control, Am. J. Occup. Ther. **34:**603, 1980.
25. McClellan, B.: Guidelines for occupational therapy treatment of the patient with upper extremity burns, Masters Thesis, Wayne State University.
26. McDougal, W.S., and others: Manual of burns, New York, 1978, Springer-Verlag New York, Inc.
27. Rivers, E.A., and others: The transparent face mask, Am. J. Occup. Ther. **33:**108, 1979.
28. Project Burn Prevention: A guide to activities for children ages 4-7, Newton, Mass., 1980, Educational Development Center, Inc.
29. Shea, P., Notes from lecture materials 1976-1982. Atlanta, Saint Joseph's Hospital.
30. Shons, A.R., and others: A rigid transparent face mask for control of scar hypertrophy, Ann. Plast. Surg. **6:**245, 1981.
31. Trygstad, L.: Simple new way to help anxious patients, R.N. **43:**28, 1980.
32. Wachtel, T.L., and others: Management of burns of the head and neck, Head Neck Surg. **3:**458, 1981.
33. Walker, L.J.S.: Psychological treatment of a burned child, J. Pediatr. Psychol. **5:**395, 1980.
34. Wernick, R.L., Brantley, P.J., and Malcomb, R.: Behavioral techniques in the psychological rehabilitation of burn patients, Int. J. Psychiatry Med. **10:**2, 1980-81.
35. Willis, B.A.: The use of orthoplast isoprene splints in the treatment of the acutely burned child: preliminary report, Am. J. Occup. Ther. **23:**1, 1969.
36. Willis, B.A.: The use of orthoplast isoprene in the treatment of the acutely burned child: a follow-up, Am. J. Occup. Ther. **24:**187, 1970.
37. Willis, B.A.: Burn scar hypertrophy—a treatment method, Galveston, Tex., 1973, Shriners Burns Institute, and Toledo, Ohio, 1973, Jobst Institute.
38. Willis, B.A.: Splinting the burn patient, Galveston, Tex., Medical Communications Department, Shriners Burns Institute.

SUGGESTED READINGS

Corlett, R.J.: The treatment of deep burns of the hand, Aus. N.Z. J. Surg. **49:**567, 1979.
Davidson, T.N., and Bowden, M.L.: Social support and post-burn adjustment, Arch. Phys. Med. Rehabil. **62:**274, 1981.
Denton, B.G., and Shaw, S.E.: Mouth conformer for prevention and correction of burn scar contractures, Phys. Ther. **56:**683, 1976.
Heembach, D.M., and others: Minor burns, guidelines for successful outpatient management, Postgrad. Med. **69:**22, 1981.
Larson, D.L., and others: Techniques for decreasing scar formation and contractures in the burned patient, J. Trauma **11:**807, 1971.
Mangus, D.J.: A simple sling method for support and aeration of burned legs, Plast. Reconstr. Surg. **68:**434, 1981.
Marvin, J.: Techniques of reaching the public with the burn prevention message, J. Burn Care Rehabil. **2:**50, 1981.
Newmeyer, W.L., and Kilgore, E.S.: Management of the burned hand, Phys. Ther. **57:**16, 1977.
Shea, P.C., and Fannon, M.: Mayonnaise and hot tar burns, J. Med. Assoc. Ga. **70:**659, 1981.
Whitaker, J., and Lamberty, B.G.: Pressure garments in the treatment of axillary burns contracture, Physiotherapy **67:**6, 1981.

22

BETTY SCANLAN SNOW

Children with visual
or hearing impairment

Hearing and vision are the distant senses that allow us to understand what is happening in the environment outside our bodies. Those of us with normal sensory function cannot truly understand the total nature of the disability but can be helped by participating in sensory awareness activities. Eating a meal blindfolded to simulate blindness or listening to records that simulate what common songs sound like to an individual with a certain type of hearing loss are examples of sensory awareness activities and are good exercises, but they do not give the total picture. Each person with normal senses has a vast wealth of visual and auditory memories to call on that people with impaired senses do not have. It is important to note that most of the children with sensory loss who are seen in occupational therapy will be congenitally impaired and therefore will have no reservoir of unimpaired information to review.

The *sense organs* (eyes, ears, skin, nose, tongue) are all extensions of the brain. The brain's primary function is to receive information from the world for processing and coding. These sensory stimuli are integrated and associated with past experiences. Since the nature and the intensity of the stimulation to the sense organs vary greatly, one may take precedence over the others, depending on the situation. If a particular sense organ is not working properly, the others do not take over and totally compensate, but another sensation may take precedence.

Ayres[4,5] developed a *hierarchy of sensory perceptual development* that helps in the understanding of sensory impairments. The senses develop and work in an inter-

active manner in all everyday activities. They do not perform in isolation, but develop in a building block manner. The *vestibular* system gives information about the body's position in space, movement or lack of movement through space, and direction of movement. The receptors for the vestibular system are located in the inner ear, and it is thought that the auditory system evolved out of the more primitive vestibular system.[4,5] The vestibular and *tactile* (touch) systems are the foundations of sensation. Visual and auditory sensations are received by the brain against a constant background of tactile stimuli and the body's position in space. It is important to think about the level of alertness required by the brain for auditory and visual perceptual processes to occur. The vestibular system and the *reticular arousal* system have a great influence on this level of alertness. Being either overly alert or not sufficiently alert can obviously have detrimental effects on visual and auditory perceptions.

Vision is the sense we use for understanding the relationships between people and objects. It puts the environment in perspective for us and precedes auditory development by building concepts and perceptual abilities. Children with visual defects often have a diminished verbal language because the relationships and associations between people and objects are not fully grasped. In discussing vision, we have to differentiate between visual acuity, visual awareness, and visual perception. Impairment can occur at any or all levels, and the child has to be assessed accurately.

In addition to its function as the building block for

speech, *audition* is the sense that conveys sound. Sound gives information on distance and direction. We can hear a dog bark and without seeing him judge where he is and how far away. Auditory perception is the attachment of meaning to sound patterns. Sound has qualities of tone and pitch that make up auditory acuity. As with vision, impairment can occur at the level of acuity, awareness, or perception. Although language development appears to be the most serious problem for a hearing impaired child, the situation is much more complex, because language is a force in the socialization and development of inner logic of the child.[60,72] Language is not innate but a product of the child's environment. As the child learns the language, she can exert greater control over her environment.

Piaget[20] discussed development in terms of periods. The first is the sensory motor period and has six stages. The first stage approximates the first month of life and is predominantly reflex behavior. Vision and audition begin to emerge out of reflexive behaviors during the second stage. The infant goes from reflexive visual response to actively following moving objects and will stop crying when he hears a noise, interrupting his activity to listen.

The problems of children with visual or hearing impairments can be enormous. Although deaf and blind children face many shared difficulties, there are also striking differences. For this reason this chapter deals separately with the hearing impaired, the visually impaired, and the multiply impaired. It is important to point out early in the chapter that the occupational therapist is usually not the primary professional for the primary problems of the visually or hearing impaired child, but instead provides critical services for the secondary complications related to the impairments.

The importance of play cannot be overemphasized for these children in particular. Play is the means by which the child learns how to solve problems, to cope with the environment, to face the unknown, and to adapt by changing behaviors.[30,46] For children whose distance senses (and therefore their abilities to perceive the environment) are limited, the development of play skills should be the highest priority.

HEARING IMPAIRMENT
Diagnostic information

It is estimated that 2% of all school-aged children have hearing losses of some degree.[38] Two out of every 1,000 children under the age of 19 are classified as deaf.[61] Approximately 30% of hearing loss is attributed to prenatal causes, and 70% to postnatal causes.[16] Total deafness is very rare and usually only happens when there is aplasia or failure of the inner ear to develop. A *deaf* person is one whose hearing is so severely impaired

that she must depend primarily on visual communication such as writing, lipreading, manual communication, or gestures. A *hard-of-hearing* person is one whose hearing is impaired but not to the extent that he must depend primarily on visual communication.[15,52]

To properly examine the subject of hearing loss, it is important to have a basic understanding of the nature of sound and the anatomy of the ear. Sound sets up a disturbance in the air. Air consists of more than 400 billion particles per cubic inch, and as we speak or make a sound these particles are set in motion, hitting against each other and forming a wave of sound energy. The ear acts as a receiver, amplifier, and transmitter.

The ear is composed of three separate sections (Figure 22-1), and the type of hearing loss that a child has will depend on where the damage is located. The outer ear includes the visible part *(pinna)* and the ear canal extending to the *eardrum (tympanic membrane)*. The function of the outer ear is to collect the sound or acoustic energy and channel it to the eardrum, which vibrates with the sound wave and changes the acoustic energy to mechanical energy. The middle ear consists of the three small bones *(hammer* or *malleus, anvil* or *incus,* and *stirrup* or *stapes)* that conduct vibrations from the eardrum to the inner ear. The stapes is inserted into the *oval window,* beyond which is the fluid-filled vestibule containing the *utricle* and the *saccule.* The motions of the bones of the middle ear result in an increase of the mechanical energy of sound so that by the time sound travels from the eardrum to the oval window, it has been many times intensified. The inner ear is composed of the hearing organ, *cochlea,* that coils off the vestibule and the *acoustic nerve* (eighth cranial nerve). The cochlea transforms the mechanical energy of the sound waves into neural energy for reception by the auditory nerve. The nerve fibers join together in the auditory nerve and follow a route to the brain through the brain stem. In the medulla some two thirds of the fibers cross over from the left to the right side, and vice versa. The hearing center of the brain is the *fissure of Sylvius* in the auditory cortex of the temporal lobe.

There are two types of hearing loss: conductive and sensorineural. In *conductive hearing loss* the problem lies in the sound-transmitting portions, that is, the outer or middle ear. Some common causes of conductive loss are wax buildup, punctured eardrum, or inability of the middle ear bones to move properly. Diagnoses with conductive hearing loss include Treacher Collins' syndrome, a hereditary underdevelopment of the external canal and middle ear, and otosclerosis, a progressive condition occurring as early as late adolescence. We hear by bone conduction as well as by air conduction, and the relationship of these two functions gives diagnostic information about the location of the hearing loss. Fortunately many conductive losses can be corrected by medical-surgical means when detected. Unfortunately,

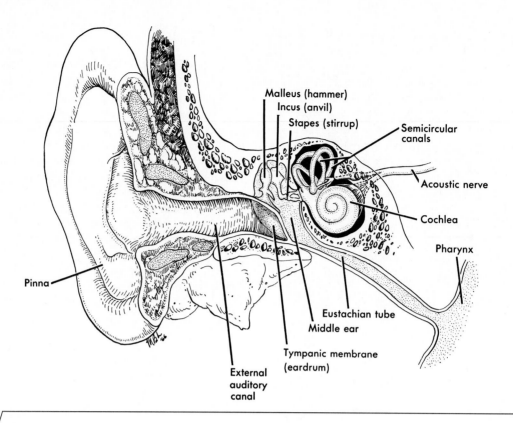

FIGURE 22-1

Cross section of the ear.

From Ingalls A.J., and Salerno, M.C.: Maternal and child health nursing, ed. 5, St Louis, 1983, The C.V. Mosby Co.

considerable impairment of the developmental process can occur before the time the child's loss is detected. Poor articulation, delayed speech development, and poor school performance can be caused by conductive hearing loss.

The *sensorineural hearing loss*, or nerve loss, problem occurs in the inner ear with damage to the cochlear hair cells or nerve fibers. A nerve loss is generally not correctable by medical-surgical means, and it requires the use of amplification (a hearing aid). This type of loss often produces problems with loudness and distortion of sound. Sensorineural hearing loss is often associated with meningitis and can be a sequela of ototoxic drugs. Several drugs used especially in early infancy to save lives can have a toxic effect on the hearing organs. Other diagnoses include tumors of the auditory nerve. These are most usually unilateral with the exception of von Recklinghausen's disease, where they are bilateral.

It is common to have a *mixed hearing loss* with both conductive and sensorineural loss present. Obviously it is important to medically treat the conductive portion of the loss as efficiently as possible to minimize the total effect. Generally speaking, if a hearing loss is measured in the "marked loss" range, it is likely to include sensorineural components.

The occupational therapist working with the hear-

ing impaired child must have an understanding of the measurement of hearing loss. This includes knowledge of the severity of the loss and its practical meaning to the child. The most common measuring device for hearing loss is the *audiogram* (Figure 22-2). This uses a gridlike score sheet to record the child's response to auditory stimuli. The audiogram has a vertical axis that measures *decibels* (dB). The decibel level is an indication of loudness or intensity of the sound or sound pressure and goes from 0 (the point at which sound is first perceived) to 140 dB (the point or threshold of pain).

The horizontal axis of the audiogram is the *hertz (Hz) level*. This is a measure of the frequency or number of sound vibrations per minute—the pitch or tone of sound. Pitch or frequency ranges from a low of 125 Hz to a high of 12,000 Hz on the audiogram. The range of 500 to 4,000 Hz is the most important because it encompasses the majority of speech sounds. On the audiogram the scores are plotted on the graph beginning with the *hearing threshold level* (where the child first begins to hear sounds). On the audiogram of a particular child, the left and right ears are differentiated by use of colors or by the symbol of a circle for right and a cross for left.

Decibel level is related to the distance that a sound moves an air particle and is measured by a particular

Frequency of tones (Hz) lows to highs

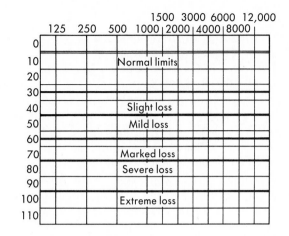

FIGURE 22-2

Audiogram indicating typical loss classifications.

standard or norm such as the 1969 American National Standards Institute (ANSI). Although it varies slightly with the norm being used, a hearing level from 0 to 25 dB is considered within normal limits. Exhibit 22-1 details typical loss classifications according to loudness or decibel loss and their respective therapy-education effects.[8] These effects as stated are general in nature and of course will vary somewhat for each individual child and program, but they will give the occupational therapist a general idea of what to expect with a certain level of hearing loss.

Although a person with a mild hearing loss may often use a hearing aid, the most benefit is derived when the hearing aid is used with a loss of up to 80 dB. Beyond that point the loss is so severe that only partial help can be obtained from the use of an aid.

The hertz level also has to be examined more closely in relationship to the child and her particular hearing loss. The hertz level, or frequency level, is related to the number of times per second the air particle moves and produces tone. In humans the hertz level goes from 20 to 20,000 Hz. Other animals have a much broader range, for example, the porpoise's range is from 150 to 150,000 Hz, and the dog's range is from 15 to 50,000 Hz. A child may have limitation in frequency, and this in turn affects hearing and language development. The hair cells inside the cochlea respond best to varied levels of frequency, depending on location, with the innermost hairs responding best to the low tone frequencies. This means that, depending on the location and extent of damage, there may be high tone loss, low tone loss, or flat loss. Frequency limitations can adversely affect syllable discrimination and understanding of speech.

A *high tone loss* means that the child can hear most

EXHIBIT 22-1

Therapy-education implications of typical hearing loss classifications

Slight loss: 25 to 40 dB
May have difficulty hearing faint or distant speech. Needs favorable seating and lighting in therapy or school settings. May need speech therapy, special attention to vocabulary, or aid in some instances.

Mild loss: 40 to 55 dB
Will understand face-to-face conversational speech (at a distance of 3 to 5 feet). May miss as much as 50% of group discussion if voices are low or not in the direct line of vision. May show limited vocabulary and speech anomalies. Will need hearing aid evaluation and training, speech therapy, help in vocabulary and reading, and favorable seating and lighting. May need special class placement or lipreading training.

Marked loss: 55 to 70 dB
Conversation will have to be loud to be understood. Will have increasing difficulty in group discussions. Will show limited vocabulary and is likely to have speech anomalies and be delayed in language use and comprehension. Will need special education services, speech therapy, lipreading instruction, special help with language skills, and hearing aids. Needs to be encouraged in therapy-education settings to pay attention to visual and auditory input at all times.

Severe loss: 70 to 90 dB
May hear loud voices about 1 foot from ear and may be able to identify environmental sounds such as a vacuum cleaner. May have speech difficulties with some ability to discriminate vowels but not all consonants. If loss is present before 1 year of age, the child will not develop spontaneous language. Will need special education services, support services, and hearing aid. Needs a comprehensive program emphasizing language and concept development, speech, and lipreading.

Extreme loss: 90 dB and more
May hear some loud sounds, such as an automobile horn, very close but is aware of vibrations more than tonal patterns. Will have to rely on vision as the primary means of communication, rather than on hearing. Speech will be deficient and will not develop spontaneously, if loss is before 1 year of age. Will need special education on a comprehensive intensive basis.

of the vowel sounds because they have a lower frequency, but he will miss the consonants. This is serious, because the consonant sounds carry most of the information needed to understand speech. If vowels are removed from a sentence, chances are that its contents will remain clear. However, if the consonants are deleted, understanding will be impossible. With a *low tone loss* the child will miss vowels but will hear many consonants. Voices will sound weak and thin but understandable if the hearing impaired child is close enough to the speaker. A *flat loss* means that all frequencies are evenly affected. Voices will sound far away, and certain strong vowels such as *a* as in *ate* will be heard best.

The audiogram will give information on both the decibel and the hertz loss of a particular child, but the therapist should consult with the other professionals involved with the individual child to get an accurate picture of the child's hearing loss.

Other services involved

Although there may be many professionals involved with a particular hearing impaired child, the most common ones are the following.[15,52]

Otolaryngologist A physician who specializes in the anatomy, physiology, and pathology of the head and neck, including the ears, nose, and throat, by using medical and surgical treatment techniques.

Otologist A physician who specializes in the anatomy, physiology, and pathology of the ear, by using medical and surgical treatment techniques.

Audiologist A specialist in the study of hearing who performs various hearing tests and provides rehabilitation and treatment, including hearing aids, for those whose hearing impairment cannot be improved by medical or surgical means.

Audiometrist A technician trained to test and measure hearing ability.

Practice settings

The occupational therapist usually encounters children with hearing impairment in hospitals at the time of diagnosis or later in the school setting. Many will be identified as "suspicious" in the neonatal unit, and others will show up for developmental testing in the clinic. The percentage of deaf children going to state institutions has decreased with the advent of more local programs, although a great number of deaf children (especially those with severe hearing losses or multiple handicaps) still do attend state schools. The occupational therapist has a strategic role in both the local and state school programs in the areas of self-help skills, socialization, fine motor, sensory integration, and perceptual motor development. The increasing number of infant programs also allows for more therapist involve-

ment in the development of the young deaf child and intervention in the all-important mother-child interaction.

Special characteristics relevant to occupational therapy

To the occupational therapist the most important characteristic of the hearing impaired child is the lack of early language development and the profound effect of this on all other areas of the child's development.[24,50,51] What appears at first to be a fairly simple problem becomes quite complicated in consideration of the importance language plays in our society. Language assists in environmental manipulation and gives the child labels for objects and concepts. It plays a critical role in socialization. The infant smiles and quiets with the sight and sounds of his mother. The deaf infant will not respond to his mother's soft voice, unless the mother is in the direct line of sight. Early intervention is imperative, but infantile deafness is often not diagnosed until later. *Babbling* is vocal play, that is, use of the vocal cords and muscles of the mouth, tongue, and larynx, and all children do this. Children who can hear get the stimulus of hearing themselves and their parents' vocalized response. The deaf child, on the other hand, gets insufficient feedback so that the babbling does not continue and progress on to language development. The deaf infant will generally babble normally up until 5 to 6 months,[62] but then, as the normal infant develops a growing repertoire of sounds, the deaf child will not keep up.

Many researchers in the field[25,42] believe that if intervention is delayed until 3 or 4 years of age, the most important formative period of language development is on the decline and permanent damage is done. If the child is denied cortical stimulation by organic means because of impaired auditory stimuli, she will need to conceptualize by other means. Provision of organized alternative stimuli should be one of the main goals of therapy and education for the hearing impaired child.

Occupational therapy assessment procedures with the hearing impaired child

The therapist can use the general scales of child development, such as the Gesell, Denver, and Bayley, with some modification of the language areas and by taking a known hearing loss into account when reporting any score. My bias is to stay away from scores as such, and instead to use the testing results for a description of the individual child's abilities and liabilities and to compare the child against himself at a later point in time. If the child is using a hearing aid, lipreading, or sign language, the therapist should be cognizant of the implications of these specialized techniques. There are some basic suggestions to follow, and these will be covered more in detail in the section on treatment techniques. If the child uses sign language, and the therapist testing the child is unable to give the commands in sign, the test results should include the information that the therapist was unable to speak the language of the child. In some instances a registered interpreter for the deaf is necessary to assure accurate scoring.

Through developmental testing the occupational therapist frequently identifies the child with a mild problem not yet diagnosed. Often a pediatrician will refer a child who is lagging for developmental testing. Part of the problem can be hearing loss. Unfortunately there are no hard and fast rules for development, and each child is an individual. However, certain findings indicate the possibility of hearing loss and suggest referral to appropriate professionals (Exhibit 22-2).

In most cases the parents are the keenest observers of their infants. Special note should be taken if the mother reports that the infant does not awaken to loud noises, does not respond when called, does not attend to noisy toys, or uses gestures to indicate wants to the exclusion of words. Also notable are the mother's complaints of the child's distractability, inattention to commands, lack of feedback to the mother, or inappropriate responses to verbal stimuli. Obviously all of these difficulties could be attributable to other causes, but hearing impairment should be considered. Also, any child with a history of recurrent ear infections or upper respiratory infections could be a prime candidate for a conductive hearing loss and should be referred to the appropriate professionals.

Other kinds of tests such as prevocational, sensory integration, and activity of daily living checklists can be administered to this population with some adaptation in instructional methods. However, written instructions should be used only if the therapist has in some way made sure that the child has the appropriate level of written comprehension. Writing is language based. We form our sentences in the same way that we form our oral statements. Although research has shown that the deaf have a normal curve on other than language-based instruments, some studies have shown 4 to 7 years lag on other written instruments.[41]

SPECIALIZED ASSESSMENTS

In the area of *psychological testing* several tests are used often with hearing impaired children. The *Hiskey Nebraska Test of Learning Abilities*[3] was developed and standardized on the hearing impaired and covers ages 2 to 17. It consists of 12 subtests selected to cover a broad span of intellectual abilities without language. It includes subtests such as bead patterns, picture associ-

---

EXHIBIT 22-2

Findings that indicate the possibility of hearing loss

Possible hearing impairment must be considered when

- A newborn does not exhibit a startle (Moro) reflex in response to a sharp clap 3 to 6 feet away
- A 3-month-old has not developed auditory-orienting responses as indicated by not becoming alert to toys that make noise
- An 8- to 12-month-old does not turn to a whispered voice
- An 8- to 12-month-old does not turn to sounds such as a rattle 3 feet to the rear
- A 2-year-old is not using words
- A 2-year-old is unable to identify an object with a verbal clue alone, such as "Show me the ball"
- A 3-year-old has largely unintelligible speech
- A 3-year-old omits beginning consonants
- A 3-year-old does not use two- to three-word sentences
- A 3-year-old uses mostly vowel sounds
- A child of any age speaks in a voice that is too loud, too soft, of poor quality, or of a quality that does not fit his age and sex
- A child always sounds as if he has a cold

---

ations, puzzle blocks, completion of drawings, and memory for digits; it is given in an untimed fashion.[9]

The *Leiter International Performance Scale* is a widely used individual IQ test administered without language with a range from 2 to 16 years. It is a performance test that was developed as a nonverbal counterpart to the Stanford-Binet. It is used with hearing impaired children as well as others, such as those who do not speak English. Directions are pantomimed, and the test is not timed. Administration begins with items below the child's estimated skill level so that the child has an opportunity to become accustomed to the testing procedure. There are numerous subtests divided into three trays for different age levels: tray 1 for 2 to 7 years, tray 2 for 8 to 12 years, and tray 3 for up to 18 years. Pattern strips and blocks are used for subtests such as matching colors, number discrimination, pattern completion, similarities, classification of animals, and spatial relations.[9]

Audiological testing is a complicated and involved process.[52] The occupational therapist should consult the professional administering the test on details of testing with the individual child. The most common method of testing requires placement of the child with earphones in a soundproof testing booth. The child indicates when she hears a sound.

There are, however, other forms of testing used with various types and ages of children about which the therapist should be aware. *Behavioral observation audiometry* (BOA) is often used with young children. The mother holds the child in her lap, and the audiologist notes different behavioral responses of the child to sounds at different levels. *Visual reinforcement audiometry* (VRA) teaches the child to orient to a sound source reinforced with light or a visual stimulus. *Tangible reinforcement operant conditioning audiometry* (TROCA) uses a token or candy for reinforcement of sounds identified. In *play audiometry* the child does a certain task, such as putting a cube in a bucket, when the sound is heard. These are all forms of behavioral observations.

There are also some forms of *objective observations* that can be helpful in the diagnosis of hearing impairment. *Evoked response audiometry* (ERA) is often done with infants or unresponsive children. It uses an electroencephalogram-type machine hooked up to a computer. Earphones are placed on a sedated or quiet child, and a series of clicks are played into the ears. The computer records the brain wave responses to these clicks and supplies information regarding the hearing mechanism response to sound. *Tympanometry* is a procedure to assess eardrum mobility or the presence of fluid in the middle ear. This requires the placement of a probe in the ear canal and can be difficult to perform on an uncooperative child. The *acoustic reflex measurement* is tested with the same instrument as the tympanogram, but measures the response of the two eardrum muscles to the presentation of sound. *Electrocochleography* measures the electrical activity of the inner ear and auditory nerve, while *electroacoustic impedance* testing measures the way sound is conducted by the middle ear to the inner ear. With the advent of newer and more sophisticated technology every day, these types of testing promise much for the future.

Objectives of intervention and treatment modalities

As mentioned earlier, the occupational therapist is usually not the primary therapist with the hearing impaired child. Therapy and educational goals must be coordinated with the special educator, the speech therapist, the audiologist, and others working with the child. Some typical occupational therapy objectives follow. These are by no means all-inclusive. Each child should be assessed as an individual by the therapist, and the treatment program should be fitted carefully into the child's total program. Typical goals are the following.

1. *To provide and enhance sensory stimulation.* The hearing impaired child is denied adequate cortical stimulation by auditory channels and must learn to perceive and conceptualize by other means. The functions of the kinesthetic, tactile, and visual systems can be enhanced by the therapist with various activities and techniques. Sensory integrative techniques are useful in developing the kinesthetic system to its fullest. The tactile and proprioceptive systems are very important in the use of sign language. Tactile activities such as having the child locate objects hidden in sand or identify objects behind a shield are among many that can be used. The visual system can be enhanced by tracking exercises, perceptual motor activities, and many games or crafts.

2. *To encourage age-appropriate self-maintenance behaviors.* The occupational therapist can act as a consultant to others for related activities. The parents and others around the child may need consultation regarding what is or what is not appropriate for a certain age. Also, self-maintenance skills involve many concepts that the child should be assisted with in whatever ways possible; for example, the idea of left shoe and right shoe can be shown visually with color coding.

3. *To encourage fine motor and hand coordination skills.* Watch the movements of the hands of a fluent signer and you can easily recognize opposition, finger and thumb flexion and extension, and finger and thumb abduction and adduction. These movements are performed by isolated digits and in total patterns but all in rapid succession and with remarkable coordination. This skill does not come naturally to a deaf child but has to be learned. Occupational therapy's emphasis on hand skills can do much for the deaf child in general and especially for those children who have an identified delay in these skills. Many games and activities can be incorporated in the treatment program.

4. *To encourage socialization.* This part of occupational therapy intervention cannot be done in isolation and is of utmost importance to the hearing impaired child. Socialization can be encouraged by involvement in groups for peer interaction. Developing skills of environmental adaptation and understanding the language-oriented points of behavior can be stressed. Deafness is not an easily visible disability, and therefore a hearing impaired child can be mistaken as being rude if he does not answer questions or respond to social overtures when in fact the child has simply not received the correct stimuli.

SPECIAL TECHNIQUES

The therapist working with the hearing impaired child is intimately involved with the special techniques used with that child. The three most commonly used techniques are lipreading, sign language, and hearing aids.

Total communication is the use of all avenues, such as oral speech, lipreading, sign language, finger spelling, gesture, and body language, simultaneously in communication. Sign language encourages communication and language development.[29,47] There has been a historical battle in the field of deafness between the *oralists* (oral language only through the use of lipreading and speech therapy) and the *sign language users*. The oralists maintain that if taught sign, the child will never learn to talk. The sign language proponents argue that the deaf child needs sign language for early concept development. Fortunately today there seems to be a softening of the lines and a general acceptance of the concept of total communication.

Lipreading would seem easy at first glance. However, consider that only one third of speech sounds are visible to the speech reader.[15] In addition, many of the sounds made in English look alike. For example, *p*, *m*, and *b* are all made with the same lip movement (lips together). Try looking in the mirror or at a friend and saying *ma*, *pa*, and *ba* without voice; the problem is readily observed. Another example of look-alike movements would be *f* and *v*, which are both formed with the teeth to the lower lip.

Sign language is not one easily understood entity, but involves many different methods. *Finger spelling* (dactylology) in the United States is done with one hand, each configuration representing a letter in the English alphabet (Figure 22-3). Finger spelling is used by itself or in conjunction with the other forms of sign language. Although it is not too difficult for the hearing person to learn to do, it is very difficult to receive. When receiving or listening, the tendency is to see the individual letter and not the words. With finger spelling it is important that the hand be close enough to the face that the hearing impaired person can see both the lip movements and the finger spelling at the same time. For fluency and readability, the hand has to be held in a comfortable position, not stiffly.

For simplification, sign language can be divided into *Ameslan* (American Sign Language) and *Signing Exact English* (SEE). Ameslan[18,40] is a language in itself and it is not directly translatable to English. Although it is not universal, Ameslan is the primary language of the prelingual deaf in the United States. It has many abbreviations and phrases contained in a single sign and does not conform to the structure of English. Signing Exact English,[31] on the other hand, does conform to the structure and form of the English language and thus is preferred by many educators. There are many arguments for and against both these types and other types of sign. The important thing for the occupational therapist to realize and understand is the philosophy of the particular unit or school that the child is a part of. It is equally important to become as fluent as possible in

that particular system. Obviously, for many it will be impossible to learn but a few of the most simple and frequently used words and phrases, but this is important to the therapy of the child. There are many good texts available.[7] However, it is best to attend a class or practice with a friend who knowns sign, since it is often difficult to correctly interpret the configuration and movement patterns of the hands.

The occupational therapist can often be involved in the initial stages of learning sign. It is usually best to select the first signs to be taught from those that represent familiar objects, real life situations, and familiar actions. Begin with what is available: things to feel, handle, or do. The parent can be given a likes-dislikes checklist to help the therapist know what is appropriate for the individual child. Often a food item is used first because of its value as a reward. The adult should work at the eye level of the child, obtain eye contact, do the sign, and then physically manipulate the child's hands through the sign. Some basic suggestions for the use of total communication are listed in Exhibit 22-3. It is hoped that with total communication, the child will demonstrate earlier development of linguistic skills, better interpersonal relationships, and understanding of self and environment.

The occupational therapist also is often involved in the initial stages of *hearing aid use.* Often a history will show that the child had a hearing aid but rejected it. This can sometimes be traced to the lack of professional support for the parents and child during the difficult adjustment period or to the professional's lack of familiarity with the aid. It is regrettable when an instrument that can be of help to the child is not used. One of the problems that occurs is that the aid does not cause the child to hear normally, it only amplifies the sounds in the environment. It does not restore hearing as glasses can restore vision. It does not localize sounds but instead amplifies all sounds in the environment, thus leading to distortion. The therapist can help the parents and child clarifying realistic expectations of the aid and what it can and cannot do for the child.

One of the main problems found in children with new aids is *tactile defensiveness.* The therapist can work on this with the parents and the child. The head is often the most sensitive portion of the body. The child must learn to think of the aid as a piece of clothing that is put on automatically in the morning along with shoes and socks. The earlier an aid is fitted to a child and put into use, the better the chances for language development.[55] The young infant learns much about language as he watches his mother's face while being held in her arms. The major need is to get used to the feel of the aid initially. It is usually best to begin wearing the aid during a quiet activity that involves the speech of just one person. The maximal benefit from an aid is ob-

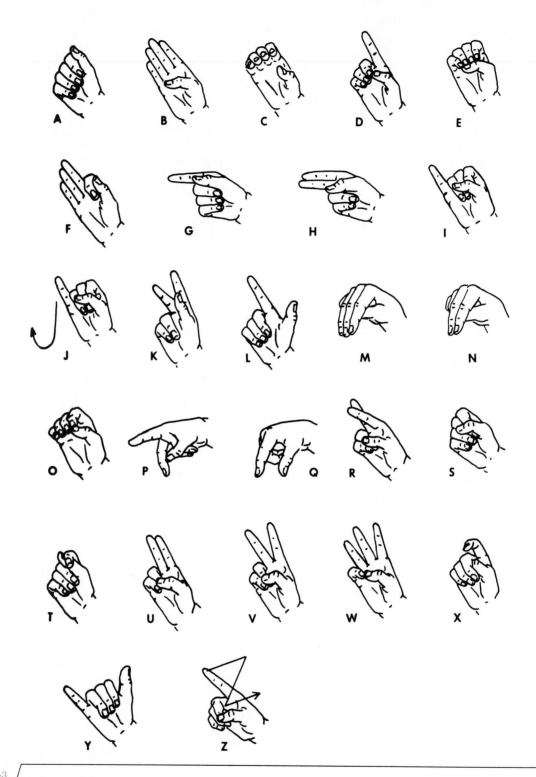

FIGURE 22-3

American one-hand manual alphabet.

Suggestions for the use of total communication

1. Face the child squarely at eye level.
2. Position yourself so that the child can see your face and hands at the same time without strain.
3. Make sure you have the child's attention.
4. Avoid light behind you. If the child has to look into the light, she may be unable to clearly see your lips.
5. Use a normal tone of voice. Do not exaggerate mouth movements, because this practice tends to confuse.
6. Speak the word and give the sign at the same time, rather than in sequence.
7. Use appropriate pauses between words, especially when finger spelling is used.
8. Better results will be obtained when you sit close to the child, rather than across the room.
9. Keep instructions simple and to the point.
10. Be consistent, especially with the young child.
11. Above all, *talk* to the child. She needs to receive the same amount of input as a hearing child, although the method may be altered.

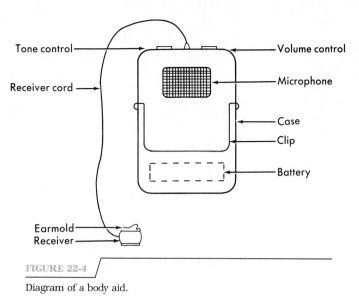

FIGURE 22-4

Diagram of a body aid.

tained in relatively quiet settings. Because the aid does not localize sounds, the following situations will present difficulties: a place with a lot of background noise; a group with three to four people speaking at once; listening to reamplification such as with a television or tape recorder; and distance listening.

The hearing aid is a sensitive piece of equipment with several parts and can often be out of order. Everyone involved with the child should be aware of some of the common problems, since an improperly working aid is useless to the child. Some of the common problems are (1) dead batteries, (2) squeal—check for looseness of the cord or earmold, (3) batteries improperly placed or corroded, and (4) opening of earmold impacted with wax.

The type of hearing aid prescribed for a particular child depends on the degree and configuration of the loss.[34] There are three major types. The *in the ear* aid is used only for very mild losses and has no external wires. The *behind the ear* aid is usually for mild to severe losses and can be built into eyeglasses. It is a small unit made up of a microphone, amplifier, and receiver located together behind the ear and connected with a short tube to an earmold. The *body aid* is by far the type most commonly used with children. It is usually prescribed for marked to extreme losses. The microphone, amplifier, and power supply are together in a case carried in a pocket or harness worn by the child. The case is connected by small wires or earmolds seated directly in the ear. A monaural aid signifies just one aid, while binaural refers to the use of two separate aids.

The parts of the body aid (Figure 22-4) are as follows:

1. *Microphone* picks up the sound waves and converts them to electrical signals. It is usually behind a protective grill. The aid should always be worn with the microphone facing away from the body.
2. *Amplifier* increases the strength of the signal and is located inside the case.
3. *Battery* provides the energy source.
4. *Receiver cord* extends from the case to the ear and is the most vulnerable part of the aid.
5. *Receiver* changes the electrical signals back to sound waves and is attached to the earmold.
6. *Earmold* is custom-formed of plastic to the shape of the individual's ear.

PREPARATION FOR ADULTHOOD

The hearing impaired adolescent must try to blend into a hearing world. Although this task is difficult, there have been many advances in social acceptance of individuals with hearing impairment. The growing technology of communication has improved future prospects. One of the important tasks of most adolescents is learning to drive a car. Most schools for the deaf have special driving training available. All students are taught by driving instructors to constantly scan the environment visually. To the deaf student this is of utmost importance.

Another important aspect of blending into the hearing world is the use of the telephone, a daily communication device often taken for granted. The telephone companies have various forms of amplification devices available. Some hearing aids have a telephone setting. If amplification alone is not sufficient to understand conversation, the Telephone Typewriter (TTY) is available. The Telephone Typewriter is a communication device that uses the telephone lines with a typewriter keyboard to "talk" and a printout device to "listen" or receive the conversation. The telephone ring is replaced with a flashing light or a fan that moves back and forth to indicate an incoming call. The obvious disadvantage is that both ends of the line need to be equipped with this system for it to work. Today technology is, however, making the system cheaper, easier to use, and more portable.

Television provides another aspect of daily life. The frequency of closed-captioned programs has increased, and in 1976 the FTC authorized the Public Broadcasting Service to develop more special programs for the deaf. The deaf use a decoding device, a "black box," to view the same programs as the regular audience but with the addition of captions. Another approach is the use of a sign language interpreter in a cameo spot, but the disadvantage is that this is difficult to read on smaller television screens.

One medical problem of deaf adolescents is of such magnitude that it should be mentioned: *Usher's syndrome.* This is a genetic disease that affects 3% to 6% of all congenitally deaf. It is marked by the progressive blindness of *retinitis pigmentosa,* a degeneration of the retina that progresses from impaired night vision, to gradual constriction of the visual field with loss of peripheral vision, to blindness, usually by 20 to 30 years of age. There is much emphasis on early screening for this problem because of the obvious changes it would make in the education and vocational choice of the deaf adolescent.

Occupational choice has always been difficult for the deaf. Schein and Belk[61] stated that the average deaf worker earns 25% less than the average hearing worker and is usually employed in skilled manual labor. Gallaudet College in Washington, D.C. was for a long time the only place available to a deaf student for higher education. There are now many programs available where deaf students are integrated with the hearing students because of the availability of special services such as interpreters and notetakers. California State University at Northridge and New York University have well-established model programs.

In addition to the obvious communication problem, there are three factors that adversely affect occupational choice for the deaf[61]: (1) psychological perception differences that affect self-perception and perception of reality, (2) restricted life space that adversely affects knowledge of areas outside of the immediate social or geographical area, and (3) limited sociocultural understanding. Although no one can make the deaf child hear normally, the occupational therapist and other professional workers can help alleviate these three blocks to fuller participation in occupation. For resources for additional study and information on hearing impairment, see the reference section of this chapter.

CASE STUDY 1

Ed is 2 years, 3 months old. He had meningitis during the neonatal period with resultant hearing loss of a severe degree. Ed is the first and only child to date of a young couple. Both parents are employed. Ed attends a local day program for children younger than 3 with handicaps of all types. He has been assessed by use of the Gesell Developmental Scale and by subjective observation. Ed performed as follows.

Motor area: Ed passed all items at the 24-month level except the cube tower of six to seven where he functioned at the 21-month level. Although he passed items such as walking up and down stairs alone, it should be noted that he often stumbled and appeared uncoordinated. However, on subjective observation, a great deal of this could be attributed to his "looking everywhere," that is, searching for visual input.

Adaptive area: Again Ed passed all items except for the cube tower and adaptation of form board. The item that requires repetition of three to four syllables was deleted from the testing. Distractability was noted.

Language area: Ed passed none of the items suitable for 24 months. He had vowel sounds and receptive total communication vocabulary of five words and no expressive vocabulary to date. He attempted to form words verbally and with sign language.

Personal-social area: Ed passed all items at the 24-month level except toileting items, communication items, and the play item of parallel play. He demonstrated domestic mimicry and would pull a person to show (21-month level).

As noted, Ed attends a day program with a teacher as the primary professional and speech therapy, audiology, and occupational therapy as supportive services. Occupational and speech therapies are available on a half-time basis, and the audiologist is employed on a consulting basis.

Treatment program

1. *Tactile desensitization* of the head and face area to promote acceptance of the hearing aid: activities such as rubbing different textures; touching different parts of face on therapist, self, dolls, and felt board (this activity also promotes body identification and sign skills); and playing dress-up with different hats.

2. *Improvement of fine motor coordination* through activities and games such as busy box, geometric form ball, putting items in containers, stacking toys, and picking up small pieces of food.

3. *Improvement of attention to activities* through activities such as mimicry games, vestibular stimulation activities such as self-regulated swinging in net and using rocker board, and use of "look" sign in gross motor playground activities.

4. *Consultation regarding toileting* to both school and home and establishment of schedule.

VISUAL IMPAIRMENT
Diagnostic information

It is estimated that 12.5% of all school-aged children have some degree of visual defect.[16] However, less than 10% of these children can be diagnosed as legally blind. Total blindness is found in only a very few children and is often a result of *anophthalmos* (absence of the eyeball). Hereditary causes account for approximately one half of all childhood blindness. *Retrolental fibroplasia* still occasionally occurs but with far less frequency. This disease is caused by giving a premature infant too high a level of oxygen. Shortly after World War II oxygen was used liberally to save the lives of premature infants, but in the middle 1950s it was discovered that because the blood vessels of the eyes of the premies were not fully developed, they were especially sensitive to the oxygen.[39] With this disease the blood vessels hemorrhage, there is retinal detachment, and there is formation of a membrane behind the lens. Today oxygen is carefully used, but even room oxygen (approximately 21%) can cause damage in an extremely undeveloped infant. Typically 26 to 31 weeks of gestation is the most involved age group. The more mature premies are usually less severely involved.

The legal definition of blindness is important to understand. In the United States the legal definition of blindness is

> Central visual acuity of 20/200 or less in the better eye after correction, or visual acuity of more than 20/200 if there is a field deficit in which the widest diameter of the visual field subtends to an angle distance no greater than 20 degrees.[36]

To put it more clearly for our understanding, this means that the legally blind child can see an object clearly at 20 feet that a normally sighted child can see at 200 feet. *Acuity* refers to central vision. The *peripheral vision*, or second part of the definition, means that the child can only see in a field of 20 degrees where a normally sighted child can see in a field of over 180 degrees. This peripheral vision is most important in mobility and general observation of the environment. There are some generally accepted gradations of acuity with correction (Exhibit 22-4). Of course, acuity is not the only factor, and two children with equal acuity can have different visual functions.

As with the ear, it is important for the occupational therapist to have a basic understanding of the anatomy and physiology of the eye to understand visual impairment. The eye (Figure 22-5) functions to transmit light to the retina. It focuses images of the environment on the retina. The eye is shaped to refract the rays of light so that the most sensitive part of the retina receives rays at one convergent point. The *cornea* is at the front of the eye and is part of the outermost layer of the eyeball. It plays a large part in focusing or bending the rays of light. Behind the cornea is the *aqueous humor*, which is a clear fluid. The pressure of this fluid helps maintain the shape of the cornea and helps in focusing the rays. The colored part of the eye, or *iris*, with its center hole, the *pupil*, is directly in back of the cornea. The iris governs the amount of light entering the eye by increasing

---

EXHIBIT 22-4

Gradations of acuity with correction

20/20 to 20/70	= Normal to slightly defective vision
20/70 to 20/100	= Mild visual limitation or good partial vision
20/100 to 20/200	= Moderate visual impairment or fair partial vision
20/200 to 20/1,000	= Legally blind with severe impairment
Over 20/1,000	= 1. Finger counting ability
	2. Form perception
	3. Hand movement
	4. Light perception (sees light and can tell where it is)
	5. Light perception (sees light but cannot locate it)

---

or decreasing the size of the pupil. The light then progresses through the *lens*, which does the fine focusing for near or far vision, and through the jellylike substance called the *vitreous humor*. The eye has three layers: the *sclera* is fibrous and elastic, helping to hold the rest of the eye structure in place; the *choroid* is primarily blood vessels that supply the eye; and the *retina* is the innermost layer. The retina layer is composed of the nerve cells that contain a chemical that is activated by light. The *fovea* (located on the retina) is the point of sharpest and clearest vision. It is most responsive to daylight and must receive a certain quantity of light before it will transmit the signal to the optic nerve. The retina has three types of receptor cells:

1. *Cones:* Used for color perception and visual acuity
2. *Rods:* Used for night and peripheral vision
3. *Pupillary:* Controls opening (dilation) and closing (constriction) of the pupil.

The *optic nerve* (second cranial nerve) transmits the visual sensory messages to the brain for processing.

Visual impairment can occur within the structures of the eyeball, at the retina, along the nerve pathway to the brain, and in the brain itself. *Refractive errors* occur when there is deviation in the course of the light rays as they pass through the eye, preventing sharp focus on the retina. The most common are the following.[54]

1. *Myopia, or nearsightedness.* This child sees most clearly at close range and much less efficiently at a distance. The eyeball is too long or refractive power is too strong so that the focus point is in front of the retina; the child has blurred vision, possibly external strabismus when looking at a distance, and often holds printed material close to his eyes.

2. *Hyperopia, or farsightedness.* This child has

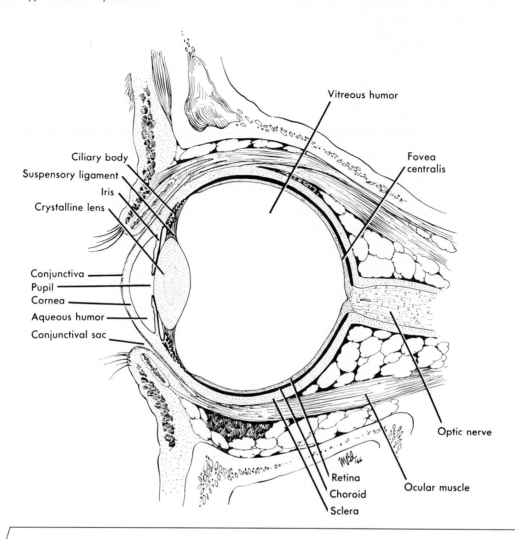

FIGURE 22-5

Cross section of the eye.

From Ingalls, A.J., and Salerno, M.C.: Maternal and child health nursing, ed. 5, St. Louis, 1983, The C.V. Mosby Co.

blurred vision and may have headaches when trying to focus. The eyeball is too short and underdeveloped, the refractive power too weak, and the focus point is behind the retina. This child sees most clearly at a distance, and with constant effort to focus at close range, will become fatigued.

These refractive errors can usually be corrected with lenses but can have a devastating effect on the development of the child in all areas if left undiagnosed or untreated during early school years.

Cataracts are often a congenital problem that give rise to poor vision. A cataract occurs when the lens of the eye changes from clear to cloudy or opaque. After removal of the lens, the child will have to wear corrective lenses. Although often the result of heredity, childhood cataracts have other common causes:

1. *Juvenile diabetes,* or other metabolic disease: Cataracts can occur as early as 3 years of age
2. *Down's syndrome:* Approximately 60% of these children develop cataracts from 8 to 17 years of age

3. *Rubella, or German measles:* Approximately 75% of infants whose mothers contracted the disease within the first trimester will have cataracts at birth.

Glaucoma is another visual problem that can occur in childhood. Glaucoma is an increase in the intraocular pressure of the eyeball resulting in hardening of the eye and damage to the cornea. The congenital type occurs in the first year of life, and the infantile type occurs between 6 and 12 years of age. It may be secondary to ocular inflammation or neurological diseases.

There are many *other eye conditions* the occupational therapist may encounter. Some of the most important of these are listed here along with common optical terms.[36,54]

Accommodation The power of altering the size of the lens to adjust the focus of the eye.
Optic atrophy Degeneration of the optic nerve fibers.
Patching Covering one eye temporarily to promote use of the other eye.

Nystagmus Rapid involuntary movement of the eyes. May be hereditary, and results in inability to fixate accurately and constantly. The movement is repetitive and may be lateral, vertical, rotary, or mixed.

Strabismus Squint or cross-eyes. Failure of the eyes to converge properly on an image, or both eyes not directed at the same point. This condition is often caused by muscle imbalance and often results in double vision. In esotropia the eye turns inward; in exotropia the eye turns outward; in vertical strabismus the eye turns up or down.

Amblyopia A condition of diminished visual acuity that usually cannot be relieved by lenses. The child may have depth perception problems and may tilt her head. Sometimes called lazy eye.

Astigmatism Unequal curvature of the refractive surfaces of the eye. This may result in focusing problems, because light is not sharply focused on the retina but spread over a more or less diffused area. Distorted images may result.

Cortical blindness The ocular structures are intact, but the child is functionally blind because of severe insult to the visual cortex of the brain. Occurs as a result of near drowning or prolonged shock, for example.

Ptosis Drooping eyelid resulting from weak or absent muscle and usually does not interfere with vision.

Retinoblastoma Malignant tumor of the retina and eye orbit, either unilateral or more often bilateral.

Toxoplasmosis Parasitic disease that can be congenital or acquired from household pets; causes scarring, usually on retina and choroid.

Visual acuity is most often tested with the use of the *Snellen chart.* This tests central visual acuity with letters, numbers, or symbols in graded sizes drawn to Snellen measurements. Each size is labeled with the distance it can be seen by the normal eye. The child stands 20 feet from the chart and indicates to the examiner what he sees line by line. Eye report terms include *OD,* which refers to the right eye, *OS* to the left eye, and *OU* to both eyes.

Other services

Visually impaired children often have a number of other professionals involved in their treatment. The most common are the following.

Ophthalmologist A physician who specializes in the diagnosis and treatment of defects and diseases of the eye, performing surgery when necessary and prescribing other types of treatment, including corrective lenses.

Optometrist A licensed specialist in vision (O.D.) who is trained in the art and science of vision care. Specializes in the examination of the eyes and the preservation and restoration of vision by optometric means; measures refractive errors and eye muscle disorders.

Optician A person who grinds lenses, fits them into frames, and adjusts frames to the wearer.

Orientation and mobility specialist An individual specialized in orientation and mobility training of the visually impaired. *Orientation* is the process of using the remaining senses to establish one's position and relationship to all other significant objects in one's environment. *Mobility* is the ability to move safely and efficiently from one point to another in the environment. This specialty began with the war blind of World War II. Today specialists in this field come primarily from graduate programs such as that started in 1960 at Boston College, although some programs are available at the undergraduate level.

Practice settings

The visually impaired child is more likely to be identified earlier in life than the hearing impaired child. The occupational therapist will encounter these children in the neonatal and acute units of the hospital. Visually impaired children will often be referred by pediatricians to outpatient clinics for developmental testing and treatment, because the effects of visual impairment on development are more medically evident than those of auditory impairment. The number of blind children going to state schools has been drastically reduced in recent years with the advent of more local programs. The therapist will be involved in both local and state school settings.

Special characteristics relevant to occupational therapy

There are many developmental deviations found among visually impaired children. Blind children have to learn about the world with their hands. Normally sighted children will develop eye-hand coordination early in life, but blind children will have to wait for ear-hand coordination to come at a later stage in development. They need good tactile system performance for exploration and concept development.[33,44] These children have to pick up a ball and feel it to tell if it is round: there is no other way to develop that concept and know what *round* means. Yet, because of their blindness these children will often exhibit tactile defensiveness. They also need to learn to move their bodies to understand how they move and that there is space (environment) for her body to move into. Blindness itself often results in fear of movement. The blind child will have difficulty progressing through the developmental sequence of random-to-purposeful movements.

Lowenfeld[43] talked about three major restrictions imposed by blindness:

1. *Restriction in range and variety of experiences with people and the environment.* Problems of physical accessibility, size, and danger impede the child's ability to interact.

2. *Restriction in ability to get about.* The child needs assurance from others to know what is out there and how to get to it, around it, or away from it.

3. *Restriction in control of the environment and self in relationship to the environment.* The child lacks information from distance sense as to form, size, position, and general orientation and is unable to read people and determine nonverbal communication.

Behavior deviations can occur, and many authors trace these to early sensory deprivation.[22,37] Blind children are deprived of adequate visual stimuli and are often secondarily deprived of tactile, vestibular, kinesthetic, and proprioceptive stimuli because of the lack of mobility. Fraiberg[22] stated that it is not uncommon for these infants to sleep or lie untouched for 14 to 18 hours a day. Also, as toddlers they walk late and are not as mobile as sighted children. Studies of animal deprivation[37] clearly show that sensory deprivation during the formative periods can result in the failure of the deprived system ever to achieve maximal development. Multisensory deprivation has an even more pronounced effect.

"Blindisms" may also develop. These include eye poking and flicking hands. Such actions appeal to children because they break up light and change what little they are able to see. However, blindisms make it impossible for them to try to use residual vision for purposeful activity. Blindisms need to be limited and activity diverted to other more productive avenues.[32,68]

Hendrickson[34a] discussed some of the implications of blindness for concept development. Vision is normally used to identify the position of things in space, to recognize shapes without feeling them, and to know the length of a room without pacing it. These concepts and many more have to be acquired by the blind child by alternate means.

Occupational therapy assessment procedures with the visually impaired child

There are some developmental differences characteristic of children with visual impairment that are important for the therapist to note. The usual developmental scales can be used with notation as to the child's impairment. Every area of development will be affected, but it should still be kept in mind that generalizations may not apply.

The sighted infant takes hold of her world with her eyes long before she learns to use her hands.[26,28] The infant has monocular fixation at first, but by the eighth week binocular vision is dominant. The infant has sustained fixation on a nearby object (that is, mother's face) during the first week and on more distant objects by the end of the first month. All of this visual grasping is a prelude to hand grasp and use. By 20 weeks the normal infant will usually pick up the pellet on the Gesell test and by 44 weeks has a neat pincer grasp. This performance contrasts sharply with the visually impaired infant who develops ear-hand coordination (the ability to locate and reach for sound), but not until almost the end of the first year. This *ear-hand coordination* begins at about the 10- to 12-month level,[22,32] but does not reach proficiency until the first year of life.

The normal child learns to associate visual experiences with symbolism, and although vision always retains a concrete core, the child learns to associate visual experiences with words. The absence of the association of words with visual experiences explains why, although the blind child receives the same auditory stimuli, *language development* will be affected.

Gross motor development will also be greatly affected by visual limitation. The blind infant will mold to her mother's shoulder like the sighted infant, but she will not spontaneously turn her head as will the sighted child.[1] The prone position without sight is not particularly interesting or comfortable. The blind child will learn to creep, if at all, only after the development of ear-hand coordination. Often the child will prefer to scoot on his back to move around. The blind child will demonstrate a delay in crawling of approximately 6 months.[1] Sitting will usually develop within sighted norms, because it is a static position, but the blind child will have to be positioned in sitting and will have difficulty with fluid movement to and from sitting. Also, time spent in this position will be limited because of the lack of the visual stimulation that motivates the child's attention. Standing is also a static position and will occur roughly within the normal age range. However, walking is a dynamic movement and may be delayed by approximately 7 months.[1] Walking involves a self-initiated movement, and the blind child will need to learn the hazards and layout of the environment. Stair climbing will also be delayed and will require a great deal of guidance. The typical climbing and exploring of the 18- to 24-month old does not take place spontaneously.

Fine motor development is strongly affected by the delay in ear-hand coordination. The blind child will sit and manipulate toys within reach, but once out of reach, the toy disappears. The sound of a familiar noise toy is not spontaneously connected with the feel of the toy. The child develops age-appropriate object transfer and hand play at midline, but manipulation of objects may well be delayed.

In the *social-emotional area* a delay in the development of play may be anticipated. A doll or a toy truck will initially have no meaning. As miniatures of visual objects, these will be difficult to perceive. Parallel play and mimicry are difficult to learn without the opportunity to see and imitate others. Feeding may well be delayed by parental apprehension about the mess and by the child's initial difficulty in coordinating the hand-to-mouth pattern. Also, many blind children have difficulty weaning away from familiar and comforting routines such as the use of the bottle.

There will be lags in *adaptive skill development.* Discrimination of shape and space, which normally appears from 12 to 18 months, does not occur in the blind child until 24 to 36 months.[58] Concept development is problematic. The blind child will have difficulty in learning that one word signifies many different tactile experiences. For example, a chair can have many different shapes, sizes, and textures, but all related forms are identified by that one word.

Exhibit 22-5 lists some observations that an occupational therapist will most likely make on a blind child. These are based on some possible problem areas.[11,14,73] The list is not all-inclusive and would have to fit the particular situation and the developmental level of the child.

The therapist may wish to administer portions of the *Southern California Sensory Integration Tests* to the child. There are several parts of the test that do not require sight and others that can be adapted. The scores should not be strictly interpreted, because the tests have not been standardized on the blind, but the test results will give important information on the child's spatial awareness or orientation, proprioception, and bilateral integration. Parts of the test that can be administered most readily include finger identification, graphesthesia, localization of tactile stimuli, standing balance, kinesthesia, and right-left discrimination. The therapist should also check for the presence of residual asymmetrical tonic neck reflex and tonic labyrinthine reflex (TLR), as well as for the presence of protective extension responses. Any interpretation of postrotary nystagmus responses would be difficult, because blind children often have ocular nystagmus as part of their visual deficit.

SPECIALIZED ASSESSMENTS

There are several tests especially adapted or devised for use with the blind. One of special interest to therapists and psychologists is the *Maxfield-Buchholz Social Maturity Scale for Blind Pre-School Children.*[45] It is an adapted version of the Vineland Social Maturity Scale and helps to obtain an accurate developmental picture of an individual child. Previously known as the Maxfield-Fjeld Adaptation, its development was initiated in 1936 shortly after Dr. Edgar Doll published the Vineland Social Maturity Scale. The Maxfield-Buchholz scale covers seven areas of the Vineland scale: self-help general, self-help dressing, self-help eating, communication, socialization, locomotion, and occupation. The only area deleted was self-direction. In the Vineland scale the first self-direction items occur at the 6-year level. The Maxfield-Buchholz scale is designed for preschoolers to

---

EXHIBIT 22-5

Observation of the visually impaired child

Posture: Is the child's head up and held at midline? Often the head is down or the child displays unusual posturing. This needs to be noted because of its relation to the prevention of back problems and the promotion of social acceptance.

Balance and stability: Can the child maintain a position well? How good is her balance on one foot? This is important for mobility training.

Ambulation and gait: Is the gait stiff? Are the steps normal in size? How does the child manage on stairs or uneven surfaces?

Strength and tone: Is the child's tone normal, and is his strength adequate for his age? Such children often have low tone because of the lack of movement.

Endurance: Can the child pursue a gross or fine motor task for an appropriate length of time?

Coordination: The dexterity of visually impaired children can be subjectively assessed on tests, such as the Minnesota Rate of Manipulation Test (MRMT). The MRMT in particular has norms for the blind.

Identification of body planes and body parts: Does the child know front from back? Can she identify body parts at an age-appropriate level? The visually impaired child needs to know "boundaries of self."

Laterality: Can the child identify right and left on himself and others and locate objects placed to either side? This is necessary in exploring the environment.

Directionality: Can the child tell which direction to go to reach an object or person, moving or stationary?

Controlled isolated body movements: Are extraneous movements present? Control is important for work and school skills, as well as social acceptance.

Tactile discrimination: Can the child use her hands and body to their fullest to explore?

Auditory discrimination: Can the child discriminate distances of sound and types of sound and identify different people by voice?

Spatial orientation: Is the child able to judge distances? This is important in mobility.

---

the 5- to 6-year level. Of the 95 items on the Maxfield-Buchholz scale, 44 are from the Vineland scale. The Maxfield-Buchholz items were all standardized with blind children and give the examiner information about how a blind child compares to other blind children. It is administered exactly as the Vineland: the parent or parent figure gives information about the usual performance of the child.

Several intelligence tests have also been adapted for

use with the visually impaired, including the Binet and the Wechsler. Other oral tests are easily adaptable. The American Foundation for the Blind publishes a comprehensive listing[63] of psychological, vocational, and educational tests appropriate for use with the visually impaired.

Visual testing has had many subjective and objective aspects. As with audiological testing, it is becoming more sophisticated with increased technology. In addition to the Snellen-type acuity examinations, there are others developed to test young children and retarded children. Sheridan[64] published a series of vision tests including such items as matching distant pictures to objects on a table. Physicians use an ophthalmoscope to view the internal structure of the eye. Electroretinography (ERG) can be done under sedation for a thorough examination of the retina and fundus. A visual evoked response (VER) test may be done with the use of an electroencephalogram. This gives as assessment of cortical response to light stimulation. If the results are good, it indicates that there is no gross defect in the eye, optic nerve, or visual cortex.

Objectives of intervention and treatment modalities

The occupational therapist may be the primary therapist for a visually impaired child, but most often works with a team that includes the special educator, the physical therapist, and the orientation and mobility specialist. Other professionals are involved as the child's needs indicate. The treatment plan is based on the individual assessment of the child. The following are some typical intervention goals for this group.

1. *To discourage blindisms and divert the child to more productive behaviors.* Blindisms are persistent stereotyped mannerisms that can seem similiar to those exhibited by autistic or retarded children. It has been shown, however, that these mannerisms in the visually impaired child are not tied to some psychological or retardation level but to the degree of blindness. As the sensory deficit increases, the need for substitute self-stimulation increases. Eye rubbing or eye poking, for example, causes excitation of the neural portion of the eye and generates impulses in the retina and through the optic nerve.[68] (People who have sight experience this in an unpleasant fashion when they poke their eyes and "see stars.") Blindisms interfere with the development of other more useful behaviors and are socially not well accepted in the sighted world. Substitution with other types of more productive stimulation seems to be the most effective therapy intervention.

2. *To encourage movement in space.* The underdevelopment of dynamic movements, such as crawling and walking, cannot be totally eliminated, but much

can be done in the therapy setting to help compensate for these. Crawling over different surfaces and movements on bolsters, therapy balls, and other objects are helpful activities. A chair or wagon can be pushed to develop security in walking. Balance activities are helpful to decrease fear of movement.

3. *To encourage sensory integration.* The blind child needs considerable vestibular stimulation from tilt boards, swings, scooters, and so on. Sensory feedback in blind children is interrupted and can cause distortion of movement.[17] It is important, however, that safety be maintained in the use of equipment and that the child be allowed to control the movement. Excessive fear of falling, poor grasp of room layout, and inability to organize or cross midline are all indications of difficulty in sensory integration.[70] Van Benschoter[70] outlined a successful summer camp experience for blind children that stressed sensory integrative programming. Children at the camp aged 6 to 21 were evaluated individually by use of the Southern California Sensory Integration Tests. Based on the results, a treatment program was developed that was found to have a positive effect on the movement skills of the children involved.

4. *To provide parental counseling.* The parents and the family of the blind child should be encouraged to handle the child as they would a normal infant and not leave the child in the crib. They need to talk to the child and explain the environment, allowing the child to do as much tactile exploration as possible. Early intervention is a must for this population.

5. *To decrease tactile defensiveness.* The blind child does not see the approach of people and objects and can exhibit a very defensive reaction to touch. Use of a firm touch is better than a light touch, which can be interpreted as being aversive, as a tickle. Allowing the child to touch textures and to play in such media as sand, water, and clay constitutes good therapy techniques.

6. *To encourage use of hands for manipulation.* At first the world has to come to the blind child. Toys should be maintained within reach, tied to the crib, walker, or tabletop. Later the child can be taught to search for and locate lost objects using a constantly expanding circle.

7. *To encourage socially acceptable behaviors.* The child should be encouraged to look at people when they speak, to smile appropriately, to keep her head up in midline, and to avoid posturing.[35,56] She must learn how others are reacting based on voices rather than gestures, facial expressions, or body language. Hill[35] in her article on intervention with blind preschoolers, stressed the area of parental and professional encouragement of socially acceptable behaviors in the visually impaired child.

8. *To maximize residual vision.* The therapist should always use whatever vision the child has in the

treatment program activities. The more a child uses visual pathways, the better his vision develops.[6] Visual awareness and discrimination activities are important, such as color or shape recognition and matching.

9. *To encourage language and concept development.* The blind child must consciously be taught to develop cognitive schemes that the sighted child picks up in a relatively casual manner. This is done with verbalization and the use of the remaining senses. Those things that cannot be touched or heard, such as clouds, need to be explained in particular.

10. *To develop self-maintenance skills at age-appropriate times.* The therapist can consult with those who work with the child about the developmental sequence of self-maintenance skills. Eating and dressing activities should be "motored through," that is, the therapist physically manipulates the child through the performance of the activity. If abnormal eating patterns develop and are not corrected, they usually do not get better. Good supportive seating is important to the self-feeding process. For dressing, differential tabs can be sewn on clothing to indicate front and back. The child will need a lot of practice time with buttons and zippers. Toilet training can be facilitated by (1) a consistent schedule, (2) an established route to the bathroom, (3) the familiar sounds and smells of the room, (4) consistent use of one or two words for toileting, and (5) establishing an association between changing wet clothes and going to the bathroom.

11. *To develop maximal tactile perceptual abilities.* The blind child obviously needs to maximize tactile abilities to learn about her environment and eventually braille, if she will need it. Activities such as finger painting, finding and identifying objects hidden in sand or beans, and identifying gradations of textures and puzzles are among those that increase tactile awareness.

12. *To develop maximal auditory perceptual abilities.* The blind child has to learn to identify sounds and their meanings and react to them appropriately. Sounds come from three basic sources: toys, speech, and the environment. Active rather than passive listening should be emphasized. Activities such as locating a squeak toy, identifying sounds such as cars and trains, and following directions from persons and recordings are helpful.

13. *To encourage knowledge of parts of the body and body planes.* The child has to know his own body before understanding how it moves and fits into the environment. Body image is important to mobility and social function.[11,73] Obstacle courses can teach the child how large his body is in relation to other objects. Touching body parts on others is helpful. Life-size dolls can also be used.

14. *To encourage laterality and directionality.* Especially for mobility skills, a blind child must know the concepts of right-left, up-down, in-out. The child must develop the awareness that things outside the body have sides and must be able to measure distance and direction.

15. *To strengthen cognitive skills such as object permanence, cause and effect, object recognition, and ability to match and sort.* Games and many simple craft activities can easily be used to accomplish these goals. The blind child needs these skills to progress intellectually and academically.

SPECIAL TECHNIQUES

Children with severe visual handicaps will usually have to rely on braille and talking books for their education. For the child who will eventually use braille in school, the importance of early tactile perceptual training cannot be overemphasized. Braille is a system of six raised dots arranged in a cell (Figure 22-6). These dots are arranged in various configurations to form the letters of the alphabet, numbers, and words.[59] Braille can be written in three levels or grades, depending on the degree of contraction used. It is read left to right with

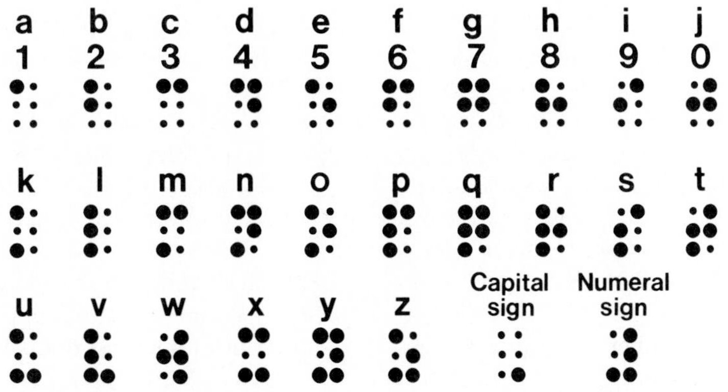

FIGURE 22-6

The braille alphabet and numbers.

one or two hands. Usually the index finger is used with a light touch. As for the child with cerebral palsy who is eating, positioning is critical to the blind child's performance with braille reading. Braille was developed by a young blind French student, Louis Braille, in 1824 and was found to be more efficient than attempting to read the raised Roman alphabet. Speeds do vary, but 104 words per minute is the average, which makes it quite useful in the educational setting. Braille is produced on a special slate or machine called a braillewriter.

Talking books are also available for almost any subject at any age level. The young blind child can be tuned in to listening with short storytelling sessions. The adult should carefully monitor the child's attention to promote good listening skills. Scratch-and-sniff books and tactile books are also available to help in early storytelling. Large print books may be used by those who can discriminate a larger typeface.

There are various types of lenses available for the visually impaired, from the relatively common ones used to correct refractive errors to telescopic and microscopic lenses that are used as low vision aids with certain types of blindness. There are also projection devices and magnifying devices such as the opticon, which converts inkprint into a readable vibrating tactile form.

In *mobility training* such techniques as using the Seeing Eye dog, sighted guides, and long canes are taught. The techniques of echo detection, trailing, and body protection are also important. Seeing Eye dogs are specially selected and expertly trained. Sighted guides usually walk a step forward of the blind person, who holds the guide's elbow. Body movement is best perceived this way. Cane technique is also a very specialized procedure that requires the training skills of a professional in the field.

Although as a rule the orientation and mobility specialist is the one who teaches trailing and body protection, there are certain basic principles that the occupational therapist should know. Trailing is the use of a wall as a guide for walking. The hand closest to the wall is extended at hip level until the outside of the little finger touches the wall, then the back of the fingertips are used to guide the person in walking. In the protection technique the upper arm is held at shoulder height and parallel to the floor with the palm facing out to meet any obstacle before the body does. The lower arm is extended downward and forward with the palm facing out. Another protection technique is to extend the arm palm out in front of the head while bending down to retrieve a dropped object.

Low vision training is another specialized technique.[6,21] Some educational personnel will specialize in this method. The basic premise is that the child can be taught to use vision. Visual acuity is by itself not really the most important part of visual ability. Through planned stimulation, visual efficiency can be increased.

Often light is used initially to increase focusing ability. Once fixation is achieved, the child can learn to discriminate global aspects of the image. When this happens, the child can move on to analyze discrete elements of the image and finally to identify form, outline, and other aspects. Obviously this method does not work with all visually impaired children, but it does have good results with others, especially when combined with a good overall program to heighten the child's levels of perception.

PREPARATION FOR ADULTHOOD

The most obvious challenge for the blind adolescent is the choice of an appropriate occupation. Options are even more limited than for the deaf adolescent, but the situation has improved with more colleges and training programs offering special services for the blind student. Almost all textbooks are available in braille or talking books. The job is to fit the personality and talent areas of the adolescent to the occupational choices. Lack of exposure to many vocational options can be a problem that the occupational therapist can address through community orientation and various activities to give the child more prevocational experiences.

There are certain mannerisms that should be discussed, because these behaviors often interfere with optimal social interaction. Again, these are things that the therapist and all the other professionals involved with the child should work to eliminate:

1. Standing too close to others
2. Rocking the body
3. Blinking, rubbing, or rolling the eyes
4. Stamping or shuffling the feet
5. Not looking at a person when speaking
6. Feeling whatever is bumped into

Daily living skills such as cooking, cleaning, and recreation become increasingly important as the child reaches adolescence. The American Foundation for the Blind puts out a comprehensive list[2] of aids and appliances. For the kitchen there are such devices as a sugar meter that dispenses one half a teaspoon of sugar at a time and an elbow-length oven mitt to prevent accidental burning. A canned goods marking kit is available, as well as self-threading needles and tools with marking gauges. For recreational activities there are braille cards and low vision cards, as well as table games such as Scrabble and Monopoly with braille markings.

Self-care can be facilitated by careful organization of the wardrobe and tactile clues for color of clothing. Handling money and shopping can be difficult tasks and require much training and assistance.

Leisure time activities are important for well-rounded adulthood. Exercise groups, weight lifting, dance classes, and bowling are all excellent physical activities that should be encouraged, since many blind adults lead very sedentary lives. Blind persons can play ball sports with sound balls and can run or jog with minimal track guidance aids. For resources for additional study and information on visual impairment, see the reference section of this chapter.

CASE STUDY 2

Bonnie is 7 years, 4 months old. She had congenital cataracts removed during her first year of life. Her resultant condition is legal blindness with form perception. Bonnie is the third and last child of a couple who have divorced since her birth. The mother works while Bonnie attends a local grammar school where she is mainstreamed into a regular second grade class. She has been assessed informally by the therapist, and parts of the Southern California Sensory Integration Tests have been administered. Bonnie performs as follows.

Motor area: Bonnie can trail in familiar settings such as home and school but needs a sighted guide for unfamiliar areas. Her gait is shuffling and hesitant, and she fears falling. Balance activities are difficult, and she can only stand on one foot momentarily. She has difficulty with motor planning. Her coordination skills, grasp, and pinch are age appropriate.

Language area: On the school testing she is 1 to 2 years behind in vocabulary. She enjoys music and talking books. Her attention span is variable and auditory discrimination poor for sound location.

Personal-social area: Bonnie was in an infant stimulation program before school placement and has acquired some play skills but remains shy and withdrawn especially in playground activities and physical education. She feeds herself, but her mother has a great deal of difficulty getting her to dress herself. The mother attributes this in part to her own inability to "let go."

As noted, Bonnie is in a regular second grade class. She receives occupational therapy on an itinerant basis, as well as visually handicapped special education services three times a week. She attends regular physical education with some adaptation of requirements.

Treatment program

1. *To increase balance, motor planning, and equilibrium skills.* Use of swing, bolster, tilt board, and scooter activities. Counseling with the teacher and the physical education instructor to provide tactile input for planning motor activities.

2. *To increase dressing skills.* Provide counseling to the mother regarding age-appropriate dressing skills. Refer mother to social worker for counseling related to "letting go" and coping with single parenthood of a handicapped girl. Practice with the child on manipulation of fasteners and use of tactile strips for clothing identification. Home visits to observe and assist in arranging clothing for ease of identification.

3. *To increase social skills.* Have the child plan and participate in group activities with small groups of her classmates. Cooking or craft projects might be used.

IEP objectives for present school year

1. Will be able to stand and balance on 1 foot for 10 seconds.

2. Will be able to manipulate buttons, snaps, and zippers 100% of the time.

3. Will plan with therapist four group activities during the school year.

MULTIPLE SENSORY IMPAIRMENT (DEAF-BLIND)
Diagnostic information

There is one important concept to understand regarding any multiple involvement, whether it is deaf-blindness, deaf-retarded, blind–cerebral palsy, or any combination of handicapping conditions: The result is not just a simple addition of the results of the handicaps, but rather a *multiplication of disability*. This combination of sensory losses with each other and with other problems presents the most devastating results, and the interaction of the problems have to be considered.

The most common problem encountered in therapy settings is deaf-blindness caused by congenital rubella. Before 1963 the number of deaf-blind children born per year was a relatively consistent 140 per year.[57] A census in 1934 indicated 379 deaf-blind persons. However, the 1963-1965 rubella epidemic in the United States affected approximately 50,000 women during the early months of pregnancy, resulting in an estimated 20,000 still-births or miscarriages and 30,000 children born with handicaps. Of these, approximately 5,000 were deaf-blind.[10,12,13]

Rubella is also known as the 3-day or German measles. It is usually a fairly mild infection with moderate fever and rash in the mother. However, rubella causes serious damage to the developing embryo. The worst damage to eyes and heart is done during the second to sixth week of pregnancy, with inner ear and hearing damage continuing until the last half of pregnancy.[12,13] Almost every system of the body can be affected, but the most common triad is congenital cataracts, sensorineural hearing loss, and congenital heart defects. The virus destroys the hair cells in the organ of Corti, causes patent ductus arteriosus and pulmonary stenosis, and interferes with the development of the eye. A viral encephalopathy after birth can continue to cause further damage, and often the heart problems cause hypoxia and sometimes cerebral palsy from lack of oxygen. These children are often small for age, hypotonic, and have abnormal electroencephalographic patterns. The eye problems are usually first diagnosed because of the cataracts, and surgery is performed early. Since the virus continues to affect fetal hearing development beyond the time it affects visual development, many of these children are not visually impaired and therefore not diagnosed until later in life.

Rubella is not the only disease that causes a combination of visual and hearing deficits. Embryological studies show that there is much similarity in the timetable of development of the eye and the ear.[66] Therefore many diagnoses involve both systems such as cytomegalovirus infections, toxoplasmosis, congenital syphilis, Hurler's syndrome, Waardenburg's syndrome, and Goldenhar's syndrome. Meningitis is the leading cause of noncongenital deaf-blindness in children.

Rubella incidence is reduced today by the live vaccine developed in 1969 and by the active antibody testing program that tests the rubella susceptibility of expectant mothers. The vaccine is often given routinely to teachers and others who work with young children with a warning against pregnancy for 3 or more months after the vaccination. However, there are still reported cases of congenital rubella, especially among the children of young adolescent mothers who contract the disease early in pregnancy and may not know they are pregnant at the time or may not have told their parents or physicians.

Before the rubella epidemic very little was known about deaf-blindness, and very few programs were available to educate or treat these children. Perkins School, a residential facility for the blind in Massachusetts, was an exception that had many deaf-blind pupils, the most famous of whom is Helen Keller.[19] A young instructor was sent in 1887 to Alabama where the 6-year-old Helen Keller lived. Helen had been deaf-blind since 19 months of age. The instruction was difficult, especially at first, but eventually the two returned to Perkins School where Helen completed her education and went on to Radcliffe College where she received a bachelor's degree. Helen Keller's success story was not often repeated, and the education of the deaf-blind did not progress much until the rubella epidemic gave it impetus. In 1968 medical professionals and educators began to anticipate the tremendous impact of the epidemic, and an amendment to the federal Elementary and Secondary Education Act of 1965 established 10 regional centers to coordinate the education of deaf-blind children. Today only a few of these centers still function, and state departments of education have taken over other programs.

Other services

All of the previously mentioned professionals may be involved, plus additional medical specialists such as cardiologists and orthopedists. As the severity of a child's disability increases, occupational therapy knowledge and skills are more frequently sought. Often an occupational therapist's initial contact with visual or hearing impairment is through a multiply involved child.

Practice settings

The number of children with multiple sensory handicaps is often too small to establish an effective local program. The number of residential placements tends to rise with the level of impairment. Also, as children grow older they need more specialized program-

ming. Although most professionals would favor local programs that allow children to live at home, there are very definite advantages to residential programs as the child matures. These are

1. No long summer or holiday breaks to lose skills
2. Continuity of program and skills training
3. Twenty-four-hour care and supervision
4. Transition for those who will always need assistance.

Special characteristics relevant to occupational therapy

There are some very characteristic behaviors of rubella deaf-blind children. Typically they show extreme tactile defensiveness. They do not like anything new or different, and changes of any type are not well accepted. There is a great deal of oral defensiveness, and the change from smooth to textured foods is quite difficult. Rubella children are usually hypotonic early in life. There is hypermobility of the joints, unless the child suffered additional brain damage from hypoxia, thereby incurring spasticity. Such children will usually learn to walk but will be delayed and cautious about giving up support. They can go from walking holding onto a wooden stick, then a smaller stick, then a piece of rope, then a piece of yarn, then a thread and still immediately fall if the thread is taken away. They often have had difficult infancy periods, setting up a cycle of negative reactions to parental handling that led to less and less parental handling. They can be "too deaf to be deaf," that is, not responding at any level. This seems to evolve because the stimuli do not make sense to the deaf-blind children, so they choose to block them out. They can have many primitive withdrawal reactions and can seem autistic. Blindisms such as eye poking, eye rubbing, flicking hands in front of eyes, head bumping, hair twirling, and rocking are often present and can become self-abusive. Perseverative behaviors are common, as are teeth grinding and masturbation. Certainly, every child is different and may manifest these behaviors to different degrees.

Occupational therapy assessment procedures with the multiply impaired

Developmental scales can be used for assessment and treatment planning. Of special interest are the prehension and tactile abilities, since almost everything will have to be taught in a "hand over hand" manner. The Callier-Azuza Scale[67] is a checklist for use with this population. It has five areas of subscales: motor development, daily living skills, language development, perceptual abilities, and socialization. It covers developmental skills up to approximately the age of 7 and is based on observations of spontaneous behaviors in structured and unstructured situations. Each subscale is further divided, for example, the daily living skills subscale consists of dressing and undressing, personal hygiene, development of feeding skills, and toileting. The directions specify that it should be administered by an individual familiar with the child. The teacher or therapist should spend a substantial period of time (at least 2 weeks is suggested) working directly with the child before attempting to use the checklist. It is also suggested that aides, parents, and others be consulted about their observations of the child to obtain the most accurate picture.

SPECIALIZED ASSESSMENTS

Psychological testing of the child with multiple sensory handicaps is challenging and must be done on an individual basis with subjective observation, rather than by standardized testing. This is also true of visual and auditory assessment, although the new technology of the evoked response testing shows much promise with these children.

Objectives of intervention and treatment modalities

Although the goals of treatment will depend on the individual assessment of the child and identified levels of functioning, some typical treatment goals follow.

1. *To minimize tactile defensiveness.* Since very little can be done with these children until they are able to accept touch, this is usually a basic goal. The child should be gradually introduced to a large variety of tactile stimulation activities and encouraged to reach out and explore independently.

2. *To provide early parental intervention.* If possible, the child and mother should be involved in an intervention program from the moment of diagnosis.[49] The cycle of diminished or negative responses from the child leading to decreased stimuli from the mother must be stopped as soon as possible. The child needs to be out of the crib and placed in the room where activity is taking place and given much gentle but firm stimulation.

3. *To maximize movement.* The child at first needs to be moved and later encouraged to move. Practice time should be allowed and new items introduced gradually. Activities with tilt boards, swings, and bolsters are useful but most important will be movement with another person such as walking (holding on) or rocking with a person. The child will need much help letting go of the supportive surface.[66] Moersch[48] detailed a treatment program that strongly emphasizes the use of meaningful activity, play, and movement in the treatment of the deaf-blind child.

4. *To improve self-maintenance skills.* As much independence as possible for the individual child should be stressed. Feeding is often a problem. Learning to accept textured foods and chewing will usually require intervention. Physically moving the child through the movements of chewing and cup placement is often needed. Toileting can be a problem, with resistance to the potty chair and difficulty in understanding what is required. Although ignoring works with many children as good behavior conditioning, deaf-blind children are often quite happy to be left alone, so this technique has little effect.

5. *To develop cause-and-effect relationships.* The child needs to learn to make things happen outside herself. Play activities such as jack-in-the-box or busy box are useful.

6. *To develop productive behaviors.* Not only must the perseverative, nonproductive behaviors be stopped, but more productive behaviors must be substituted. Otherwise, equally undesirable behaviors will be established. The child will need consistency and continuity. If tactile signs are used, they should be simple initially and consistent from one person to the next. The development of interpersonal and play skills is crucial.

SPECIAL TECHNIQUES

Many of the specialized techniques used with these children deal with the development of some form of communication. *Clueing* is a system that was developed primarily by the mother of a rubella child in England.[23] It is a signal-type of language (one-way communication) between the mother and child. In this technique the daily activities of the child must be analyzed for clues or signals that can be picked up by the child. These signals tell the child what is happening or about to happen and form the beginning of communication. For example, the mother might rub the child's arms with a warm wet cloth before putting him into the bath.

TADOMA is a method of teaching speech and speech reading by placing the child's hand on the speaker's face and throat and thereby having the child pick up the vibrations that are made by sound. Children usually place the thumb on the speaker's lips and spread the fingers over cheek and neck.

Coactive movement is a system developed by Dr. J. Van Dijk in Holland.[71] He began the system with what he called the "resonance phenomenon": the therapist goes with the child's action, rocking or crawling, or whatever it is. This is to develop a rapport at the child's level. In the next stage of coactive movements, the therapist moves with the child in a prearranged sequence. This leads to nonrepresentational reference with such activities as identifying body parts on self and others, and then to imitation. *Imitation* uses body movements or positions and leads to natural gesture, a system that describes the object according to what is done with it; for example, a toothbrush would be identified by making toothbrushing movements with the hand. This system is developed for very low functioning children and is based on the premise that the rubella child will not naturally explore and that the world outside herself does not exist.

There are other more sophisticated communication techniques that are often used by people who developed the double handicap later in life, such as the blind child who has lost her hearing, the meningitis child with the double handicap, or the deaf adolescent with Usher's syndrome. These are methods such as the following.

1. Printing in the palm. The block letters of the alphabet are traced in the palm of the person's hand.
2. Alphabet glove. A thin glove with the letters of the alphabet placed on different parts of the hand is worn by the deaf-blind person; the interpretor simply spells out the words.
3. Tellatouch machine. The interpreter uses a machine with a standard typewriter keyboard on one side and a space for the deaf-blind person's index finger on the other side. As the keys are hit on the typewriter, the letters pop up in braille under the index finger of the deaf-blind person.

Other techniques that can be very helpful in the treatment of this population are task analysis and behavior modification. *Task analysis* is used to teach activity of daily living and vocational skills. The total task, such as buttering a piece of bread, is broken down into its smallest components, and then backward or forward chaining of steps is used. In forward chaining the object is to teach the first step until it is mastered, then the second, and so on. In backward chaining the last step is taught until mastered, then the next to last, and so on. It is important to fade out assistance, but still give as much as needed. Each time a repeated error is corrected, enough information to correct the error should be provided but not as much as before.[27]

Behavior modification is a systematic approach to alter the child's behavior through environmental programming. Reinforcement is often used, and detailed records of the child's responses are kept. Often a positive trait needs to be reinforced, such as urinating when placed on the potty, or a negative trait such as eye poking needs to be extinguished. These behaviors are charted, and positive reinforcement is given for the desired behavior.

PREPARATION FOR ADULTHOOD

The multiply handicapped child is usually prepared for sheltered employment rather than for independent living. Approximately 75% of the rubella children will need sheltered living and employment.[65] There are four levels of independence to consider:

1. Custodial care–sheltered living: Not capable of taking care of own needs, although may have some self-help skills and may participate in recreation programs.
2. Sheltered employment–sheltered living: Capable of working with close supervision and living in group home situation with supervision and assistance in some tasks.
3. Sheltered employment–semisheltered living: Capable of working in sheltered workshop and living with some support services available.
4. Self sufficient: Employed and competent in daily living skills.

Some of the behaviors that the adolescent will have to develop for more self-sufficient living are (1) communication of at least basic emergency/survival words such as stop, eat, more, no, and finish; (2) social skills; (3) self-care skills; (4) telling time; (5) cooking and shopping skills; (6) home management; (7) travel and mobility; and (8) housekeeping. Workshop activities are manipulative for the most part and can include folding, stamping, collating, counting, gluing, bending, sorting, assembling, wrapping, stuffing, filing, measuring, stapling, and clipping.

If the child has remained at home with the family unit through school, adolescence is often the time when a move must be made to a residential facility. Both the family members and the child must be prepared for this.[69] Also, the emerging sexuality of the child has to be dealt with at the level of the child's understanding. For resources for additional study and information on multiple sensory impairment, see the reference section of this chapter.

CASE STUDY 3

Mary is 17 years, 3 months old. She had congenital rubella syndrome with cataracts, with resultant severe hearing loss and markedly delayed development. Mary is presently in a state residential facility for the blind that has a deaf-blind treatment unit. She is gradually being transferred from the school program into the sheltered workshop program. She has been at the state facility since the age of 10 when her parents could no longer maintain her at home because of self-abusive behaviors and the need for constant supervision. Since her placement, she has been placed on a behavior modification program that has markedly reduced her self-abusive behaviors. She was assessed with the Gesell scale and a self-help skills checklist used by the school. She has difficulty with cup placement in eating, with fasteners in dressing, and with rigidity in walking. She understands and uses some tactile sign language and is functioning overall on a level of about a 3- to 4-year-old.

Treatment goals

1. *To increase coordination and manipulative skills for workshop experience.* Include activities such as sorting nails by size and shape, folding letters, and stamping envelopes.

2. *To improve eating skills.* Reinforce techniques to locate tabletop and to place cup upright with gradually fading physical assistance.

3. *To improve dressing skills.* Practice fasteners on self, practice boards, and dolls.

4. *To decrease rigidity in walking.* Movement through space activities such as trampoline, swimming, tilt board, and scooter board.

SUMMARY

This chapter has provided an overview of occupational therapy intervention with the child with visual or hearing impairment. Degrees of impairment have been investigated, as well as typical causes of impairment. Eye and ear anatomy has been reviewed to give information on the dynamics of a sensory loss. Emphasis in occupational therapy assessment has been placed on the interruption in the developmental process caused by the loss of one or both of these distance senses. General treatment goals have been given, stressing provision of activities and experiences to allow the child to develop adaptive behaviors and to develop to her fullest potential. Brief explanations have been given regarding specialized techniques used with these children, including the use of hearing aids, sign language, braille, and low vision aids. It is my hope that the profession of occupational therapy will become increasingly involved with these children because of its emphases on adaptation, activity analysis, and developmental sequence.

REFERENCES

1. Adelson, E., and Fraiberg, S.: Gross motor development in infants blind from birth, Child Dev. **45:**114, 1974.
2. American Foundation for the Blind: Aids and appliances for the blind and visually impaired, New York, 1970.
3. Anastasi, A.: Psychological testing, London, 1969, Macmillan Co.
4. Ayres, A.J.: The influence of the vestibular system on the auditory and sensory systems, new techniques for working with deaf blind children, Denver, 1973, Mountain Plains Regional Center.
5. Ayres, A.J.: Sensory integration and learning disorders, Los Angeles, 1973, Western Psychological Services.
6. Barraga, N.: Impaired visual behavior in low vision children, New York, 1964, American Foundation for the Blind.
7. Basic pre-school signed English, Washington, D.C., 1973, Gallaudet College Press.
8. Bernero, R.J., and Bothwell, H.: Relationship of hearing impairment to educational needs, Springfield, Ill., 1966, Illinois Department of Public Health and Office of the Superintendent of Public Instruction.
9. Buros, O.K.: The sixth mental measurement yearbook, Newark, N.J., 1965, Gryphon Press.
10. Chess, S.: Behavioral study of children with congenital rubella, New York, 1967, New York University Rubella Project.
11. Cohen, J.: The effects of blindness on children's development, New Outlook Blind **60:**150, 1966.
12. Cooper, L.Z.: Rubella: clinical manifestations and management, Am. J. Dis. Child. **18:**142, 1969.
13. Cooper, L.Z.: Congenital rubella in the United States in infections of the fetus and newborn infant, New York, 1975, A.A. Gershon.
14. Cratty, B.J.: Movement and spatial awareness in blind youth, Springfield, Ill., 1971, Charles C Thomas, Publisher.
15. Davis, H., and Silverman, S.R.: Hearing and deafness, New York, 1970, Holt, Rinehart and Winston.
16. Davison, W.C., and Davison, J.D.: The compleat pediatrician, Durham, N.C., 1961, Duke University Press.
17. deQuiros, J.: Neuropsychological fundamentals in learning disorders, San Rafael, Calif. 1976, Academic Therapy Publications.
18. Fant, L.J.: Ameslan—an introduction to American sign language, Silver Springs, Md., 1971, National Association for the Deaf.
19. Fish, A.G.: Perkins Institute and its deaf-blind pupils, Watertown, N.Y., 1934, Perkins School for the Blind.
20. Flavell, J.H.: The developmental psychology of Jean Piaget, New York, 1963, D. Van Nostrand Co.
21. Fonda, G.: Management of the patient with subnormal vision, St. Louis, 1970, The C.V. Mosby Co.
22. Fraiberg, S.: Parallel and divergent patterns in blind and sighted infants, Psychoanal. Study Child **23:**264, 1968.
23. Freeman, P.: Parent's guide to early care of a deaf-blind child, London, 1966, National Association for Deaf-Blind and Rubella Children.
24. Furth, H.G.: Deafness and learning: a psychological approach, Belmont, Calif., 1973, Wadsworth Publishing Co., Inc.
25. Furth, H.G.: Thinking without language: psychological implications of deafness, New York, 1966, The Free Press.
26. Gesell, A., Ilg, F.L., and Bullis, G.E.: Vision: its development in infant and child, New York, 1967, Hafner Publishing, Inc.
27. Gold, M.: Try another way, Washington, D.C., 1977, National Childrens Center.
28. Gregory, R.L.: Eye and brain—the psychology of seeing, New York, 1972, McGraw-Hill Book Co.
29. Grinnel, M.F., Dentamore, K.L., and Lippke, B.A.: Sign it successful—manual English encourages expressive communication, Teach. Except. Child. Spring, p. 123, 1976.
30. Gunn, S.L.: Play as occupation—implications for the handicapped, Am. J. Occup. Ther. **25:**285, 1971.
31. Gustafson, G., Pfetzing, D., and Zawalkow, E.: Signing exact English, Silver Springs, Md., 1975, Modern Sign Press.
32. Halliday, C.: The visually impaired child: growth, learning, development—infancy to school age, Louisville, Ky., 1970, American Printing House for the Blind.
33. Haupt, C.: Improving blind children's perceptions, New Outlook Blind **58:**172, 1964.
34. Hearing aids for children, Lansing, Mich., 1966, Michigan Department of Public Health.
34a. Hendrickson: In Orem, R.C.: Montessori and the special child, New York, 1969, G.P. Putnam's Sons.
35. Hill, L.: Working with blind pre-schoolers, Am. J. Occup. Ther. **31:**417, 1977.
36. Illinois Society for the Prevention of Blindness: Definition of words relating to vision, Springfield, Ill., 1964.
37. Jastrzembska, Z.S.: The effects of blindness and other impairments on early development, New York, 1976, American Foundation for the Blind.
38. Kempe, C.H., Silver, H.K., and O'Brien, D.: Pediatric diagnosis and treatment, Los Altos, Calif., 1976, Lange Medical Publications.
39. Kinsey, E.: Retrolental fibroplasia—cooperative study of the use of oxygen and RLF, Arch. Ophthalmol. **56:**481, 1956.
40. Klima, E.S., and Bellugi, U.: The signs of language, Cambridge, Mass., 1978, Harvard University Press.
41. Kohl, H.R.: Language and education of the deaf, New York, 1966, Center for Urban Education.
42. Leenenberg, E.H.: Biological foundation of language, New York, 1967, John Wiley & Sons, Inc.
43. Lowenfeld, B.: Our blind children, Springfield, Ill., 1969, Charles C Thomas, Publisher.

44. Lydon, W.T., and McGraw, L.M.: Concept development for the visually handicapped child, New York, 1973, American Foundation for the Blind.

45. Maxfield, K.E., and Buchholz, S.: A Social Maturity Scale for Blind Pre-school Children, New York, 1957, American Foundation for the Blind.

46. Michelman, S.: The importance of creative play, Am. J. Occup. Ther. **25:**285, 1971.

47. Mindel, E.D., and Vernon, M.: They grow in silence—the deaf child and his family, Silver Springs, Md., 1971, National Association for the Deaf.

48. Moersch, M.: Training the deaf-blind child, Am. J. Occup. Ther. **31:**425, 1977.

49. Moucka, S.: The deaf-blind infant in the family, parent counseling and infant stimulation, Denver, 1973, Mountain Plains Regional Center.

50. Myklebust, H.R.: Auditory disorders in children, New York, 1954, Grune & Stratton, Inc.

51. Myklebust, H.R.: The psychology of deafness: sensory deprivation, learning, and adjustment, New York, 1964, Grune & Stratton, Inc.

52. Newby, H.: Audiology, New York, 1972, Appleton-Century-Crofts.

53. Reference deleted in proofs.

54. Perera, C.A.: May's disease of the eye, Baltimore, 1957, The Williams & Wilkins Co.

55. Pollack, D.: Educational audiology for the limited hearing infant, Springfield, Ill., 1970, Charles C Thomas, Publisher.

56. Preschool learning activities for the visually impaired, Springfield, Ill., 1972, Illinois Office of Education.

57. Robbins, N., and Stenquist, G.: The deaf-blind rubella child, Watertown, N.Y., 1967, Perkins School for the Blind.

58. Robbins, N.: Educational beginnings with deaf-blind children, Watertown, N.Y., 1960, Perkins School for the Blind.

59. Rugers, C.T.: Understanding braille, New York, 1969, American Foundation for the Blind.

60. Sapir, R.: Culture, language and personalilty, Los Angeles, 1966, University of California Press.

61. Schein, J.D., and Delk, M.T.: The deaf population of the United States, Silver Springs, Md., 1975, National Association for the Deaf.

62. Schlesinger, H.S., and Meadow, K.P.: Sound and sign: childhood deafness and mental health, Berkeley, Calif., 1972, University of California Press.

63. School, G., and Schaun, R.: Measurement of psychological, vocational, and educational functioning in the blind and visually handicapped, New York, 1976, American Foundation for the Blind.

64. Sheridan, M.D.: Manual for the STYCAR Vision Tests (Screening Tests for Young Children and Retardates), Berks, England, 1969, NFER Publishing Company, Ltd.

65. Smith, B.: Potentials of rubella deaf-blind children, 1980 is now: a conference on the future of deaf-blind children, Sacramento, Calif., 1974, John Tracy Clinic and Southwestern Regional Center.

66. Smith, D.W.: Recognizable patterns of human malformation, Philadelphia, 1970, W.B. Saunders Co.

67. Stillman, R.D.: The Callier-Asuza Scale, Dallas, 1973, Callier Speech and Hearing Center.

68. Thurnell, R.J., and Rice, D.G.: Eye rubbing in blind children: application of a sensory deprivation model, Except. Child. **36:**325, 1970.

69. Tretaloff, M.: Counseling parents of handicapped children, Ment. Retard. **7:**231, 1969.

70. Van Benschoter, R.: A sensory integration program for blind campers, Am. J. Occup. Ther. **29:**617, 1975.

71. Van Dijk, J.: The non-verbal deaf-blind child and his world: his outgrowth towards the world of symbols, St. Michielsgestel, Holland, 1965, Instituut Voor Doven.

72. Van Riper, C.: Teaching your child to talk, New York, 1950, Harper & Row, Publishers.

73. Wolff, P.: Developmental studies of blind children, New Outlook Blind **60:**179, 1966.

RESOURCES FOR ADDITIONAL STUDY AND INFORMATION ON HEARING IMPAIRMENT

Alexander Graham Bell Association for the Deaf, 3417 Volta Place, N.W., Washington, D.C. 20007. (Publishes *The Volta Review.*)

American Speech and Hearing Association, 19801 Rockville Pike, Rockville, Md. 20852. (Information on deafness, audiology, and speech therapy.)

California State University, Northridge, National Center on Deafness, 18111 Nordhoff, Northridge, Calif. 91324.

Conference of American Instructors of the Deaf, 5034 Wisconsin Ave, N.W., Washington, D.C. 20016. (Publishes *American Annals of the Deaf.*)

Deafness Research and Training Center, New York University, 80 Washington Square East, New York, N.Y. 10003.

Gallaudet College, 7th and Florida Ave, N.E., Washington, D.C. 20910.

John Tracy Clinic, 806 West Adams Blvd., Los Angeles, Calif. 90007. (Correspondence course for parents of deaf preschoolers. Information on oral approach.)

National Association for the Deaf, 814 Thayer Ave., Silver Springs, Md. 20910. (Publishes *The Deaf American*, clearing house of information.)

National Captioning Institute, P.O. Box 57064, Washington, D.C. 20037. (Information on tv and film captioning.)

National Hearing Aid Society, 24261 Grand River, Detroit Mich. 48219. (Information on hearing aids and dealers.)

National Technical Institute for the Deaf, 1 Lomb Memorial Dr., Rochester, N.Y. 14623.

Professional Rehabilitation Workers of the Deaf, 814 Thayer Ave., Silver Springs, Md. 20910. (Publishes *Journal of Rehabilitation of the Deaf.*)

RESOURCES FOR ADDITIONAL STUDY AND INFORMATION ON VISUAL IMPAIRMENT

American Academy of Ophthalmology and Otolaryngology, 15 Second St. S.W., Rochester, Minn. 55901. (Information on low vision aids and ophthalmology.)

American Academy of Optometry, 1506-1508 Forshey Towers, Minneapolis, Minn. 55402. (Information on low vision aids and optometry.)

American Association for the Blind, 15 West 65th St., New York, N.Y. 10011. (Publishes *Journal of Visual Impairment and Blindness.*)

American Foundation for the Blind, 15 West 16th St., New York, N.Y. 10011. (Disseminates information, research, films, publications. Publishes *New Outlook for the Blind.*)

American Printing House for the Blind, 1839 Frankfort Ave., Louisville, Ky. 40206. (Publications, talking books, large print and braille publications.)

Association for the Education of Visually Handicapped, 919 Walnut St., 4th Floor, Philadelphia, Pa. 19107. (Publishes *Education of the Visually Handicapped.*)

Division for the Blind and Physically Handicapped, Library of Congress, 1291 Taylor St. N.W., Washington, D.C. 20542. (Regional libraries of large print, braille, and talking books.)

Howe Press, Perkins School for the Blind, Watertown, Mass. 02172. (Games, writing, and educational aids publications.)

National Association of the Visually Handicapped, 305 East 24th St., New York, N.Y. 10010. (Large print publications and information.)

National Society for the Prevention of Blindness, Inc., 79 Madison Ave., New York, N.Y. 10016. (Studies the causes of blindness, clearing house of information.)

Recording for Blind, Inc., 215 East 58th St., New York, N.Y. 10022. (Taped and recorded educational material.)

RESOURCES FOR ADDITIONAL STUDY AND INFORMATION ON MULTIPLE SENSORY IMPAIRMENT (DEAF-BLIND)

Centers and Services for Deaf-Blind, Special Services Branch, Bureau of Education for the Handicapped, U.S. Office of Education, Donohue Bldg. Rm. 4046, 400 Maryland Ave. S.W., Washington, D.C. 20202. (List of regional centers and state educational agencies working with the deaf-blind.)

Helen Keller National Center for Deaf-Blind Youths and Adults, 111 Middle Neck Rd., Sands Point, N.Y. 11051. (Information on the deaf-blind, especially vocational training.)

John Tracy Clinic, 806 West Adams Blvd., Los Angeles, Calif. 90007. (Correspondence learning program for parents of preschool deaf-blind children.)

23

DIANA P. BURNELL

Children with severe emotional or behavioral disorders

Well over 1 million American children demonstrate severe emotional or behavioral disorders. Such conditions may be unique to childhood and adolescence, such as conduct disorder, attention deficit disorder, or identity disorder. On the other hand, the condition may be a major illness that may occur at any time during a lifetime, such as schizophrenia, depression, and substance abuse. However, the symptoms may vary according to the age of the individual. The schizophrenic child may appear withdrawn and unable to relate to others but does not have the hallucinations and delusions seen in the adult with this diagnosis. Temper tantrums and hyperactivity may mask depression in children. Similarly, delinquency and underachievement may mask depression in adolescents.

CAUSES OF EMOTIONAL DISORDERS

The cause-and-effect relationship is not simple in human behavior. In general, emotional disorders may have primary, predisposing, precipitating, and reinforcing causes. A primary cause may be a neurological deficit. A predisposing cause could be a failure to learn adaptive behaviors. A precipitating cause, such as a stressful situation in the home, may trigger a maladaptive behavior. A reinforcing cause may be the circumstances that help to continue a pattern of maladaptive behavior.

Most theorists agree about two major factors that contribute to emotional disorders in children and adolescents: (1) inadequate family patterns and (2) disturbed family patterns. Inadequate family patterns lay the foundation for early deprivation. Limited tactile stimulation, overprotection, restricted movement, faulty discipline, poor communication, and aversive stimulation, such as loud noises and an overcrowded environment, produce stress in the child. The disturbed family, with its pattern of quarreling and emotional conflicts, rejection, and physical abuse, provides poor personality models for the child. Emotional difficulties are soon apparent in children from these families.[15]

Despite the agreement about the importance of environmental stress as a cause of emotional disorders, there are five divergent viewpoints about the cause of emotional disorders. Each approach focuses on particular characteristics related to the overall problem: (1) biophysical, (2) behavioral, (3) phenomenological, (4) psychoanalytic, and (5) sociocultural. The biophysical view emphasizes the various organic conditions that can impair mental function. The behaviorists discuss the lack of learning adaptive behaviors and the learning of maladaptive behaviors. The phenomenological theories trace the course of emotional disorders to a person's perception of, and reaction to, environmental stress. The psychoanalytic approach identifies the conflict between the id, ego, and superego of the individual and the demands of the environment. And finally, the sociocultural view sees the person as simply responding to a pathological social condition. Each of these five theoretical views influences models for describing, assessing, and treating emotional disorders.[36]

CLASSIFICATION OF EMOTIONAL AND BEHAVIORAL DISORDERS

There are two compatible resources that may be used to recognize and describe emotional and behavioral disorders arising in infancy, childhood, and adolescence: the *International Classification of Diseases*, ed. 9, published in 1977 by the World Health Organization (ICD-9),[54,55] and the *Diagnostic and Statistical Manual of Mental Disorders*, ed. 3, published by the American Psychiatric Association in 1980 (DSM-III).[53]

The ICD-9 is a statistical classification of all diseases, injuries, and causes of death. It was designed for use in gathering worldwide data and for indexing and retrieval of medical records. After the ICD-9 was published, psychiatrists in the United States complained that the classification system was not specific. Therefore a revised version was developed, the ICD-9-CM. This classification system includes all mental disorders found in the DSM-III, as well as many other codes and terms; however, the DSM-III is generally employed as the resource for coding diagnosis in most mental health facilities.

The DSM-III uses a multiaxial organization and description of mental disorders. This means that each individual is assessed through different categories of information called axes. There are five axes in the DSM-III assessment classification. Axes I and II include all classifications of mental disorders. Mental disorders are generally thought to be patterns or syndromes associated with behavioral, psychological, or biological dysfunction. A clear boundry between the various syndromes is not believed to exist. It is important to understand that the term *mental disorder* in the DSM-III is used to classify behavior patterns observed in the individual, not the person himself.

Axis I: Applies to clinical syndromes or focus of treatment

Axis II: Records personality or developmental disorders

Axis III: Provides the clinician with a category to define any physical disorders that may accompany the mental disorder

Axis IV: Describes the severity of psychosocial stressors that may have caused the mental disorder

Axis V: Codes the highest level of adaptive functioning manifested during the past year

The last two axes are especially important for occupational therapists. It is in these areas that the therapist's expertise may be best used by the treatment team.

The following two examples are provided to illustrate how this classification system is used with emotional disorders in children and adolescents.

A child of 5 who has been accepted into a program for autistic children might have the following DSM-III diagnoses and their respective codes:

Axis I: 313.89 Reactive attachment; 299.00 Disorder of infancy with autistic features

Axis II: 315.90 Atypical specific developmental disorder

Axis III: Rule out neurological dysfunction

Axis IV: 4-5 Moderate to severe psychosocial stressors

Axis V: 4-5 Fair to poor adaptive development

An adolescent admitted to an acute psychiatric hospital might have the following DSM-III diagnoses:

Axis I: 309.00 Separation anxiety disorder with mixed emotional features; 305.30 Substance abuse, hallucinogens; drug-induced psychosis

AxisII: Deferred

Axis III: Mild physical symptoms

Axis IV: Fair psychosocial stressors

Sometimes the psychiatrist will code one syndrome, or several, on an axis; while at other times the coding will be deferred until further information is available on the patient. It is not unusual to find in a long case history one or two additional DSM-III diagnoses that reflect either an update of the condition of the patient or a difference of opinion between clinicians. Occupational therapists should regard the most recent diagnosis for planning treatment.

A simple method of remembering the different classes of emotional disorders of childhood and adolescence used on Axes I and II is by separating them into five groups according to the predominant symptom of the condition:

1. Intellectual
   a. Mental retardation
2. Behavioral
   a. Attention deficit disorder
   b. Conduct disorder
3. Emotional
   a. Anxiety disorders of childhood or adolescence
   b. Other disorders of infancy, childhood, or adolescence
4. Physical
   a Eating disorders
   b. Stereotyped movement disorders
   c. Other disorders with physical manifestations
5. Developmental
   a. Pervasive developmental disorders
   b. Specific developmental disorders

This outline will be useful to the occupational therapist when planning treatment goals and selecting treatment modalities. However, it is oversimplified and impractical for understanding the diagnostic information in the case records. For this purpose, one must have the following numerical coding and subcategories available to review.*

Mental retardation (subaverage general intellectual functioning, impaired adaptive behavior, onset before 18 years) The symbol (x) reserves space for identification of other behavioral symptoms that require treatment: 1 = With symptoms; 2 = Without symptoms.

317.0(x) Mild mental retardation, IQ is 50 to 70
318.0(x) Moderate mental retardation, IQ is 35 to 49
318.1(x) Severe mental retardation, IQ is 20 to 34
318.2(x) Profound mental retardation, IQ is 0 to 19
319.0(x) Unspecified mental retardation, child is untestable

Attention deficit disorder (inappropriate impulsivity and inattention)

314.00 Without hyperactivity
314.01 With hyperactivity
314.80 Residual type

Conduct disorder (persistent and repetitious pattern of violating social conventions or the rights of others, corresponds to antisocial personality disorder in the adult)

312.00 Undersocialized, aggressive
312.10 Undersocialized, nonaggressive
312.23 Socialized, aggressive
312.21 Socialized, nonaggressive
312.90 Atypical

Anxiety disorders of childhood or adolescence (unrealistic worry, physical symptoms, social withdrawal)

309.21 Separation anxiety disorder
313.00 Overanxious disorder
313.21 Avoidant disorder of childhood or adolescence, corresponds to avoidant personality disorder in the adult

Other disorders of infancy, childhood, or adolescence

313.22 Schizoid disorder of childhood or adolescence (inability to form social relationships, no interest in activities, corresponds to schizoid personality disorder in the adult)
313.23 Elective mutism (refusal to speak in most situations, may communicate by gestures or monosyllabic utterances)
313.81 Oppositional disorder (disobedient, negativistic, and provocative to authorities, corresponds to passive-aggressive personality disorder in the adult)
313.82 Identity disorder (distress resulting from the inability to form an acceptable sense of self, corresponds to borderline personality disorder in the adult)
313.89 Reactive attachment disorder of infancy (failure to thrive before 8 months, apathetic mood, excessive sleep, lack of interest in environment)

Eating disorders (gross disturbances in eating behavior)

307.10 Anorexia nervosa (fear of becoming obese, disturbance of body image and weight loss)
307.50 Atypical eating disorder
307.51 Bulimia (episodical binge-eating terminated by induced vomiting, sleep, or abdominal pain)
307.52 Pica (persistent eating of nonnutritive substances)
307.53 Rumination disorder of infancy (repeated regurgitation of food without nausea)

Stereotyped movement disorders (abnormal gross motor movements)

307.20 Atypical tic disorder
307.21 Transient tic disorder (recurrent, involuntary, purposeless, rapid movements)
307.22 Chronic motor tic disorder (same as above, lasting over 1 year)
307.23 Tourette's disease (same as above, with vocal tics)
307.30 Atypical stereotyped movement disorder

Other disorders with physical manifestations

307.00 Stuttering (frequent repetition or prolongation of sounds, syllables, or words that disrupt the rhythmic flow of speech)
307.46 Sleepwalking disorder (repeated episodes of arising from bed and walking for several minutes while sleeping)
307.60 Functional enuresis (involuntary voiding of urine)
307.70 Functional encopresis (involuntary, inappropriate passage of feces)

Pervasive developmental disorders (a distortion, not a delay, in adaptive functioning) The symbol (x) is reserved for state of condition: O = Full syndrome; l = Residual state.

299.0(x) Infantile autism (lack of responsiveness to others, gross impairment in communication skills, bizarre responses, onset before 30 months)
299.8(x) Atypical in communication skills, bizarre responses, onset before 30 months
299.8(x) Atypical
299.9(x) Childhood onset pervasive developmental disorder (oddities of behavior, disturbance in social relationships after 30 months)

Specific developmental disorders (coded on Axis II)

315.00 Developmental reading disorder (dyslexia)
315.10 Developmental arithmetic disorder
315.31 Developmental language disorder
315.39 Developmental articulation disorder
315.50 Mixed specific developmental disorder
315.90 Atypical specific developmental disorder

---

*From Williams, J.B.W., editor: Diagnostic and statistical manual of mental disorders, ed. 3, Washington, D.C., 1980, The American Psychiatric Association.

GENERAL PSYCHOLOGICAL MODELS FOR TREATMENT
Five treatment approaches

In the first part of this chapter the five general theoretical approaches[36] that guide the manner in which the clinician views emotional disorders were introduced. These models are now expanded to demonstrate how they may guide the treatment environment in which the occupational therapist functions.

Why do occupational therapists have to learn general theories of psychological treatment when they have their own professional theories? It is necessary for several reasons. First, the occupational therapist's practice is primarily within mental health facilities where one general psychological frame of reference (or a combination of) will guide the admittance, treatment, and discharge of the patients. Second, the occupational therapist needs to be able to understand and communicate in a common language with the treatment team: psychiatrist, nursing staff, social worker, psychologist, and others. Third, the therapist must be able to read the case histories and understand the emotional disorder within the context of the particular theory so that he or she may contribute appropriate therapeutic activities. Fourth, the therapist must be able to adjust or adapt the occupational therapy models that guide the systematic application of activity for treatment to each specific treatment environment, as well as to each specific patient. The occupational therapist cannot expect the treatment team to learn the professional language of occupational therapy before the therapist learns the language of the facility in which he or she has found a job. When the therapist is working in a behavioral treatment environment with autistic children, he or she must be able to discuss positive reinforcement. If the therapist works in a psychiatric hospital in which the psychoanalytic model predominates, than he or she must define the goals as strengthening ego functions. These are examples of two completely different psychological languages. It is expected that an occupational therapist, like other mental health professionals, should be able to understand and communicate in the language of the five major models.

BIOPHYSICAL TREATMENT APPROACH

In the biophysical treatment approach most psychiatrists, believing that abnormal behavior has a biochemical or anatomical cause, use methods that directly affect the physiology of the person. Tranquilizers, antidepressants, sedatives, stimulants, and anticonvulsants are some of the psychopharmacological techniques used by most psychiatrists to treat abnormal or maladaptive behavior. This approach is usually used in conjunction with other theoretical approaches in psychiatric hospitals.

The literature shows several occupational therapy programs that fit into this approach. King[29] used sensory integration methods to stimulate and improve neurological symptoms in chronic schizophrenics. Ayres and Heskett[2] applied their sensory integration theories successfully with autistic children.

BEHAVIORAL TREATMENT APPROACH

Clinicians who practice the behavioral treatment approach agree that objective, observable actions and events are the target of their therapeutic intervention. Treatment is systematically applied. Based on experimentally derived principles, it attempts to modify maladaptive and asocial behavior usually seen as preventing the client from living a satisfying life. Therapists view abnormal behavior as learned, and they proceed to teach the individual to unlearn old patterns and to learn new, more adaptive ones.

Occupational therapists often work in the behavioral treatment approach with children and adolescents and the mentally retarded. The successful treatment of patients by using this approach is well documented. Occupational therapists have predominantly used behavioral observation scales to gather data about patients within various treatment environments. A complete list of performance and occupational areas that can be observed may be found in Reed and Sanderson.[44] The Mosey model[40] fits into this approach fairly well. Mosey also provided some specific examples of observational scales that are useful in psychiatry.

PHENOMENOLOGICAL TREATMENT APPROACH

The phenomenological treatment approach is used by therapists who employ a variety of different techniques. Two factors link their therapy methods: all believe that the internal processes influence behavior, and they attempt to treat the individual through his or her conscious perceptions and attitudes. Self-actualization, cognitive learning, and reality integration are phenomenological concepts.

Occupational therapy has moved in the direction of this model since Watanabe[51,52] presented her ideas on psychiatric occupational therapy in the home. Life tasks in the home are evaluated by the occupational therapist. Present habitual patterns of adaptive functioning are compared to past performance. The patient and occupational therapist plan treatment goals together to improve mastery of the environment and responsibility for decisions and actions. As in all techniques using this approach, the therapist must understand the strengths and weaknesses of the patient's ego to guide the treatment process.

PSYCHOANALYTIC TREATMENT APPROACH

The psychoanalytic treatment approach is based on Freudian theory. The psychiatrist attempts to help the client be more aware of unconscious conflicts and drives. The focus is on the relationship between early developmental experiences and the client's present functioning. Therapy is used to reconstruct the client's personality rather than remove a symptom. Techniques used are classical psychoanalysis, ego analysis, character analysis, interpersonal analysis, transactional analysis, and other adjunctive procedures such as hypnotherapy, art therapy, and play therapy.

This psychoanalytic approach influenced much of the practice of occupational therapy in psychiatry, especially during the years when mental patients were hospitalized for long periods of time. Fidler and Fidler's model[20] of psychiatric occupational therapy is appropriate for this model. In occupational therapy, therapists have used the Draw-A-Person Test and the Buck House-Tree-Person Test assessments for many years to determine the underlying dynamics of a patient's emotional disorders. Art therapy and other creative techniques have been used as therapeutic activities to work out the emotional conflicts felt by the patients.

SOCIOCULTURAL TREATMENT APPROACH

The sociocultural treatment approach tries to improve mental disorders by changing the individual's life situation. Many methods are used in this approach: changing parental behavior; foster home care; special school programs; hospitalization (crisis intervention, short-term care, long-term care); correctional institutions; and community mental health programs.

Most occupational therapy models have traditionally considered the effects of the sociocultural environment on the behavior of the patient. Therapeutic activities are designed in all practice settings to reflect the patient's environmental and interpersonal needs. Group activities within the institution take advantage of the current life situation to promote improved emotional and behavioral symptoms.

Assessment procedures reflecting the five treatment approaches

The occupational therapist working with children who have psychological problems should know how to interpret information gathered on various psychological instruments (Chapters 9-11). There are three purposes of assessments in therapy: (1) to reflect a theory, (2) to describe a person, and (3) to design a treatment plan. Those assessments that reflect a specific theory are generally used as screening tools for the selection of individuals who would benefit from the particular treatment program. Those tools that are used to evaluate the attributes of an individual are used for the purpose of establishing the baseline performance level when entering the program and measuring change after treatment. The treatment plan is designed to analyze activity stages so that the process of therapy can progress. According to Sundberg,[49] there are five categories of assessments, and all should be used for a comprehensive clinical analysis.

BIOPHYSICAL TECHNIQUES

Biophysical techniques fall into four categories: genetic, anatomical, physiochemical, and neurophysiological. Usually most patients are given a physical examination that includes analysis of blood, urine, and x-ray films. Other assessments can be made by use of the polygraph, the electrocardiograph, and the electroencephalograph, as well as paper-and-pencil tests such as the Wechsler Memory Scale, the Bender Visual-Motor Gestalt Test, and the Halstead-Reitan Neuropsychological Test Battery. If appropriate, the physician or treatment team may request the Ayres' Southern California Sensory Integration Tests.

BEHAVIORAL TECHNIQUES

Behavioral techniques are used by many professionals to objectively structure the observation of children and adolescents with emotional disorders. The purpose is to determine the antecedents and consequences of behavior. Usually information is obtained by observing behavior in either natural or contrived situations, (such as interviews), and then determining the plan for intervention. Because behavioral assessment is individualized for specific treatment of symptoms, there are very few standard devices. There is, however, a standard procedure in designing these scales. The therapist should define the target behavior to be examined, develop a measuring device, decide when and where to gather data, and address the reliability of the rater.

OBJECTIVE TECHNIQUES

Objective techniques characterize the phenomenological approach and are used to develop a self-presentation of the individual. There are two types of tests: those that reveal interest and values, and those that are designed to reveal maladjustment. The tools consist of interviews, paper-and-pencil inventories and scales, self-ratings, intelligence tests, and other measurements of behavioral and physiological performance. Responses to these tests are believed to correlate with personal characteristics and are used to predict future behavior. Extensive statistics have been developed for these techniques to reduce the amount of subjectivity influencing the results. Interpretation by the clinician is made only after the data has been processed. Examples of objective tests are the Minnesota Multiphasic Personality Inventory, the California Psychological Inventory, and the Strong Vocational Interest Blank.

PROJECTIVE TECHNIQUES

Projective techniques have developed as part of the psychoanalytic approach. Clinicians who use these assessments believe that questionnaires and inventories have little value, because important, unconscious psychic material may remain hidden. The purpose of using projective techniques is to elicit material that reveals the inner dynamics of the personality. These techniques are usually ambiguous and open-ended so that the individual may reveal his or her predispositions, conflicts, and dynamics indirectly. Information gathered by means of these assessments must be interpreted by the use of psychoanalytic theory. There are five types of projective techniques: association, construction, choice, ordering, and expression. Examples of these tests are the Rorschach, Thematic Apperception Test (TAT), Draw-A-Person Test, and Buck House-Tree-Person Test.

SOCIOCULTURAL TECHNIQUES

Sociocultural techniques focus on the person within the system. Characteristics of the group and its effect on the individual are identified. Environmental limitations and influences; structure and organization; function; tasks; and communication patterns are all investigated. The groups can be the family, school, occupation, recreation, community organizations, and special groups such as hospitalized patient encounter or occupational therapy groups. Instruments include field observations, interviews, sociograms, and interaction analysis matrices.

HISTORY OF OCCUPATIONAL THERAPY FOR CHILDREN WITH EMOTIONAL DISORDERS 1947 to 1968

The treatment of children with emotional problems has been considered to be a complex and highly specialized branch of occupational therapy from the late 1930s through the 1950s, according to Gleave.[26] Her writing in 1947 guided the learning of many occupational therapy students during those decades. The training of the occupational therapist involved learning the "dynamic factors" responsible for the disorder. The psychoanalytic approach defined these factors as either mismanagement of the erotic drive, or misdirected, destructive energy. Activities could be used as a means to (1) permit aggression, (2) foster positive identifications, (3) allow the atonement of guilt, (4) obtain love, (5) act out fantasies, and (6) be creative.

Activities in occupational therapy were selected for developmental, as well as therapeutic value. A healthy child was expected to develop physically, emotionally, socially, and intellectually. Any child having difficulty with the development of any of these areas was expected to become insecure and therefore maladjusted. Many of these children with conduct disorders often found themselves institutionalized after committing misdemeanors. Occupational therapy in correctional facilities was designed to stimulate habit training, work habits, social development, and self-confidence. Musical, recreational, and manual arts and crafts were the general activity classifications used with children and adolescents.

Developmental guidelines were used for applying musical activities. In the early years rhythm was stimulated through simple tunes and folk songs. Singing and playing instruments was recommended for later childhood, while the adolescent was encouraged to attend live performances of orchestras to counteract the "musical trash" on the radio.

The purpose of recreational activities, such as games, sports, and parties, was to develop play interests, perception, social interaction, self-confidence, good sportsmanship, and training of the will, which probably meant motivation to perform well.

Manual activities were used not only for therapeutic value as a supplement to psychoanalytic therapy, but also as an opportunity to learn fine motor skills, proper care of equipment, and an appreciation for good workmanship. These are some of the work skills that are still important for children and adolescents to learn in any prevocational program.

From 1947 to 1968 therapists published a variety of articles and some books about their practice environments. Documentation about the nature of occupational therapy with children and adolescents with emotional disorders covered a wide area of concerns. For the therapist of today to understand the professional growth of this specialty area, some of these reports are summarized here.

In 1953 Edelman[17] described a comprehensive treatment program for children ages 6 to 14, some of whom had emotional disorders, who were neurotic, schizophrenic, and neglected. A team approach was used to establish goals of treatment, and the occupational therapist provided specific objectives for each condition. The *neurotic child*, who might have many different symptoms such as depression, anxiety, guilt, and aggressive acting-out, was provided with a structured environment and clear limits. The occupational therapist used this setting to help the child reduce anxiety and encourage function at the highest capacity. The *schizophrenic child*, anxious and unsure of his own identity and with a limited ability to relate to others, experienced a one-to-one relationship with the occupational therapist in a consistent and routine environment. The goals of the program were to furnish warmth and security as a foundation for growth. Therapeutic activities could include any structured craft. Creative activities were not used, because they were thought to encourage fantasy instead of reality. The *neglected child*, who was trained as a good learner, was given love and affection and patterning of social behavior. A structured environment with rules and limitations helped discipline the child. Everyday living activities were used as therapeutic modalities.

In 1956 Piper and LeGrows[43] suggested tutoring as an appropriate modality in a comprehensive occupational therapy program for hospitalized adolescents. There were no teachers assigned to the hospital at that time. Cognitive skills of the adolescents were exercised and in part maintained while they experienced the emotional disturbance. Six case studies were presented. The individuals were able to return to their educational studies after discharge.

Rousos[47] discussed the occupational therapy treatment program used in a ward of 30 boys who had different conditions: schizophrenia, character disorders, and psychoneurosis. The boys were divided into the following four groups according to (1) performance level and (2) occupational therapy objectives.

1. Group 1, ages 8 to 12: Schizophrenic, nonverbal, noneducable, overtly psychotic, performance level approximately 3 to 4 years.
   a. Weekly schedule: Twice a week for 30 minutes.
   b. Occupational therapy: To increase awareness and attention span and to stimulate interest in play, socialization, self-expression, and self-control.
   c. Treatment activities: Play activities with building blocks, musical toys, balls, puppets, toy telephones and beads; occasional visits to a gymnasium for exercise, basketball, and punching bag; guided creative activities such as drawing and painting for communication purposes; and structured activities and paper and woodworking crafts.
2. Group 2, ages 7 to 11: Schizophrenic, verbal, able to relate to others, educable, performance level of approximately 5 to 6 years.
   a. Weekly schedule: Three times a week for 45 minutes.
   b. Occupational therapy objectives: To improve the same functions as Group 1 and to stimulate group awareness and increase expectations of self-control.
   c. Treatment activities: Same as for Group 1
3. Group 3, ages 9 to 12: Schizophrenic and behavioral problems, educable, performance level approximately 6 to 8 years.
   a. Weekly schedule: Four times a week for 50 minutes.
   b. Occupational therapy objectives: To increase group's awareness, sociability, and self-control; stimulate interest in community environment and learning.
   c. Treatment activities: Group decorative and art projects; group games in the gymnasium or occupational therapy room; structured crafts, such as leather, wood, metal, ceramics, paper crafts, paper mache figures, kites, and masks; and some guided creative activities.
4. Group 4, ages 9 to 13: Schizophrenic and behavioral problems, sociopathic, educable, performance level approximately 11 to 12.
   a. Weekly schedule: Three times a week for 60 minutes.
   b. Occupational therapy objectives: To stimulate independence and group belongingness through masculine activities, crafts, and cooperative projects.
   c. Treatment activities: Woodworking and metal work; games with art emphasis once a week; occasional group decorative projects; horticulture and cooking (with caution by the physician not to make it appear feminine).

In 1960 Llorens[31] stressed the importance of the therapist's giving the emotionally disturbed child a wide variety of evaluations in order to assess intelligence, emotional functioning, performance, sociability, and interests before planning treatment goals. The psychologist's battery of formal tests and the occupational therapist's informal observations of the child doing activities may be used together to form a complete picture of the patient. Occupational therapy goals should take into account all possible sources of information about the child. The value of psychological assessments for establishing these goals is discussed for three examples of emotional disorders: the immature child, the neurotic child, and the psychotic child.

The *immature child* is unable to handle excessive stress. Frequent loss of self-control and low frustration tolerance produces hyperactivity, aggression, and hostile behavior. The psychological tests may be used to indicate intelligence level, level of impulse control, direction and level of hostility, commonly used defense mechanisms, and probable course and outcome of treatment. The occupational therapy goals are directed toward gratifying infantile needs, accepting hostility, providing an outlet for aggression, and promoting independence. The *neurotic child* is restless, frightened, and hyperactive. Anxiety leads to crying, clinging, and acting-out behavior. The psychological tests are able to reveal reaction to stress, intellectual level, creativity, capacity for insight, and ego strengths. The occupational therapy environment should be consistent, warm, and accepting with firm limits. Therapeutic activities are used for the expression of creativity, the increase of self-esteem, and an outlet for aggression. The *psychotic child* is withdrawn from the environment and is unresponsive to others. The psychological testing establishes the level of fantasy-reality orientation and perseverative thinking through the projective techniques. Channelization of fantasy material into reality-oriented activities may be accomplished in occupational therapy. Gratification of needs and impulse release opportunities within a structured setting are suggested goals.

Llorens and Rubin[32] reported on a graded activity program with children ages 6 to 12 who had a variety of diagnoses, including adjustment reaction of childhood, psychoneurotic reaction, infantile autism, and schizophrenia. Psychotherapy, chemotherapy, school therapy, recreational therapy, and occupational therapy were offered to the children at the clinic. The occupational therapy program used a directive educational approach in small groups. The children were grouped according to needs, level of skill, motivation, and behavior. In group 1 basic skills of coordination and manipulation were emphasized. Painting, drawing, cutting, and pasting activities were used. Typical behavior problems included loss of control, distractibility, low frustration, and inhibited and hyperactive behavior. In Group 2 intermediate skills development was emphasized. Art and paper crafts were used to stimulate participation interest, attention span, and motivation. These children demonstrated some distractibility, immaturity, and poor motivation. Group 3, designed for the older children of 10 to 12 years, provided activities for the practice of self-organization and constructive independence. Art, leather, and metal crafts; graphic arts; ceramics; and sculpture were used as therapeutic modalities. The children, already having good skills, were encouraged to cooperate with peers and take responsibility for their own behavior.

Babcock, Gross, and Gohl[4] reported on a special occupational therapy program for adolescents institutionalized in a state hospital. The daily program included 1 hour of occupational therapy, 1½ hours in the hospital industry, and 2 hours of recreation. Once a week the adolescents had 1 hour with the hospital chaplain, 1 hour of psychodrama, and 1 hour of library activities. No teacher was available in the hospital. The adolescents were categorized as neurotic, psychotic, or delinquent. The occupational therapy program objectives were the following:

1. The program must be consistent.
2. The occupational therapy clinic should be safe and accepting.
3. The therapist should be understanding.
4. The adolescent should learn acceptable social limits within the environment.
5. There should be an opportunity for creativity.
6. The therapist should help the adolescent build a sense of accomplishment, self-esteem, and self-confidence.
7. Activities should be used to help redirect sexual and hostile feelings into socially acceptable channels.
8. Activities should be used that encourage male and female identification.
9. Good work habits and work tolerance should be part of the learning environment.
10. Possessive dependent behavior of the adolescent should be channeled into healthy relationships with the therapists.
11. Vocational and avocational interests should be pursued.
12. Observations of the adolescents should be communicated to the treatment team by the occupational therapists.

In 1964 Finn[21] discussed the occupational therapy treatment of an 18-year-old with a severe character disorder. Finn explained the emotional disorder in psychoanalytic language. At the anal stage of 18 months to 3 years when the child begins to strive for autonomy or independence, the child with a character disorder is unable to assert himself. A sense of shame and self-doubt are substituted for a healthy ego. Later this extends into a poor body image, poor self-concept, lack of role identity, and poor reality orientation. Persons with a character disorder are still concerned with what their bodies can or cannot do. They have no clear sense of who they really are. Occupational therapy for this condition is especially appropriate, because it can be nonverbal. The patient learns who he or she is by doing activities. A variety of arts and crafts experiences can be used to satisfy the basic needs of this psychosocial level of development. The therapist should enter into the treatment situation with an unconditional acceptance of the patient. Warmth and support, together with a total lack of demand, will encourage the patient to begin to explore the treatment environment.

After 6 years of developing an effective program, Llorens and Rubin[33] published in 1967 their view of treating emotional disorders of childhood. This was the first in-depth description of the treatment of the emotionally disturbed child. The goals of the program were to (1) improve motor skills and coordination, (2) assist in the development of positive social relationships, (3) modify maladaptive behavior, (4) teach how to fulfill psychological and emotional needs, (5) work through psychodynamic conflict, and (6) improve cognitive-perceptual-motor function. For more information, the reader should refer to Llorens and Rubin.[33]

1969 to present

Mosey[39] described an occupational therapy program directed toward the minimization of body image distortion in adolescents. Symptoms of this distortion are clumsy movements, unkempt apearance, accidental injuries, and the tendency to dress inappropriately. Corrective experiences provided in occupational therapy included vestibular and sensory stimulation, rhythmic movements, and cooperative and competitive peer group activities structured to help the adolescents compare themselves to others. Sculpture and drawing the human body assisted the patients in accepting the sexual body components. Verbalization and guidance by the therapist replaced their fears with more realistic concepts.

In 1970 Fahl[19] studied the effects of cooperative and competitive activity on peer interaction in emotionally disturbed children. She found that cooperative activity promoted socialization.

A treatment program for hyperactive children was reported by Cermak, Stein, and Abelson[12] in 1973. The occupational therapy goal was to facilitate self-regulation by using other children as monitors. In a special education setting, by use of a great deal of behavior modification, the children learned cooperation, appropriate interaction with peers, and concentration through games and skits.

Rider[46] studied sensory-integration deficits in emotionally disturbed children. She designed a study in which 20 emotionally disturbed children were compared with 23 normal children. The children's ages were from 6½ to 12½. All children were enrolled in regular school. There were no special classes for emotionally disturbed children in the community. Rider used the Purdue Perceptual-Motor Survey, the Southern California Sensory Integration Tests, and the Reflex Testing Survey for Evaluating CNS Development. Scores for the disturbed children were all lower than those of the normal children. Twelve out of sixteen scores on the Purdue Perceptual-Motor Survey were significantly lower, and the emotionally disturbed children had significantly more abnormal reflex responses. The results of this study supported the hypothesis that emotionally disturbed children are likely to be integrating environmental stimuli poorly and should be referred to occupational therapy for sensory integration evaluation and treatment.

Hand-gesturing in psychotic children was studied in 1973 by Masagatani.[35] Eighteen hospitalized children, ages 2½ to 13, were observed for 15 months. It was found that each child had different personal gestures: fixed finger patterns, clapping, rubbing, pinching, and flapping. Some gestures were associated with communication. Speech delays were also noted. Incoherent sounds were found in four children. Three children made sounds resembling speech. Six used echolalic speech, and only four children had spontaneous normal speech. Fixed finger patterns were seen in 16 out of the 18 children. It was found that more gesturing behavior was apparent when the child was upset or interrupted. Hand-gesturing behavior in psychotic children can interfere with the development of basic skills. Through the process of self-stimulation, the child is able to screen out the reality of the environment and thus withdraw into his or her own inner private reality. The hands seem to be used to discharge emotions or to substitute for speech, rather than to be used to perform routine tasks. Poorly developed egos are the result of such behavior.

In 1974 Loveland and Little[34] described the role of an occupational therapist in a mobile multidisciplinary clinic that was organized to serve the needs of children in a juvenile correctional system. The occupational therapist's role was to identify, assess, and treat juveniles with sensory-integrative and visual-motor problems; consult about the development of a vocational training program in child care for institutionalized girls; and coordinate the recreational-crafts program for several institutions.

A program for low-achieving adolescents (12 to 14 years) that used behavior modification techniques for the management of behavioral problems was reported by Christiansen and Davidson[13] in 1974. The objectives of the program were to increase self-esteem, improve

social behavior, and develop appropriate values. A symbolic contract was used to define behavioral expectations. Occupational therapy tokens were earned for punctuality, appropriate language, and satisfactory work. The tokens were made from poker chips with holes drilled in them. They could be used to purchase special items such as record albums. Therapeutic activities were limited to those that could be structured and easily completed, such as leather, ceramic, and beadwork crafts.

Reese[45] described in 1974 a program that forced adolescent alcohol and drug abusers into a treatment program. The program was organized in two stages: (1) the 30-day inpatient phase and (2) the long-term outpatient habilitation phase. The problems in the adolescent's life, such as self-medication, self-concept, feelings, parents, school, friends, and the law, were used as a measure of the need for hospitalization. Three or more problems were considered criteria for admission. The inpatient program had eight goals:

1. To take the adolescent out of the noxious environment.
2. To help the adolescent gain control over self-destructive behavior.
3. To evaluate the problems of the adolescent.
4. To involve the adolescent in a self-help process.
5. To motivate each adolescent to find healthy self-expression.
6. To include the parents in the program.
7. To prepare the adolescent for the second phase.
8. To place the adolescent in a residential treatment program outside the hospital.

This program was designed in a therapeutic community model with an orthopsychiatric team. Education, arts and crafts, and sports supplemented the counseling. The adolescents were classified as (1) character disorders (used drugs to violently defy authority), (2) neurotic-depressive (used drugs for suicide attempts), (3) addictive personality (dependent on drugs for becoming unconscious), (4) psychotic (used drugs for control of anxiety), (5) mild personality disorders (used drugs for defiance, but no violence), and (6) below average intelligence (used drugs for peer acceptance). In this model the occupational therapist was codeveloper and cotherapist with the physician. Both served as surrogate parents to the adolescents. A follow-up of 48 of these adolescents demonstrated a 79% success rate.

Ayres and Tickle[3] in 1980 studied the relationship between specific sensory processing deficits in autistic children and the outcome of sensory integration therapy. Ten children, ages 3½ to 13, were tested for sensory reaction to stimuli in the tactile, proprioceptive, vestibular, visual, auditory, olfactory, and pain areas. The children were then treated for 1 year and evaluated in five areas: awareness, self-stimulation, language, purposeful activity, and social-emotional behavior. Progress of each child was measured qualitatively and differentially. It was found that children with normal or hyperreactive postrotary nystagmus responded better to the treatment program than children with hyporeactive nystagmus.

In 1983 Clark[14] discussed the implications of underlying neuropathophysiological processes in autism. Recent studies indicated that there is dysfunction in the arousal mechanisms, the left temporal horns of the limbic system, and other vestibular and auditory areas of the left temporal lobe. The autistic child seems to prefer to process information through the right hemisphere. Current therapeutic-educational programs are not completely successful. Therefore Clark suggested that occupational therapists develop treatment procedures based on neurobiological research.

Implications for the pediatric occupational therapist

The treatment of emotional and behavioral disorders of children and adolescents is still considered a complex and highly specialized area of pediatric occupational therapy. In the last 50 years many psychological approaches have been used successfully. Between 1930 and 1954 the psychoanalytic approach guided most of the treatment of psychotic children. Adolescents with conduct disorders who were institutionalized in correctional facilities were treated by use of an unstructured behavioral approach. During the 1950s and 1960s psychoanalytic theories still regulated most of the goals and treatment modalities used in occupational therapy. However, the phenomenological approach was used to justify tutoring, skill development, and work programs. From the 1960s the biophysical approach was included with other current approaches in a therapeutic milieu environment. Vestibular and sensory stimulation were used to improve cognitive-perceptual-motor functions. Some programs were reported to have used several theories for establishing goals. The behavioral approach began to replace the psychoanalytic model as the guide for occupational therapy with disturbed children and adolescents in the 1970s. The sociocultural approach influenced the design of therapeutic community programs for adolescents with drug and alcohol abuse problems. In the 1980s a renewed interest in the treatment of autism brought forth the recommendation that occupational therapists working in this area look for answers to treatment in the neurobiological literature. Occupational therapists in this specialty area used all the general psychological approaches as a means of assessing, planning, and documenting treatment intervention with children and adolescents. Knowledge of these approaches is necessary for the understanding of past treatment, communication with other professionals, and future practice. The case histories that follow will demonstrate how this knowledge is helpful for the occupational therapist.

THE CONCEPT OF OCCUPATIONAL THERAPY WITH DISTURBED CHILDREN AND ADOLESCENTS

In 1982 Moersch[37] stated that the mental health practice area of occupational therapy had previously assumed responsibility for the treatment of the mentally retarded population. Today retarded individuals may occasionally be included in programs designed primarily for normal children and adolescents with emotional disorders. Generally there are separate programs available. The DSM-III includes categories of mental retardation with emotional and behavioral disorders. Level of intelligence may be considered a factor in diagnosis.

Mental health practice also overlaps with the sensory integration practice area of occupational therapy. It is not unusual to find psychosis and behavioral problems occurring with learning disabilities and sensory integration lags. But this chapter will only briefly refer to sensory integrative treatment.

Professional intervention

What is the meaning of professional intervention? It means that occupational therapists present themselves to the public as possessing a specialized body of knowledge and skill. Through extensive education and clinical experiences, the occupational therapy student prepares to take over the responsibility of making decisions on treatment intervention. These decisions are based on the documentation of successfully used treatment techniques in the field of occupational therapy: our professional body of knowledge.[41] This section examines the process of occupational therapy through the example of case studies.

CASE STUDY 1

Twelve children, ages 5 to 12 with emotional and behavioral problems, are treated at a day treatment center. It is difficult for these children to adjust at home, in their neighborhood, and in school. Symptoms of their disorders are disruptive, acting-out behavior; behaving like a victim; being easily frustrated with poor peer relationships; and exhibiting below normal ability in academics. Developmental disabilities are observed in some, but not all, of the children.

The day treatment center is located in several classrooms in a local elementary school. One classroom is designated for academic work and one room is for multiple activities. Two classrooms have been subdivided into several smaller rooms that are used for family counseling, play therapy, staff preparation, and office space. The program uses the school playground and takes field trips into the community for swimming, horseback riding, and other experiences. The overall purpose of the program is to assist the children in the successful adaptation to their home and social environments.

An eclectic or combination of treatment approaches is used by the staff. A sociocultural approach is used by the family counselor. The art therapist applies a Jungian psychoanalytic approach when planning and interpreting the creative productions of sand table and art projects. The therapists most often use a phenomenological treatment approach in individual counseling. However, psychoanalytic theories are sometimes used to justify play therapy techniques. A behavioral approach is used to control children when they are participating in group activities. Time-out in a chair may help a child gain control of his or her emotional behavior. At other times a therapist may have to physically hold the child to prevent self-abuse or harm to others. Special privileges are used as rewards (positive reinforcement for desired behaviors). The occupational therapist uses a biophysical approach as a frame of reference for planning therapeutic activities. Therapeutic activities are selected to stimulate different systems of the brain and body.

A van brings the children to school at 9 AM. The ride from home takes up to 1½ hours. The children often fight and become upset before school begins. The driver gives the offensive children a warning in the van at the time of the problem. Later in school the children must take the consequences of their behavior. Punishments of time-out in a chair and the loss of recess, field trips, or lunch are the usual results of the lack of self-control. If the behavior is extreme, the child may be asked to stay off the van for several days.

Personal grooming is evaluated each day. The children are checked for clean hair, combed hair, brushed teeth, clean body, and clean clothes. Points are received for each good evaluation and may be used to "buy" toys, ice cream, or field trips.

Each day the children participate in a sharing circle. The staff and children sit on pillows in a large circle and share feelings and experiences with each other. The leadership of the group is rotated among the children on a daily basis. Paper stars are given by the staff members to various children who have performed well the previous day. Rocks are put into a large jar for sharing difficult feelings. When the jar is filled, all the children have a treat. The child leader gives warnings for inappropriate behavior in the circle. Lack of attention, talking out of turn, and loss of control may result in time-out in a chair away from the group.

During recess the children and staff members play together in a relatively unstructured session. If several children ask to play basketball or baseball with the staff, then a game is arranged. Otherwise, the children do as they wish: swing, run, talk, and play together. Usually other children in the school do not have recess at the same time so that there is minimal contact with them during the day.

Class periods are organized into 40-minute periods. There are two periods in the morning and two periods after lunch. The children are divided into two groups. Six go to academic class first, and six participate in occupational therapy, art therapy, or other group activities, depending on the day of the week. After the first period the groups change classes. An educational handicap (EH) teacher and assistant provide the academic work. Child therapists (children chosen to help) assist the occupational therapist and art therapist during the morning and organize creative activities for the afternoon periods.

CASE STUDY 2

Warren is an 8-year-old boy who was referred to the day treatment center by the school psychologist. Warren is an obese child with long, stringy blond hair that looks uncombed and unwashed. His clothes fit poorly and are often torn and dirty. He has been referred for evaluation because of emotional problems at home and school. He lives with his mother and stepfather in a middle-class neighborhood of a large city. His father left the family when Warren was 2 years old, and Warren has not seen him since that time. Warren has had difficulties in school since kindergarten. At home Warren is either withdrawn and pouting, or clinging to his mother. He has difficulty following directions. He is disobedient and rejective toward his stepfather. Both mother and stepfather have full-time jobs and seem to lead their own lives with minimal commitment to building a family life for themselves and Warren. At school Warren provokes fights with older boys and is beaten up regularly during recess. He has no friends. In class he refuses to work on assignments and disrupts the class. When the teacher requests his attention, he will put his head down on his desk and cry. Warren has been on methylphenidate (Ritalin) for 1 year to control his behavior.

The diagnostic team summary, dated 7 months after Warren came to the center, showed the following:
  I. Speech and language report: No therapy needed
 II. Psychology report: Uneven intellectual development; overanxious disorder, dysrhythmic disorder
III. Pediatric neurologist: Some signs of minimal neurodysfunction
IV. Occupational therapist
    A. Lincoln-Oseretsky Motor Development Scale
       1. Gross motor subtests
          a. Running speed and agility (6.8 years)
          b. Balance (6.5 years)
          c. Bilateral coordination (6.11 years)
          d. Strength (8.2 years)
       2. Gross and fine motor combined
          a. Upper limb coordination (9.2 years)
          b. Response speed (5.8 years)
          c. Visual-motor control (6.11 years)
          d. Upper limb speed and dexterity (8.5 years)
    B. Southern California Sensory Integration Tests: selected subtests
       1. Space visualization (normal)
       2. Figure-ground (normal)
       3. Position in space (normal)
       4. Design copying (low −1.5)
       5. Motor accuracy, revised right hand (low −2.0)
       6. Motor accuracy, revised left hand (normal)
       REMARKS: Motor performance is 6½- to 7-year level. There is difficulty in visual-motor tasks because of delayed motor development, rather than visual perceptual difficulties. Occupational therapy or adaptive physical education is recommended.
 V. Psychiatrist
    A. Axis I: 299.90—Pervasive developmental disorder onset after 30 months.
    B. Axis II: 299.90
    C. Axis III: —
    D. Axis IV: 3 Mild stressors
    E. Axis V: 5 Poor adaptive skills

When Warren arrived at the day treatment center, the staff members observed him for several days, and then at a team meeting they decided to give Warren individual treatment goals and family therapy goals.

Individual treatment goals

1. Find more appropriate ways of relating to peers and making friends. Develop sportsmanship behavior.
2. Become more independent, less needy.
3. Come to terms with angry feelings and find more appropriate ways of expressing them.
4. Learn to handle disappointment and pain. Act less like a baby, and stop whining.
5. Decrease tattling on other children.
6. Improve self-confidence, increase risk-taking.
7. Improve personal appearance.
8. Work on learning problems and auditory discrimination.

Family therapy goals

1. Parents should define and establish the commitment to each other.
2. Improve parenting skills and set clear-cut limits and structure for Warren.
3. Help Warren build his self-esteem.
4. Help Warren express his feelings in an appropriate way.

Warren was in the program 2 months before the occupational therapist and art therapist were hired for the program. These goals were not included until later.

Treatment program: general progress notes

Month 1 Two green stars for good behavior
Month 2 One green star for good behavior
Month 3 Six green stars for good behavior

Participation in classes remains poor, but is good in family therapy. Disconnected thought patterns, easily frustrated; whining "poor me" image invites other children to ridicule him; no progress in self-concept.

Month 4 Six green stars for good behavior (1 in occupational therapy)

Occupational therapist and art therapist each participate in the program 2 mornings a week. The goal of the occupational therapist is to exercise and stimulate development of adaptive skills appropriate for a 9-year-old boy through his participation in games and sports. The goal of the art therapist is to encourage the expression of feelings through art, ceramics, and sandbox designs.

Month 5 Two green stars

Warren is unable to cooperate or compete in any occupational therapy activities (games and sports) without losing control of his emotions. Crying and fighting occur many times during the day in the total program. He verbalizes that every activity is arranged so that he cannot do it. He feels that the staff members are picking on him.

Month 6 Four green stars

Warren is putting on weight. He takes little interest in his appearance. He has no friends in the program and continues to act like a victim. He has poor impulse control. His mother has just delivered a new baby brother.

Month 7 Four green stars

Warren is making an effort to learn many new skills such as throwing a basketball, racing a scooter board, bowling, putting golf balls, playing marbles, and other gross motor activities. He is better able to handle the frustration of not winning.

Month 8 Three green stars
Month 9 One green star (in occupational therapy)

Participation in activities is fair. Attendance is excellent. There is a slight improvement in self-awareness and frustration level. Warren is attempting to lose weight.

Month 10 Two green stars (one in occupational therapy)

Warren is very affectionate with the occupational therapist. He asks to be hugged each day.

Month 11 Six green stars, two gold stars (one in occupational therapy)

Older children have left the program. Warren is now one of the leaders. He has lost weight during the summer and now has much better motor coordination.

Month 12 Eight green stars, one gold (one in occupational therapy)

Participation in all classes is improved. Warren mixes better with the other children. He is more assertive; acts less like a victim. He is less frustrated when things do not turn out the way he wishes. He attempts to play all games in occupational therapy, even when he is doing poorly.

Month 13 One green star (in occupational therapy)

Mother is acting like a victim in family therapy. Warren has not been able to control his emotions in classes. He is overaggressive with the other children.

Month 14 Five green stars (one in occupational therapy)

Warren is appropriately aggressive in sports. He enjoys competiton and cooperative activities.

Month 15 Seven green stars, three gold (one in occupational therapy)

Participation is improved again. Warren is in control and able to communicate his feelings.

Month 16 Four green stars, two gold (one in occupational therapy)

Warren continues to improve. He helps teach younger children how to do the activities he knows.

Month 17 Nine green stars (one in occupational therapy)
Month 18 Eight green stars

The treatment team has decided to send Warren back to regular school in September. Goals of the program have been reached. He is now able to control his anger and has appropriate ways of expressing anger. He is able to accept disappointment and deal with frustration. He shares attention with adults and has an excellent personal appearance. Occupational therapy visual-motor skill development has reached normal functioning level.

DISCUSSION OF CASE STUDY

There were three realistic limitations placed on the occupational therapist working with Warren in Case Study 2.

1. Therapy was limited to 1 hour, twice a week, because of the financial constraints of the center.

2. Warren was treated in an activity group. Therefore the dynamics of the daily group process often affected Warren's progress in therapy. Mosey[40] described the factors that contribute to maintaining a therapeutic group environment. She stated that the goal of a therapeutic activity group is to develop basic skills, rather than to accomplish a particular task. Activities for this occupational therapy program were selected on the basis of the developmental needs of all children in the program, not just Warren. In some activities Warren supplied information and helped orient and encourage others; while in other activities he sought information and followed. Each minipractice game was considered a competitive or a cooperative project group involving short-term tasks.

3. The rules of the program regulating the behavior of the children were relatively more important than the individual treatment objectives. Often emotional outbursts and loss of control interfered with the planned activity. The therapist needed to design game rules that allowed flexibility, were fair and consistent, and yet promoted the exercise and development of brain-body functional skills. In the beginning of Warren's involvement in occupational therapy he could not participate in the games without many episodes of loss of control.

The goal of the occupational therapy program at the center is to develop normal brain-body functions and to improve performance skills for all children. A biophysical frame of reference is used to provide a systematic description of treatment intervention.[8,9,10] Luria's theory[27] of three functioning systems of the brain determines behavior observed, techniques, and modalities used in occupational therapy. The central postulates of Luria's theory place systems of brain function at three levels:

Level I: This system is located in the brain stem and limbic system. It controls attention and emotional arousal.

Level II: The posterior lobes of the right and left hemispheres contain this functional system. The dominant side is responsible for comprehension of language. The nondominant side is responsible for sensory (proprioception, auditory and vestibular, and visual) integration.

Level III: The frontal lobes are the highest level of the cortex. They direct and monitor all behavior through numerous connections. The dominant side controls speech, slow logical thinking, and fine motor skills. The nondominant side controls

fast (fight or flight) emotional decisions. It controls movement through space and automatic skills.

Using this frame of reference with children provides several strategies for treatment intervention: (1) direct training of a functional area by repeated activity, (2) simplifying a functional skill into subskills and teaching these consistently, and (3) tapping into a higher, more complex level of thinking to find alternative ways of solving the skill deficit.

Three objectives were selected for Warren:

Objective 1: Exercise the frontal lobes of both hemispheres and thereby improve fine and gross motor performance as recommended by the occupational therapy assessment.

Objective 2: Stimulate the left posterior lobe integration of the notions of sportsmanship, assertiveness, leadership, skill learning, friendship, and more appropriate ways of relating to peers as recommended by the treatment team assessment.

Objective 3: Stimulate the posterior lobes of the right hemisphere with sensory integrative activities leading toward a better body image, improved self-confidence, and increased risk-taking as recommended by the team assessment.

Games were judged to be the best modalities to fit the needs of the majority of children in the center. Classifications of play development by Takata[50] and Florey[22] have been useful to define developmental changes in human and nonhuman play skills. Games promote both physical and emotional growth and development. They are the natural means used by children to assimilate adaptive skills. There are four categories of play according to Piaget:[42]

1. Exercise play: Sensorimotor repetitive action
2. Symbolic play: A self-expressive language
3. Games with rules: Social interaction
4. Games of construction: Adaptations or solutions to problems and intelligent creations

All of these types of games have been used in the program. However, the games with rules have been the most successful in occupational therapy. Games with rules produce significant changes in peer relationships. Mastering game rules helps to build self-identity. At first children have difficulty in following rules, then they become fascinated by them. Finally they are able to adhere to the rules and make up their own for new games.[50] Children can regularly be observed going through these stages at the center. Minigames[38] are designed around floor and mat skills; running, jumping, and hopping; movement in space; tactile discrimination and visual memory; target skills; and manual dexterity. Each day a new minigame is introduced by the occupational therapist. The children are required to learn new rules and exercise different skills. No child is an expert in all areas, so they must learn to lose, as well as win.

Warren has learned to be very flexible in his play behavior. He knows his strengths and his weaknesses and is a good sport when he loses. In areas of his strength, he will teach other children his skills. He verbalizes the changes in his own behavior and attitudes. He predicts he will do well back in regular school.

CONTACT WITH PARENTS

Being a good parent is not easy. No one is born with special knowledge about becoming a good parent. We learn parental skills from watching our own parents, trial-and-error methods with our own children, and professional assistance. If we are trying to provide a healthy environment for our children while undergoing severe stress ourselves, such as divorce, we sometimes fail. If one of our children has emotional or behavioral problems, it may add excessive stress to the family.

What can the parent do to help the child with an emotional disorder? Ayres[1] suggested several steps for parents to take: (1) observe the child's behavior carefully. Is there tactile defensiveness, motor performance delay, speech delay, or other symptoms that accompany the emotional disorder? (2) Help the child understand his emotions and behavior. There are many resources available to assist in this effort. (3) If there are signs of sensory integration deficits, explain to the child that his behavior is a reaction to a physical problem. For example, the child may be sensitive to too much environmental stimulation. The parent may need to reduce stimulation by withdrawing the child from the situation and providing soothing stimulation in the form of favorite toys or rocking. (4) Try to provide a consistent, structured, active environment in the home. Lower expectations, reward good behavior, and take away privileges for inappropriate behavior. Be sure, however, that the child has opportunity for sensory stimulation and vestibular and proprioceptive experiences. (5) Help the child learn to play.[48] Encourage the child to express his or her own inner drive for activity that will lead to mastery over body and environment. The occupational therapist is able to provide resources for the parents. (6) Locate appropriate professional help in the community. All sources should be investigated. Occupational therapists can be useful in referring parents to community programs, if contacted by parents.

How can the occupational therapist help the parent of an emotionally disturbed child? The therapist can provide a parent-oriented treatment program such as that discussed by Knickerbocker.[30] Parents are included in the program as observers of occupational therapy on a regular basis. Resources on understanding the emotional problem may be given to the parent.* Parents can be encouraged to record and report changes in the child's behavior. Therapeutic activities can be recommended for the home that maximize the effect of treatment.[5-7] And, the occupational therapist can refer the parent to other professionals for problems outside the expertise of the therapist (Chapter 8).

SUMMARY

This chapter reviewed the scope and causes of emotional disorders in children and adolescents as viewed from five different psychological approaches. Current nomenclature used to define the diagnoses of patients and to categorize mental disorders in the DSM-III and ICD-9-CM have been examined. The history of occupational therapy in this special area of the field from 1930 to the present time was summarized. Two case studies were presented. One presented an 8-year-old boy being treated by a multidisciplinary team. The team's occupational therapist used an eclectic treatment approach, including aspects of all five different psychological approaches and biophysical (neuropsychological) frame of reference. Assessments from all approaches were summarized. Recommendations for parents with an emotionally disturbed child were discussed, as well as suggested contacts between therapists and parents.

---

*References 11, 16, 18, 23-25, 28.

REFERENCES

1. Ayres, A.J.: Sensory integration and the child, Los Angeles, 1980, Western Psychological Services.
2. Ayres, A.J., and Heskett, W.M.: Sensory integrative dysfunction in a young schizophrenic girl. In Henderson, A., and others: The development of sensory integrative theory and practice, Dubuque, Iowa, 1974, Kendall/Hunt Publishing Co.
3. Ayres, A.J., and Tickle, L.S.: Hyper-reponsivity to touch and vestibular stimuli as a predictor of positive response to sensory integration procedures by autistic children, Am. J. Occup. Ther. **34:**375, 1980.
4. Babcock, P., Gross, D., and Gohl, A.: Occupational therapy for disturbed adolescents, Am. J. Occup. Ther. **16:**176, 1962.
5. Borba, M., and Borba, C.: Self-esteem: a classroom affair, Minneapolis, 1978, Winston Press, Inc.
6. Borba, M., and Borba, C.: Self-esteem: a classroom affair, vol. 2, Minneapolis, 1982, Winston Press, Inc.
7. Braga, J., and Braga, L.: Children and adults, Englewood Cliffs, N.J., 1976, Prentice-Hall, Inc.
8. Burnell, D.P.: A cognitive frame of reference for curriculum planning with mentally retarded adults based on the psychological literature, Ph.D. Dissertation, 1973, Wright Institute.
9. Burnell, D.P.: Egocentric speech: an adaptive function applied to developmental disabilities in occupational therapy, Am. J. Occup. Ther. **33:**169, 1979.

10. Burnell, D.P.: Stimulus nutriment model of adaptation: treatment intervention. In American Occupational Therapy Association Continuing Education Conference Neurophysiology Review: treatment application to adult, pediatric and mental health populations, June-July, 1982, American Occupational Therapy Association, Inc.

11. Canter, L.: Assertive discipline for parents, Santa Monica, Calif. 1982, Canter and Associates, Inc.

12. Cermak, S.A., Stein, F., and Abelson, C.: Hyperactive children and an activity group therapy model, Am. J. Occup. Ther. **27:**311, 1973.

13. Christiansen, C.H., and Davidson, D.A.: A community health program with low-achieving adolescents, Am. J. Occup. Ther. **28:**346, 1974.

14. Clark, F.: Research on the neuropathophysiology of autism and its implications for occupational therapy, Occup. Ther. J. Res. **3:**3, 1983.

15. Coleman, J.C.: Abnormal psychology and modern life, ed. 5, Glenview, Ill., 1976, Scott, Foresman and Co.

16. Dinkmeyer, D., and McKay, G.D.: The parent's handbook—STEP, Circle Pines, Minn., 1982, American Guidance Service.

17. Edelman, A.M.: Some observations on occupational therapy with disturbed children in a residential program, Am. J. Occup. Ther. **8:**113, 1953.

18. Faber, A., and Mazlish, E.: How to talk so kids will listen and listen so kids will talk, New York, 1980, Avon Books.

19. Fahl, M.A.: Emotionally disturbed children: effects of cooperative and competitive activity on peer interaction, Am. J. Occup. Ther. **24:**31, 1970.

20. Fidler, G.S., and Fidler, J.W.: Occupational therapy: a communication process, New York, 1963, Macmillan, Inc.

21. Finn, G.L.: Severe character disorders: treatment through occupational therapy, Am. J. Occup. Ther. **18:**185, 1964.

22. Florey, L.: Development through play. In Schaefer, C., editor: The therapeutic use of child's play, New York, 1979, Jason Aronson, Inc.

23. Freed, A.M.: TA for tots, vol. II, Sacramento, Calif., 1980, Jalmar Press, Inc.

24. Freed, A.M.: TA for tots, Sacramento, Calif., 1981, Jalmar Press, Inc.

25. Freed, A., and Freed, M.: TA for kids, Sacramento, Calif., 1980, Jalmar Press, Inc.

26. Gleave, G.M.: Occupational therapy in children's hospitals and pediatric services. In Willard, H.S., and Spackman, C.S., editors: Principles of occupational therapy, Philadelphia, 1947, J.B. Lippincott Co.

27. Golden, C.J., and Anderson, S.: Learning disabilities and brain dysfunction, Springfield, Ill., 1979, Charles C Thomas, Publisher.

28. Hetherington, E.M., and Parke, R.D.: Child psychology: a contemporary viewpoint, New York, 1975, McGraw-Hill Book Co.

29. King, L.J.: A sensory-integrative approach to schizophrenia, Am. J. Occup. Ther. **28:**529, 1974.

30. Knickerbocker, B.M.: A holistic approach to the treatment of learning disorders, Thorofare, N.J., 1980, Charles B. Slack, Inc.

31. Llorens, L.A.: Psychological tests in planning therapy goals. Am. J. Occup. Ther. **14:**243, 1960.

32. Llorens, L.A., and Rubin, E.Z.: A directed activity program. Am. J. Occup. Ther. **16:**287, 1962.

33. Llorens, L.A., and Rubin, E.Z.: Developing ego functions in disturbed children: occupational therapy in milieu, Detroit, 1967, Wayne State University Press.

34. Loveland, C.A., and Little, V.L.: Juvenile correctional system. Am. J. Occup. Ther. **28:**537, 1974.

35. Masagatani, G.N.: Hand-gesturing behavior in psychotic children, Am. J. Occup. Ther. **27:**24, 1973.

36. Millon, T.: Disorders of personality: DSM-III: axis II, New York, 1981, John Wiley & Sons, Inc.

37. Moersch, M.S.: The issue: developmental disabilities, an ambiguous term, Am. J. Occup. Ther. **36:**111, 1982.

38. Morris, G.S.D.: How to change the games children play, Minneapolis, 1976, Burgess Publishing Co.

39. Mosey, A.C.: Treatment of pathological distortion of body image, Am. J. Occup. Ther. **23:**413, 1969.

40. Mosey, A.C.: Activities therapy, New York, 1973, Raven Press.

41. Mosey, A.C.: Occupational therapy: configuration of a profession, New York, 1981, Raven Press.

42. Piaget, J., and Inhelder, B.: The psychology of the child, New York, 1969, Basic Books, Inc., Publishers.

43. Piper, B.J., and LeGrow, D.: Tutoring for behavioral delinquents, Am. J. Occup. Ther. **10:**147, 1956.

44. Reed, K., and Sanderson, S.R.: Concepts of occupational therapy, Baltimore, 1980, The Williams & Wilkins Co.

45. Reese, C.C.: Forced treatment of the adolescent drug abuser, Am. J. Occup. Ther. **28:**540, 1974.

46. Rider, B.A.: Perceptual-motor dysfunction in emotionally disturbed children, Am. J. Occup. Ther. **27:**316, 1973.

47. Rousos, I.C.: Planning occupational therapy for schizophrenic children, Am. J. Occup. Ther. **14:**137, 1960.

48. Singer, D.G., and Singer, J.L.: Partners in play, New York, 1977, Harper & Row, Publishers.

49. Sundberg, N.D.: Assessment of persons, Englewood Cliffs, N.J., 1977, Prentice-Hall, Inc.

50. Takata, N.: Play as a prescription. In Reilly, M., editor: Play as exploratory learning: studies in curiosity behavior, Beverly Hills, Calif., 1974, Sage Publications, Inc.

51. Watanabe, S.G.: The developing role of occupational therapy in a psychiatric home service, Am. J. Occup. Ther. **21:**353, 1967.

52. Watanabe, S.G.: Four concepts basic to the occupational therapy process, Am. J. Occup. Ther. **22:**439, 1968.

53. Williams, J.B.W., editor: Diagnostic and statistical manual of mental disorders, ed. 3, Washington, D.C., 1980, The American Psyciatric Association.

54. World Health Organization: Manual of the international statistical classification of diseases, injuries, and causes of death, ninth revision, vols. 1 and 2, Geneva, 1977, The Organization.

55. World Health Organization: Mental disorders: glossary and guide to their classification in accordance with the ninth revision of the international classification of diseases, Geneva, 1978, The Organization.

24

LINDA C. STEPHENS

Occupational therapy in the school system

All children are required to spend considerable time in an educational setting in preparation for adult roles in life. Education has been defined as "a continuous process by which individuals learn to cope with their environments" (p. 1,257).[15] The occupational therapist who works in a school setting has the unique opportunity to help children become more functional in their own environments. This chapter discusses the educational environment as it relates to the occupational therapist, as well as the therapist's roles and functions in this setting.

LEGISLATION

The Education of All Handicapped Children Act of 1975 and Section 504 of the Rehabilitation Act of 1973 dramatically changed the focus and availability of education for handicapped children in the United States. Before the enactment of this federal legislation many handicapped children were excluded from public schools, received education in private schools (at their parents' expense), were institutionalized, or remained at home. In 1975, when the Education of All Handicapped Children Act was enacted, approximately 1.75 million handicapped children in the United States were receiving no education at all, and 2.5 million were receiving inadequate services.[16]

The Education of All Handicapped Children Act[4,p.42474] and its regulations have four main purposes:

1. To assure that all handicapped children have available to them a free appropriate public education;
2. To assure that the rights of handicapped children and their parents are protected;
3. To assist states and localities to provide for the education of handicapped children;
4. To assess and assure the effectiveness of efforts to educate such handicapped children.

Section 504 of the Rehabilitation Act of 1973 was enacted to prohibit discrimination against handicapped persons in programs or activities receiving federal funds. This act states that "no otherwise qualified handicapped individual . . . shall, solely by reason of his handicap, be excluded from the participation in, be denied the benefits of, or be subjected to discrimination under any program or activity receiving federal financial assistance" (p. 22676).[14] This legislation also provides for a free appropriate education for handicapped children and requires that nonacademic services and extracurricular activities be available to handicapped students on the same basis as nonhandicapped students.

Federal legislation provides for the use of certain "developmental, corrective, and other supportive services as are required to assist a handicapped child to benefit from special education" (para. 121a.13).[4] Occupational therapy is identified as one of these related services. As a result, greater numbers of occupational therapists are being employed by school systems to provide this related service to children in special education. Public schools are mandated to develop programs to provide adequate education for all handicapped children. Consequently, a significant portion of the practice of occupational therapy has shifted from medical settings to public schools.

THE EDUCATIONAL ENVIRONMENT
Systems theory

The educational environment can be analyzed and undertstood in terms of systems theory. A system is a functional unit that consists of a structuring of events or happenings rather than physical parts; it describes a pattern of relationships. Every system is made up of a number of subsystems and is also part of larger intercting suprasystems. All systems have definite boundaries, or limits, and are interdependent with surrounding systems.

The occupational therapist can be considered a subsystem interacting with other subsystems within larger systems and suprasystems. Figure 24-1 shows some of these interactions. In this example the occupational therapist interacts with other subsystems, such as special education, speech therapy, physical therapy, and the student. As various schools have contact with one another, they represent interacting systems within the larger suprasystem—the educational organization and school administration. The suprasystem has an infinite number of contacts and interactions with other suprasystems, such as the State Board of Education, the community, and the state, local, and federal governments.

Many occupational therapists working in school settings are itinerant, that is, they are expected to travel among several schools to provide services to handicapped children. It is important for these therapists to realize that they are moving from one system to another within the same suprasystem. Each system and subsystem has "its own distinctive function, develops its own norms and values, and is characterized by its own dynamics" (p. 99).[10] The effective itinerant therapist is one who recognizes the differences between systems and adapts to each unique environment.

Each occupational therapist, as an individual, can be considered a unique subsystem with different combinations of background, training, professional experience, personality, race, values, perceptions, and childhood experiences. Figure 24-2 illustrates the components of the individual as a subsystem and the

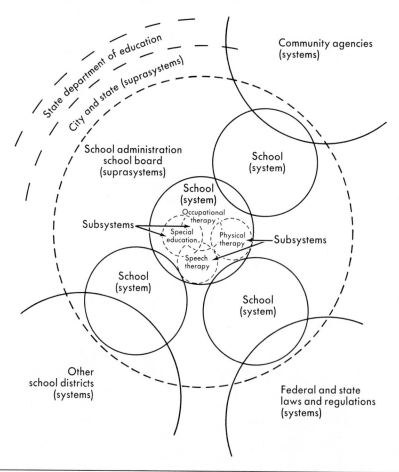

FIGURE 24-1

Systems, subsystems, and suprasystems in the schools.

interactions with other subsystems. These components are sometimes taken for granted when an individual interacts with individuals from similar backgrounds. When there are substantial differences, these must be examined so that interpersonal relationships can be developed for the therapist to be effective on a professional level. Some examples are the white middle-class therapist working in an inner-city black school, or an urban therapist working in a rural area.

A public school is a system made up of elements from the community reflecting the culture, traditions, and values of that community. It is a relatively open system, accepting any child within its geographical boundaries and usually encouraging participation from families and other community members. The system itself develops its own values and traditions, establishes channels of communication, and bestows power on certain individuals. As a system of interacting elements with a purpose of education, the school sometimes becomes inflexible and resistive to change.

Regan[17] described the characteristics of a rural school system and its suprasystems. Rural areas often have a high incidence of poverty, resulting in substandard housing, poor nutrition, and inadequate medical care. The rural schools are likely to have fewer funds and less modern equipment than urban schools. Rural persons often have more conservative religious and moral values and live in more homogeneous communities than do urban persons. Regan[17] stated that "not until the population's needs and resources, as well as the school administrative structure are understood can therapists deliver their services with the cooperation and support of the community and the administrative hierarchy" (p. 88).

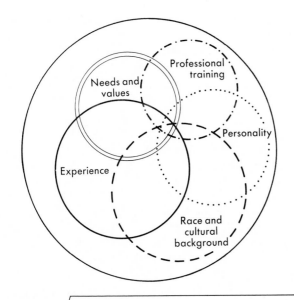

FIGURE 24-2

The occupational therapist as a subsystem.

Medical and educational models

The occupational therapist typically receives training and experience in a system referred to as the medical model. In this model, dysfunction or disease is identified, and strategies are developed, to increase function and to alleviate disease and dysfunction. The occupational therapist, as a subsystem working within the medical model, interacts closely with other medical subsystems (nurses, physical therapists, and so on) under the direction of the physician. Treatment may end once the patient is considered cured or has reached a "maintenance" level. The patient enters the system voluntarily at any point in time, receives services, and then leaves the system.

The educational system is concerned primarily with the "normal" child who is expected to gain increasing skill, knowledge, and competency in moving through the system. Although educators are increasingly working in interdisciplinary teams, there is no one recognized leader, and the close interaction found in the medical model is not required (for example, the educational planning team does not have the same type of interdependence and need for a leader that a surgical team has). The consumer in the educational model is the student who enters the system at a predetermined time (typically age 5 or 6) and remains within the system for a set length of time (usually 12 or 13 years). A comparison between the hospital and school, as examples of the medical and educational systems, is found in Table 24-1.

Role conflict

The occupational therapist, as a member of a health profession working in an educational setting, may experience role conflict. Role conflict occurs when there is an inability to reconcile inconsistencies between two or more simultaneous sets of expected role behaviors. The therapist, trained in a medical model, might have a perception of the occupational therapist's role that is different from the educator's perception of that role. "Providing services that are medically and behaviorally oriented to programs that are designed to enhance student's learning may cause further confusion in the occupational therapists' perception of their roles and functions as a related service" (p. 6).[5]

As an example, an occupational therapist received referrals for students in a class for the severely mentally handicapped. The therapist, after assessing the students, determined that the students needed maintenance programs that could be carried out by the teacher and the aide. The occupational therapist perceived her role as an indirect one, instructing the teacher and the aide and returning periodically to check the students' progress. The teacher's perception of the occupational

TABLE 24-1	Comparison of medical and educational systems	
	Hospital	**School**
Function	Saving lives, caring for the sick, curing or healing the injured	Instruction and development, preparation for life
Type of system	Relatively closed; must have credentials to participate; restricted areas; may be located at a distance from consumer; must pay fee or make appointment to enter	Relatively open; public has general knowledge and experience; building open to all; part of community; records accessible; parents and others urged to participate
Contact with system	Intermittent; contact when problem arises; consumer chooses when and where to enter system	Constant; continues through age 16+; admittance and attendance required by law
Barriers to consumer provider interaction	Medical mystique; lack of understanding of terminology, clothing (nametags, uniforms, patient's gowns); inaccessible records; accessible only through receptionist or answering service	Teachers' lounge; teachers' dining area
Delivery of services	Cooperative team headed by physician; consumer usually not part of team	Individual professionals or collaborative and consensual decision making by team; consumer (parent) is team member
Administration	Appointed board members (prestigious citizens); board meetings usually closed with little consumer input	Board members elected by public (members of community); board meetings open with frequent consumer input
Funding	Private pay; insurance; federal funds; grants; taxes; fee for service; salaries usually not public	Property taxes; state and federal funds; indirect pay for service; salaries public knowledge

therapist's role was different. The teacher thought that the therapist should take the students out of class for a half hour twice each week and give them therapy. These differences in role perceptions resulted in confusion and friction. The teacher thought that the therapist was "not doing her job," and the therapist thought the teacher was "uncooperative."

Another source of role conflict is derived from the nature of the occupational therapist's role in an educational environment. The occupational therapist deals with students with problems and frequently must be creative in finding solutions to those problems. The educational organization is often a bureaucracy that resists change and does not know how to handle the unusual situation. The system that has no difficulty in purchasing hundreds of desks for students may be stymied by a request to build an adapted desk for one handicapped student. "The degree to which a given role demands innovative activity is associated significantly and positively with both the degree of role conflict and the amount of tension the role occupant experiences on the job" (p. 127).[10]

Role conflict for the occupational therapist also oc-

curs when the therapist is in a position requiring a liaison or boundary-spanning function. The occupational therapist working in a school setting may perform this function between the educational and medical systems with different role expectations from both systems.

There are several strategies the occupational therapist can employ to deal with role conflict to reduce tension and frustration. First, the therapist should expect role conflict to be a part of the job. It is unrealistic to expect all persons in an educational setting to have an accurate perception of the functions of an occupational therapist. Demands for innovative solutions to problems and for liaison functions are necessary parts of the occupational therapist's role, but they tend to increase role conflict. A second strategy is to develop support systems with other occupational therapists in neighboring school systems or in professional organizations. Third, the presence of role conflict can be considered an opportunity to develop innovative ideas and to act as a change agent in the resolution of conflicts. This gives the occupational therapist an opportunity to be creative and to derive satisfaction from successful problem solving.

ROLES OF THE OCCUPATIONAL THERAPIST
Description of roles

What does an occupational therapist do in the school system? The occupational therapist is concerned with improving functional skills and developing coping behavior through the use of purposeful activity. The basis of occupational therapy intervention is a functional inability to perform.[21] Occupational tasks for the child in an educational setting are those tasks necessary for adequate performance in the classroom. It is the occupational therapist's role to provide intervention to enable the child to overcome or compensate for his or her functional inability in order to benefit from special education.

Five major roles were identified by Gilfoyle and Farace[7] and have been officially adopted by the American Occupational Therapy Association:

1. Evaluation: The identification of the student's deficits and needs to plan an occupational therapy program
2. Program planning: The determination of an appropriate occupational therapy program that is coordinated with the student's total education program
3. Program delivery: The implementation of an occupational therapy program designed to enhance the student's functioning and to enable the student to benefit from special education
4. Consultation: To provide training and information for school personnel and parents, which enables them to be more effective with the student
5. Management and supervision: To plan, supervise, and direct others as needed to implement occupational therapy services for the school or school system

The American Occupational Therapy Association has developed standards for each of these roles[20] (Appendix A).

Assessment role and evaluation procedures

SCREENING

The first step in developing or implementing occupational therapy services in an educational setting is to identify those children who need occupational therapy services. The occupational therapist needs to be involved in screening programs so that this can be accomplished. Screening involves setting certain criteria for a particular population and identifying those children who do not meet the criteria and who therefore need further evaluation. A determination of the need for occupational therapy services is not made in the screening process, only the determination that further evaluation is needed.

There are several ways in which an occupational therapist can be involved in the screening process in a school. Many school systems have established educational or health screenings of certain age groups, especially of children who are entering school for the first time in kindergarten or first grade. It is appropriate for the occupational therapist to become involved as a member of the educational team charged with the responsibility to identify children who deviate from the norm.

The occupational therapist might choose to screen certain populations of children, such as classes for the mentally handicapped, physically handicapped, or learning disabled. The teachers of such classes are valuable sources of information for identifying those children who have problems or whose performance deviates from that of other children in the class. Information can be obtained through record review, teacher checklist, teacher interview, and observation.

Screening instruments need to be chosen that are "appropriate to the chronological, educational and/or functional level of the student and shall not be racially or culturally discriminatory" (p. 900).[20] It is appropriate for the school-based occupational therapist to screen in one or more of the following areas: self-care, occupational tasks (school, leisure, play, or home), prevocational or vocational skills, developmental levels, neuromuscular functioning, and psychosocial functioning. By using information obtained through the screening process, the therapist can determine if a referral for a full evaluation is appropriate (Chapter 9).

REFERRAL

The referral for an occupational therapy evaluation is usually the initial step in obtaining occupational therapy services for a student. This is step 1 of the flowchart found in Figure 24-3. The referral should follow guidelines established by the American Occupational Therapy Association Statement on Referral.

The student who is initially identified as possibly needing special education placement is usually referred by a teacher or principal to an educational evaluation team or educational planning committee. This team determines which educational or related service evaluations are needed and makes appropriate referrals. If an occupational therapy evaluation is requested, the occupational therapist contributes data to the educational team to help determine a student's special education placement and need for related services.

In the case of a child already placed in a special education setting, referrals may come from a variety of sources. Screening programs may identify students who need occupational therapy evaluations; parents and teachers might have concerns about problems that in-

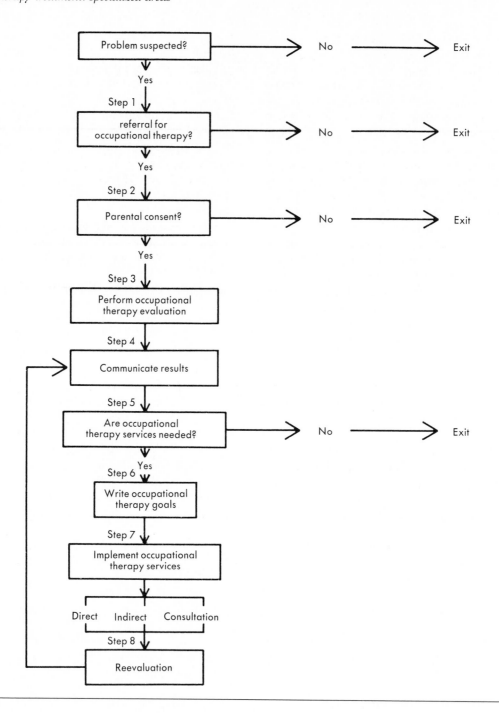

FIGURE 24-3

Flowchart for occupational therapy in educational settings.

terfere with the child's ability to function in the special education setting; or requests might come from physicians or community agencies. When a problem is suspected or a request made, the referral for occupational therapy evaluation should be generated through the educational planning team that follows procedures established by the local school system for referrals to related services.

Usually the major criterion for referral to occupa-

tional therapy is the functional inability to perform, which interferes with the child's ability to benefit from special education. The functional inability may relate to occupational performance (self-care activities, home-school-work activities, play-leisure activities, prevocational activities) or to dysfunction in neuromuscular development, sensory-integrative development, emotional development, social development, or cognitive development. However, some children might have a dysfunction in one of these areas, which does not interfere with their ability to benefit from special education. For example, a mentally handicapped child might have a developmental age of 3 years, which is significantly below the chronological age. In the areas of social development, cognitive development, and self-care activities the child may perform consistently on a 3-year level. In the absence of any neuromuscular or sensory-integrative impairment, occupational therapy might not be indicated. In this case the child's dysfunction does not interfere with the ability to benefit from special education, which is geared to the child's developmental level.

Licensure laws in some states or policies established by some local education agencies may require a physician's referral before occupational therapy services are initiated. Every school-based occupational therapist must be cognizant of local laws and regulations. Even when a physician's referral is not required, it is the occupational therapist's professional responsibility to seek medical management when indicated. The occupational therapist should counsel the parent or guardian regarding the need for medical services and should secure permission to contact the physician to obtain needed medical information and guidance.

EVALUATION

Step 2 in the flowchart (Figure 24-3) is to obtain parental consent for evaluation. The parents or guardian of a child have a right to be informed of any special evaluations or procedures given to their child at school, and they also have a right to give or withhold permission for evaluations. Parental permission for evaluation must be in writing and becomes part of the confidential records maintained by the school.

Step 3 is the occupational therapy evaluation. The evaluation process consists of data gathered from several sources. Examples are educational and medical records, interviews with teacher and parents, observation of the student, and administration of standardized and nonstandardized tests. The occupational therapist should choose tests and evaluation instruments that are appropriate for the chronological and functional levels of the student, and should take care that they are administered in such a manner so as not to be culturally or racially discriminatory. The therapist should use test results and clinical judgment in assessing the student's abilities and dysfunction (Chapters 10 and 11).

Once the evaluation is complete, the therapist must communicate results and make recommendations to parents, teachers, and other involved persons (step 4). Often this reporting is done orally in a parent or teacher conference or in the educational planning meeting. Results also must be documented in writing in the occupational therapy evaluation report (Exhibit 24-1). At this time the occupational therapist determines if the student or family

---

EXHIBIT 24-1

Outline for evaluation report for school-based occupational therapist

1. General information
   a. Relating to student: Name, age, school, birthdate, educational placement, summary of developmental-medical history
   b. Relating to referral: Referral source, presenting problems, diagnosis
   c. Relating to evaluation: Date of evaluation, tests administered, other sources of data
2. Psychosocial skills
   a. Relationships: Peer relationships, dyadic interaction, family relationships
   b. Behavior: Coping skills in classroom, behavior during evaluation, self-expression, self-control
   c. Self-concept—self-identity
   d. Play and leisure interests; extracurricular activities
3. Developmental skills
   a. Performance levels for physical-emotional-social components
   b. Manipulative hand skills
4. Daily living skills
   a. Daily personal care: Grooming, hygiene, feeding-eating, dressing, functional communication, use of adapted equipment
   b. Prevocational skills: Work process skills and performance, work product quality
   c. Use of environment: Functional mobility, restrictions imposed by environmental barriers
5. Sensorimotor skills
   a. Neuromuscular: Reflex integration, range of motion, gross and fine motor coordination, strength and endurance
   b. Sensory integration: Sensory awareness, visual-spatial awareness, body integration
6. Cognitive skills: Orientation, concentration, attention span, memory, generalization, problem solving
7. Preventive measures taken or needed: Energy conservation, joint protection, body mechanics, positioning
8. Conclusions: Summary of student's functional levels, including strengths and weaknesses; identification of areas of dysfunction needing intervention
9. Recommendations: Need for other services; need for occupational therapy intervention, including type of intervention, service delivery model, frequency, duration, and goals
10. Name and signature of occupational therapist

needs additional services in the community (rehabilitation, medical, vocational, counseling, and so on) and makes appropriate referrals. A determination is then made as to whether the student needs occupational therapy services in the school setting (step 5).

Program planning

The second role identified for occupational therapists in the school system is concerned with program planning. The occupational therapist, using results of the occupational therapy evaluation, determines expected outcomes following intervention and establishes long-term and short-term goals related to these outcomes. These goals are coordinated with goals from special education and other educational or related services the student receives and are included in the student's Individualized Education Program (IEP). Detailed planning is done by the occupational therapist by outlining methods and activities to be used to reach goals.

WRITING GOALS

A statement of present levels of performance describes a child's function at a particular time in a particular setting. When used as a reason for referral or as data gathered from an interview or observation, it is compared to the expected level of performance for a child of similar chronological or developmental age. When the described level of performance does not meet the expected level of performance, then a functional inability to perform exists. It is this functional inability to perform occupational tasks that provides the basis for occupational therapy intervention.

After a determination has been made that occupational therapy intervention is needed, goals are written (step 6). Occupational therapy, a related service, provides intervention to assist the child in benefiting from special education. The occupational therapy goals, then, should reflect the impact of this service on the child's special education through clearly stated long- and short-term goals describing expected outcomes in occupational therapy intervention. The following is an example of occupational therapy goals in an educational setting.

CASE STUDY

Present level of performance: Mary slumps over her desk, rests her head on her arm, and tilts her head when writing. She frequently turns sideways in her chair or sits half off the chair when doing seat work.

Long-term goal: Mary will remain in an appropriate position when doing seat work in class.

Short-term goal 1: When doing written work at her desk in the classroom (condition), Mary will demonstrate the ability to cross the midline of her body by writing from left to right, maintaining an erect posture (behav-

ior), turning sideways in her chair no more than one time in 15 minutes (criterion).

Short-term goal 2: When doing written work at her desk in the classroom (condition), Mary will demonstrate greater postural stability by maintaining an erect posture, with feet on floor, left hand holding paper (behavior), slumping over the desk no more than one time in 15 minutes (criterion).

PLANNING OCCUPATIONAL THERAPY ACTIVITIES

The purpose of the occupational therapy evaluation is to determine reasons for the inability to perform and to establish baseline data for performance levels. The occupational therapist then draws on his or her knowledge of abnormal and normal functioning along with various theoretical frameworks for ameliorating the inability to function to devise a plan of intervention and to predict its effect. The therapist then plans specific activities and methods to be used in working toward the established goals. The following is an example of an occupational therapy program plan using the previously cited case.

CASE STUDY

Functional inability to perform: Mary does not maintain acceptable posture at her desk. Her writing is messy and slow; she does not finish her work.

Causes of functional inability: Lack of integration of righting reaction causes entire body to follow when head turns; inability to maintain prone extension pattern indicative of hypotonic postural muscles; lack of integration of two sides of body; poor eye tracking (tendency to use one eye only); inability to inhibit or screen out inappropriate auditory or visual stimuli (involuntarily turns toward noise or movement in the classroom); poor eye-hand coordination aggravated by postural instability.

Methods of occupational therapy intervention: Sensory integrative treatment emphasizing vestibular and tactile input and adapted responses to enhance postural stability, integration of the two sides of the body, and normal movement patterns.

Occupational therapy program objectives: (1) Normalize response to vestibular and tactile stimuli, (2) develop ability to maintain prone extension position for 10 seconds, (3) demonstrate ability to cross midline of the body, (4) demonstrate integration of neck on body righting reaction when tested by the arm extension test, (5) maintain sitting position without external support.

Occupational therapy program activities: Spinning in net hammock (seated and prone); riding scooter board down ramp (prone); wheelbarrow-walking across room; reaching for beanbags while gliding on scooter board; rolling across rug with one arm up and one arm down; throwing Velcro darts across midline while sitting on T-stool.

INDIVIDUALIZED EDUCATION PROGRAM (IEP)

The Individualized Education Program is a written plan for a handicapped child required by federal regulations. It must be written and in effect before special education and related services are provided to a student. It is usually developed at a staffing or Individualized Education Program meeting by a team made up of a supervisory person, the child's parents, the child (where appropriate), and other individuals involved with the child. The latter could include an occupational therapist who has evaluated or provided services to the child.

According to federal regulations for Public Law 94-142, the Individualized Education Program must include the following[4]:

1. Present levels of functioning
2. Goals and short-term objectives
3. Special education and related services to be provided
4. Dates for initiation and duration of services
5. Criteria for evaluating the achievement of goals and objectives (para. 121a.346)

The Individualized Education Program is the vehicle by which interdisciplinary team planning is accomplished to meet the individualized needs of the handicapped child. The Individualized Education Program meeting is an opportunity for all involved, including parent, to communicate with each other and to make contributions from their perspectives of the child. The occupational therapist, as part of this team, can contribute valuable information regarding the child's performance and in turn can benefit from information provided by other team members.

The occupational therapy goals are included as a part of the Individualized Education Program and, along with other goals in the program, are reviewed at least once a year and revised or rewritten as needed. These long- and short-term goals relate to the child's improved function in the environment and are written without the use of professional jargon. In this way the occupational therapist shows how occupational therapy intervention can improve the child's functional abilities in the classroom to enhance his or her ability to benefit from special education.

Program delivery

IMPLEMENTATION OF THE OCCUPATIONAL THERAPY PROGRAM

The third role identified for school-based occupational therapists is that of implementing an intervention program (step 7, Figure 24-3). There are several aspects to consider in the implementation of occupational therapy services: (1) determining the appropriate service delivery model, (2) balancing the needs of the child with available resources, (3) determining the maximum and minimal frequency of service, and (4) determining the duration of the program, including the appropriate time to discontinue.

Service delivery models. The two major models for service delivery are those of direct and indirect services.[18,19] According to Gilfoyle,[18] *direct services* are "those related services within a student's educational program for which the occupational therapist has the primary responsibility" (p. 2). Direct service can be conducted on an individual or a group basis, but it must be implemented personally by the therapist or assistant. Weekly contact is usually considered the minimal frequency of intervention. *Indirect service* is programming planned by a therapist and administered by another person. This could be a parent, teacher, or aide who is periodically monitored by the occupational therapist. Indirect services may include instruction to classroom personnel in procedures required for daily management of a specific student. Examples are handling, positioning, use of equipment, and techniques used to adhere to medical precautions.

Methods of providing services. Either of the service delivery models can be implemented on a centralized or a decentralized basis. The centralized system can be compared to the occupational therapy clinic in a hospital or rehabilitation center in which all clients are physically located in one building and are transported to the occupational therapist in a space established primarily for that purpose. Some advantages of this system include more efficient use of the therapist's time, greater flexibility in scheduling and grouping, permanent establishment of equipment, easy accessibility to stored supplies, and greater accessibility of the occupational therapist to students and staff.

In the decentralized system the occupational therapist is itinerant, traveling to the students' locations. It can be compared to the home health model of providing occupational therapy services. Often it is necessary for the occupational therapist to carry equipment and supplies from place to place and to set up temporary therapy areas for providing services. While this system is less efficient for the therapist, it has definite advantages for the student. Students may be able to attend their neighborhood schools and attend some classes with nonhandicapped peers (mainstreamed), thus giving them greater opportunity for normal life-styles than if they were transported to a special school that housed only handicapped students. Even severely mentally and physically handicapped children can benefit from the stimulation of contact with nonhandicapped children in the school.

In one city several classes for severely mentally handicapped children were located within an urban elementary school. Even though these children were not capable of participating in classes with nonhandicapped children, they did attend assemblies and other special school functions. The children enjoyed the music and activities on these occasions and benefited by the change from their classroom routine. In turn, the nonhandicapped children became accustomed to the sight of children in wheelchairs or children whose behavior deviated from the norm. Some of the non-handicapped children made a habit of stopping to speak or touch a hand of a handicapped child and enjoyed the handicapped child's delight at this special attention.

The trends toward mainstreaming handicapped children and providing itinerant therapy pose challenging problems for the therapist, especially in rural areas. Some school systems have equipped special therapy vans as mobile therapy rooms. One project in New York made use of a converted bus to provide transdisciplinary services to children in rural areas.[13]

Duration of intervention. It is often difficult to determine the appropriate duration of occupational therapy intervention for a handicapped child in a school setting. The medical model of treatment is oriented to the care of acute problems, often with limitations imposed by the high cost of medical care or by guidelines established by third-party payers. In the educational model, on the other hand, a child is expected to remain and progress within the educational system, usually for at least 12 years. The occupational therapist, drawing from both models, has the freedom and opportunity to plan and implement long-range programs to improve the functional abilities of a handicapped child, but also has the responsibility to terminate services when the child has obtained maximal benefit from therapy.

For example, a child with cerebral palsy will improve with therapy but will always have a physical disability. It is the occupational therapist's responsibility to determine the point at which the child can no longer benefit from therapeutic intervention, but must rely on home programs or other special programs in the special education setting.

THE SETTING FOR THE OCCUPATIONAL THERAPY PROGRAM

Once the occupational therapist has evaluated children, established a caseload, and determined the type of program needed, it is necessary to locate an appropriate place to carry out the occupational therapy program. In schools with a relatively large number of children needing occupational therapy, there may be a room designated for therapy. However, the trend is toward mainstreaming handicapped children into local schools, so the occupational therapist may find it necessary to see one or two children in a school that has never had occupational therapy services.

If an empty classroom is available, this may be an ideal space for an occupational therapy program. Another satisfactory solution is to share a room with other itinerant staff members, such as the speech therapist or

music teacher, and arrange schedules to use the room at different times. In crowded schools or in schools with an open classroom–type of construction, the occupational therapist sometimes must be innovative and creative, as well as flexible, in finding and using space. Some therapists have used the auditorium, cafeteria, stage, storage room, hallway, or stairwell. One occupational therapist used the stage in the auditorium very satisfactorily until one day she walked in to find it full of voting machines and neighborhood people coming in to vote. The occupational therapy program was moved to the hall that day. Another therapist, using a stairwell, created a number of activities for proprioceptive input, spatial awareness, and motor planning by using the steps.

ADAPTED EQUIPMENT IN THE CLASSROOM

The occupational therapist can make a valuable contribution to the educational process by providing or fabricating adapted equipment needed by the child to function in the classroom. This includes equipment needed for seating or other positions in the classroom, as well as adapted equipment for managing classroom materials, writing, eating, dressing, and toileting.

The ambulatory, physically handicapped child may lack adequate labyrinthine or optical righting reactions to maintain a seated position without external support.

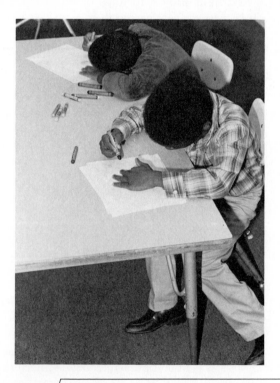

FIGURE 24-4

Although initially seated correctly, these children make increasing use of the table to provide trunk support as they become absorbed in the activity. Note position of the child's legs.

Courtesy Atlanta Public School, Atlanta, Ga.

This is the case with the children pictured in Figure 24-4. Obviously when a child must exert a great deal of effort to remain in his seat, he will lack the proximal stability necessary for control of distal musculature necessary for writing. When an occupational therapist developed adapted seating to provide external support for one child, the child's writing improved dramatically (Figure 24-5).

The nonambulatory child may need wheelchair adaptations or special adapted seating to increase functional abilities. Such adaptations should aid in normalizing body alignment, neutralize primitive reflexes, facilitate appropriate motor behavior, and provide comfort and security[6] (Figure 24-6).

Some therapists have used thick corrugated cardboard (Tri-wall) for fabricating adapted seating for physically handicapped children. This material is lightweight and less expensive than plywood, yet adequately meets the adapted seating needs of the young child whose rapid growth makes frequent changes necessary.

Devising functional positioning for the severely involved physically handicapped child may require some ingenuity on the therapist's part. One therapist made a seat by cutting out portions of a plastic kitchen garbage can, adding padding and supports where needed.[8] This therapist also devised a sidelying positioner from a cardboard box.

Adapted equipment, such as prone standers, corner chairs, bolster chairs, and sidelying positioners, is commercially available from a number of sources. It is the occupational therapist's responsibility to choose or make equipment to meet each child's needs, based on the occupational therapy evaluation.

The physically handicapped child who is capable of performing academic work in a regular classroom may challenge the problem–solving abilities and the creativity of the therapist. An adapted device (Figures 24-7 and 24-8) must meet at least three criteria to be satisfactory:

1. It must increase the child's functional abilities for the intended task. If the child can do just as well without the device, leave it off.
2. It must be accepted by the child, other students in the classroom, and the teacher.
3. It must be simple. Elaborate adapted devices often require too much effort to set up and need frequent adjustment or repair.

It must be kept in mind that the occupational therapist's role in the school setting is to assist in the special education of the child. Any adapted devices must be for that purpose and become the property of the school system, not the child. If an adapted wheelchair is sent home with the child, the adaptations may be altered or even missing when the child returns to school. It may be more effective to devise classroom seating and use the wheelchair only for transportation to and from school. The occupational therapist can, however, consult with the family regarding wheelchair adaptations and other adapted equipment for the home and guide the family to available resources for obtaining needed equipment.

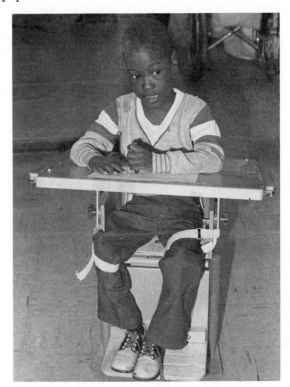

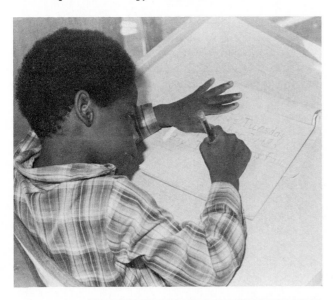

FIGURE 24-5

The use of a cutout table tilted to 45 degrees provided the support this child needed for writing.

Courtesy Atlanta Public Schools, Atlanta, Ga.

FIGURE 24-6

The use of an adapted classroom chair with tilted lap tray and adequate foot-leg support helps this child inhibit abnormal reflexes to maintain a functional position.

Courtesy Atlanta Public Schools, Atlanta, Ga.

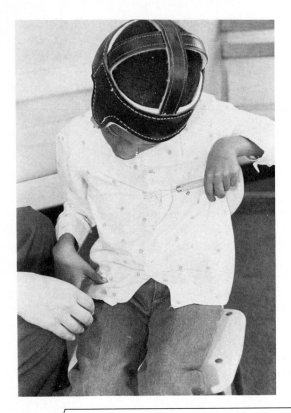

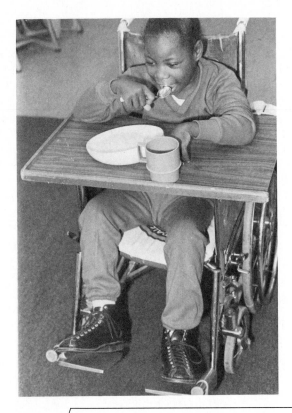

REEVALUATION

The eighth, and final, step in the flowchart in Figure 24-3 is reevaluation. This can be done whenever the therapist determines it is appropriate, but should be done at least once a year. When reevaluating a student, the therapist determines if goals have been met and if there is a further need for occupational therapy services. Reevaluation results are communicated to the parent and teacher (step 4) and are documented. If occupational therapy services continue to be needed, goals are revised or rewritten, the Individualized Education Program is reviewed and revised, and appropriate intervention is given.

Consultation

The fourth role identified for occupational therapists in the school setting is to consult with school personnel and parents regarding occupational therapy for the child. The consulting role can be carried out on a one-to-one basis, in formal in-service training for groups of parents or teachers, or as a liaison between the school system and community agencies. The areas of consultation identified in the Standards of Practice for Occupational Therapists in Schools[20, p. 905] are summarized here:

1. Consultative functions
   a. Develop and coordinate occupational therapy programs with the total educational curriculum
   b. Collaborate with the educational team regarding the student's progress, including the individualized education program
   c. Provide consultation and training for school personnel and parents
2. Areas of consultation
   a. Classroom or home environmental adaptations
   b. Special needs of students
   c. Appropriate programs outside the school program
   d. Preventive health education and activities to enhance the educational environment and learning potential of students

Gilfoyle[3] described a consultant as "a person who has expertise in a profession and can communicate this expertise to help others achieve identified goals and objectives" (p. 19). According to West,[22] a consultant is an individual who is "a change agent, a catalyst in decision-making, an enabler and a helper/adviser" (p. 51). The consultant and the consultee are involved in an unusual problem-solving relationship in which there is no obligation for the consultee to accept the help, suggestions, or recommendations offered. To be effective, the consultative relationship should be based on mutual trust and respect.

The effective consultant is one who listens to the needs, concerns, and problems of the clients and guides them in developing skills to meet those needs or solve their problems. The ineffective consultant tries to apply solutions or give advice without developing a helping relationship or taking the time to understand the client's real concerns.

There are a number of barriers to effective consultation. A major barrier is difficulty in communication resulting from the lack of mutual trust and respect. Establishing rapport is especially difficult if there are cultural differences between consultant and client, or if the consultant is much younger or less experienced than the client. To be effective, the consultant must have respect for the client's expertise and experience and have some understanding of that person's needs, values, and perceptions. Communication takes place only after two persons have developed some common or shared expectations and attach similar meanings to messages exchanged.[1]

An example of the difficulty in developing shared meaning might be the difficulties encountered by a therapist from a large northern city who is employed by a rural mountain southern school system. The therapist, seeking to consult with families of handicapped children, might find real differences in perceptions and values based on cultural differences in life-styles, traditions, and religion that result in lack of understanding and communication. There may also exist a distrust of the "outsider," regardless of how well-meaning the therapist might be. The therapist will need to develop communication and shared meaning on a personal level before it will be possible to develop a helping relationship on a professional level. This often takes time to develop—months or even years.

Other barriers to effective consultation may be attitudinal ones. Here are some examples:

1. Hostility: "Don't try to show me anything!"
2. Anger: "I don't want to be here."
3. Dependency: "You do it for me."
4. Apathy: "Who cares?"
5. Indifference: "Why change?"
6. Frustration: "Whenever I want to try something new, I can't get supplies."
7. Discouragement: "We tried that before, and it didn't work."
8. Denial: "Everything is fine; we don't have any problems."
9. Passive aggression: Verbally accepts suggestions, but later finds reasons not to carry them out.
10. Defensiveness: Gives excuses; excessive need to explain action or lack of action.

Another form of consultation is in-service training for school personnel, which is often done in a group setting with an organized presentation of material. Teaching methods might include lecture, discussion, demonstration, role-playing, and use of audio-visual aids. Lemerand[12] listed four kinds of in-service programs: (1) concept exploration, (2) skill demonstration, (3) material adaptation, and (4) case study analysis.

Topics for in-service training should be planned to meet the needs of the group receiving the training. Some appropriate topics for teachers and aides include lifting and handling techniques for physically handicapped students; techniques for teaching self-help skills to mentally handicapped students; feeding techniques for children with oral-motor problems; and how sensory integrative problems of learning disabled children affect their performance in the classroom. When the in-service training is completed, the therapist should request formal and informal evaluation of its effectiveness from the participants (Chapter 17).

The occupational therapist may be called on to act as a liaison between community health agencies and the school system or parents. The occupational therapist's experience and knowledge of the medical system are valuable in helping to bring understanding between groups that are sometimes divergent. The therapist, working in a consulting role as a liaison, may work with physicians, hospitals, rehabilitation agencies, vocational counselors, or community occupational therapists in helping the handicapped child receive complete health or rehabilitative services.

Administration and management

The fifth, and final, role of the occupational therapist in a school-based program is managing and supervising the occupational therapy program. This role includes developing and maintaining the occupational therapy program, managing occupational therapy personnel, documentation, and time management.

DEVELOPING THE OCCUPATIONAL THERAPY PROGRAM

The occupational therapist charged with the responsibility of developing an occupational therapy program in a school system uses exactly the same process as the occupational therapist charged with the responsibility of providing occupational therapy service to an individual child. This process includes needs assessment, program planning, implementation, and reevaluation.

The needs assessment, or evaluation phase, includes data collection and identification of needs, problems, and priorities. The therapist will find it helpful to collect data regarding the number of schools in the district, the number of handicapped students, the types of handicaps, the geographical locations of schools with handicapped children, and other related services available to students. In performing a needs assessment, the occupational therapist considers the occupational therapy needs of the school system. Have some children already been identified as needing therapy? What are high priority needs identified by school administrators for in-service training, consultation, and direct service? What needs have been identified by special education teachers? What are the expectations of parents regarding occupational therapy services? Are there particular problems to be addressed by the occupational therapist?

Once needs and priorities have been identified, the occupational therapist can design an occupational therapy program to meet these needs. Timelines should be established as guides for implementing the program. The program plan should include screening programs, service delivery models, types of therapy needs, recommendations for staff, anticipated caseloads, and budget for equipment and supplies.

The implementation phase includes the process of carrying out the established program plan. The occupational therapist evaluates, plans, and carries out intervention for individual students, as well as performs consultative and administration functions.

Reevaluation is concerned with assessing the effectiveness of the occupational therapy program. Goals and objectives of the program are reviewed along with the criteria for judging the effectiveness and efficiency of the program. Peer review or record review could be used in assessing the quality of occupational therapy services provided to individual children. As a result of the reevaluation process and quality review, weaknesses can be identified, and new needs may emerge. The circular process continues with additional program planning, implementation, and reevaluation.

PERSONNEL

The occupational therapist in the school system is required to maintain certification and state licensure, if applicable. Some states also require teacher certification for therapists employed in school systems. The occupational therapist has a professional responsibility to maintain competency with current professional knowledge and skills. Some states require continuing education units as a part of licensure or teacher certification requirements.

Occupational therapists in the school system may have the responsibility for supervising other personnel, such as paraprofessionals (aides) or volunteers. This re-

sponsibility may include informal or formal training, assigning duties, overseeing the performance of these duties, and evaluating employee performance.

Certified occupational therapy assistants can make a valuable contribution to the provision of occupational therapy services in the schools. Requiring consultation from the occupational therapist, not direct supervision, the certified assistant can implement occupational therapy programs for some students, which releases the occupational therapist for evaluation and consultation. When a certified occupational therapy assistant is employed by the school system, roles and responsibilities should be carefully defined.

DOCUMENTATION

Many therapists groan at the thought of paperwork and consider it a burden, but it is necessary to document services given. Reporting requirements vary from one school system to another, but in general the following are the types of records that should be kept:

1. General information
   a. Caseload data: Names, ages, and educational placement
   b. Number of times each student received occupational therapy and type of intervention (direct or indirect)
   c. Consultation and in-service training given
   d. Number and names of schools served by the itinerant therapist
   e. Use of the therapist's time in hours for direct service, travel, consultation, and meetings
2. Individual student information
   a. Evaluation report and parental consent for evaluation
   b. Medical information and physician's referral, if indicated
   c. Goals and objectives of occupational therapy in Individualized Education Program
   d. Frequency, service delivery model, and duration of service in Individualized Education Program
   e. Indication of child's progress toward goals
   f. Discharge report for occupational therapy

CASELOADS AND TIME MANAGEMENT

Determination of an appropriate caseload and allocation of the therapist's time are subject to many variables: frequency of services needed by the child based on the therapist's evaluation, number of schools in which children are located, geographical distribution of schools, and time required for travel. Other variables are the amount of time required for meetings and staffings, amount of consultation requested, need for community contacts, time required for documentation, number of requests for in-service programming, and availability of paraprofessionals.

In a situation in which the therapist has a large caseload, it is helpful to use a systematic and objective method to prioritize services and to determine the maximal number of children that one therapist can serve effectively. As a result of data gathered from a number of school-based therapists, some criteria were developed by the Georgia Alliance of School Occupational and Physical Therapists[19] to identify children having the greatest need for therapy. These included the following:

1. Younger children
2. Children with a potential for independent functioning
3. Children who have received little or no previous therapy
4. Children with a potential to be mainstreamed
5. Children who need therapy to increase function rather than to maintain function
6. Children with recent disabilities
7. Children who are unable to perform schoolwork tasks without therapy intervention

As a practical matter, the therapist must also consider some negative aspects. The child who has no follow-up at home or in the classroom sometimes will progress more slowly than another child with similar problems. This is especially true if the child has had intensive therapy in the past and has regressed because of lack of follow-up. Perhaps the child who is consistently uncooperative or unable to attempt activities should receive therapy less frequently. And finally, the therapist must weigh the needs of the child against the time available to provide service. If it takes 2 hours to see one child in an isolated school, then that is less efficient use of the therapist's time than seeing three children in 2 hours at another school. Perhaps the isolated child could be seen less frequently with greater reliance on home and classroom follow-up programs.

These priority factors were combined to form the caseload data sheet in Exhibit 24-2. A numerical score is obtained for each child to determine the relative need for therapy (severe, moderate, mild, indirect, or consultation). Note that the data sheet is not used to determine whether a child needs therapy; it is used to determine the relative amount of therapy needed based on functional disability and potential for function. A number of units is assigned per category.

The occupational therapist next determines the total number of hours available in the week for implementation of occupational therapy programs and the time unit to be used for determining maximal caseload. For many full-time therapists, the total time available is 20 hours per week, but this number will depend on the variables listed at the beginning of this section. The time unit is typically one-half hour but could be any available unit of time. The number of units per hour is multiplied by the number of hours per week to determine total number of units available for direct and indirect therapy. For example, a unit of one-half hour results in two units per hour, giving a total of 40 units per week for the therapist having 20 hours of therapy time. The weekly therapy time per student can be calculated by using the number of units per category. When the unit is one-half hour the times are as follows:

EXHIBIT 24-2

Caseload data sheet

Caseload rating

Severe need for therapy: 5 to 7 points
Moderate need for therapy: 3 to 4 points
Mild need for therapy: 1 to 2 points
Indirect therapy: 0 to 1 point
Consultation: 0 or less

Part A (give 1 point for each criterion met)

1. Child is under 10 years of age _____
2. Disabling injury or surgery related to disability within 1 year _____
3. Child has received 1 year or less of therapy _____
4. Potential for functional improvement as a result of therapy _____
5. Continues to make progress, noticeable change each month _____
6. Treatment of child's problem would better enable him or her to function with normal peers (mainstreamed) _____
7. School performance depends on therapy intervention _____

Part B (give ½ point for each criterion met)

1. Little or no family support or follow-up after repeated attempts to involve family _____
2. History of lack of follow-up in classroom; therapy recommendations not followed _____
3. Child unable or unwilling to follow directions or attempt therapy activities _____
4. No other children receive therapy in child's school _____

PART A SCORE _____

MINUS PART B SCORE _____

TOTAL SCORE _____

Severe need	3 units	1½ hours
Moderate need	2 units	1 hour
Mild need	1 unit	½ hour
Indirect therapy	¼ unit	½ hour per month

If the above figures are used, then the therapist whose caseload consists entirely of high priority students has a maximum caseload of 13 students (3 units × 13 students = 39 total units). On the other hand, the therapist having only low priority students can handle a caseload of 40 students. Examples of figuring mixed caseloads follow:

Time unit: ½ hour; Total units: 40 (20 hours per week)

4 high priority students	= 4 × 3 units	= 12
10 moderate priority	= 10 × 2 units	= 20
8 low priority students	= 8 × 1 units	= 8
22 students	=	40 units (maximum)

or

2 high priority students	= 2 × 3 units	= 6
10 moderate priority	= 10 × 2 units	= 20
10 low priority	= 10 × 1 unit	= 10
16 indirect	= 16 × ¼ unit	= 4
38 students	=	40 units (maximum)

CASE STUDY

Initiation of special education

Parent request. Brian, age 5 years, 6 months, entered kindergarten in an urban elementary school in January of the school year after having attended a private nursery school. Brian's mother requested a staffing to explore the need for special education, and she obtained reports of recent evaluations for the in-school team to review.

Record review. Psychological, medical, occupational therapy, and physical therapy evaluations had been completed on an outpatient basis at a local hospital. According to the psychological reports, Brian had a low normal IQ, showed low self-esteem, was easily frustrated (especially with motor tasks), displayed acting-out and aggressive behaviors, and was depressed. The therapists reported these problems: crossing the midline of the body, equilibrium, fine and gross motor planning, graphic skills, prehension, and visual perception. It was reported that Brian was considerably delayed in language development and that his speech was difficult to understand. Medical reports indicated a normal physical examination with a history of ear infections and allergy. Hearing and vision were within normal limits. In addition to the services received from the hospital, the family participated in counseling sessions with a local agency.

Initial staffing. The in-school team, made up of the classroom teacher, speech therapist, occupational therapist, resource teachers for behavior disorders and learning disabilities, school pychologist, and parent, met on Brian's second day of school. The purpose of the meeting was to recommend evaluations and to decide on a 30-day interim placement while those evaluations were being completed. As a result of this meeting, Brian was placed in a regular kindergarten class with daily resource help from the behavior disorders teacher. Referrals were made for speech, occupational therapy, learning disabilities, and behavior disorder evaluations. Based on reports of previous evaluations and classroom observations, some goals were developed for the 30-day period. These were concerned with developing appropriate classroom behaviors and decreasing aggressiveness and fighting.

Occupational therapy assessment

Preevaluation data collection. The data collection for the occupational therapy assessment began with a review of the records, especially that of the previous occupational therapy evaluation. After consulting with the occupational therapist who had worked with Brian previously, the present therapist decided to use the following in assessing Brian: parent and teacher interviews, informal observation, the Southern California Sensory Integration Tests, clinical observations, and informal assessment of play and developmental skills.

An interview was conducted with Brian's mother by use of a questionnaire of developmental and sensory behaviors. Responses to the questionnaire revealed a possible tactile problem. Brian has a habit of touching everything in sight; he frequently withdraws from touch, bumps and pushes other children, and wears a coat when not needed. Brian's mother also described coordination problems, possible auditory perception problems, and slowness in reaching developmental milestones. Brian turned over at 7 months, was slow talking, and, according to the mother, had trouble walking.

Brian's kindergarten teacher described an active, talkative child who pushed and hit other children and had difficulty attending to class activities. He lagged behind his classmates in readiness skills for reading and writing. Classroom observation during show-and-tell revealed that Brian sometimes watched and listened, but more often played with a toy car or wandered around the room.

Occupational therapy evaluation

Psychosocial skills. In the one-to-one testing environment Brian was lively and restless, sometimes refusing to attempt tasks presented to him. Although his behavior was often stubborn and manipulative, he appeared to have a desire to gain approval from adults. He responded well to a reward system that used a brightly colored sticker for appropriate behavior. However, in an unstructured group situation Brian had difficulty following rules, disobeyed adults, and antagonized his peers. When observed with his mother, Brian seemed rebellious and hostile.

Although Brian appeared aggressive and rebellious, he may have been using these behaviors to hide a low self-esteem and feelings of insecurity. His refusal to attempt tasks could be a defense mechanism to avoid failure. Brian refused to draw a boy, but did finish a drawing of an incomplete man. The therapist talked to Brian about this drawing, asking, "How does he feel inside?" Brian's only response was to scribble vigorously on the stomach of the man in the drawing. When asked, "Is he happy or sad?" Brian replied, "He's angry, angry at you!"

Brian enjoyed playing with small cars and trucks and toy guns, but avoided drawing and coloring, as well as toys that required fine motor skills. His play was often destructive in nature. He made pretend bombs, destroyed towns made of blocks, or had cars and trucks engage in massive wrecks. Brian's play was usually solitary; he had not yet developed interpersonal skills needed to play cooperatively with other children.

Developmental skills. Gross motor skills that did not require a great deal of balance, such as jumping, hopping, and skipping, were developmentally on age level. The abilities to balance on one foot and to walk heel-to-toe were 1 to 2 years below his chronological age. Upper extremity gross motor planning, as measured by the Imitation of Postures Test, was above the norm.

Brian's ability to manipulate small objects was on age level, although he would not remain on task for more than a few minutes. Eye-hand coordination, as measured by the Motor Accuracy Test, was above the norm for the right hand but significantly below the norm for the left. Brian is right-handed, but his left eye is dominant for sighting. He tended to use each hand on its own side of space, rather than crossing the midline of his body. Visual-motor integration, as indicated by the Design Copying Test, is significantly above the norm.

Although Brian's behaviors seem extreme, they must be viewed in light of normal emotional development. The 5½- to 6-year-old child is typically emotional, with aggresiveness and a false sense of self-confidence.[9] Brian's emotional difficulties appear to magnify and intensify the negative aspects of normal 6-year-old behavior.

Daily living skills. Brian was independent in age-appropriate feeding, dressing, and grooming skills, although his mother described his eating as sloppy. Occupational skills needed for the classroom were on the whole adequate. Brian could manipulate scissors to cut straight lines; he made jerky circular cuts when cutting a circle. He was learning to print letters of his name and displayed immature, but adequate, prehension patterns with pencils and crayons. Visual perceptual tests showed average functioning.

Sensorimotor skills. Sitting balance was poor with a dependence on external support. Brian was hypotonic and was unable to assume the prone extension position or maintain the flexed supine position. Brian was very unstable in a quadriped position and objected to having the therapist put her hands on his head to test for reflexes. He giggled and pulled away when he was touched and did not want his sleeves rolled up. There were indications of residuals of the symmetrical tonic neck reflex and lack of integration of righting reactions.

In addition to the clinical manifestations of tactile defensiveness, Brian scored poorly on tests for graphesthesia and localizing tactile stimuli. There were irregularities in diadochokinesia, rapid thumb to finger movement, and eye tracking. He was observed to avoid crossing the midline of the body in hand activities and in eye tracking. He also showed deficiencies in coordinating the two sides of his body.

The occupational therapist suspected vestibular problems because of Brian's low muscle tone, lack of postural stability, eye tracking problems, and difficulty with bilateral integration. However, Brian could not maintain a sitting position on a moving nystagmus board, and overhead hanging equipment for a net hammock was not available at his school. Therefore duration of nystagmus was not measured.

Evaluation summary. The occupational therapy evaluation indicated that Brian has a sensory integrative dysfunction in the areas of bilateral and postural integration, which could be a result of ineffective processing of the tactile system and possibly the vestibular system. There is also a disorder in psychosocial functioning in that the child displays maladaptive methods of coping with his environment and in developing relationships both with adults and peers.

The following summary was written for the in-school team: This evaluation shows moderate sensory integrative dysfunction primarily in the areas of tactile functioning and bilateral motor integration. Significant findings are evidence of tactile defensiveness (avoidance of touch), difficulty in coordinating the two sides of the body (including avoidance of the midline and poor performance of nondominant hand), and unstable gross motor movement patterns.

The presence of tactile defensiveness has been linked with behavioral problems in some children who display aggressiveness and hyperactivity. Brian's tendency to overreact to tactile stimuli (fight-or-flight pattern) may account for some of his behavioral problems in the classroom.

Brian's inability to stabilize large postural muscles make his movements appear clumsy and uncoordinated. When he is seated in a chair, his motor planning with his arms is adequate, but when he is seated in a cross-legged position on the mat, he can be pushed over easily. It is very important for Brian to have a chair of the proper size in the classroom so that his feet can be firmly on the floor. Round tables are not recommended, as they do not give enough surface for arm support.

Placement staffing

Review of evaluation data. The in-school team reconvened after the 30-day evaluation period to write goals and determine placement for Brian. Evaluation results were discussed. The speech therapist found no language deficits, but indicated that there were some articulation errors that interfered with the intelligibility of Brian's speech. Speech therapy was recommended twice a week. Testing in the area of learning disabilities showed that Brian did not meet the state requirements for this exceptionality and therefore would not need help from the learning disabilities teacher. The behavior disorders teacher found significant deficiencies in accepting authority from adults, relating to peers, and in developing acceptable behavior patterns. The occupational therapist reported on the results of the occupational therapy assessment and recommended occupational therapy on an individual basis two times a week.

Development of the Individualized Education Program. All of the evaluation results were used in developing statements of present levels of performance for the Individualized Education Program. These were in the following areas: academic achievement, social-emotional adjustment, communication skills, psychomotor skills, career-vocational areas, self-help skills, and physical-medical considerations. Next, goals were written for each of the identified deficit areas needing intervention from special education and support services. The occupational therapy goals were as follows:

Annual goal: To improve sensory integration and postural stability.

Objectives:
1. When working on a pencil-and-paper task at the table, Brian will remain in his chair and cross the midline of his body 80% of the time without verbal reminders.
2. When touched on the arm, leg, or face without visual cues, Brian will locate the touch accurately without withdrawing four out of five times.
3. Brian will play a game requiring him to balance on three extremities without falling 70% of the time.

Special education placement. Based on the information gathered and the needs that had been identified, the team agreed that Brian's primary exceptionality was behavior disorders. The next task was to decide on the most appropriate and least restrictive educational placement for Brian. The team agreed that Brian's needs could be met with placement in a regular kindergarten class with a resource class for behavior disorders 2 hours daily and itinerant services from the speech therapist and occupational therapist. All of these services were available at the present school, so no change in school placement was needed. Brian's mother agreed to this placement.

Occupational therapy intervention

Frequency of service. Brian was considered to have high priority for occupational therapy services. However, when Brian entered school in January, the therapist already had more than the maximum number of children on her caseload. Consequently Brian received occupational therapy only one time a week.

Occupational therapy activities. A sensory integrative approach was used, with an emphasis on tactile and vestibular input. Brian participated eagerly and responded positively to the tasks presented, but sometimes continued his manipulative behaviors. As a result, it was necessary to provide therapy sessions that were structured, yet included opportunity for movement exploration and experimentation.

Therapy activities included numerous scooter board activities and games that challenged balance in quadruped and sitting positions. Tactile input was given by rubbing the extremities with various textures and by rolling up in a rug. Brian especially enjoyed the latter, which probably indicated a need for the moving touch-pressure stimulus it provided. Spinning was used cautiously, as Brian sometimes complained of nausea or headache following this stimulation. Proprioceptive input was given with activities such as the wheelbarrow walk.

Review staffing

In June of the school year the in-school team met again to review goals and objectives in the Individualized Education Program and to write a program for the next school year. The team agreed that Brian had made tremendous progress during the year. Some of the goals for improving behavior and interpersonal skills had been met, and his kindergarten teacher felt he was ready for first grade. The occupational therapist's progress report read in part:

"Brian has shown a great deal of improvement in the short time he has received occupational therapy. He is better able to tolerate tactile (touch) stimuli and has much better control of large muscle movements. Although Brian sometimes acted in a manipulative, demanding, or stubborn manner, he always responded to firm limits and completed the task. He appeared to enjoy the sessions, and on a one-to-one situation, his behavior was controllable. However, on at least one occasion he verbalized hostile, destructive feelings toward the school and adults, saying, 'I'm going to put bombs in the school,' and 'I want to shoot arrows in all the teachers.' "

The occupational therapist recommended continuation of occupational therapy for the next school year in a group of two or three children. Previous goals for occupational therapy had not yet been achieved, so they were carried over to the next year's Individualized Education Program. In addition, the occupational therapist and behavior disorders teacher agreed to work jointly to develop appropriate group behavior and classroom coping skills. The following goals were added:

Annual goal: To improve classroom behavior and coping skills
Objectives:
1. When working on an activity in a group of three children, Brian will remain in his place and allow the other children to participate in the activity without interruption 70% of the time.
2. Brian will take turns while playing a game with another child without adult direction 80% of the time.
3. When frustrated with a task, Brian will ask for assistance without destroying materials four out of five times.

A new Individualized Education Program was completed with goals for behavior disorders, speech therapy, and occupational therapy. It is anticipated that Brian will continue to improve with these services so that eventually he can participate fully in a regular educational environment.

SUMMARY

This chapter described occupational therapy in the school system and the roles of the occupational therapist within that setting. These roles are evaluating, program planning, implementing services, consulting, managing, and supervising. The occupational therapist, in carrying out these roles, provides occupational therapy services in eight steps: (1) obtain referral, (2) obtain parental consent, (3) perform evaluation, (4) communicate results of the evaluation, (5) determine need for services, (6) write goals, (7) implement intervention, and (8) reevaluate students.

The function of the occupational therapist in the school system is to provide related services to students with impairments in functional abilities in the classroom. The purpose of occupational therapy intervention is to increase functional levels of students so that they are able to benefit from special education.

REFERENCES

1. Baskin, O.W., and Aronoff, C.: Interpersonal communication in organizations, Santa Monica, Calif., 1980, Goodyear Publishing Co., Inc.
2. Binder-Macleod, C., and Walden, G.: Adaptive equipment construction with Tri-wall cardboard, Dev. Disabil. Spec. Interest Sec. Newsletter **5:**3, 1982.
3. Consultation. In Gilfoyle, E., editor: Training: occupational therapy educational management in schools, vol. 3, module 5, Rockville, Md., 1980, American Occupational Therapy Association, Inc.
4. Education of handicapped children: implementation of part B of the Education of the Handicapped Act, Fed. Reg. **42:**163, 1977.
5. Educational/medical models and occupational therapy as a related service. In Gilfoyle, E., editor: Training: occupational therapy educational management in schools, vol. 4, module 8, Rockville, Md., 1980, American Occupational Therapy Association, Inc.
6. Farber, S.D.: Neurorehabilitation: a multisensory approach, Philadelphia, 1982, W.B. Saunders Co.
7. Gilfoyle, E., and Farace, J.: The role of occupational therapy as an education-related service, Am. J. Occup. Ther. **35:**811, 1981.
8. Houston, J.: Inexpensive adaptive positioning equipment for a multiply handicapped child, Dev. Disabil. Spec. Interest Sec. Newsletter **5:**2, 1982.
9. Ilg, F.L., and Ames, L.B.: The Gesell Institute's child behavior, New York, 1981, Harper & Row, Publishers.
10. Kahn, R.F., and others: Organizational stress: studies in role conflict and ambiguity, New York, 1964, John Wiley & Sons, Inc.
11. Katz, D., and Kahn, R.: Social psychology of organizations, New York, 1966, John Wiley & Sons, Inc.
12. Lemerand, P.: Inservice training packet. In Gilfoyle, E., editor: Training: occupational therapy educational management in schools, vol. 4, module 7, Rockville, Md., 1980, American Occupational Therapy Association, Inc.
13. Magrum, W.M., and Tigges, K.N.: A transdisciplinary mobile intervention program for rural areas. Am. J. Occup. Ther. **36:**90, 1982.
14. Nondiscrimination on basis of handicap: programs and activities receiving or benefiting from federal financial assistance, Fed. Reg. **42:**86, 1977.
15. *PARC vs Commonwealth of Pennsylvania*, 344 F. Supp. 1257, 1971.
16. Rebell, M.A.: Implementation of court mandates concerning special education: the problems and the potential, J. Law Educ. **10:**335, 1981.
17. Regan, N.N.: The implementation of occupational therapy services in rural school systems, Am. J. Occup. Ther. **36:**85, 1982.
18. Service delivery. In Gilfoyle, E., editor: Training: occupational therapy educational management in schools, vol. 3, module 5, Rockville, Md., 1980, American Occupational Therapy Association, Inc.
19. Service delivery patterns, Georgia Alliance of School Occupational and Physical Therapists, Unpublished, 1982.
20. Standards of practice for occupational therapy in schools, Am. J. Occup. Ther. **34:**900, 1980.
21. Task force on target populations, Am. J. Occup. Ther. **28:**158, 1974.
22. West, W.F.: The principles and process of consulation. In Llorens, L.A., editor: Consultation in the community: occupational therapy in child health, Dubuque, Iowa 1973, Kendall/Hunt Publishing Co.

SUGGESTED READINGS

Creighton, C.: The school therapist and vocational education, Am. J. Occup. Ther. **33:**373, 1979.
Gilfoyle, E., editor: Training: occupational therapy educational management in schools, vols. 1-4, Rockville, Md., 1980, American Occupational Therapy Association, Inc. (Supported by Grant #G007801499, U.S. Dept. of Education, Office of Special Education and Rehabilitative Services.)
Gilfoyle, E., and Hays, C.: Occupational therapy roles and functions in the education of the school-based handicapped student, Am. J. Occup. Ther. **33:**565, 1979.
Kinnealey, M., and Morse, A.B.: Educational mainstreaming of physically handicapped children, Am. J. Occup. Ther. **33:**365, 1979.
McCormick, L., and Lee, C.: PL 94-142:mandated partnerships, Am. J. Occup. Ther. **33:**586, 1979.
Mitchell, M.M.: Occupational therapy and special education, Children **18:**183, 1971.
Mitchell, M.M., and Lindsey, D.: A model for establishing occupational therapy and physical therapy services in public schools, Am. J. Occup. Ther. **33:**361, 1979.
Ottenbacher, K.: Occupational therapy and special education: some issues and concerns related to PL 94-142, Am. J. Occup. Ther. **36:**81, 1982.
Punwar, A., and Wendt, E.: Certification of occupational therapists in the public schools: the Wisconsin experience, Am. J. Occup. Ther. **34:**727, 1980.

25

PEGGY BARNSTORFF

The dying child

On a pediatric ward in a large medical center, I met two people who challenged me to learn more about death, especially children's perceptions of death.

Jan was an 11-year-old girl with a distorting facial malignancy that had been in progress for over 2 years. She had been seen periodically in various outpatient clinics, interspersed with hospital stays both in her hometown and in the regional medical center. The treatment she received, as well as the disease process, was extremely painful.

Finally, when Jan was dying in the medical center, she was in a private room that was darkened at all times. Her contacts with the outside world were few. The medical staff rarely visited her room, except to administer medications or during rounds.

Donna, a nursing student, was Jan's only meaningful contact with the outside world. Jan looked for Donna's visits, asked for her when she was not there, and allowed only Donna to spend extended periods of time with her. It was a relationship full of meaning for both, and it sparked my interest in the problems of dying children.

THE SCOPE OF THE PROBLEM

One hundred years ago, childhood deaths were very common, and many families had to learn to accept the loss of a child. Today, children's deaths are more unusual and often unexpected, even though a child may have a terminal disease.[10] Our beliefs in the medical system and its ability to cure us leave us unprepared for death. Therefore children's deaths grievously affect all of those around the child: the family, the medical staff, and the community of friends and professionals.

In the United States it is expected that tens of thousands of children will die annually. The most prevalent cause of childhood deaths is accidents; however, neoplastic disease is the second major cause of death. These chronic neoplastic diseases include leukemia; solid tumors such as lymphomas, neuroblastomas, Wilms' tumor, or rhabdomyosarcomas; and tumors of the brain, bone, and eye.[36]

When a child is terminally ill, with an acute or chronic situation, there are various people who will care for that child: the medical staff, consisting of the child's primary care physician and the many specialists who work together to provide diagnosis and treatment; and the nursing staff, dealing with the dying child on a daily basis, taking care of the child, administering the medications, charting the course of the disease, and providing opportunities for the child to use daily living skills. Allied health personnel also may be involved in the child's care and include the social worker, the physical therapist, the occupational therapist, the dietitian, and the medical technician.[39]

Children who are dying also have the concern of parents, grandparents, aunts and uncles, siblings and cousins, as well as members of the community, such as teachers and family friends. All of these individuals are affected by, and may be involved in the care of, the dying child.

It is typical for a child who is an accident victim to die in the hospital. However, children with terminal illnesses are now more often involved in home care programs, where they are followed by home care nurses, physical therapists, occupational therapists, aides, and hospice volunteers.[24,26,37] Children with more chronic diseases are seen in outpatient clinics until they become too ill. Then they are admitted to the hospital and wait

490

for a remission so that they may be released to go home. In the last 10 years a trend has developed to allow the child for whom treatment fails to have the option to die at home, rather than in a hospital. This has been fostered through programs such as the hospice and individually developed programs at various medical centers.[24,26]

CHILDREN'S PERCEPTION OF DEATH

Depending on one's frame of reference for understanding children, there are either three or four stages in the development of a child's understanding of death. Nagy,[29,30] one of the earliest individuals to study this topic, suggested three stages: (1) from birth to 5 years the child believes that death is a reversible process in which life activities such as growing, hearing, and feeling can take place, (2) from the ages of 5 to 9 years the child personifies death as a distinct personality, and (3) from the age of 9, onward, death is understood to be a cessation of corporeal life and is a universal phenomenon.[35]

Kane[18] and Koocher[19,20] related the development of a child's perception of death to Piaget's stages of development during the preoperational, concrete operations, and formal operations states. Their research suggested that as a child's mind matures, the cognitive stages will be reflected in the child's understanding of death.

Childers and Wimmer[5] studied children's perceptions of death, and their results indicated that differential awareness of death is a universal function of age. Among the subjects of their study, the understanding of death as being irrevocable was not demonstrated systematically until age 10.

Meliar[28] suggested that there are four stages to the development of the concept of death: (1) the majority of 3- and 4-year-olds demonstrate a relative ignorance of the meaning of death, (2) among 4- to 7-year-olds death is seen as a temporary state, (3) 5- to 10-year-olds appear to function in a transitional state: these children believe that death is final, but that the dead function biologically, (4) to most older children death is a cessation of all biological functioning.

Infants

As a child matures from infancy to adulthood, his or her concepts of self, life, and eventual death parallel Erikson's and Piaget's developmental theories. The postpartum infant facing death reacts only physiologically, using all of his strength to continue living. As the child reaches the end of the period of bonding at around 6 months of age, he reacts to the physical process of the disease symptoms and the resulting treatment procedures. At this age the infant is capable of recognizing that he disturbs people, especially his parents. The infant equates this with being bad. The infant may respond to treatment with anxiety and fear, which is further aggravated by separation anxiety.[8] These reactions continue throughout the ages of 2 and 3. It is also during this period that the child learns the word *death*, but the word has little or no meaning for the toddler.

Preschool children

Egocentricity diminishes as the child is introduced to a world larger than the one known during the toddler years. At 4 years of age the child is beginning to conceptualize himself or herself as an individual; however, this conception is accompanied by that of "not me" as well. Feelings of being and not being must be dealt with by a preschooler. The thought of not being is very anxiety-producing, because if one is no longer being, that means separation from family and also loss of all the independence that has so far been acquired. The child focuses on the single dimension of comparing objects at a given time. Therefore the child focuses on life, which means being with others on earth as compared to death, which means separation from loved ones. Death also means that one becomes immobile, unable to move.[41] Thus thoughts of dying suggest dependency and loss of the self-control that a child of this age has just begun to acquire. Disease then threatens a child's very psychosocial existence.

Although children of 4 and 5 approach death with fantasy reasoning and magical thinking,[19,47] they can begin to appreciate the meaning of a diagnosis, and this greatly influences their reactions to the world around them. Television, radio, magazines, books, and communications with others disclose many ideas. They hear words, view the responding emotions, and develop associations that can be applied to later experiences. Children begin this application process as they come to identify with others. Concurrently they develop an increased curiosity about burial, dead animals and flowers, and the accidental features of death.[8]

For 3- to 5-year-olds death means absence or going away and is a temporary, impermanent state.[17,28] Death is seen as a continuation of life, but in a different place. Preschool children are not capable of cognitively understanding the process as being irreversible; such a concept is indicative of the ability to abstract thought. This is also true of retarded children who function cognitively at the preoperational level. Neither are these children realistic about the permanence or timing of death.[46] The most painful aspect of dying is the realization of separation. Denial is processed to overcome feelings of helplessness and the sense of loss. Narcissism develops with the threat to life and the recognition of the reality of the situation.[6]

School children

The prognosis and its significance are understandable to children of 5 to 7 years of age.[8] Although children may realize that death is imminent, thoughts about this are seldom vocalized. They perceive absence and death with a sense of impending tragedy. By this time the concept of time has been mastered. School children can think of an object as a whole, as well as consider its parts. With the vivid imagination that is also present at this time, the physical change and deterioration that occurs with death can be visualized. Death is specific and concrete and has both internal and external causes.[41] The prognosis becomes absolute and creates such anxiety that the child can no longer cope.[8] As increasing age brings increased emotional and intellectual capability; it also brings greater meaning to a child's own death. This leads to needing more help in coping.

Going to school full time adds to the child's continually changing social role and relationships within it. A 6- or 7-year-old realizes that with death there comes a change in previously established relationships. Again, death symbolizes separation from loved ones. This breeds anxiety. The child now understands that separation cannot be avoided, and because of this knowledge he learns to be a "good patient": death is not mentioned and feelings of pain and emotions are repressed.[8] The rules of life are learned. At this time there is an emotional shift from anxiety to fear of physical injury and mutilation, operations, body intrusions, and needles.[44]

From 5 to 9, death is personified and thought of as a contingency. Death as a personality is usually invisible, either having no form or going through the night so that it cannot be seen.[6] This is the time of life when children may have difficulty going to bed at night in the dark for fear that they may not wake the next morning. There is much talk at this age about the boogeyman. Death is remote, it exists outside of one's self, and through careful living it can be kept at a distance. This is also a period of interest in animate and inanimate things, which evolves into a transition period of superstitions and rituals around death, being uncertain as to whether death is funny or fearful—"Don't step on the crack, it will break your mother's back."[17]

It is not until children become 8 or 9 that play and verbal expressions come to terms with each other. Weininger[48] found that previous to this age, when children were told that a doll was sick and going to die, they tended to talk about the doll's death as being permanent, but continued on in the play situation to have the doll return to life, recovering.

Egocentricity is decreased in the 9- and 10-year-old, while mature concepts of time, space, quantity, and causality are emerging. These children appreciate living and begin to understand death as the physical finality of living.

Adolescents

Adolescence is the bridge from childhood to adulthood; it is a period of transition. These transitions occur not only in the physiological, but also in the cognitive, psychodynamic, and sociocultural aspects of development.[15] Cognitively adolescents move into the world of abstract thought. They learn to speculate on possibilities beyond reality and what might occur, as well as what does occur.[34,41] In this exploration adolescents will delve into the limits of life and the meaning of death[33]

Adolescents appreciate the reality of death.[5,19,20] However, personal death is not accepted.[27] The adolescent tends to assume the attitude of "Everyone else but me can die."[14] Adolescence is a period of intense present, with the immediate life situation being important, and past and future being pallid. More structure is given to the past than to the future, but the past represents a period of confusion. Attitudes toward the future are subjective and distinctly negative. Often the future is viewed as being risky and devoid of any positive values.[6] Even if imminent, death is thought of as remote, because it distorts the importance of the present.

Adolescence represents the drive for complete independence and self-sufficiency. It is a time of group identity with peers and the development of personal ideas and behavior, usually through the peer group relationships. Guilt and vague feelings of badness are felt during rejection of parental control. This rejection bothers the adolescent. As most deaths in this age group occur secondarily to trauma or accidents (frequently resulting from the breaking of rules), death becomes a confirmation of badness and is perceived as punishment that is meted out by the unforgiving parent. This idea leads to fear of the authority figure and eventual bitterness and resentment, deepening the adolescent's guilt and accentuating his or her depression.[8]

Death also means rejection by the gang, as it emphasizes the vulnerability of the individual, as well as the difference between individuals. The rejection cannot be tolerated by an emerging independent individual. Death then becomes a function of dependency in isolation.

As the child gets older, there is an increase in expressed death anxiety in relation to illness. Before the age of 9 this anxiety is expressed in terms of separation or mutilation fears. After 9 it is expressed in the younger patients as anxiety demonstrated through symbolization and physiological expression. Older boys tend to act out, while older girls are prone to depression.[6] This expression appears to be directly related to our society's role models and the inability on the part of men to actively express emotion. Anxiety may also appear as

TABLE 25-1	Developmental stages: children's perception of death compared with Erikson's psychosocial and Piaget's cognitive stages		
Erikson's psychosocial stages	**Piaget's cognitive stages**	**Perception of death**	

Erikson's psychosocial stages

1. *Trust vs mistrust* (birth to 1 year)
   Development of the sense of trust through the pairing of the infant's actions with pleasant events.
2. *Autonomy vs doubt, shame* (1 to 3 years)
   The terrible twos. Beginning development of control over one's body, self, and environment.
3. *Initiative vs guilt* (3 to 5 years)
   Beginning exploration of the physical environment through senses and the social, physical worlds through language.
4. *Industry vs inferiority* (5 to adolescence)
   Begins to be a worker.
   Wants to please.
   Learns the meaning of rules and uses them.
5. *Identity vs role diffusion*
   Merging of past identity with future expectations (bodily, societal, and one's own).

Piaget's cognitive stages

1. *Sensorimotor period* (birth to 2 years)
   Based on the formation of action schemas for skilled movement, language, visual perception, and object permanence.
2. *Preoperational period* (birth to 7 years)
   The ability to symbolize through language, thought, drawing, and play.
   Egocentricity.
   Asks questions and *why?* Is more able to employ past events and to consider more than one aspect of an event at a time.
3. *Concrete operations* (7 to 11 years)
   Time of real, concrete thought.
   Orders, counts, and thinks in terms of cause and effect.
   Beginning to compare own views and ideas.
4. *Formal operations*
   Beginning of abstract thought and reasoning. Ability to form hypotheses and test them.

Perception of death

1. *Birth to 1 year*
   Reacts physiologically.
   Without bonding there is little desire to live (failure to thrive).
2. *One to four years*
   Responds with fear and anxiety to treatment.
   Death has little or no meaning.
3. *Four to six years*
   Has the concept of "me" and "not me." Fantasy reasoning with an increased curiosity about dead animals, flowers, burial, and so on.
   Death is temporary.
4. *Six to eight years*
   Death means being separated from loved ones and causes anxiety.
   The child learns to be a good patient.
   Superstitions about death predominate.
5. *Eight to eleven years*
   Death is realized to be permanent.
6. *Adolescence*
   Speculates about what occurs after death. Death is perceived in terms of loss of independence and identity.

regression to an earlier stage of development.

It may be concluded that children at any age perceive their own death according to their developmental level and through the catalyst of some crisis event, such as a catastrophic illness (Table 25-1).

THE IMPACT OF HOSPITALIZATION

At some time a dying child will be hospitalized for medical intervention. Even to the most carefully briefed child, the hospital represents something fearful, simply by virtue of its difference and newness in a child's repertoire of experiences.

The *toddler* views home as the seat of security, safety, and guidance. When hospitalized, the toddler experiences separation anxiety, separated from his familiar surroundings, routine, and family. Compounding the strangeness of the hospital setting, the treatment personnel cause the child pain and discomfort. The child, in turn, reacts to the physical pain and his perceptions of his parents' discomfort rather than to any understanding of the end of his own existence.[8]

Erikson pointed out that with increasing age, increasing independence develops. The preschool child does not separate thinking from concrete reality. Thus hospitalization is thought of as punishment for bad thoughts.[8,36] The child reacts with guilt and noncomprehension of the treatment. He is angry with the hospitalization process, and the treatment he receives he views as a form of punishment. Anger is usually directed toward the treatment team or other patients. In addition to anger and guilt such a child also must deal with loneliness.

The awareness of self increases as children develop. They begin to think in terms of "me" and "mine" versus "not me" and "not mine." The thought of not being produces anxiety, thus children react through the process of denial. Denial allows them to deal with more tolerable and productive subjects that will ultimately lessen the anxiety. These children avoid speaking of death. Often their play behavior centers around accidents and disasters as they attempt to prove to themselves that existence can be controlled just as toys are controlled.[8]

The *grade-school child* is busy learning rules and is expected to exert some self-control and cooperation. Intellectually the child of this age is able to solve problems through thoughts, as well as by action. They child develops increased self-awareness, leading to independence from parents. Meanwhile, parental beliefs are internalized. By late grade school, the child has developed special friends, and the children teach and help each other.

Studies suggest that children in this stage are aware of the seriousness of their disease, even though they may not be capable of speaking about it,[45] and even though no one has told them how ill they are.[44]

Smallness, vulnerability, and inadequacy characterize the grade-school child. Such a child deals with these feelings through the use of denial and reaction formation.[8] For example, he or she may try to act fearless.

Grade-school children are also aware of their own identity. This allows them to think beyond self boundaries and to imagine. They understand about past and future concepts and fantasize about death and the idea of their own deaths. Thus they develop an alternative to death, seen in such forms as heaven, paradise, and hell.[8] Children want their existence to continue. Through learning rules, they pattern themselves after other individuals, leading to the realization that their parents are not perfect. Children therefore seek alternative heroes, groping for something to believe in and worship. These beliefs allow them to organize their worlds methodically, including a cause and purpose behind every action. This is then followed by a reward or punishment. Death being perceived as a punishment causes religious guilt.[25] Secondary to this perception of punishment, dying children may reject the idea of heaven, which then represents only separation from family. Understanding of death increases throughout this stage, but these children tend to think that death comes suddenly and quickly. They may blot out feelings of death and in turn rely on parental authority (God, physicians, or teacher) for final protection from death.

Hospitalization involves various degrees of separation from family and friends. The grade-school child is lonely, scared, and sad, as well as fearful of the unknown. A study by Spielberger and others[43] indicated strong support for the hypothesis that terminally ill children show greater awareness of their hospital experience than do children who are chronically ill. These same children also expressed more hospital and non-hospital-related anxiety. Homesickness, anger, frustration, and anxiety are usually expressed to the treatment staff in the form of refusing to cooperate.[8] Some children might withdraw and become obviously depressed; however, the usual course of behavior is one of regression. They learn quickly from others and become sensitive to the feelings of the team. When involved with the hospital through the use of activities, children may become happier, and their self-image tends to improve. As death approaches, they may become sad and bitter, not wanting to leave. They feel lonely from the realization that this is one trip that must be made alone. Thus comfort and security are sought.

In dealing with death the *adolescent* progresses through the stages outlined by Dr. Elisabeth Kübler-Ross[23]: (1) denial, (2) anger, (3) bargaining, (4) depression, and (5) acceptance. Emotions in adolescents are more likely to be expressed than in younger children. Death is representative of loneliness and passivity. Hospitalized adolescents fear being returned to the dependent role and may overtax their strength through continued independence. Although they long for warmth and caring, they reject support and thus force people to withdraw from them, even while dreading loss of control. With approaching death, they become weakened and allow themselves to be loved and cared for. At this point they rationalize that control will be regained as strength is. The adolescent wants to live, but at the same time may be fascinated with the concept of death.[8]

Death in the middle teens defeats the newly developed self-control, self-confidence, and self-direction that all led to the enjoyment of self. Older grade-school children and adolescents who know they are dying and accept death's finality prepare their families for the event. They gradually withdraw their expectations from the family and seemingly reject them. It is as if they are trying to comfort their families and ease them through the final phase of death with as little pain as possible.

On the whole, then, most children recognize the severity of their own illness whether or not they have been presented with the diagnosis.[45] They react according to their stage of development, as well as their sociocultural expectations. For the most part a terminal illness and the resulting thoughts of death are recognized by the children as the removal of independence. This and the intense feelings of separation affect their response to their own deaths.

ASSESSING THE CHILD'S UNDERSTANDING OF DEATH

Assessing the child's understanding of death is important when working with a terminally ill child. This process helps the therapist to know how to deal with the child's understanding of what is happening to him or her. Therefore it is helpful to assess what stage of Piaget's cognitive and Erikson's psychosocial development the child evidences (Table 25-1). This gives a fairly accurate assessment of the child's understanding of death. It is also easier than trying to get a child to talk about death, since most children tend to avoid this subject with someone they have just met.

A second consideration in assessing the child's understanding is to record the parents' understanding of death and any relevant sociocultural ideas they have. These sociocultural aspects will color a child's perception of death and may differ from the occupational therapist's. When working with terminally ill children, one should also ask what expectations the parents have, whether they are willing to have their child told that he or she is terminally ill, and what approach they are using with the child.

OBJECTIVES FOR OCCUPATIONAL THERAPY INTERVENTION

Determining objectives for the terminally ill child is often very difficult for the staff. The staff members realize this is a child who will not get well and who is different from the usual pediatric patient for whom they can set goals and develop long-term expectations. Therefore their objectives are mainly psychological in nature, with less emphasis on physical aspects.[1,7,38,49] They are to

1. Understand the origin and intensity of the child's anxiety
2. Allow thoughts or reactions to death to come into the open
3. Encourage expression of grief
4. Provide support
5. Facilitate and maintain independence
6. Facilitate and maintain participation in activities of daily living

TREATMENT MODALITIES

The underlying principle when providing occupational therapy care for terminally ill children is to add quality to their remaining days. Two modalities are available to occupational therapists for terminally ill children: play activities and activities of daily living.

Until the age of 5, children learn exclusively about their world through play. They learn and practice activities before incorporating them into practical application. Once they go to school, play and teaching help them learn. The more playful and interesting the subject, the more likely they are to learn. Therefore the use of play is encouraged when dealing with terminally ill children.

Activities that are appropriate for the child's developmental level, physical level (including endurance and tolerance), intellectual level, and emotional state should be chosen. Play will allow the child to work through some of the feelings that he either has no words for, or cannot express. It also will allow the child to focus his interests on something other than himself, something in the world around him. The occupational therapist can also suggest appropriate activities to the family.

The second treatment modality that is useful in treating terminally ill children is activities of daily living. Too often adults take away the independence that a sick child has acquired. Parents and staff often jump to perform an activity such as bedmaking, dressing, or eating to save the child's strength. However, by doing so they take away the vestiges of independence that remain for the child and imply that there are no more decisions the child can make. Encouraging the continuation of routine activities of daily living allows a child to look forward to consistency and to know and have some control over what is coming. As the child becomes weaker, energy conservation methods can be taught to parents and introduced to children, allowing them to continue functioning independently. These modifications can be as simple as changing from metal to plastic utensils, using Velcro fastenings on clothing, and using pushcarts so that the child does not have to carry objects as weakness progresses. These modifications allow the child to continue functioning and to feel useful, rather than force the child to spend numerous hours on the sofa or bed watching countless television programs.[16]

WORKING WITH THE FAMILY OF THE DYING CHILD

Parents must deal with the loss of their child throughout the process of the illness. They must also deal with the idea that they will continue to survive after their child's death.

Parents often suspect the severity of the child's illness and anticipate the news.[13,21,31] Their reaction on hearing the diagnosis may range from loss of control to outward calm.[3] Those who display a lack of affective response do so as a defense mechanism to allow themselves to deal realistically with the problems at hand. Clinical observers, as well as parents, report that it takes several days or weeks for the realization of the diagnosis to sink in.[13,32] Typically both parents are eager to hospitalize the child once it is suggested, as this renews their hope that the diagnosis is faulty and that treatment will cure their child.

With the realization of the diagnosis and the major decisions made as to treatment, the parents are then free to react to the situation. Initially the reaction appears as shock or denial contaminated by guilt.[31] This guilt takes the form of the parents' thinking either that they are the cause of the illness of that they had not paid enough attention to the child.[4] This, combined with questioning of the medical staff, represents an attempt to search for meaning or understanding of the situation.[12] A problem occurs, however, if feelings of guilt become prolonged in nature and lead to overindulgence or to lack of discipline.

Denial is seen as the underlying reason for seeking other opinions,[9] representing the hope that the diagnosis is wrong and that the physician and medical staff have been in error. Binger and others[3] studied 23 families of terminally ill children and found this reaction is not usually shown by the immediate family, but rather by the grandparents and friends of the family.

Intellectualization also occurs. Parents seek information about the disease and cures, especially from other parents on the hospital ward and in support groups. This behavior is healthy up to a point. It gives the family an intellectual understanding of the disease to help them deal with the situation and the decisions that surround the treatment.[12] However, the increasing numbers of questions usually indicate increasing anxiety and guilt, which are not resolved by more information[17] and should be dealt with realistically.

Throughout the course of the child's illness, hostility and anger are expressed by parents.[12] Initially this reaction appears as a fight to reverse the diagnosis. Next, parents often feel resentment that they should suffer in such a manner. This may be complicated by guilt over their feelings of resentment. Resentment is usually channeled outward, often directed toward the treatment team. Third, anxiety of the unknown produces feelings of anger and hostility. Further, in the course of an illness, sick children often do not act sick, which reinforces the parents' denial.[8]

Parents often want to stay with their child during the course of his or her hospitalization. Urging the parents to return home may add to feelings of distress and guilt. Most often other children at home are neglected, thus increasing sibling rivalry and resentment toward the sick child.[4] Seeking to cheer a child is a constant need felt by the parents. However, this does not acknowledge a child's true feelings. Hospitalization promotes feelings of separation and anxiety on the part of the parent and the child. The parents are eager to hospitalize the child, but are fearful to let the child go. Hospitalization represents a loss of control. No longer is the parent in charge; the authority is transferred to the medical personnel, and eventually the parents come to depend on the strength and support of the hospital.[12,13]

Resentment is increased if the physician is unable to provide a curative treatment. This is complicated by the child's feelings. The child expects his parents to ease the pain and make him well. The parents are unable to do this, and the child becomes angry. This leaves the parents confused with feelings of failure.

A remission is anticipated eagerly until the child is allowed to return home.[12] The child's parents then realize that they are in sole care of the child, and this increases their anxieties. Overprotective behavior displayed by the parents leads to resentment by others and affects all family matters.[31]

A relapse confronts the parents with the cold reality of the situation. They may react as if they had just learned of the diagnosis. A relapse causes great stress, and effective coping behavior is needed. There is a dynamic balance of emotional states, and transient episodes of ineffective coping are not uncommon.[12] Successful coping behavior protects the parents from being overwhelmed by environmental and psychological stress while they continue to function in the medical and psychological care of their child.

Anticipatory grief is the gradual occurrence of mourning behavior, precipitated by the first acute critical phase of a terminal illness.[6] It is typically characterized by somatic symptoms: apathy, weakness, preoccupation with thoughts of the ill child, sighing, occasional crying at night, and appearing depressed. At other times, there is increased motor behavior and increased talk about the child. These symptoms help to reintegrate the feelings with the gradual redirection of external energies.[12]

Physical complaints are gradually replaced by resignation and the desire to have it over with. Parents turn their energies to other matters. Visits become a duty; the parents seem detached from their own child and more interested in the remaining children on the ward.[6] This is indicative of acceptance. Mourning energies are being converted to more constructive means.

Exhaustion of treatment options accelerates the grieving. The child's parents may experience decreasing understanding and become more prone to anger.

In chronic terminal cases the parents have had time to rehearse how they will act. They usually control their expressions of grief, taking death calmly. However, if the parents have expressed denial continually throughout the course of their child's illness, death will be a shock, an experience of immediate loss. The parents will often need many months before they can speak about the child without distress.

Finally, death is experienced with relief, and guilt is tinged with remorse.[25] Mourning may deepen feelings of self-value through thoughts of death. Also, the love and warmth felt for the dead child may lead to a greater sense of self-worth. Three to six days after the child's death, the parents' mourning becomes less pronounced. However, there tends to be a continued interaction with the hospital through such things as gifts, initiation of research foundations, and library donations. After the child's death there is a tendency of the parents to reverbalize the guilt, which is bound up with the feelings of relief.

Binger and others[3] found that in half of the 23 families they studied, one or more members required psychiatric help after a child's death, although none had required it before. This finding makes it important to understand the three types of unhealthy family protective maneuvers that can occur. The first is the *conspiracy of guilt* that occurs when the parents feel the death was preventable. Communication about the lost child is shrouded and evasive to protect the living members of the family. This tends to support the idea that if the parents had acted differently, the child would still be alive. Therefore guilt is maintained, and there is no chance for the exploration of the event for fear that someone will be blamed.[22] Surviving children in such a family live in a world of distrust and in constant fear of what may be in store, and they are hesitant to ask for clarification. A second unhealthy coping mechanism is the *preciousness of the survivor.* This leads to overprotection and shielding of the surviving children with fantasied attributes and expectations placed on them. This may lead to implications of specialness and good fortune placed on the survivors. Survivors may be filled with feelings of omnipotence and the desire to test fate, which limits their ability to develop practical coping mechanisms.[22] The last type of unhealthy coping is the *substitution for the lost child* in one of the survivors or a new child. The chosen child is likely to be vulnerable and forced to live a dual life: one of his own, and one of the dead sibling's. Because of this, the child is not likely to develop a secure sense of identity.[22] Unhealthy coping strategies used by families require outside intervention from mental health professionals.

After their experiences, families of dying children have made the following suggestions to health professionals. Listening seems to be the most valuable asset of a medical staff.[31,42] This is followed in importance only by offering reassurance, which often calms a parent's guilt feelings. Knowledge presented at the parents' level of understanding is calming. Questions should be answered patiently, kindly, and realistically. Families may be grateful, as well as angry. These angry feelings are dealt with best if the treatment team does not react to them as a personal insult or attack, and if the anger can be channeled productively.[42] If information is available on support groups, the staff members should make it known to parents.

General components of good management include the following[2]:
1. Competence of staff
2. Availability of staff
3. Continuity of care
4. Personalized care
5. Well prepared procedures
6. Active treatment role for the child
7. Questions encouraged
8. Supportive actions and discussions

WORKING WITH PERSONNEL CLOSE TO THE DYING CHILD

Among the personnel who treat the dying child and counsel the family, there may be a feeling of ambivalence in which compassion struggles against repulsion inherent in the threat of death. The degree of success in resolving this conflict determines the degree of success of the health care worker.[40] Therapists should be aware of this ambivalence in their colleagues and in themselves as well.

Since the primary goal of a health care worker is to help the sick child get well, a dying child prevents reaching this goal, thus causing feelings of frustration and anger. However, one cannot get angry with a sick child, so instead this situation often leads to feelings of guilt and even greater anger toward the one causing the guilt. This emotional state may become cyclic.[40,42]

Reactions of the personnel toward the child are influenced by previous experiences with death. The health care personnel may take the approach of being overprotective toward the child. This overprotectiveness often leads to overt or covert reactions of anger by the child. On the other hand, the staff members may be overindulgent, and thereby put an added burden of guilt on the child; after all, what has the child done to deserve this special treatment? When both types of behaviors are shown by the staff, there is inconsistency and confusion within the child, who then may not know how to behave.[40]

When treatment fails, workers may accuse each other of failure, thus redirecting toward each other the anger, frustration, and irritation they feel because they were unable to help.[40]

One staff member reacted to a dying child by hopping into his sports car and racing the highways until he had worked through his distressed feelings. This is one method of coping; however, in this case it produced anxiety in the rest of the staff until he returned. More constructive methods can channel anger and irritation into productive actions, whether oriented to motor release or to talking. Some of the methods currently used by staff members to deal with a child's death include individual counseling, team support group meetings, and case conferences where a child's course of treatment and eventual death is discussed.[11,49]

Although a child's death is painful to all, it can also be a time of learning about life, love, and the appreciation of others. The best advice is often the hardest to take. Parents recommend trying to live each day as it comes, and with each day enjoying one's child.[3] Occupational therapists are able to provide aid and support to these very special children and their families.

CASE STUDY

When Jan, the 11-year-old girl described at the beginning of this chapter, first had treatment, her facial cancer was hardly noticeable. She often came down to the playroom. In the playroom, occupational therapists worked with the children, allowing them to express their feelings about the medical procedures through the use of play, for example, playing nurse and doctor with a doll and actual nonharmful medical items, and encouraging the children to play with age-appropriate toys.

After several admissions and subsequent surgery, Jan began to withdraw to her room. The staff initially tried to get her to come out, but eventually obeyed her wishes and went to her in her room. By this time, Jan preferred quieter activities, such as painting, drawing, sewing, and crafts. These activities offered recognizable end products and allowed her to feel purposeful, able to accomplish a task from the beginning to the end. As she became weaker because of the disease and the treatment for it, the activities often consisted only of talking and reading. Now Jan was being bathed primarily by the nursing staff, although she was encouraged to perform at least part of the routine. She could still feed herself most of her meals, although her intake was supplemented with intravenous feedings. She continued to refuse to leave her room. At the same time she began to draw away from the majority of the staff, as well as her parents—as if to spare them the pain of death. She allowed only a few within her realm, thus adding to her life an element of control respected by the staff. It was during this time that Donna, the nursing student, became important to her. Donna and Jan talked together as Jan grew weaker and lost her ability to perform activities. Treatment eventually failed to produce a response, and Jan grew weaker and died.

CASE STUDY

John was an 8-year-old who entered the hospital semicomatose after having the flu. He evidenced depressed neurological functioning, was diagnosed as having Reye's syndrome, and was placed in the pediatric intensive care unit. He was referred to the occupational and physical therapists for maintenance of joint mobility and for general stimulation activities aimed at raising his conscious level. At the time, hospital policy allowed parents to visit 10 minutes each hour. Instead of using the pediatric waiting room, John's parents stayed just outside the intensive care unit, waiting anxiously for any news of their son.

The occupational and physical therapists worked together with the nursing staff by exchanging ideas for tactile, auditory, and olfactory stimulation. The parents were counseled to touch and speak to their son when they visited him. The nursing staff also left a radio or television on during the child's normal waking hours.

The therapists performed range of motion exercises three times a day, while the nursing staff took the responsibility for changing John's position in the bed to prevent decubitus ulcers. The staff also maintained his hygiene. Positioning was taken into account after a discussion with his neurologist and neurosurgeon.

Eventually the nursing staff placed chairs for John's parents outside the intensive care unit, and the occupational ther-

apists would stop and report to them about John's therapy. Often his parents asked medical questions that the therapists either did not know how to answer or ethically could not answer. This dilemma was solved by honestly admitting inability to answer and arranging for further information from the physicians.

After a week in the intensive care unit, never having gained consciousness, John died.

SUMMARY

In working with dying children, occupational therapists must be aware of developmental differences in the way children view death. These differences, added to the impact of hospitalization, affect children's responses to treatment and to surrounding people. Therapists can be effective with play activities and activities of daily living. It is important to understand the positive and negative emotions affecting parents, staff, and self.

REFERENCES

1. American Occupational Therapy Association: The objectives and functions of occupational therapy, Dubuque, Iowa, 1958, Kendall/Hunt Publishing Co.
2. Bergman, A.B.: Psychosocial aspects in the care of children with cancer, Pediatrics **40**(3):492, 1967.
3. Binger, C.M., and others: Childhood leukemia: emotional impact on patients and family, N. Engl. J. Med. **280:**414, 1969.
4. Bozeman, M.F., and others: The adaptation of mothers to the threatened loss of their children through leukemia, Cancer **8:**1, 1955.
5. Childers, P., and Wimmer, M.: The concept of death in early childhood, Child Dev. **42:**1299, 1971.
6. Cook S.S., and others: Children and dying: an exploration and a selected bibliography, New York, 1973, Health Sciences Publishing Corp.
7. Duff, R.S.: Guidelines for deciding care of critically ill or dying patients, Pediatrics **64**(1):17, 23, 1979.
8. Eason, W.M.: The dying child: the management of the child or adolescent who is dying, Springfield, Ill., 1970, Charles C Thomas, Publisher.
9. Evans, P.R., and others: The management of fatal illness in childhood, Proc. R. Soc. Med. **62:**549, 1969.
10. Fischoff, J., and O'Brien, N.: After the child dies, J. Pediatrics **88**(1):140, 1976.
11. Fox, S.: The death of a child, Nurs. Times **68:**1322, 1972.
12. Friedman, S.B.: Care of the family of the child with cancer, Pediatrics **40:**498, 1967.
13. Friedman, S.B., and others: Behavioral observations on parents anticipating the death of a child, Pediatrics **32:**610, 1963.
14. Gibson, J.E.: How much do you know about what other people believe? Gainesville Sun, p. 19, Dec. 2, 1973.
15. Hankoff, L.D.: Adolescence and the crisis of dying, Adolescence **10**(39):373, 389, 1975.
16. Hays, C.: General medicine and surgery. In Hopkins, H.L., and Smith, H.D., editors: Willard and Spackman's occupational therapy, Philadelphia, 1978, J.B. Lippincott Co.
17. Howarth, R.V.: The psychiatry of terminal illness in children, Proc. R. Soc. Med. **65:**1039, 1972.
18. Kane, B.: Children's concepts of death, J. Gen. Psychol. **134:**141, 1979.

19. Koocher, G.P.: Childhood, death, and cognitive development, Dev. Psychol. **9**(3):369, 1973.

20. Koocher, G.P.: Talking with children about death, Am. J. Orthopsychiatry **44:**404, 1974.

21. Koop, C.E.: The seriously ill or dying child: supporting the patient and the family, Pediatr. Clin. North Am. **16:**555, 1969.

22. Krell, R., and Rabkin, L.: The effects of sibling death on the surviving child: a family perspective, Fam. Process **18**(4):471, 1979.

23. Kubler-Ross, E.: On death and dying, New York, 1969, Macmillan, Inc.

24. Lauer, M.E., and Camitta, B.M.: Home care for dying children: a nursing model, J. Pediatrics **97**(6):1032, 1980.

25. Lewis, M., and Lewis, D.O.: The crisis of death: a child dies, Curr. Probl. Pediatr. **3:**1, 1973.

26. Martinson, I.M., and others: Home care for children dying of cancer, Pediatrics **62**(1):106, 1978.

27. McDonald, R.T., and Carroll, J.D.: Appropriate death: college students' preferences vs. actuarial projections, J. Clin. Pychol. **37**(1):28, 1981.

28. Meliar, J.D.: Children's conception of death, J. Gen. Psychiatry **123:**359, 1973.

29. Nagy, M.: The child's theories concerning death, J. Gen. Psychiatry **73:**3, 1948.

30. Nagy, M.: The child's view of death. In Feifel, W.H., editor: The meaning of death, New York, 1959, McGraw-Hill Book Co.

31. Noland, R.L.: Counseling parents of the ill and the handicapped, Springfield, Ill., 1971, Charles C Thomas, Publisher.

32. Oakley, G.P., and Patterson, R.B.: The psychologic management of leukemic children and their families, N.C. Med. J. **27:**186, 1968.

33. O'Brien, C.R., and others: Death education: what students want and need, Adolescence **13**(52):729, 1978.

34. Orbah, I., and Glaugman, H.: Children's perception of death as a defensive process, J. Abnorm. Psychol. **18**(4):471, 1979.

35. Orbach, I., and Glaubman, H.: The concept of death and suicidal behavior in young children, J. Am. Acad. Child Psychiatry **18**(4):668, 1979.

36. Oremland, E.K., and Oremland, J.D.: The effects of hospitalization on children, Springfield, Ill., 1973, Charles C Thomas, Publisher.

37. Picard, H.B., and Magno, J.B.: The role of occupational therapy in hospice care, Am. J. Occup. Ther. **36**(9):597, 1982.

38. Plank, E.N., and Plank, P.: Children and death: as seen through art and autobiographies, Psychoanal. Study Child **33:**593, 1978.

39. Richmond, J.B., and Waisman, H.A.: Psyhological aspects of management of children with malignant diseases, Am. J. Dis. Child. **89:**42, 1955.

40. Rothenberg, M.B.: Reactions of those who treat children with cancer, Pediatrics **40**(3):507, 1967.

41. Salladay, S.A., and Royal, M.E.: Children and death: guidelines for grief work, Child Psychiaty Hum. Dev. **11**(4):203, 1981.

42. Solnit, A.J., and Green, M.: Psychologic considerations in the management of deaths on pediatric hospital services, Pediatrics **24:**106, 1959.

43. Spielberger, C.D., and others: Children's state-trait anxiety inventory, Palo Alto, Calif., 1972, Consulting Psychologist's Press.

44. Spinetta, J.J.: The dying child's awareness of death: a review, Psychol. Bull. **81**(4):256, 1974.

45. Spinetta, J.J., and others: Anxiety in the dying child, Pediatrics **52**(6):841, 1973.

46. Sternlicht, M.: The concept of death in preoperational retarded children, J. Gen. Psychol. **137**(2): 157, 1980.

47. Von Hug-Hellmuth, H.: The child's concept of death, Psychoanal. Q. **34:**499, 1965.

48. Weininger, O.: Young children's concepts of dying and dead, Psychol. Rep. **44:**395, 1979.

49. Whit, J.K., and others: Pediatric liaison psychiatry: a forum for separation and loss, Int. J. Psychiatry Med. **11**(1):59, 1981-1982.

Appendixes

Standards of Practice for Occupational Therapy Services

Standards of practice for occupational therapy services for clients with physical disabilities

PREFACE

These standards are intended for internal use by the AOTA as guidelines to assist members in the practice of their profession. These standards by themselves cannot be interpreted to constitute a standard of care in any particular locality.

STANDARD I

The Referral for Occupational Therapy Services Must Be Based Upon the Provisions Outlined in the Statement on Occupational Therapy Referral.

1. When a referral is received, the therapist shall document:
   a. the date of receipt and referral source
   b. the services requested
   c. the above (a & b) within one working day of the receipt of the referral

STANDARD II

The Occupational Therapist Shall Evaluate the Client's Performance.

1. The therapist shall orient the client, family and/or significant others to the purposes and procedures of the occupational therapy evaluation.
2. An initial evaluation shall be completed at least five working days after acknowledgment of referral receipt.
3. The initial evaluation shall include an initial assessment of the client's goals, and functional abilities and deficits in:
   a. occupational performance (ADL)
      1) self-care skills
      2) home-work-school skills
      3) play/leisure skills
   b. motor skills
   c. sensory integration
4. If the results of the above evaluation indicate possible deficits in psychological/social and/or cognitive skills, the therapist should evaluate these areas and document any functional deficits; or should refer the client to the appropriate service.
5. If any of the above evaluation results indicate the client's need for referral to community services or programs, the therapist should determine the availability of such community resources; or should refer the evaluation to the appropriate service.

6. The therapist should obtain information about the client's medical history, education, work history, avocational interest, family, and cultural background. This information may be obtained through client interview, record review, and/or discussion with informed sources.

STANDARD III

The Therapist Shall Prepare and Document a Program Plan Based Upon an Analysis of the Occupational Therapy Evaluation Data and the Client's Expected Prognosis.

1. The therapist shall document the program plan within six working days after the acknowledgment of the referral receipt.
2. The documented program plan should consist of a statement of:
   a. achievable program goals
   b. methods to achieve the goals
3. The program plan goals and methods should be consistent with:
   a. the evaluative results and expected prognosis
   b. the goals of the client and/or family
   c. the program plans of other health care practitioners
4. The program plan methods may include, but need not be limited to, the use of:
   a. adaptive equipment and techniques
   b. passive, assistive, active and/or resistive activities and exercises
   c. counseling techniques
   d. facilitation/inhibition techniques
   e. joint protection techniques
   f. orthotic and/or prosthetic devices
   g. work simplification techniques

STANDARD IV

The Therapist Shall Implement the Occupational Therapy Program According to the Program Plan.

1. The therapist shall routinely document the occupational therapy services provided, the frequency of the services, and the client's progress toward goals. The timing of documentation shall be based upon frequency of contact with the patient/client and the significance of change in the client's condition.
2. The therapist shall periodically re-evaluate and document the changes in the client's occupational performance and/or performance component skills.
   a. if the client's program exceeds a three-month period, the client should be re-evaluated at least every two months.
   b. if the client's program is less than three months, the client should be re-evaluated at least once per month
3. The therapist shall formulate, document and implement program changes consistent with changes in the client's occupational performance and performance-component-skills.

STANDARD V

The Therapist Shall Prepare and Document the Occupational Therapy Discharge Plan.

1. The discharge plan shall be consistent with the client's goals, functional abilities and deficits, community resources, and expected prognosis.
2. The discharge plan shall be consistent with the discharge plans of the other health care practitioners.
3. In preparation of the discharge plan, the therapist should allow enough time for coordination, acceptance, and effective implementation of the discharge plan.
4. The therapist shall document within two days following discharge, the client's functional abilities and deficits in occupational performance and performance component skills at time of discharge.
5. The therapist shall recommend discontinuation of occupational therapy services when the client has achieved the program goals and/or has achieved maximum benefit from the services.

STANDARD VI

The Therapist Should Re-evaluate the Client with Chronic Conditions at an Appropriate Time Interval Following Discharge.

1. The re-evaluation results shall be documented.
2. If the client needs further service, the therapist shall refer the client to the services needed.

STANDARD VII

The Occupational Therapist Shall Systematically Review the Quality, Including Outcomes, of their Services, Using Predetermined Criteria Reflecting Professional Consensus and Recent Developments in Research and Theory.

1. If actual care does not meet the criteria, it may be justified by peer review.
2. If justification by peer review fails, a program to improve care shall be planned and implemented.
3. Patient care review will be repeated to assess the success of the corrective action.

Standards of practice for occupational therapy services in a mental health program

PREFACE

These standards are intended for internal use by the AOTA as guidelines to assist members in the practice of their profession. These standards by themselves cannot be interpreted to constitute a standard of care in any particular locality.

STANDARD I

A Referral for Occupational Therapy Must Be Based Upon the Provisions as Outlined in the Statement on Occupational Therapy Referral.

1. When a referral is received, the therapist shall:
   a. document the date of receipt and referral source
   b. document the occupational therapy services requested in the referral

STANDARD II

The Occupational Therapist Shall Evaluate the Client's Performance.

1. The therapist shall evaluate and document the client's goals, functional abilities and deficits in occupational performance (activities of daily living):
   a. self-care skills
   b. work skills
   c. play/leisure skills
2. The therapist shall evaluate and document the client's goals, functional abilities and deficits in the following performance component areas:
   a. psychological/intrapersonal skills
   b. social/interpersonal skills
   c. cognitive skills
3. If the results of the occupational performance evaluation indicate possible deficits in the client's motor and/or sensory-integrative skills, the therapist should evaluate these areas and document any functional deficits; or should refer the client to another practitioner for evaluation.
4. If any of the above evaluation results indicate the client's need for referral to community services or programs, the therapist should determine the availability of such community resources; or should refer the evaluation to another.

STANDARD III

The Therapist Shall Prepare and Document a Program Plan Based Upon an Analysis of the Occupational Therapy Evaluation Data and the Client's Expected Prognosis.

1. The documented program plan shall consist of a statement of achievable program goals and the methods to achieve the goals.
2. The program plan goals and methods shall be consistent with the evaluation data on the client's goals, functional abilities and deficits, community resources, and expected prognosis.

3. The program plan goals and methods shall be compatible with the program plans of the other health care practitioners.

STANDARD IV

The Therapist Shall Implement the Occupational Therapy Program According to the Program Plan.

1. The therapist shall periodically document the occupational therapy services provided and the frequency of the services.
2. The therapist shall periodically re-evaluate and document the changes in the client's occupational performance and performance component skills.
3. The therapist shall formulate, document and implement program changes consistent with changes in the client's occupation, performance and performance component skills.

STANDARD V

The Therapist Shall Prepare and Document the Occupational Therapy Discharge Plan.

1. The discharge plan shall be consistent with the client's goals, functional abilities and deficits, community resources, and expected prognosis.
2. The discharge plan shall be consistent with the discharge plans of the other health care practitioners.
3. Sufficient time should be allowed for coordination, acceptance and effective implementation of the discharge plan.
4. The therapist shall document the client's functional abilities and deficits in occupational performance and performance component skills at time of discharge.
5. The therapist shall terminate occupational therapy services when the client has achieved the goals, or when the client has achieved maximum benefit from occupational therapy.

STANDARD VI

The Therapist Should Re-evaluate the Client with Chronic Conditions at an Appropriate Time Interval Following Discharge.

1. The re-evaluation results shall be documented.
2. If the client needs further service, the therapist shall refer

STANDARD VII

The Occupational Therapist Shall Systematically Review the Quality, Including Outcomes, of their Services, Using Predetermined Criteria Reflecting Professional Consensus and Recent Developments in Research and Theory.

1. If actual care does not meet the criteria, it may be justified by peer review.
2. If justification by peer review fails, a program to improve care shall be planned and implemented.
3. Patient care review will be repeated to assess the success of the corrective action.

Standards of practice for occupational therapy services for the developmentally disabled client

PREFACE

These standards are intended for internal use by the AOTA as guidelines to assist members in the practice of their profession. These standards by themselves cannot be interpreted to constitute a standard of care in any particular locality.

STANDARD I

A Referral for Occupational Therapy Must Be Based Upon the Provisions as Outlined in the Statement of Occupational Therapy Referral.

1. A client should be referred to the occupational therapist for evaluation when the client has or appears to have a dysfunction, or has a predisposition towards dysfunction in any of the following areas:
   a. occupational performance (activities of daily living):
      1. self-care activities
      2. home-school-work activities
      3. play/leisure activities
   b. performance components:
      1. neuromuscular development
      2. sensory-integrative development
      3. psychological development
      4. social development
      5. cognitive development
2. When a referral is received, the therapist shall document:
   a. the date of receipt and referral source
   b. services requested in the referral

STANDARD II

The Occupational Therapist Shall Evaluate the Client's Performance.

1. The occupational therapy evaluation shall include an assessment of the developmental level, as well as the functional abilities and deficits in the following areas:
   a. occupational performance (activities of daily living):
      1. self-care skills
      2. home-work-school skills
      3. play/leisure skills
   b. motor skills
   c. sensory integration
2. If the results of the above evaluation indicate possible deficits in psychological/social and/or cognitive skills, the therapist should evaluate these areas and document any functional deficits; or should refer the client to the appropriate service.
3. If any of the above evaluation results indicate the client's need for referral to community services or programs, the therapist should determine the availability of such community resources; or should refer the evaluation to the appropriate service.
4. All evaluation methods shall be appropriate to the chronological age and functional level of the client. The methods may include, but need not be limited to, observation of activity performance, interview, record review and testing.

5. If standardized evaluative tests are used, the tests should have normative data for the age range of the client. If normative data are not available for the age range of the client, the standardized test results should be expressed in relation to the normative data that are available.
6. The therapist shall document the evaluation results in the client's record, indicating evaluation tools.

STANDARD III

The Therapist Shall Prepare and Document a Program Plan Based Upon an Analysis of the Occupational Therapy Evaluation Data and the Client's Expected Prognosis.

1. The documented program plan shall consist of a statement of achievable program goals and the methods to achieve the goals.
2. The program plan goals and methods shall be consistent with:
   a. established principles of normal growth and development
   b. the evaluative results and expected prognosis
   c. the goals of the client, the client's family and significant others
   d. the program plans of the other health care practitioners
3. When the occupational therapy program goal is to prevent or diminish dysfunction in occupational performance (activities of daily living) or to enhance occupational performance, the program plan shall include the use of one or more of the following types of activities:
   a. self-care activities; may also include instruction in the use of adapted methods and/or equipment
   b. home-work-school activities; may also include instruction in the use of adapted methods and/or equipment
   c. play/leisure activities; may also include instruction of family in play activities appropriate for child's developmental level; instruction in the use of adapted methods and/or equipment
4. When the goal is to prevent or diminish neuromuscular dysfunction or enhance neuromuscular development, the program plan shall include (but need not be limited to) the use of one or more of the following types of activities:
   a. activities which maintain or increase range of motion and/or muscle strength
   b. activities which facilitate integration of developmentally appropriate reflex behavior
   c. activities which provide appropriate sensory stimulation
   d. activities which promote the development of normal movement patterns and motor control
   e. activities which maintain or increase coordination
   f. instruction in use of proper positioning techniques
   g. provision of and instruction in the use of adaptive equipment and/or orthotic devices
5. When the goal is to prevent or diminish sensory-integrative dysfunction or to enhance sensory-integrative development, the program plan shall include (but need not be limited to) the appropriate use of:
   a. sensory input techniques for visual, auditory, gustatory, olfactory tactile, proprioceptive/kinesthetic, and vestibular stimulation

b. facilitation techniques
c. inhibition techniques
d. activity to promote adaptive motor response

6. When the goal is to prevent or diminish psychological dysfunction or to enhance psychological development, the program plan shall include (but need not be limited to) the use of activities which assist the client in learning to:
   a. experience and cope with competition, frustration, success, failure
   b. identify and respond appropriately to feelings
   c. develop or refine self-esteem; self-identity

7. When the goal is to prevent or diminish social dysfunction or to enhance social development, the program plan shall include (but need not be limited to) the use of activities which assist the client in learning to:
   a. initiate and develop appropriate social behavior
   b. listen and communicate
   c. develop sensitivity to other person's feelings and behavior

8. When the goal is to prevent or diminish cognitive dysfunction or to enhance cognitive development, the program plan shall include (need not be limited to) the use of the following activities which assist the client in developing:
   a. concentration/attention span
   b. memory/recall
   c. decision-making and problem-solving skills

STANDARD IV

The Therapist Shall Implement the Program According to the Program Plan.

1. The therapist shall periodically document the occupational therapy services provided and the frequency of the services.
2. The therapist shall periodically re-evaluate and document the changes in the client's occupational performance and performance components.
3. The therapist shall formulate, document and implement program changes consistent with changes in the client's occupational performance and performance components.

STANDARD V

The Therapist Shall Prepare and Document the Occupational Therapy Discharge Plan.

1. The discharge plan shall be consistent with the client's goals, functional abilities and deficits, expected prognosis, and the goals of the client's family. Consideration should be given to community resources and other environmental factors.
2. The discharge plan shall be consistent with the discharge plans of the other health care practitioners.
3. Sufficient time should be allowed for coordination, acceptance and effective implementation of the discharge plan.
4. The therapist shall document the client's functional abilities and deficits in occupational performance and performance components at time of discharge.
5. The therapist shall terminate occupational therapy services when the client has achieved the goals; or when the client has achieved maximum benefit from occupational therapy.

STANDARD VI

The Therapist Should Re-evaluate the Client with Chronic Conditions at an Appropriate Time Interval Following Discharge.

1. The re-evaluation results shall be documented.
2. If the client needs further service, the therapist shall refer the client to the services needed.

STANDARD VII

Occupational Therapist Shall Systematically Review the Quality, Including Outcomes, of Their Services, Using Predetermined Criteria Reflecting Professional Consensus and Recent Developments in Research and Theory.

1. If actual care does not meet the criteria it may be justified by peer review.
2. If justification by peer review fails, a program to improve care shall be planned and implemented.
3. Patient care review will be repeated to assess the success of the corrective action.

Standards of practice for occupational therapy in schools

These guidelines are to assist AOTA members and school administrators in the management of occupational therapy in the school systems. These standards by themselves cannot be interpreted to constitute a standard of care in any particular locality.

The occupational therapist shall manage the therapy program in accordance with all available STANDARDS OF PRACTICE, as defined by the American Occupational Therapy Association, Inc.

The purpose of the Occupational Therapy program in the school system is to enable the student to gain optimum benefit from the educational program.

DIRECT SERVICES

Direct services include screening, referral systems, evaluations, program planning, program implementation, re-evaluation and termination of services.

STANDARD I: SCREENING

The Occupational Therapist Should be Involved in the Screening Process.

1. The screening process should allow the therapist to identify those students who need further educational and/or related service evaluation.
2. All screening methods shall be appropriate to the chronological, educational and/or functional level of the student, and shall not be racially or culturally discriminatory.
3. The occupational therapist should refer the results and recommendations to the appropriate school educational planning committee.

STANDARD II: REFERRAL

A Referral for Occupational Therapy Must Comply with the AOTA Statement on Referral.

1. A student should be referred to the occupational therapist for evaluation when the student has or appears to have a dysfunction in any of the following areas:
   a. occupational performance (activities of daily living); self-care activities; home-schoolwork activities; play/leisure activities; and/or pre-vocational/vocational activities/skills.
   b. performance components: neuromuscular development; sensory integrative development; psychological development; social development; and/or cognitive development
2. A referral may originate through the individual education plan or educational planning committee (including teachers, other student services staff, parents, physicians, etc.).
3. When a referral is received, the therapist shall document:
   a. the date of receipt and referral source; and
   b. services requested in the referral.

4. If in the therapist's judgment there is the need for medical management of the student, the therapist shall immediately apprise the student's parent/guardian or appropriate person and recommend physician involvement, or the therapist shall, after parental/guardian written permission or release has been obtained, contact the physician.

STANDARD III: EVALUATION

The Occupational Therapist Shall Evaluate the Student's Performance.

1. The initial occupational therapy evaluation shall be completed and results documented according to the time frames established by federal and/or state rules and regulations.
2. The occupational therapy evaluation shall include assessment of the developmental level as well as the functional abilities/capacities and deficits/limitations as related to the student's educational level and needs in the following areas:
   a. occupational performance: self-care activities; home-school-work activities. prevocational/vocational activities/skills, and/or play/leisure activities.
   b. performance components: neuromuscular development; sensory integrative development; psychological development; social development and/or cognitive development.
3. If the results of the above evaluation indicate possible deficits in psychological/social, cognitive, physical/medical, speech/language areas, the therapist should refer the student to the appropriate service and/or request consultation if necessary.
4. All evaluation methods shall be appropriate to the chronological age and/or functional level of the student and identify baseline behaviors. The methods may include, but need not be limited to, observation of activity performance, interview, record review, testing and individual/group screening.
5. If standardized evaluative measurements are used, the tests should have normative data for the age range of the student. If normative data are not available for the age range of the student, the results should be expressed in a descriptive report and standardized scales not used.
6. Tests and other evaluation material used in placing handicapped students will be prepared and administered in such a way as not to be racially or culturally discriminatory, and they will be presented in the child's native tongue.
7. As part of the evaluation process, the therapist may make clinical judgments based on observations and recorded progress during intervention programs.
8. The therapist shall document evaluation results in the student's record, indicating evaluation instruments and procedures and also communicate these findings via written reports, oral conferences, and staffings to the appropriate persons and/or community resources.

STANDARD IV: PROGRAM PLANNING AND/OR INDIVIDUAL EDUCATION PLAN

The Therapist Shall Prepare and Document a Program Plan Based upon an Analysis of the Data from the Occupational Therapy and Other Educational Planner's Evaluation Results.

1. The initial program plan shall be prepared and documented according to the time frames established by federal and/or state rules and regulations.
2. The therapist shall utilize the results of the evaluation process to prepare an occupational therapy program that is:
   a. stated in practical outcomes applicable to the student's needs and educational goals,
   b. consistent with principles and concepts of growth and development; and
   c. consistent with expected behavior/progress for the student's defined educational/health problems and needs.
3. The planning process shall include:
   a. identifying short term and long term (annual) goals;
   b. collaborating with child/family/staff to establish appropriate goals to enhance education;
   c. participation in staffings to coordinate the occupational therapy program with the other programs within the educational setting;
   d. documenting of practical outcomes to be achieved;
   e. selecting the media, methods, environment and personnel to accomplish goals; and
   f. monitoring and modifying the program to meet the established goals.
4. The documented educational program plan shall consist of a statement of when these services will be provided and how long they will last.
5. When the occupational therapy program goal is to prevent or diminish dysfunction in occupational performance and learning or to enhance occupational performance, the program plan shall include the use of one or more of the following types of activities:
   a. self-care activities; may also include instruction in the use of adapted methods and/or equipment, energy conservation, joint protection techniques.
   b. home-work-school activities; may also include instruction in the use of adapted methods and/or equipment.
   c. pre-vocational/vocational activities/skills may also include improvement of standing or sitting tolerance, general endurance, or awareness and utilization of community resources; and
   d. development play/leisure activities; may also include instruction of family in activities appropriate for student's developmental level; instruction in the use of adapted methods and/or equipment.
6. When the goal is to prevent or diminish neuromuscular dysfunction or enhance neuromuscular development and learning, the program plan shall include, but need not be limited to, the use of one or more of the following types of activities:
   a. activities which maintain or increase range of motion and/or muscle strength;
   b. activities which facilitate integration of developmentally appropriate reflex/reaction behavior;

c. activities which provide appropriate sensory stimulation;
d. activities which promote the development of normal postural tone, movement patterns and motor control;
e. instruction in the use of proper positioning and handling techniques;
f. provision of and instruction in the use of adapative equipment; and/or
g. fabrication/recommendation of splints or orthotic devices/equipment.

7. When the goal is to prevent or diminish sensory integrative dysfunction or to enhance sensory integrative development, the program plan shall include, but need not be limited to, the appropriate use of:
   a. sensory facilitation and/or inhibition techniques for vestibular, tactile, proprioceptive/kinesthetic, visual, auditory, gustatory and olfactory stimulation; and/or
   b. activities to promote adaptive sensorimotor response.
8. When the interdisciplinary educational evaluation results indicate goals to prevent or diminish psychological or social dysfunction, or enhance psychological or social development, the occupational therapy program shall include, but need not be limited to, the appropriate use of activities which assist the student in learning to:
   a. experience and cope with competition, frustration, success and failure;
   b. identify and respond appropriately to feelings;
   c. develop or refine self-esteem or self-identity;
   d. imitate and develop appropriate social behaviors;
   e. listen and communicate; and
   f. develop sensitivity to other persons' feelings and behaviors (interpersonal relationships).
9. When the interdisciplinary education team evaluation results indicate goals to prevent or diminish cognitive dysfunction or to enhance development in the cognitive areas, the occupational therapy program shall include, but need not be limited to, the appropriate use of activities which assist the student in developing:
   a. concentration/attention span;
   b. memory/recall;
   c. decision making and/or problem solving.

The purposes of the occupational therapy program in the above stated areas, (#8 and #9), are not intended to replace academic or other programming. The purposes are to assist the child to receive maximum benefit from educational programming.

STANDARD V: PROGRAM IMPLEMENTATION

The Therapist Shall Implement the Program According to the Program Plan.

1. The therapist shall periodically and on an ongoing basis document the occupational therapy services provided (including techniques utilized and the results) and the frequency of the services.
2. The therapist shall periodically re-evaluate and document the changes in the student's occupational performance and performance components.
3. The therapist shall formulate, document and implement program changes consistent with changes in the student's occupational performance and performance components.

STANDARD VI: RE-EVALUATION

The Therapist Shall Re-evaluate the Student Receiving Occupational Therapy on a Yearly Basis.

1. The re-evaluation results shall be documented.
2. If the client needs further service, the therapist shall make appropriate recommendations.
3. A re-evaluation does not necessarily constitute a referral for services.

STANDARD VII: TERMINATION OF SERVICES

The Therapist Shall Prepare and Document the Occupational Therapy Discharge Plan.

1. The discharge plan shall be consistent with the student's goals, functional abilities and deficits, expected prognosis and the goals of the educational planners. Consideration should be given to appropriate community resources for referral and environmental factors/barriers that may need modification.
2. The discharge plan shall be consistent with the discharge plans of the other educational planners and appropriately documented through the individual educational planning process.
3. The therapist shall document the comparison of the initial state of functional abilities and deficits in occupational performance and performance components and the current state of these abilities and deficits at the time of discharge.
4. The therapist shall terminate occupational therapy services when the student has achieved the goals, or has achieved maximum benefits form occupational therapy.
5. Recommendations for follow-up or re-evaluation, if appropriate, shall be documented.

INDIRECT SERVICES

With the provision of indirect services the occupational therapist in a school-based program performs supervision, consultation and administration/management roles.

STANDARD VIII: ADMINISTRATION/MANAGEMENT

The Occupational Therapist Shall Provide Appropriate Management and Administrative Services.

The management and administrative functions for the school-based therapist shall include:

1. Supervision of other personnel as assigned.
   a. informal and formal training of personnel and volunteers assigned to occupational therapy.
   b. reviewing performances (self and others) and providing evaluations.
2. Design of the occupational therapy program with periodic reviews of all aspects of the total occupational therapy program to determine its effectiveness and efficiency.
3. Occupational therapists shall systematically review the quality, including outcomes, of services delivered, using predetermined criteria reflecting professional consensus and recent developments in research and theory.
   a. To determine if actual service may be justified by peer review.
   b. If justification by peer review fails, a program to improve service shall be planned and implemented.

   c. Review will be repeated to assess the success of the corrective action.
4. Maintaining current certification as required by state regulations and AOTA.
5. Maintaining current records and files to meet school requirements and professional standards.
6. Participating in budget planning and is responsible for budget implementation.
7. Responsibility for knowledge, including use of, and utilizing community resources.
8. The therapist shall maintain and update professional knowledge and skills and seek consultation/supervision from others when necessary to assure continued competency.

STANDARD IX: CONSULTATION

The Therapist Shall Provide Consultation Services When Appropriate

In the consultation role, the therapist is one member of an interdisciplinary educational team collaborating with a variety of professional personnel to assist students with special needs. The practice of consultation shall include when appropriate:

1. Developing and coordinating occupational therapy programs with the total educational curriculum.
2. Provide consultation for classroom environmental adaptation to enhance the learning potential of students.
3. Provide consultation to teachers and staff regarding the identified special needs of students.
4. Collaborate with the educational team regarding the student's program including the IEP (Individualized Education Program).
5. Provide inservice education.
6. Provide consultation for appropriate programs outside the school program.
7. Provide consultation and education to parents to help them understand the special needs of their child.
8. Provide consultation for home environmental adaptation to enhance independent functioning.
9. Provide consultation to school administrators and staff regarding preventive health education and activities to enhance the educational environment and learning potential of students.

STANDARD X: LEGAL/ETHICAL COMPONENTS

The Occupational Therapist Shall Provide all Aspects of Direct and Indirect Services According to Legal Regulations and Ethical Standards.

1. The occupational therapist shall practice and manage occupational therapy programs as defined by federal and state laws or legal principles as they apply to issues or situations when relevant to students or themselves in school systems.
2. The therapist shall observe the ethical practices as defined by the American Occupational Therapy Association Standards and Ethics Commission.
3. The therapist should be familiar with and abide by the ethical practices of the specific school district or system in which the therapist serves.

Glossary of terms used in the occupational therapy standards of practice

Abnormal patterns of motion (synergies): certain primitive patterns of motion which typically appear to varying degrees in the C.N.S. damaged individual when isolated movement is attempted. These patterns may be seen in the extremities in stereotyped flexion and extension patterns as distinguished from normal, coordinated, voluntary motion which is also synergistic in nature.

Activities of daily living: the components of everyday activity including self-care, work and play/leisure activities.

Activity restriction: the exclusion of certain activities, or restrictions in method or duration of performance.

Assistive/adaptive equipment: a special device which assists in the performance of self-care, work or play/leisure activities or physical exercise.

Cognitive skills: the level, quality and/or degree of comprehension, communication, concentration, problem solving, time management, conceptualization, integration of learning, judgement, time-place-person orientation.

Community services, programs or resources: vocational, social, religious, recreational, health, education and transportation services or programs that may be available in the community.

Coordination: the ability to perform motions in a smooth concerted way.

Dexterity: skill and ease in performing physical activities.

Document: the written recording of information in the client's overall record/chart and/or in the occupational therapy record/chart.

Evaluate/evaluation: the process of collecting and interpreting data obtained through observation, interview, record review, or testing.

Environmental adapatations: structural or positional changes designed to facilitate independent living and/or increase safety in the home, work or treatment setting; i.e., the installation of ramps, bars; change in furniture heights; adjustments of traffic patterns.

Facilitation techniques: selection, grading and modification of sensory input which attempts to encourage motion in a nonfunctioning muscle or muscle group.

Inhibition techniques: selection, grading and modification of sensory input which attempts to decrease muscle tone or excess motion that interferes with function.

Joint protection/preservation: the principles or techniques of minimizing stress on joints. Includes the use of proper body mechanics; avoidance of excessive weight-bearing, static, or deforming postures.

Kinetic activities: those activities requiring motion. Can include activities of daily living and isometric, assistive, resistive exercises.

Life space: an individual's cultural background, value orientation, and environment.

Life style: the degree, range and balance of self-care, work, and play/leisure activities.

May: indicates an acceptable method that is recognized, but not necessarily preferred.

Motor skills: the level, quality and/or degree of range of motion, gross muscle strength, muscle tone, endurance, fine motor skills, and functional use.

Occupational performance: the performance of self-care, work and play/leisure activities, the activities of daily living. The performance of these activities requires self-care, work and play/leisure skills. The concept of occupational performance is further described in the delineation of roles and functions in Appendix V.

Performance components: the learned and developmental patterns of behvior which are the prerequisite foundations of self-care, work, and play/leisure skills. The performance components include:

a. motor skills

b. sensory integration

c. cognitive skills

d. psychological/intrapersonal skills

e. social/interpersonal skills

Periodically: occurring at regular intervals of time.

Play/leisure skills: those skills necessary to perform and engage in activities such as games, sports, and hobbies.

Positioning: the placing of body parts in proper alignment.

Psychological/intrapersonal skills: the level, quality and/or degree of self-identity, self-concept, and coping skills.

a. *self identity* and *self-concept:* the ability to perceive self needs and expectations from those of others; identify areas of self-competency and limitations; accept responsibility for self; perceive sexuality of self; have self-respect; have appropriate body image; view self as being able to influence events.

b. *coping skills:* includes the ability to sublimate drives, find sources of need gratification, tolerate frustration and anxiety, experience gratification, and control impulses.

Reality orientation: the treatment approach aimed at reinforcement of reality; i.e., the use of simple structured activities for orientation to time, place, and person.

Self-care skills: skills such as dressing, feeding, hygiene/grooming, mobility, and object manipulation.

a. *mobility:* skills such as getting in or out of bed, chair, wheelchair, vehicles and using transportation.

b. *object manipulation:* skills such as the handling of common objects such as telephone, keys, money, light switches, doorknobs.

Sensation: reception of stimuli, includes touch, pain, temperature, stereognosis, proprioception/kinesthesia, vestibular, taste, smell, vision, hearing.

Sensory integration: the level, quality or degree of development and integration of somatosensory functions, reflected in reflex and sensory status, posture, motor activity and praxis, form and space perception, body schema and self-concept.

Shall or must: indicates a mandatory statement; the only acceptable method.

Should: indicates the commonly accepted method, yet allows for the use of effective alternatives.

Significant others: persons who have an important relationship to the client. This could include the client's family, friends, employer, teacher, or other health care providers.

Social/interpersonal skills: the level, quality, and/or degree of dyadic and group interaction skills.

   a. *dyadic interaction skills:* abilities in relationships to peers, subordinates, and authority figures; demonstrating trust, respect, and warmth; perceiving and responding to needs and feelings of others; engaging in and sustaining interdependent relationships; communicating feelings.

   b. *group interaction skills:* abilities in performing tasks in the presence of others; sharing tasks with others; cooperating and competing with others; fulfilling a variety of group membership roles; exercising leadership skills; perceiving and responding to needs of group members.

Splinting: the provision of dynamic and/or static splints for the purpose of: relieving pain, maintaining joint alignment, protecting joint integrity, improving function, and/or decreasing deformity.

Structuring environment: the organization of the client's time, activities, and/or physical environment in order to enhance performance (see environmental adaptations).

Work simplification: the streaming of the performnce of an activity in order to minimize energy output.

Work skills: skills such as habits, workmanship, actual skills related to specific job tasks. The skills may refer to the work of the student, home manager, or paid employee. Home manager skills include such skills as cooking, budgeting, shopping, clothing maintenance, house-cleaning and maintenance.

Children's Hospital at Stanford Occupational Therapy Time–oriented Record Activities of Daily Living Assessment

CHILDREN'S HOSPITAL AT STANFORD

ACTIVITIES OF DAILY LIVING ASSESSMENT *

Name of patient _____ Hospital no. _____

Diagnosis _____ Onset _____

Birth date _____

Sex: M   F   Handedness: R   L

Assessor's signature   **Date**

1. _____

2. _____

3. _____

4. _____

5. _____

6. _____

7. _____

8. _____

Subtests utilized:

Basic ADL	Communication	Adolescent self-care	Transfers
Wheelchair	Household activities	Equipment list	

*From Bleck, E. E., and Nagel, D. A., editors: Physically handicapped children: a medical atlas for teachers, New York, 1975, Grune & Stratton, Inc. By permission.

CHILDREN'S HOSPITAL AT STANFORD

OCCUPATIONAL THERAPY

TIME-ORIENTED RECORD

ACTIVITIES OF DAILY LIVING ASSESSMENT

addressograph stamp

Key to scoring: 4 . . . Independent
3 . . . Independent with equipment and/or adaptive technique
2 . . . Completes but cannot accomplish in practical time
1 . . . Attempts but requires assistance or supervision to complete
0 . . . Dependent—cannot attempt activity
— . . . Nonapplicable

The **Year-Month** vertical column represents the Order of developmental sequence or approximate age when the child accomplishes the activity; the horizontal column represents the chronological age of the child being assessed.

	Visit number	Yr. Mo.	1		2		3		4		5		6		7		8	
	Julian date		R.	L.	R.	L.	R.	L.	R.	L.	R.	L.	R.	L.	R.	L.	R.	L.
	BED	Order of dev. seq.																
1	Supine position	Birth																
2	Prone position	Birth																
3	Roll to side	1-4 wk.																
4	Roll prone to supine	0.6																
5	Roll supine to prone	0.7																
6	Sit up	0.10																
7	Propped sitting	0.6																
8	Sitting/hands props	0.7																
9	Sitting unsupported	0.10-0.12																
	Reaching																	
10	To midline	0.5																
11	To mouth and face	0.6																
12	Above head	—																
13	Behind head	—																
14	Behind back	—																
15	To toes	1.3																
	FEEDING																	
16	Swallow (liquids)	Birth																
17	Drooling under control	1.0																
18	Suck and use straw	2.0																
19	Chew (semisolids, solids)	1.6																
20	Finger foods	0.10																

ACTIVITIES OF DAILY LIVING

Continued.

CHILDREN'S HOSPITAL AT STANFORD

OCCUPATIONAL THERAPY

TIME-ORIENTED RECORD

ACTIVITIES OF DAILY LIVING ASSESSMENT

Key to scoring: 4 . . . Independent

3 . . . Independent with equipment and/or adaptive technique

2 . . . Completes but cannot accomplish in practical time

1 . . . Attempts but requires assistance or supervision to complete

0 . . . Dependent—cannot attempt activity

— . . . Nonapplicable

The **Year-Month** vertical column represents the [Order of developmental sequence] or approximate age when the child accomplishes the activity; the horizontal column represents the chronological age of the child being assessed.

Visit number		1		2		3		4		5		6		7		8	
	Yr. Mo.																
FEEDING—cont'd	Order of dev. seq.	R.	L.	R.	L.	R.	L.	R.	L.	R.	L.	R.	L.	R.	L.	R.	L.
Utensils																	
21 Bottle	0.10																
22 Spoon	3.0																
23 Cup	1.6																
24 Glass	2.0																
25 Fork	3.0																
26 Knife	6.0-7.0																
TOILETING																	
27 Bowel control	1.6																
28 Bladder control	2.0																
29 Sit on toilet	2.9																
30 Arrange clothing	4.0																
31 Cleanse self	5.0																
32 Flush toilet	3.3-5.0																
HYGIENE																	
33 Turn faucets on/off	3.0																
34 Wash/dry hands/face	4.9																
35 Wash ears	8.0																
36 Bathing	8.0																
37 Deodorant	12.0-																
38 Care for teeth	4.9																
39 Care for nose	6.0																

<table>
<tr><td colspan="2"></td><td colspan="4">**CHILDREN'S HOSPITAL AT STANFORD OCCUPATIONAL THERAPY**

TIME-ORIENTED RECORD

ACTIVITIES OF DAILY LIVING ASSESSMENT</td></tr>
</table>

Key to scoring: 4 . . . Independent
          3 . . . Independent with equipment and/or adaptive technique
          2 . . . Completes but cannot accomplish in practical time
          1 . . . Attempts but requires assistance or supervision to complete
          0 . . . Dependent—cannot attempt activity
          — . . . Nonapplicable

The **Year-Month** vertical column represents the [Order of developmental sequence] or approximate age when the child accomplishes the activity; the horizontal column represents the chronological age of the child being assessed.

Visit number		Yr. Mo.	1		2		3		4		5		6		7		8	
HYGIENE—cont'd		Order of dev. seq.	R.	L.	R.	L.	R.	L.	R.	L.	R.	L.	R.	L.	R.	L.	R.	L.
40	Care for hair	7.6																
41	Care for nails	8.0																
42	Feminine hygiene	Puberty																
	UNDRESSING																	
	Lower body																	
43	Untie shoe bow	2.0-3.0																
44	Remove shoes	2.0-3.0																
45	Remove socks	1.6																
46	Remove pull-down garment	2.6																
	Upper body																	
47	Remove pull-over garment	4.0																
	DRESSING																	
	Lower body																	
48	Put on socks	4.0																
49	Put on pull-down garment	4.0																
50	Put on shoe	4.0																
51	Lace shoe	4.0-5.0																
52	Tie bow	6.0																
	Upper body																	
53	Put on pull-over garment	5.0																

ACTIVITIES OF DAILY LIVING

Continued.

CHILDREN'S HOSPITAL AT STANFORD
OCCUPATIONAL THERAPY

TIME-ORIENTED RECORD

ACTIVITIES OF DAILY LIVING ASSESSMENT

Key to scoring: 4 . . . Independent
3 . . . Independent with equipment and/or adaptive technique
2 . . . Completes but cannot accomplish in practical time
1 . . . Attempts but requires assistance or supervision to complete
0 . . . Dependent—cannot attempt activity
— . . . Nonapplicable

The **Year-Month** vertical column represents the Order of developmental sequence or approximate age when the child accomplishes the activity; the horizontal column represents the chronological age of the child being assessed.

Visit number		1	2	3	4	5	6	7	8
	Yr. Mo.								
FASTENERS	Order of dev. seq.								
Unfastening									
54 Button: front	3.0								
55 side	3.0								
56 back	5.6								
57 Zipper: front	3.3								
58 separating front	3.6								
59 back	4.9								
60 Buckle: belt	3.9								
61 shoe	3.9								
62 Tie: back sash	5.0								
Fasten									
63 Button: large front	2.6								
64 series	3.6								
65 back	6.3								
66 Zipper: front, lock tab	4.0								
67 separating	4.6								
68 back	5.6								
69 Buckle: belt	4.0								
70 shoe	4.0								
71 insert belt in loops	4.6								
72 Tie: front	6.0								
73 back	8.0								
74 necktie	10.0								
75 Snaps: front	3.0								
76 back	6.0								
Assessor's initials:									

ACTIVITIES OF DAILY LIVING

addressograph stamp		**CHILDREN'S HOSPITAL AT STANFORD** **OCCUPATIONAL THERAPY** **TIME-ORIENTED RECORD** **ACTIVITIES OF DAILY LIVING ASSESSMENT**															

Key to scoring:
- 4 . . . Independent
- 3 . . . Independent with equipment and/or adaptive technique
- 2 . . . Completes but cannot accomplish in practical time
- 1 . . . Attempts but requires assistance or supervision to complete
- 0 . . . Dependent—cannot attempt activity
- — . . . Nonapplicable

	Visit number	1		2		3		4		5		6		7		8	
	Julian date																
	COMMUNICATION	R.	L.	R.	L.	R.	L.	R.	L.	R.	L.	R.	L.	R.	L.	R.	L.
	Writing																
1	Sharpen pencil																
2	Print																
3	Write																
4	Erase																
	Typing																
5	Insert paper																
6	Press space bar																
7	Press key																
8	Turn carriage																
9	Remove paper																
	Telephone																
10	Remove receiver																
11	Hold receiver																
12	Dial																
13	Speak																
14	Replace receiver																
15	Take message																
16	Use telephone book																

ACTIVITIES OF DAILY LIVING

	Visit number	1		2		3		4		5		6		7		8	

CHILDREN'S HOSPITAL AT STANFORD OCCUPATIONAL THERAPY

TIME-ORIENTED RECORD

ACTIVITIES OF DAILY LIVING ASSESSMENT

addressograph stamp

Key to scoring: 4 . . . Independent
3 . . . Independent with equipment and/or adaptive technique
2 . . . Completes but cannot accomplish in practical time
1 . . . Attempts but requires assistance or supervision to complete
0 . . . Dependent—cannot attempt activity
— . . . Nonapplicable

	Visit number	1		2		3		4		5		6		7		8	
	Julian date																
	ADOLESCENT SELF-CARE	R.	L.	R.	L.	R.	L.	R.	L.	R.	L.	R.	L.	R.	L.	R.	L.
	UNDRESSING																
1	Remove nylons/panty hose																
2	Remove girdle/garter belt																
3	Remove brassiere																
4	Remove necktie																
	DRESSING																
5	Put on nylons/panty hose																
6	Put on girdle/garter belt																
7	Put on brassiere																
8	Put on necktie																
	AIDS																
9	Put on eyeglasses																
10	Remove eyeglasses																
11	Put on hearing aid																
12	Remove hearing aid																
	HYGIENE																
13	Shampoo hair																
14	Set hair																
15	Shave face																
16	Shave underarms																
17	Shave legs																
18	Apply deodorant																
19	Apply makeup																
20	Groom fingernails																
21	Groom toenails																

ACTIVITIES OF DAILY LIVING

	CHILDREN'S HOSPITAL AT STANFORD					
	OCCUPATIONAL THERAPY					
	TIME-ORIENTED RECORD					
addressograph stamp	**ACTIVITIES OF DAILY LIVING ASSESSMENT**					

Key to scoring: 4 . . . Independent
3 . . . Independent with equipment and/or adaptive technique
2 . . . Completes but cannot accomplish in practical time
1 . . . Attempts but requires assistance or supervision to complete
0 . . . Dependent—cannot attempt activity
— . . . Nonapplicable

	Visit number	1	2	3	4	5	6	7	8
	Julian date								
	TRANSFERS								
	Specify: ambulatory								
	with crutches								
	with wheelchair								
1	To bed								
2	From bed								
3	To toilet								
4	From toilet								
5	To bathtub								
6	From bathtub								
7	To shower								
8	From shower								
9	To regular chair								
10	From regular chair								
11	To car								
12	From car								
13	To bus								
14	From bus								

ACTIVITIES OF DAILY LIVING

CHILDREN'S HOSPITAL AT STANFORD
OCCUPATIONAL THERAPY

TIME-ORIENTED RECORD

ACTIVITIES OF DAILY LIVING ASSESSMENT

addressograph stamp

Key to scoring: 4 . . . Independent
3 . . . Independent with equipment and/or adaptive technique
2 . . . Completes but cannot accomplish in practical time
1 . . . Attempts but requires assistance or supervision to complete
0 . . . Dependent—cannot attempt activity
— . . . Nonapplicable

Visit number	1		2		3		4		5		6		7		8	
Julian date																
WHEELCHAIR SKILLS	R.	L.	R.	L.	R.	L.	R.	L.	R.	L.	R.	L.	R.	L.	R.	L.
1 Sitting balance																
2 Fasten belt																
3 Unfasten belt																
4 Lock brakes																
5 Unlock brakes																
6 Propel forward																
7 Propel backward																
8 Propel corners																
9 Open doors																
10 Close doors																
11 Go up ramp																
12 Go down ramp																
13 Raise footrests																
14 Lower footrests																
15 Swing footrests to side																
16 Remove arms																
17 Replace arms																
18 Pick up object from floor																
19 Sitting push-ups (10)																
20 Adjust position																
21 Reach crutches, holder																
22 Place crutches, holder																

		CHILDREN'S HOSPITAL AT STANFORD
		OCCUPATIONAL THERAPY
		TIME-ORIENTED RECORD
addressograph stamp		ACTIVITIES OF DAILY LIVING ASSESSMENT

Key to scoring: 4 . . . Independent
              3 . . . Independent with equipment and/or adaptive technique
              2 . . . Completes but cannot accomplish in practical time
              1 . . . Attempts but requires assistance or supervision to complete
              0 . . . Dependent—cannot attempt activity
              — . . . Nonapplicable

	Visit number	1	2	3	4	5	6	7	8
	Julian date								
	HOUSEHOLD ACTIVITIES								
	Food preparation								
1	Open: milk								
2	packaged food								
3	bottles, capped								
4	screw lids								
5	Pour: liquids								
6	dry ingredients								
7	Mix: with spoon								
8	egg beater, manual								
9	electric mixer								
10	Sift flour								
11	Break egg								
12	Peel vegetables/fruit								
13	Cut vegetables/fruit								
14	Use: measuring spoons								
15	cups								
16	can opener								
17	rolling pin								
	Range								
18	Operate: burner controls								
19	oven controls								
20	Place pans on range								
21	Remove hot pans from range								

ACTIVITIES OF DAILY LIVING

Continued.

| | | CHILDREN'S HOSPITAL AT STANFORD
OCCUPATIONAL THERAPY

TIME-ORIENTED RECORD

ACTIVITIES OF DAILY LIVING ASSESSMENT | | | | | | | |

Key to scoring: 4 . . . Independent
3 . . . Independent with equipment and/or adaptive technique
2 . . . Completes but cannot accomplish in practical time
1 . . . Attempts but requires assistance or supervision to complete
0 . . . Dependent—cannot attempt activity
— . . . Nonapplicable

	Visit number	1	2	3	4	5	6	7	8
	Julian date								
	Range—cont'd								
22	Oven: open								
23	place pans (2-4 lb.)								
24	remove pans (2-4 lb.)								
25	Broiler: in								
26	out								
27	Storage areas: open								
28	close								
	Refrigerator								
29	Open								
30	Close								
31	Food: in								
32	out								
33	Handle ice trays								
	Sink								
34	Dishes, utensils: wash								
35	dry								
36	store								
37	Faucets: reach								
38	turn on/off								
39	Wash sink								

	CHILDREN'S HOSPITAL AT STANFORD **OCCUPATIONAL THERAPY** **TIME-ORIENTED RECORD** **ACTIVITIES OF DAILY LIVING ASSESSMENT**

Key to scoring: 4 . . . Independent
3 . . . Independent with equipment and/or adaptive technique
2 . . . Completes but cannot accomplish in practical time
1 . . . Attempts but requires assistance or supervision to complete
0 . . . Dependent—cannot attempt activity
— . . . Nonapplicable

	Visit number	1	2	3	4	5	6	7	8
	Julian date								
	Table								
40	Set								
41	Clear								
42	Serve food								
	Shopping								
43	Make list								
44	Travel to store								
45	Carry parcels								
46	Handle money								
47	Store purchases								
	Cleaning								
48	Use: dust cloth								
49	dust mop								
50	broom								
51	dust pan								
52	Clean: stove								
53	wash bowl								
54	toilet								
55	Empty waste basket								
56	Floors: wash								
57	polish								
58	vacuum								

ACTIVITIES OF DAILY LIVING

Continued.

		CHILDREN'S HOSPITAL AT STANFORD OCCUPATIONAL THERAPY TIME-ORIENTED RECORD ACTIVITIES OF DAILY LIVING ASSESSMENT

Key to scoring: 4 . . . Independent
3 . . . Independent with equipment and/or adaptive technique
2 . . . Completes but cannot accomplish in practical time
1 . . . Attempts but requires assistance or supervision to complete
0 . . . Dependent—cannot attempt activity
— . . . Nonapplicable

	Visit number	1	2	3	4	5	6	7	8
	Julian date								
	Cleaning—cont'd								
59	Furniture: polish								
60	vacuum								
61	Bed: change								
62	make up								
	Laundry								
63	Clothes: wash								
64	hang								
65	dry								
66	fold								
67	Ironing: dampen								
68	set up board								
69	set up iron								
70	put away clothes								
	Sewing								
71	Thread needle								
72	Tie knot								
73	Use straight pins								
74	Use scissors								
75	Sew button								
76	Mend								
77	Use sewing machine								

ACTIVITIES OF DAILY LIVING

CHILDREN'S HOSPITAL AT STANFORD **OCCUPATIONAL THERAPY** **TIME-ORIENTED RECORD** **ACTIVITIES OF DAILY LIVING ASSESSMENT**								

Key to scoring: 4 . . . Independent
3 . . . Independent with equipment and/or adaptive technique
2 . . . Completes but cannot accomplish in practical time
1 . . . Attempts but requires assistance or supervision to complete
0 . . . Dependent—cannot attempt activity
— . . . Nonapplicable

Visit number	1	2	3	4	5	6	7	8
Julian date								
Child care								
78 Bathe								
79 Dress								
80 Undress								
81 Feed								

ACTIVITIES OF DAILY LIVING

Georgia Retardation Center Occupational Therapy Service Assessment Instruments

Georgia Retardation Center Occupational Therapy Service screening tool

Student: _____ Social Security no.: _____

Unit and section: _____ Birthdate: _____

Evaluator: _____

Key for I and II:
1 = Cannot do at all
2 = Can do partly with assistance
3 = Can do all, but needs assistance
4 = Can do alone with spoken directions
5 = Can do alone

Hand preference: L   R
Color-blind: Yes   No

I. *Gross motor skills* (Check one.)

1	2	3	4	5	Skills	Comments
					1. Sits down and gets up from floor	
					2. Rolls over (log roll)	
					3. Gets on hands and knees	
					4. Crawls	
					5. Crawls reciprocally	
					6. Walks	
					7. Runs	
					8. Balances on one foot—seconds: ( )L; ( )R	
					9. Hops on left foot	
					10. Hops on right foot	
					11. Skips	
					12. Jumps over stick (both feet)	

I. *Gross motor skills*—cont'd

1	2	3	4	5	Skills	Comments
					13. Rolls ball	
					14. Catches ball (two hands)	
					15. Catches beanbag (left)	
					16. Catches beanbag (right)	
					17. Throws ball (two hands)	
					18. Throws ball (left)	
					19. Throws ball (right)	
					20. Bounces ball (dribble): ( ) times	
					21. Jumps rope (turns his own): ( ) times	
					22. Other	

Comments: _____

_____

_____

_____

_____

_____

II. *Hand coordination* (Check one.)

1	2	3	4	5	Skills	Comments
					1. Looks at objects	
					2. Reaches for object	
					3. Grasp (left)	
					4. Grasp (right)	
					5. Lateral pinch (paper) preferred hand: L R	
					6. Palmer pinch (straight fingers) preferred hand: L R	
					7. Three-finger pinch (peg)	
					8. Tip prehension (small bead)	
					9. Holds crayon—how:	
					10. Scribbles with crayon	
					11. Traces with crayon	
					12. Transfers block from one hand to other	
					13. Puts block in box	
					14. Puts peg in hole (½-inch)	
					15. Strings large bead	
					16. Other	

Comments: _____

_____

_____

_____

Continued.

III. *Eye coordination* (Use *x* or * under each.)

Left	Both	Right	Skills	Comments
			1. Focus: ( ) seconds	
			2. Track ←——→	
			3. Track ↕	
			4. Track ↘	
			5. Track ↙	
			6. Track ○	
			7. Track toward nose	
			8. Track from nose	
			9. Two point •——•	
			10. Two point ╎	
			11. Two point ╲	
			12. Two point ╱	
			13. Two point to and from nose	

Comments: _____

IV. *Perceptual motor skill* (Check *yes* or *no*.)

Yes	No	Skills	Comments
		1. Matches ○	
		2. Matches □	
		3. Matches △	
		4. Copies ———	
		5. Copies │	
		6. Copies ╲	
		7. Copies ╱	
		8. Copies ○	

Comments: _____

V. *Imitation* (Do not give spoken instructions except to tell a student to do what you are doing. Check *yes* or *no*.)

Yes	No	Skills	Comments
		1. Raise two arms out straight, shoulder high	
		2. Clap hands	
		3. Wave good-bye	
		4. Pick up object	
		5. Touch the floor	
		6. Raise one hand over head.	

Comments: _____

VI. *Cooperation and following directions* (Check one.)

	1. Will not hold still, pay attention, or listen to directions
	2. Does not usually follow directions
	3. Tries to follow directions, but needs help
	4. Tries but needs reminders or encouragement
	5. Follows directions usually

Comments: _____

VII. *Self-feeding* (Use * in *Yes* column for initial evaluation if they can; use *x* in *No* column for initial evaluation if they cannot; use date in *Yes* column later when they master the skill.)

Hand preference: L   R

Yes	No	*(If no, explain problem, present method, and present equipment.)*
		1. Lip closure
		2. Sucking (straw)
		3. Swallowing
		4. Chewing
		5. Finger feeding
		6. Grasp (spoon)
		7. Arm control (scoop and spoon to mouth)
		8. Feeds self
		9. Regular food
		10. Regular plate or tray
		11. Regular glass or paper cup
		12. Regular spoon
		13. Regular fork
		14. Cuts food with spoon
		15. Cuts food with fork
		16. Cuts food with knife
		17. Uses napkin
		18. Special diet
		19. Other

Problems (Use same directions as specified in *Self-feeding*.)

Yes	No	
		1. Tongue thrust
		2. Drooling
		3. Bad appetite
		4. Does not want to feed self
		5. Messy eater
		6. Throws food
		7. Other

Continued.

Other information and equipment: _____

Georgia Retardation Center Occupational Therapy Department ADL in food preparation skills

Student names:

1. _____
2. _____
3. _____
4. _____
5. _____
6. _____
7. _____

Session no.: _____

Date: _____

Staff: _____

		Student No.
		1	2	3	4	5	6	7
Preparing to cook	Washes hands							
	Dries hands							
	Puts on apron							
	Sits at table							
Utensil recognition	Recognizes cutting knife							
	Large spoon							
	Frying pan							
	Bowl							
	Saucepan							
Kitchen appliances recognition	Locates oven							
	Sink							
	Refrigerator							
Fine motor	Spreads with knife							
	Stirs batter with spoon							
	Cuts with knife							
Setting table	Puts silver at place							
	Puts plates							
	Puts glasses							
Eating	Waits for others to begin							
	Serves self food							
	Passes food							
	Uses napkin							
	Uses condiments							
Clean up	Cleans off table							
	Washes dishes							
	Dries dishes							
	Puts dishes away							
	Vacuums							

Georgia Retardation Center Occupational Therapy Department ADL in area of food preparation

Name: _____ Birthdate: _____ Unit: _____

Diagnosis: _____

Precautions: _____ Examiner: _____

Hand preference: _____ Eye dominance: _____ Eye level: _____

Wheelchair: _____ Walker: _____ Ambulatory: _____

Other adaptive devices: _____

Food restrictions: _____

	Right UE	*Left UE*		*Right UE*	*Left UE*
Vertical reach:					
Comfortable—up	_____ inches	_____ inches	Maximal	_____ inches	_____ inches
Comfortable—down	_____ inches	_____ inches	Maximal	_____ inches	_____ inches
Horizontal reach:					
Comfortable—forward	_____ inches	_____ inches	Maximal	_____ inches	_____ inches
Comfortable—sideways	_____ inches	_____ inches	Maximal	_____ inches	_____ inches

Two-handed control: Gross-grade _____   Fine-grade _____
                        (poor, fair, good, normal)   (poor, fair, good, normal)

One-handed control: *Right UE* (poor, fair, good, normal)   *Left UE* (poor, fair, good, normal)
                        Gross-grade _____   Gross-grade _____
                        Fine-grade _____   Fine-grade _____

Rating values:

1. No comprehension; student is unable to function in this area.
2. Student is unable to perform in this area because of physical limitations.
3. Student exhibits some difficulty with regard to this area, but with assistance task can be completed.
4. Student is able to complete activity independently.

Student is exposed to each activity by spoken directions or demonstrations for a minimum of four times.

	Date	Date	Date	Date	Assistive devices	Comments
Cooking activities						
Blend ingredients by hand						
Stir ingredients by hand						
Scoop						
Clean vegetables with a brush						
Measure dry ingredients using measuring spoons						
Measure dry ingredients using measuring cups						
Measure wet ingredients using measuring spoons						
Measure wet ingredients using measuring cups						
Pare or peel vegetables and fruit						
Grate						
Toss						
Pour cold liquids						
Pour hot liquids						
Pour batter into container						
Sift						
Break eggs						

Ratings

	Ratings					
	Date	Date	Date	Date	Assistive devices	Comments
Slice with knife						
Chop with knife						
Melt						
Simmer						
Boil						
Broil						
Ladle						
Drain using collander or slotted spoon						
Pan fry						
Roll cookie dough or pie crust						
Able to read simple recipe						
Cooking mechanics Turn faucet on and off						
Wash and dry hands						
Apron on and off						
Open and close refrigerator door						
Place and remove items from refrigerator						
Open and close overhead cupboard doors						
Remove and store items in overhead cupboards						
Open and close bottom cupboard doors						
Remove and store items in lower cupboards						
Turn range off and on at proper setting						
Turn oven off and on at proper setting						
Put container in oven						
Take container out and place on counter						
Use toaster						
Use electric mixer						
Open packages						
Open and use wax, plastic wrap and aluminum foil boxes						
Use can opener						
Open and close bottles and jars						
Knows hot from cold						

Continued.

	Ratings					
	Date	Date	Date	Date	Assistive devices	Comments
Table activities Set table						
Serve the table						
Clear the table						
Clean the table						
Scrape dishes						
Stack dishes						
Wash dishes						
Dry dishes						
Clean up area						
Wipe up spills						
Dispose of garbage						

Recipes used

1.
2.
3.
4.
5.
6.
7.
8.
9.
10.

Georgia Retardation Center outline for occupational therapy evaluations

Occupational therapy evaluation

Date: _____

Diagnosis: (EXAMPLE: This is an 11-year-old female with the medical diagnosis of profound mental retardation secondary to cranial-cerebral injury sustained in an automobile accident, spastic quadriplegia, major motor seizures, visual
handicaps.)

Summary of previous therapy:

General behavior:

Tests used: (could include these or others)

        Range of motion

        Gross and fine motor

        Developmental

        Unit feeding evaluation

Gross motor:

Fine motor:

Handedness:

Sensory integration:

Self-help:

Adaptive equipment: positioning, feeding, wheelchair

Summary:

Recommendations for placement:

Recommendations for training

1. a. Occupational therapy services are not appropriate for this student.
   b. Indirect occupational therapy services are appropriate for this student. (These services will be indicated on the
      student activity and staff functions list in his program, since these activities are not appropriate for behavioral
      objectives.)
   c. Direct occupational therapy services are appropriate for this student. These services are appropriate for behav-
      ioral objectives.
   d. Direct occupational therapy services are appropriate for this student. These services will be indicated on the
      student activities and staff functions list in his program, since these activities are not appropriate for behavioral
      objectives.

2. Discipline specific goals: None

             or

   Discipline specific goals: Student will increase wrist range of motion 15 degrees by Dec., 1981 through exercise
   program 3 times a week and wearing of wrist splint 16 hours daily.

   Discipline specific goals: Student's adaptive equipment will be reviewed quarterly and repaired as needed.

3. General recommendations for program team:

   Self-help skills: Student will learn to place button through buttonhole.

4. If occupational therapy services are not currently appropriate: The next occupational therapy evaluation will be
   done at the request of the primary physician or the program team.

   If indirect or direct occupational therapy services are appropriate: The next occupational therapy evaluation will
   be done for the annual review of this student on _____

                                           _____

                                                Signature

Georgia Retardation Center adaptive equipment-rehabilitation survey

Key: Unit _____   Date _____
  RS = Rehabilitative support
  MS = Mechanical support
  PD = Protective device
  AD = Adaptive equipment
W/C = Wheelchair

Student	Device	Type	Justification	Application

Index